Psychotropic Drugs

Psychotropic Drugs

NORMAN L. KELTNER, Ed D, RN

Associate Professor, Graduate Program,
University of Alabama School of Nursing,
University of Alabama at Birmingham,
Birmingham, Alabama

DAVID G. FOLKS, MD

Professor of Psychiatry and Behavioral Neurobiology,
University of Alabama School of Medicine,
University of Alabama at Birmingham,
Birmingham, Alabama

Illustrated

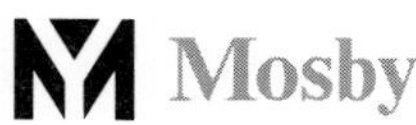

St. Louis Baltimore Boston Chicago London Philadelphia Sydney Toronto

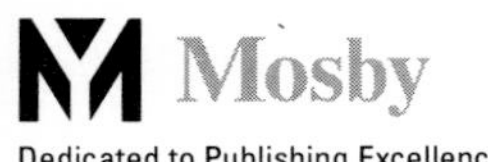

Editors: Linda L. Duncan and Jeff Burnham
Developmental Editors: Teri Merchant and Becky Sweeney
Project Manager: Patricia Tannian
Production Editor: Mary McAuley
Designer: Liz Fett
Manufacturing Supervisor: John Babrick

Printed in the United States of America

Mosby–Year Book, Inc.
11830 Westline Industrial Drive
St. Louis, Missouri 63146

Library of Congress Cataloging in Publication Data

Keltner, Norman L.
Psychotropic drugs / by Norman L. Keltner, David G. Folks. — 1st ed.
p. cm.
Includes bibliographical references.
ISBN 0-8016-5840-3
1. Mental illness—Chemotherapy. 2. Psychotropic drugs.
3. Psychopharmacology. I. Folks, David G. II. Title.
[DNLM: 1. Mental Disorders—drug therapy. 2. Psychopharmacology.
3. Psychotropic Drugs—pharmacology. QV 77 K29p 1992]
RC483.K45 1992
616.89'18—dc20
DNLM/DLC
for Library of Congress 92-48501
CIP

93 94 95 96 97 CL/RRD 9 8 7 6 5 4 3 2 1

Contributors

CLEVELAND F. KINNEY, MD, Ph D
Assistant Professor of Psychiatry,
School of Medicine, University of Alabama at Birmingham,
Birmingham, Alabama

RICHARD A. SUGERMAN, Ph D
Professor of Anatomy,
College of Osteopathic Medicine of the Pacific,
Pomona, California

Reviewers

STEVEN M. PEPIN, BS, Pharm D
Director of Pharmacy, Shakopee, Minnesota;
Assistant Clinical Professor of Pharmacy,
University of Minnesota College of Pharmacy,
Minneapolis, Minnesota

KENNETH W. RENTON, Ph D
Professor and Head, Department of Pharmacology,
Dalhousie University, Halifax, Nova Scotia

Preface

Psychotropic Drugs was written in response to the need clinicians have for immediate, accurate, and complete psychopharmacologic information. The book is divided into two parts, each uniquely contributing to an overall comprehensive discussion of chemical interventions in psychiatric care.

Part One, "Clinical Psychopharmacology," provides a narrative presentation in 17 chapters that will enable both the recent graduate and the experienced clinician to better integrate the wide-ranging nature of psychopharmacology into practice. Part One is further divided into four units, each organized around a significant conceptual theme.

Unit I introduces the reader to psychotropic drugs and provides a brief historical perspective of these agents. In addition, chapters reviewing neuroanatomy and neurotransmitter mechanisms are so presented as to immerse those a bit "rusty" and challenge those who are more conversant with brain biology.

Unit II, "Drugs Used in the Treatment of Mental Disorders," focuses on the major categories of drugs used in psychiatric care. Each chapter begins with an introductory review establishing the need for the drug, followed by a discussion of pharmacokinetics, administration and dosage, side effects, and clinical implications. Clinical implications include therapeutic versus toxic serum levels, use in pregnancy, interventions for side effects, drug interactions, and patient education considerations.

Unit III, "Drug Issues Related to Psychopharmacology," reviews electroconvulsive therapy, drugs of abuse, central nervous system stimulants, and drugs used to treat extrapyramidal side effects of psychotropic drugs.

Unit IV, "Developmental Issues Related to Psychotropic Drugs," includes chapters on the psychopharmacologic treatment of children, adolescents, and elderly persons.

Part Two, "Psychotropic Drug Profiles," contributes the additional feature of quick, handy drug profiles for 96 psychotropic drugs. Each drug is profiled according to several selected categories such as drug classification, indications, contraindications, pharmacokinetics, and interactions. The combination of this feature with the extensive narrative explanation in Part One is unique among books written on this topic.

This book has two purposes. It can be used as a textbook and as a reference book. The reader can use the drug profiles when quick information is required and then, by noting the referent chapter listed at the beginning of each profile, can follow up with more concentrated study as time permits. The book is designed to meet the needs of the on-duty clinician as well as the student of psychopharmacology.

Acknowledgments

This book was written with the help of several key individuals. For their critical yet careful review of our work, the authors are indebted to Drs. Cleveland Kinney and Stanley K. Wong. Additionally, for their patient and meticulous typing of this manuscript we are particularly grateful to Mary Ann Bailey, Charlene Bender, Karen Buckner, Joyce Lowe, Judy Mason, Amanda Miller, Vicki Moon, Nida Treet, and Melissa Williams. Finally, a special thank you to Carol Shaffhouser, an education coordinator, and to our library support staff.

NLK and DGF

I wish to thank my colleagues at the University of Alabama School of Nursing for their helpfulness during the writing of this book. I am also appreciative of the support of my family: my wife, Bette, a source of strength for over 25 years; my children, Sara, Amanda, and Alex; and brother Hode and sister Jennifer.

NLK

I would like to thank my wife, who hung the moon, Diane Baker, RN, BSN.

DGF

Contents

CLINICAL PSYCHOPHARMACOLOGY

PART ONE

UNIT I

Introduction to Psychotropic Drug Use

CHAPTER 1

Psychiatric Care and Contemporary Treatment

The modern era of psychiatric care, including the discovery and use of psychotropic drugs, can be traced from events occurring near the end of the eighteenth century. The work of several individuals, including Philippe Pinel (1745-1826) in France, William Tuke (1732-1822) in England, and Dorothea Dix (1802-1887) in the United States, is particularly noteworthy because their efforts laid the foundation for compassionate and scientific treatment of the mentally ill. This era of treatment is referred to as the period of enlightenment and is considered the first of four significant benchmarks in the historical development of psychiatric care. Before this time the mentally ill were frequently abused or neglected, or both.

Rosenblatt (1984) writes of the assistance, banishment, and confinement (the ABCs) of the preenlightenment era. Assistance included efforts to help families cope with the problems of living with a mentally disordered family member. Banishment, driving the mentally ill away from the "healthy," was a more common approach to the mental illness and led to wandering bands of "lunatics" who frightened the public and stole or begged from them for survival. Just as often, however, these wandering bands were victimized by "sane" society. Confinement was the most calculated approach of the preenlightenment era. The mentally ill were often chained indiscriminately, the old to the young, men to women, the insane to the criminal or pauper, and by some accounts the living to the dead. Confinement and the natural progression of this practice led to a variety of distorted and uninformed views of mental illness, for example, the mentally ill were thought to be immune from normal biologic stressors such as cold, heat, and hunger (Foucault, 1973). Whether such thinking was representative of the times or merely a rationalization for withholding the investment of resources is not documented. Nonetheless, the mentally ill suffered greatly; they were deprived of basic biologic needs, that is, shelter, clothing, and food, while their basic emotional needs were also being violated. Confined mental patients, for example, were placed on display for the paying public and forced to oblige their keepers in many vile and inhumane ways. This widespread abuse and neglect of the mentally ill ultimately stimulated a reaction among those who were enlightened—Pinel, Tuke, and Dix—that led to the first of the four significant benchmarks in psychiatric care.

BENCHMARKS IN PSYCHIATRIC CARE

Benchmarks in psychiatric care are significant time periods when converging forces led to a unique view of mental illness. The four benchmarks are the period of enlightenment, the period of scientific study, the period of psychotropic drugs, and the period of community mental health care. Each period represents a definite change in the public perception of mental health or psychiatric problems; these changes in perception have led to new strategies and interventions in the treatment of mental illness. A thorough investigation of these benchmarks is beyond the scope of this book. However, a brief description of the relationship between important events and the advent and use of psychotropic drugs is provided.

Period of Enlightenment

The period of enlightenment is so named because reformers, Pinel, Tuke, Dix, and others, rejected the common reasoning of the day and substituted a humane approach to the care of the mentally ill. Affected individuals were no longer considered animal-like but instead were to be treated as fellow humans deserving of adequate shelter, clothing, and food, which would be provided in a dignified manner. Pinel became superintendent of the French institutions Bicêtre for men and, later, Salpêtriére for women, where, dismayed by the living conditions, he unchained the shackled, clothed the naked, fed the hungry, and disposed of whips and other instruments of cruel treatment. Tuke, on the other hand, developed a private institution to care for the psychiatric needs of his English Quaker brethren. He established the York Retreat in 1796, a facility in which moral treatment was instituted and maintained to help the mentally ill. Dix, an American reformer, visited the York Retreat and, on returning to the United States, launched an effective campaign to change the treatment of the mentally ill. She played a direct role in the opening of 32 public mental hospitals.

The period of enlightenment was significant because the first evolutionary step toward a humane and scientific way of thinking was accepted, paving the way for the discovery of contemporary treatments, including psychotropic drugs. The mentally ill were now included in the human family, no longer to be chained and beaten but to be accorded dignity and access to humane treatment. This period also set the stage for the period of scientific study.

Period of Scientific Study

The second benchmark in the evolution of psychiatric care was the period of scientific study. The period of enlightenment represented a change in the way people perceived the mentally ill, that is, the perception emerged that "these poor souls are part of the human family and should be cared for in a humane manner." During the period of scientific study clinicians such as Kraepelin (1856-1926), Freud (1856-1939), and Bleuler (1857-1939) made significant contributions to the knowledge of mental illness. These individuals not only were concerned with providing a humane atmosphere but also wanted to study mental illnesses and develop treatment strategies. The thrust of this period, therefore, was moving beyond caring to curing. Kraepelin, a gifted and thorough neurologist, carefully studied the course of serious mental illness. *Kraepelin, it could be said, laid the groundwork for those who study mental illness from a biologic perspective.* Freud, through years of observation and treatment, developed an approach to working with patients, the psychoanalytic approach, that is still used and, more importantly, is the foundation for many other psychodynamic and psychotherapeutic approaches. Bleuler and others provided unique contributions to our understanding of mental illness, including etiology, prognosis, and treatment. *Freud, Bleuler, and others laid the groundwork for those who study mental illness from a psychologic perspective.*

The significance of the period of scientific study was the concerted effort to identify causes and cures for emotional disturbances. The predominant approach that evolved from the work of Freud and his followers was a therapy based on dialogue with patients, such as psychoanalysis, individual therapy, and group therapy, which is still used, studied, and refined in the modern era. The predominant approach that evolved from the work of Kraepelin and other neurologists was somatic, including the development of drug therapy, electroconvulsive therapy, and other nonpsychotherapeutic interventions.

Period of Psychotropic Drugs

The milieu of theory development and scientific advances superimposed on a humane regard for the mentally ill further led toward the discovery of psychotropic drugs. In 1949 John Cade, an Australian physician, discovered lithium to be an effective drug treatment for bipolar illness. In the early 1950s chlorpromazine (Thorazine) was developed and found effective in the treatment of schizophrenia and other psychoses. In 1958 Kuhn published the first article on antidepressant therapy with imipramine (Tofranil). Hence within one decade three major classes of psychotropic drugs were discovered, antimanic, antipsychotic, and antidepressant drugs; these compounds were a significant advance in the approach to the treatment of bipolar illness, psychosis, and depression, respectively.

The significance of this period of psychotropic drugs was particularly noted as patients began to consistently take these drugs; the demand for observation, food and shelter, and ongoing treatment by a professional staff decreased. For example, in 1955, shortly after the introduction of chlorpromazine, state hospitals reached a peak census of 560,000 patients but by 1986 that population had dropped to 120,000. Many mental health professionals believe the single most significant factor affecting this decrease was the introduction of psychotropic drugs. The concept of least restrictive alternative was a by-product of this period, and the fourth benchmark period evolved, the period of community mental health care.

Period of Community Mental Health Care

If the first three periods represent the evolution of psychiatric care, the fourth represents a revolution. A multitude of converging factors resulted in public demand for reforms in the mental health care system: films and books depicted an isolated, leaderless, and often cruel state hospital system that was, perhaps, contributing to the cause and perpetuation of mental illness; the promise of "talking" patients back to health was losing appeal as the public began to demand and expect faster results; and new emphasis on patient rights began to significantly affect the infrastructure of the public hospital, which previously had been immune to outside interference and criticism. However, the most influential factor contributing to the closing of many state hospital beds was the development of psychotropic drugs. As previously mentioned, patients were helped tremendously by these drugs insofar as patients were more amenable to psychodynamic treatment and other less restrictive formats. Behaviors necessitating inpatient care and locked units, that is, agitation, withdrawal, delusions, hallucinations, suicidal ideations, and the like, were significantly "relieved" by the introduction or institution of psychotropic drugs that enabled patients to respond more appropriately, to cooperate, and to comply with physicians, nurses, psychologists, and social workers. Dialogue with professionals occurred only a few times per week; thus an economical alternative to hospital care that had been conceptualized and desired, outpatient care, was now possible.

Although the concept of community mental health care provides a five-pronged approach to treatment modalities and levels of care, the outpatient dimension has been the most widely used. The development and success of psychotropic drugs were largely responsible for the advent of this fourth benchmark in psychiatric care. Today many affected individuals, who only forty years earlier would have been committed to a state hospital for treatment, are able to lead productive lives in or near their own homes because of the efficacy of psychotropic drugs and community-based care.

The significance of the period of community mental health care has not yet been fully revealed. Neither the promise of psychotropic drugs nor the dream of community mental health care has been realized. The consequences of depopulating state hospitals, often referred to as "deinstitutionalization," and the subsequent rise in mental illness among an ever-growing homeless population, the overuse of emergency psychiatric services, and the flight of professionals from the community mental health arena remind us that, to accomplish the objectives of the community approach, much work remains. Since the promise of psychopharmacology is not yet realized, researchers continue to pursue the development of new drugs. This ongoing research and development of drugs remain critical elements in the care of individuals with mental illness or psychiatric disturbances.

REMARKS

The foregoing discussion is meant to serve as a historical foundation for the remainder of this book and to describe, albeit briefly, social and scientific factors associated with the development and use of psychotropic drugs today. The four benchmarks in psychiatric care have been chosen to illustrate the steady movement by the psychiatric community to develop humane (benchmark 1), scientific (benchmark 2), treatment (benchmark 3) in an optimal therapeutic environment (benchmark 4). Those who have discovered and developed psychotropic drugs owe a conceptual debt to Pinel and Tuke for changing the world's view of the mentally ill and to Freud and the early scientists who studied mental illness and were determined to find a cure. The community mental health movement has demonstrated to the psychiatric community and to the lay public that drug therapy alone is insufficient for many psychiatrically disordered individuals. Continuing research is needed to identify more effective treatment approaches and to refine existing therapeutic interventions and techniques, including the research and development of new psychotropic agents.

REFERENCES

Foucault M: *Madness and civilization,* New York, 1973, Vintage.

Kuhn R: Treatment of depressive states with G22355 (imipramine hydrochloride), *Am J Psychiatry* 115:459, 1958.

Rosenblatt A: Concepts of the asylum in the care of the mentally ill, *Hosp Community Psychiatry* 35:685, 1984.

CHAPTER 2

Review of Functional Neuroanatomy

RICHARD A. SUGERMAN
CLEVELAND F. KINNEY

The nervous system is artificially divided into the central nervous system (CNS) and the peripheral nervous system (PNS). A careful review of Figure 2-1 will improve the reader's understanding of this chapter. The CNS (Figure 2-2) is composed of the brain, which fills the cranial vault, and the spinal cord, which lies within the vertebral canal. The CNS is frequently presented as if the brain and spinal cord were separate entities; however, they are logically viewed as one functional unit. Motor information is transmitted from the telencephalon (forebrain) down the spinal cord and ultimately to body musculature; sensory information from the body and muscles ascends the spinal cord to higher levels. Integration of information takes place throughout the CNS.

The CNS may be divided into three sections based on embryologic development: the prosencephalon, the mesencephalon, and the rhombencephalon. The prosencephalon, or forebrain, is further separable into the telencephalon and the diencephalon. The telencephalon consists of two cerebral hemispheres that constitute the bulk of the nervous system; these are composed of the cerebral cortex, certain limbic structures, the corpus striatum, and a multitude of nervous system pathways. The cerebral cortex (Figure 2-3) is divided into four lobes, the frontal, temporal, parietal, and occipital lobes. The insular cortex (Island of Reil) is buried deep to the frontal, parietal, and temporal lobes and lies at the depth of the lateral fissure. The cingulate gyrus is associated through its length with frontal, parietal, and temporal lobes. The corpus striatum (Figure 2-4) is made up of the caudate nucleus and the lentiform nucleus (putamen and globus pallidus). It is involved in motor functions and is described later in this chapter. The pathways formed by axons from neurons in the cerebral cortex transmit information throughout the CNS. Some of these pathways form the corpus callosum (Figures 2-3 and 2-4), which interconnects the two cerebral hemispheres, internal capsules (Figure 2-4), and the corona radiata through which pass motor and sensory information, as well as many other pathways interconnecting the four cerebral lobes.

The diencephalon (Figure 2-5) is made up of (1) the epithalamus, which is composed of several small nuclei and the pineal gland, (2) the dorsal thalamus, which is the major sensory relay nuclear area to and from the cerebral cortex, (3) the hypothalamus, which maintains homeostasis, and (4) the ventral thalamus, which functions primarily with the basal ganglia. The hypothalamus (Barr and Kiernan, 1988) is a tiny structure inferior to the dorsal thalamus, which is a major sympathetic-parasympathetic visceral integration center. It functions in part as a chemoreceptor by "sampling" cerebrospinal fluid and blood. The hypothalamus controls and influences such functions as body temperature regulation, food and water intake, gastrointestinal activity, and respirations, as well as cardiovascular and endocrine functions. The hypothalamus has two modes of affecting the pituitary gland. The *first* mode is by

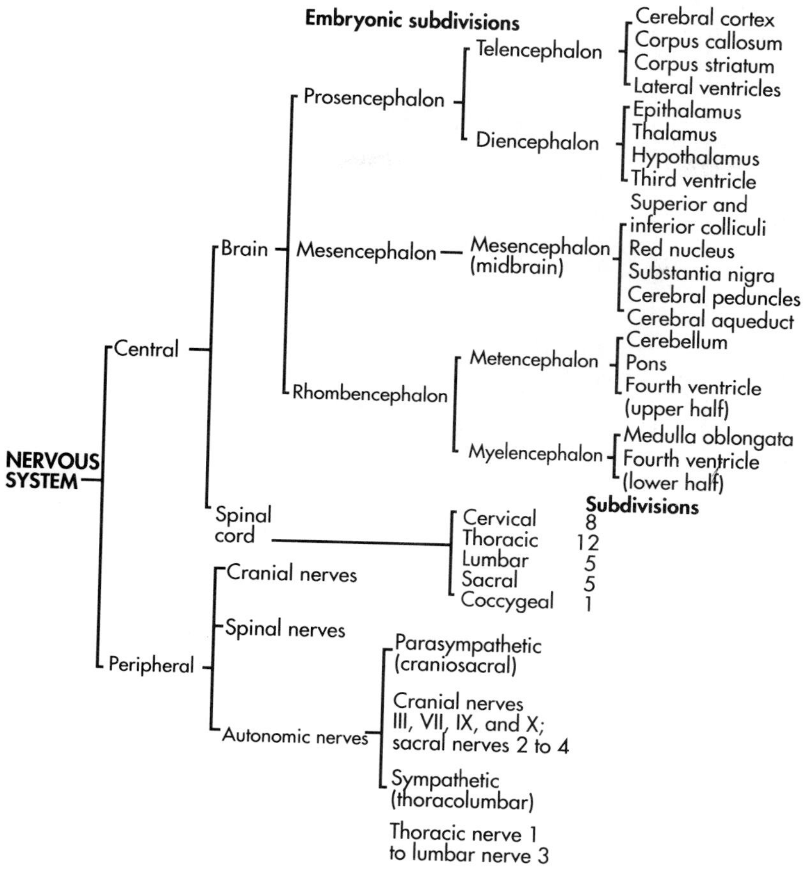

Figure 2-1 Major divisions of the nervous system.

the production of releasing or inhibiting factors that pass into the pituitary portal system, that is, capillary beds in the hypothalamus and pituitary gland, which are interconnected by a portal vessel. These factors are thus transmitted to the anterior pituitary, where they cause the release or inhibition, or both, of anterior pituitary hormones into the blood. The *second* mode is by the direct projection of hypothalamic neurons upon the posterior pituitary, where the neurons directly release their hormones into the pituitary blood supply (portal system).

Beneath the forebrain resides the brain stem, cerebellum, and spinal cord. The brain stem is a collective term for the midbrain, pons, and medulla oblongata. The cerebellum is an expansive area attached to the posterior surface of the pons and resembles its Latin name, "little brain." The most caudal portion of the CNS is the spinal cord.

The midbrain (Figure 2-6) is the caudal (inferior) continuation of the CNS below the forebrain. It is about 1.5 cm long and is significantly narrower than the forebrain. The midbrain consists of the tectum, the tegmentum, the cerebral peduncles, and the associated substantia nigra. The red nuclei and substantia nigra are large structures

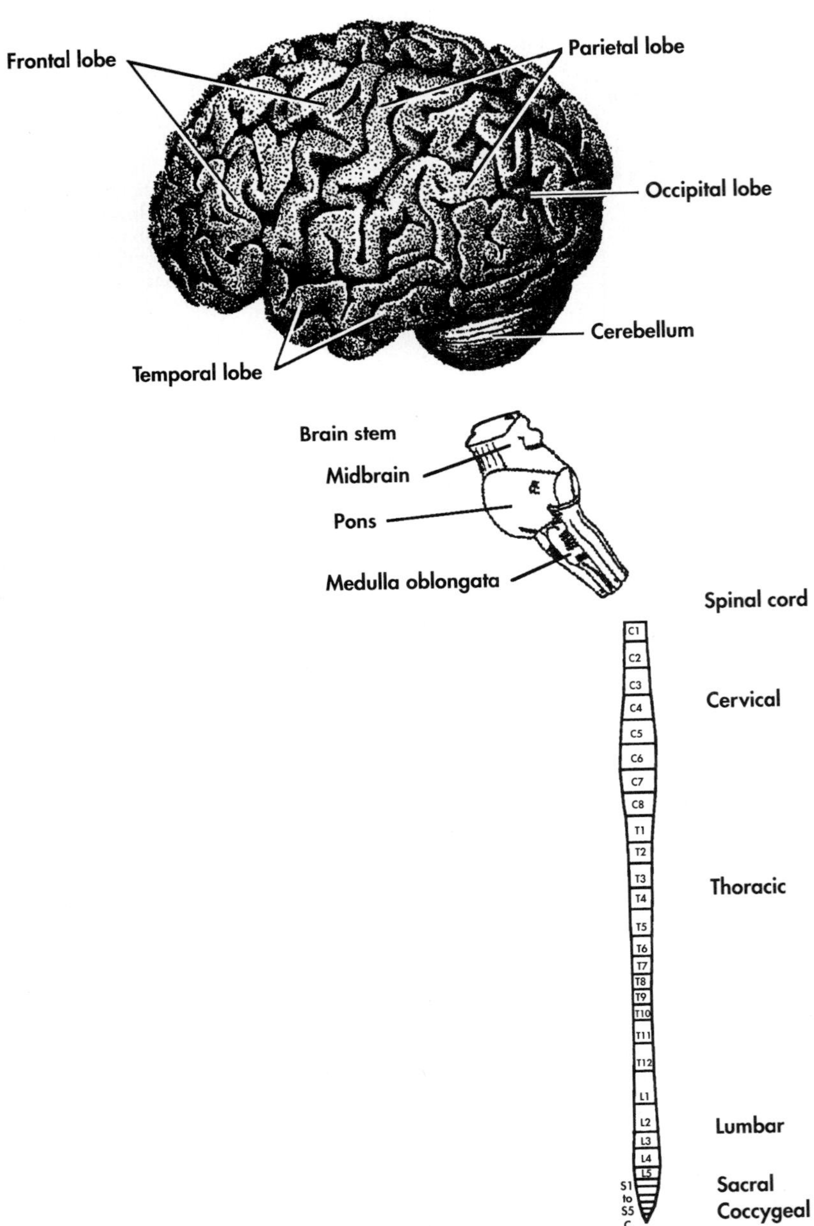

Figure 2-2 Expanded view of the central nervous system showing the major components. (From Berne RM, Levy MN: *Physiology*, ed 2, St Louis, 1988, Mosby.)

Frontal lobe
Cingulate gryus
Parietal lobe
Cerebral aqueduct
Parieto-occipital sulcus
Occipital lobe
Calcarine sulcus
Cerebellar hemisphere
Vermis of cerebellum
Fourth ventricle
Corpus callosum
G
R
S
Interventricular foramen
Temporal lobe
Diencephalon (forming wall of third ventricle)
Midbrain Medulla Pons
Brain stem

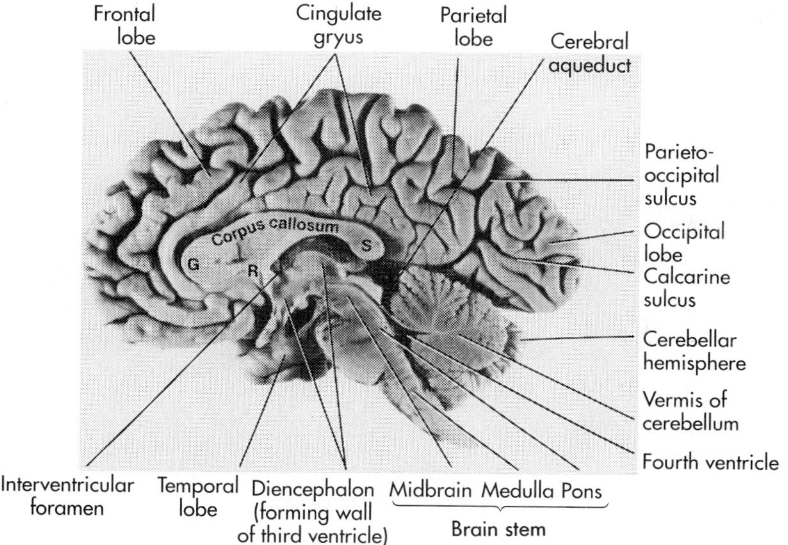

Figure 2-3 Major regions of the cerebrum, cerebellum, and brain stem as seen in the saggital plane. *R*, *G*, and *S* indicate the rostrum, genu, and splenium, respectively, of the corpus callosum. (From Nolte J: *The human brain*, ed 3, St Louis, 1992, Mosby.)

Head of caudate nucleus
Genu of corpus callosum
Lateral ventricle (anterior horn)
Internal capsule (anterior limb)
Septum pellucidum
External capsule
Extreme capsule
Claustrum
Ventral tier nuclei
Putamen
Dorsomedial nucleus
Globus pallidus
Pulvinar
Tail of caudate nucleus

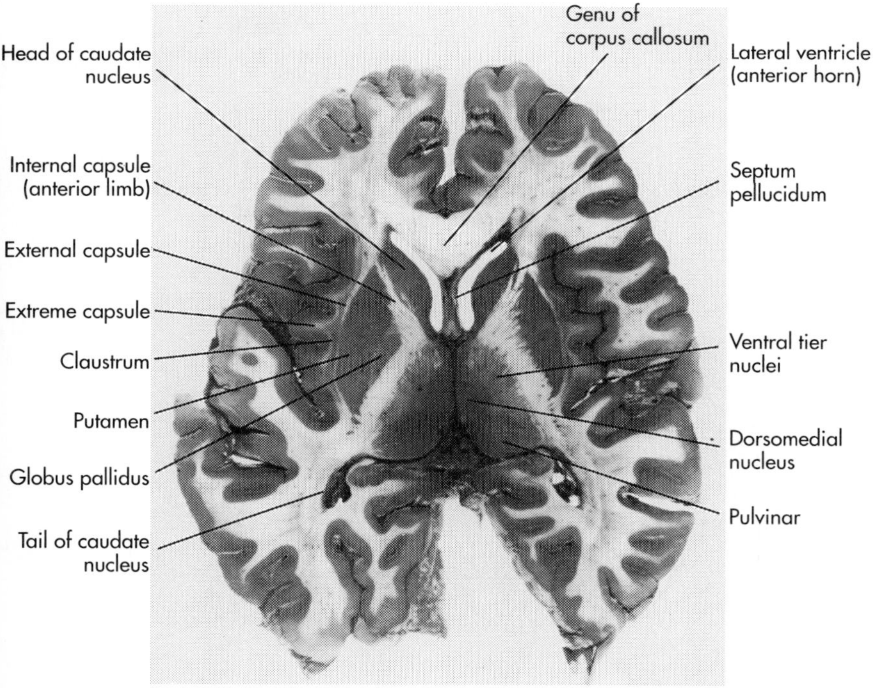

Figure 2-4 Basal ganglia and surrounding structures as seen in an approximately horizontal section. (From Nolte J: *The human brain*, ed 3, St Louis, 1992, Mosby.)

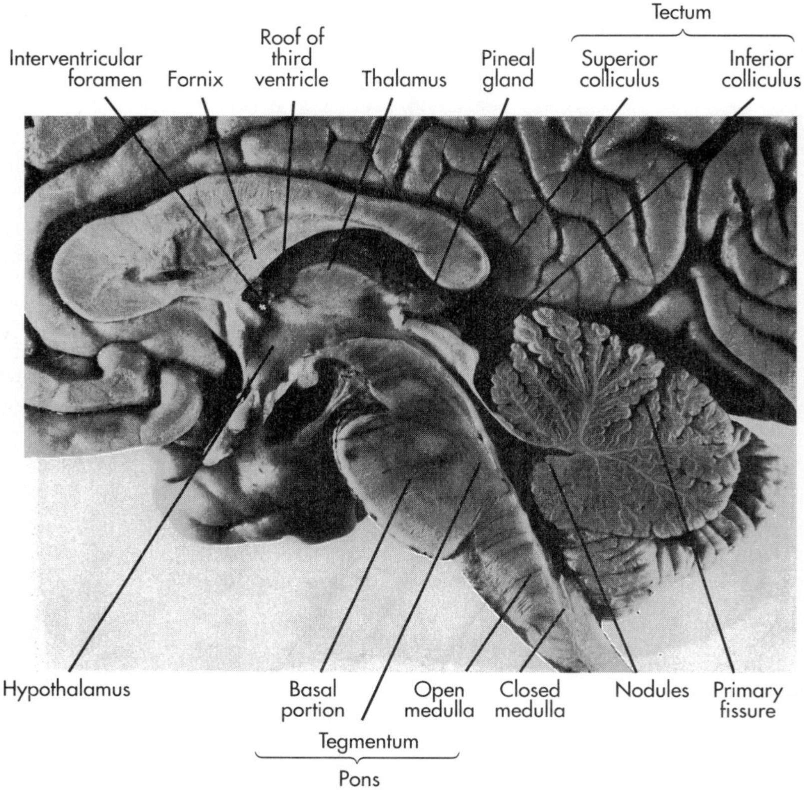

Tectum
Interventricular foramen
Fornix
Roof of third ventricle
Thalamus
Pineal gland
Superior colliculus
Inferior colliculus
Hypothalamus
Basal portion
Open medulla
Closed medulla
Nodules
Primary fissure
Tegmentum
Pons

Figure 2-5 Major features of the diencephalon, brain stem, and cerebellum as seen in the sagittal plane. (From Nolte J: *The human brain,* ed 3, St Louis, 1992, Mosby.)

Superior colliculus (of tectum)
Periaqueductal gray
Cerebral aqueduct
Cerebral Peduncle
Red nucleus
Substantia nigra
Basis pedunculus

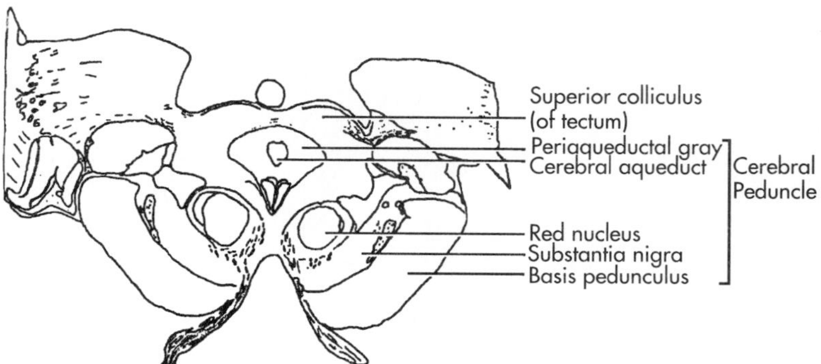

Figure 2-6 Cross section through superior colliculus of the midbrain.

in the midbrain that can be seen by the naked eye on examination. The red nuclei may be seen on freshly cut brains as large, vaguely reddish, round circles; the substantia nigra, as its name implies, is black. The black coloration is due to melanin pigment found in neurons within the substantia nigra. More is said about these nuclei in the discussion of the motor systems. The basis pedunculi (cerebral peduncles) are basically a continuation of axons from motor neurons that project from the cerebral cortex through the corona radiata and internal capsule. The pedunculi form prominent bulges on the anterior (ventral) surface of the midbrain.

The hindbrain is composed of pons, medulla oblongata, and cerebellum. The pons is an expansive area approximately 2.5 cm long that lies between the midbrain and the medulla oblongata. Some of the fibers in the basis pedunculi continue into the pons near the ventral surface of the brain stem, where many of them synapse in pontine nuclei. The pontine nuclei in turn project their axons to the cerebellum.

The medulla oblongata is about 3 cm long and narrows until it is continuous with the cervical spinal cord at the level of the foramen magnum. On the anterior surface of the medulla oblongata is located the continuation of motor fibers (from the cerebral cortex); these fibers are known collectively as the pyramids. (They form two pyramidal bulges.) The decussation of the pyramids, that is, the crossing of the motor pathways contralaterally (to the opposite side), takes place at the lower level of the medulla oblongata. The pons and the medulla oblongata contain the central nuclei associated with the last 8 of the 12 cranial nerves and also contain autonomic control centers.

The cerebellum consists of two hemispheres separated by a central portion called the vermis. The cerebellar hemispheres and most of the vermis simultaneously receive (through complex ascending pathways from the spinal cord) sensory input from muscles and joints. Also, they receive motor signals from the cerebral cortex indicating how the muscle is being directed. The various areas of the cerebellum then communicate with the cerebral cortex to coordinate the final motor activity. These cerebellar areas function in coordinating muscle synergy and activity, but they do *not* initiate movements. The second function of the cerebellum is the maintenance of equilibrium. The central processing of balance information occurs in a small part of both the vermis and each cerebellar hemisphere.

Within the brain stem resides the reticular formation. It comprises a discontinuous series of large nuclei located within the mesencephalon that extend interiorly through the pons and the medulla oblongata, as well as many multisynaptic ascending and descending neural pathways. The reticular formation may be conceived of as a primitive brain buried deep within the brain stem. Input from most sensory pathways passes into the reticular formation, where it is integrated and then projected to the thalamus or the hypothalamus, or both. There are also descending reticulospinal tracts to the spinal cord. The reticular formation is a polysynaptic integration area that affects motor, sensory, and visceral functions. The functional relationship between cell bodies that arise from the reticular formation and are involved in norepinephrine, serotonin, acetylcholine, and dopamine synthesis is fundamental in understanding the neuroanatomy of behavior. These systems and projection fields are further discussed in Chapter 3.

The spinal cord is approximately 42 to 45 cm in length and 1 cm in diameter. In the normal adult the spinal cord ends between lumbar vertebrae L1 and L2. Internally the spinal cord (Figure 2-7, *A*) is divided into gray and white matter, cell bodies, and cell processes. The gray matter is in the shape of an H and fills the central portion of the cord. The posterior (dorsal) part of the H, or posterior (dorsal) horn, is concerned with sensory information, and the anterior (ventral) part of the H, or anterior (ventral) horn, is related to somatic (skeletal muscle) and visceral motor actions. The white matter is divided into posterior, lateral, and anterior areas (funiculi). In general the posterior area contains ascending sensory pathways; the lateral and anterior areas transmit both ascending sensory and descending motor pathways. According to all theories on pain pathways, pain information ascends in both the anterior and the lateral areas.

The spinal cord is organized in segments. There are 8 cervical, 12 thoracic, 5 lumbar, and 5 sacral segments and 1 coccygeal segment. This arrangement is reflected in the dermatomes of the body (Figure 2-8). For example, sensory nerves from the fourth and twelfth thoracic vertebrae (T4 and T12) subserve a narrow band of skin at the level of the nipples and the umbilicus, respectively. A transection of the spinal cord at the fourth cervical vertebra (C4) results in a total loss of motor and sensory functions from the level of the superior surface of the shoulders and below, that is, quadriplegia.

The peripheral nervous system is composed of 31 pairs of spinal nerves and 12 pairs of cranial nerves. The peripheral nervous system can be divided into a "motor nervous system" and an "autonomic nervous system." The spinal nerve is considered a prototype for the entire peripheral nervous system. The spinal nerve (Figure 2-7, *A*) contains motor and sensory neurons. The motor axons originate from neurons in the ventral horn, pass through the ventral root into the spinal nerve, and terminate in skeletal (somatic) muscle, cardiac muscle, smooth (visceral) muscle, or glands. The spinal cord receives sensory information from exteroceptors, proprioceptors, and interoceptors. This information travels from sensory organs through the spinal nerve

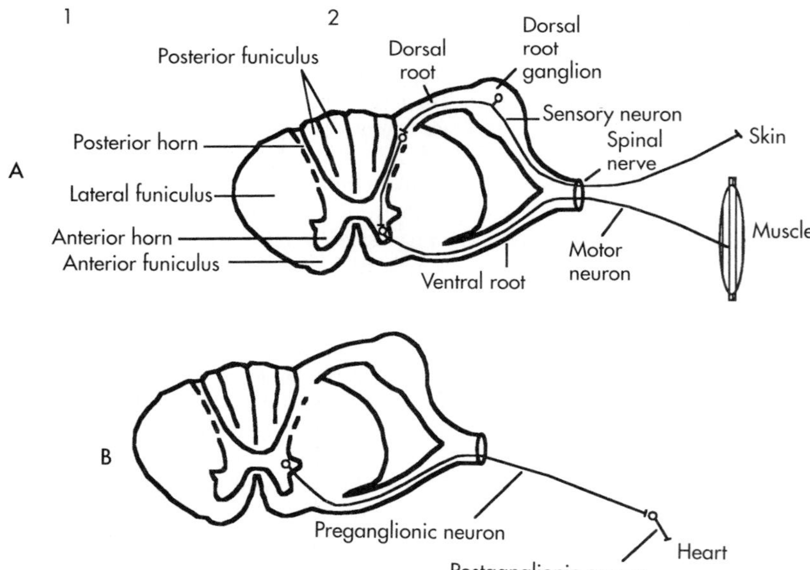

Figure 2-7 **A,** Cross section through a sacral segment of spinal cord. *1,* Basic subdivisions of horns and funiculi columns. *2,* Somatic components of a spinal nerve. **B,** Cross section through a sacral segment of spinal cord. Parasympathetic (visceral) motor components.

and dorsal root before synapsing in the dorsal horn of the cord. The exteroceptors transmit sensations of pain, touch, and temperature, the proprioceptors are responsible for joint, muscle, and tendon perceptions. These sensory modalities are consciously perceived. All these receptors are transducers, that is, they change sensory modalities into action potentials, which are generated by the receptive neurons. The cranial nerves may be considered practically as modified spinal nerves. Some cranial nerves are primarily motor, others are mainly sensory, and still others are a mixture of somatic and visceral, motor and sensory.

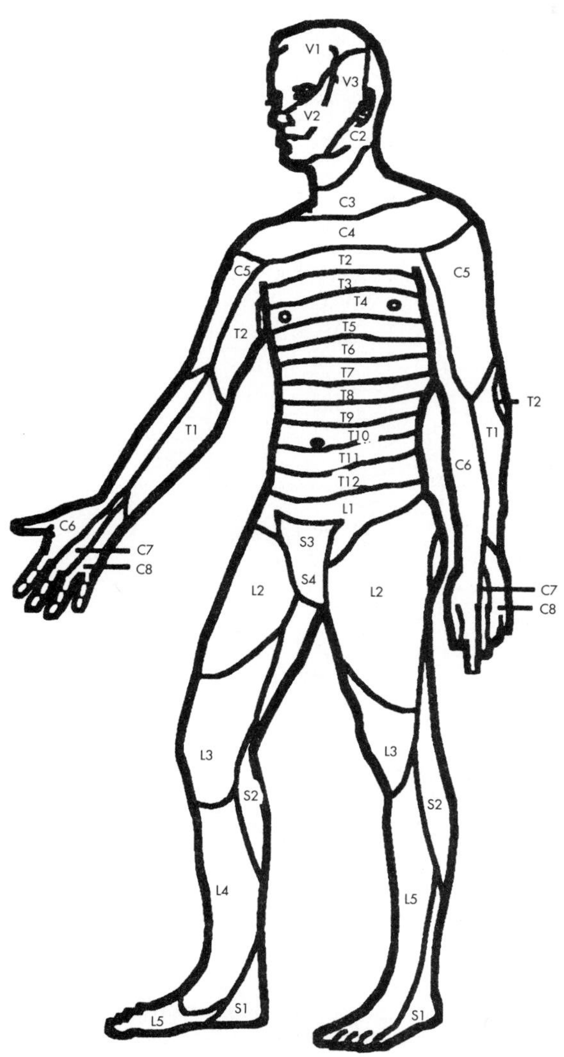

Figure 2-8 Dermatomes. Cutaneous distribution of spinal nerves.

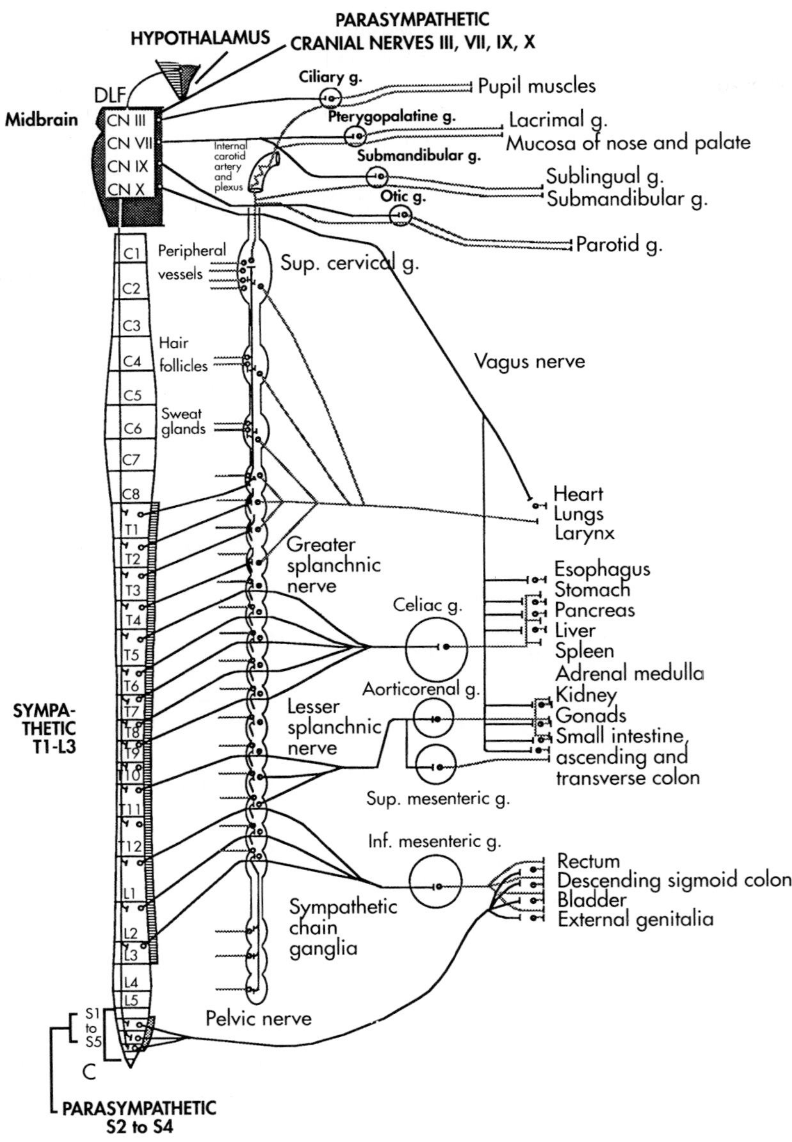

Figure 2-9 Diagram of the entire autonomic nervous system. Sympathetic portions of the central nervous system are shown as horizontally lined areas; the parasympathetic portions are shown as stippled areas. Preganglionic neurons are represented as solid lines, and postganglionic neurons are represented as dashed lines. The dorsal longitudinal fasciculus *(DLF)* interconnects the hypothalamus.

The autonomic nervous system (Figure 2-9) receives interoceptor input and transmits visceral motor output. The autonomic nervous system is further divided into the parasympathetic (craniosacral) and the sympathetic (thoracolumbar) nervous systems. The parasympathetic nervous system is divided into cranial and sacral portions. The cranial part has neuronal components within the oculomotor, facial, glossopharyngeal, vagus, and spinal accessory nerves, whereas the sacral part is composed of neuronal elements located in the second through fourth sacral nerves. The sympathetic nervous system is associated with the spinal nerves in a continuous column from the first thoracic nerve to the third lumbar nerve. Although sympathetic neurons originate within the thoracic portion and part of the lumbar portion of the spinal cord, sympathetic neurons innervate effector organs throughout the body. The anatomy of the visceral motor portion of the autonomic nerves is different from that of the somatic motor nerves. Each somatic motor neuron projects its axon out of the spinal cord and innervates a skeletal muscle. Each neuron has its cell body in the anterior (ventral) horn of the spinal cord. The visceral nerve is made up of two neurons that are referred to as the preganglionic and postganglionic neurons (Figure 2-7, *B*). The preganglionic neurons of the autonomic nervous system have their cell bodies in the gray matter of the spinal cord and brain stem but are located for the most part slightly dorsal to somatic neurons. In the spinal cord the myelinated axon of the preganglionic neuron joins with the axons of the somatic motor neurons in the ventral root but soon leaves the spinal nerve to enter the sympathetic chain ganglia. The axon of the preganglionic neuron synapses on the dendrites or cell body of the postganglionic neuron. The cell bodies of the postganglionic neurons are organized into either ganglia or plexuses. When many neuronal cell bodies are in a connective tissue capsule outside the CNS, these are called a ganglion. If the cell bodies are spread out,

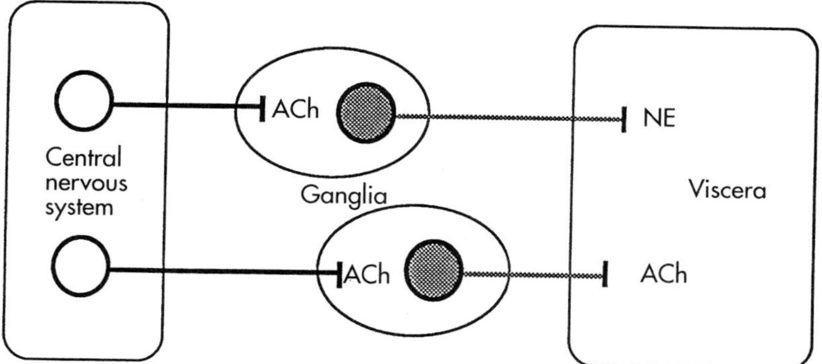

Figure 2-10 Major differences between the sympathetic and parasympathetic systems. The axons of preganglionic sympathetic neurons end in ganglia near the spinal cord, whereas those of preganglionic parasympathetic neurons travel a longer distance and reach ganglia near the innervated organ. The preganglionic neurons of both systems use acetylcholine (ACh) as their neurotransmitter, but at the synapses of postganglionic neurons the parasympathetic system uses ACh and the sympathetic system uses norepinephrine (NE). (From Nolte J: *The human brain,* ed 3, St Louis, 1992, Mosby.)

as in the wall of the gut, they are called a plexus. The sympathetic chain ganglia, the largest of the autonomic structures, run parallel to the vertebral column and extend from the base of the skull to the end of the coccyx.

Preganglionic neurons utilize acetylcholine as their neurotransmitter (Figure 2-10). The postganglionic neurons send their lightly myelinated axons to their effector organs, smooth muscle cardiac muscle, or glands. In general the parasympathetic postganglionic neurons utilize acetylcholine and the sympathetic postganglionic neurons utilize norepinephrine as their neurotransmitters.

SUPRASPINAL MOTOR PATHWAYS

The term "supraspinal motor pathways" refers to pathways concerned with motor activity that involve cortical and subcortical (including brain stem nuclei) structures. The motor aspects of peripheral nerves and spinal reflexes are not discussed in this section. The three major motor systems traditionally include the corticospinal tracts (pyramidal system), corticobulbar pathways, and the basal ganglia system (extrapyramidal system). These systems function as an integrative whole in accomplishing motor activity.

The corticospinal tract originates primarily in the precentral gyrus, the most caudal gyrus of the frontal lobe, with contributions from adjacent cortical areas. The motor strip located within the precentral gyrus is often called the primary motor cortex and has an inverted body pattern in the form of a homunculus *(little man)* (Figure 2-11). The foot and leg muscles are represented on the medial surface of the precentral gyrus, and in order, descending over the lateral surface of the gyrus, are the buttock, thorax, arm, hand, and facial muscles. This somatotopic organization is maintained throughout the CNS. Motor and sensory information are both organized throughout the nervous system in specific patterns.

The cortical neurons (Figure 2-12) project from the precentral gyri ipsilaterally (same side) through the corona radiata, the internal capsule, and the middle three fifths of the cerebral peduncles (basis pedunculi), thence they are interspersed within the basal pons and ultimately form the pyramids at medulla oblongata levels. In the inferior medulla oblongata most (about 70%) of the pyramidal fibers decussate (cross) contralaterally, forming the lateral corticospinal tract, which ultimately synapses either directly or indirectly on alpha motor neurons in the spinal cord. Therefore the right cerebral cortex gives rise to the left lateral corticospinal tract and vice versa. This pathway controls voluntary, precise motor movements.

The corticobulbar pathways synapse on brain stem motor nuclei associated with the cranial nerves. The pathways have their origin in the precentral gyrus or immediately adjacent areas and descend through the corona radiata, the genu of the internal capsule, the cerebral peduncles, the basal pons, and the medulla oblongata.

The vestibular nuclei and their associated ascending and descending connections help coordinate conjugate eye movements, balance, and primarily extensor muscle groups of the body. The descending pathway from the vestibular nuclei (located in the caudal pons and medulla) is called the lateral vestibulospinal tract, and descends ipsilaterally (on the same side) in the brain stem and spinal cord, synapsing ipsilaterally on extensor motor neurons. This pathway functions to help keep us standing erect and to maintain balance.

The basal ganglia give rise to the extrapyramidal system; these projections do not pass through the pyramidal tracts. The extrapyramidal system is composed of a group of nuclei (deep within the telencephalon) and their projection pathways, which

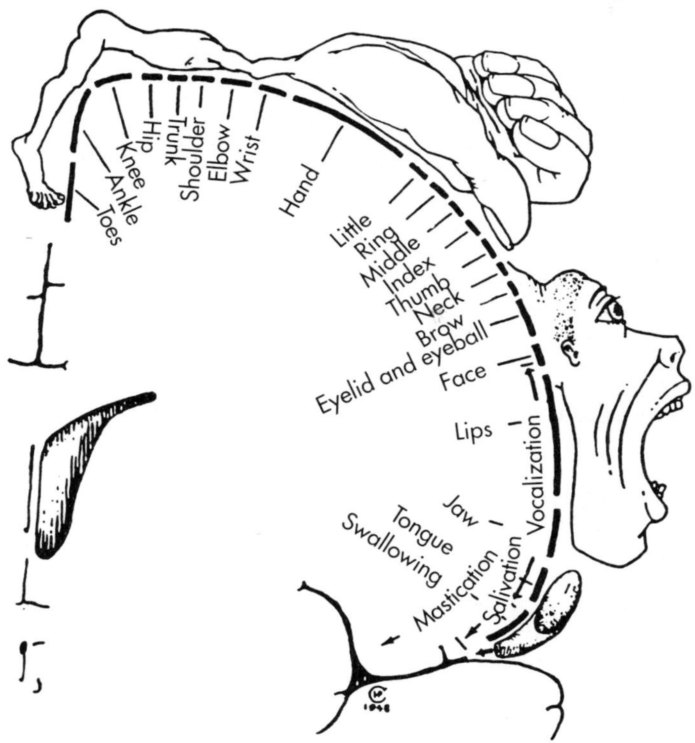

Figure 2-11 Homunculus of the precentral gyrus. This is a frontal section depicting the relative amount of cortex subserved in controlling the motor functions of various body areas. (From Penfield W, Rasmussen T: *The cerebral cortex of man,* New York, 1950, Macmillan.)

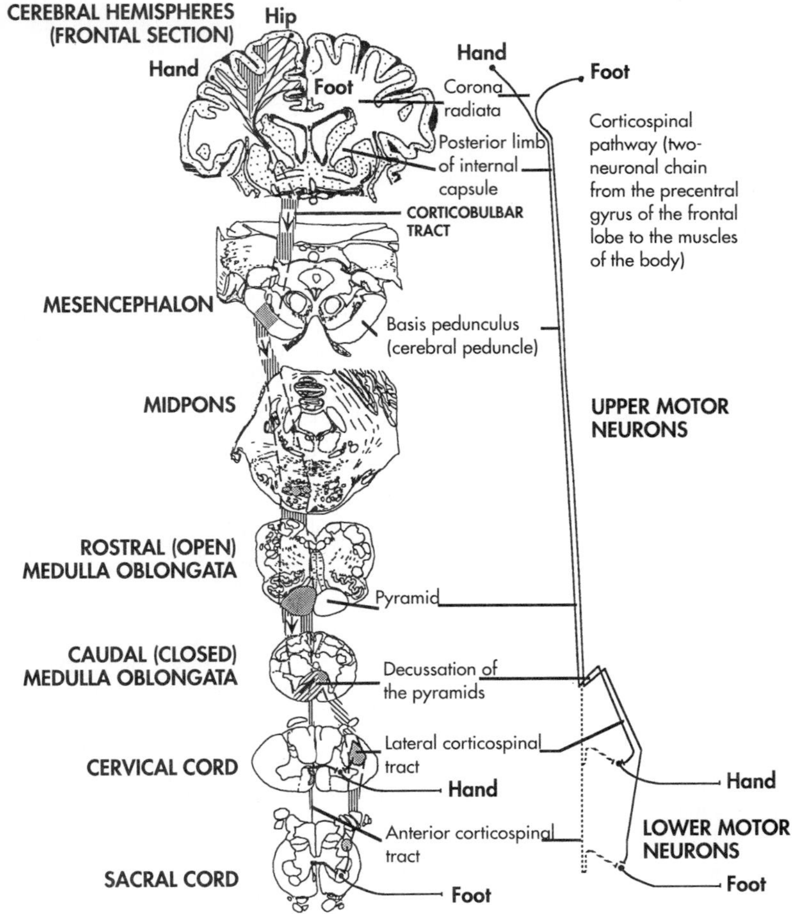

Figure 2-12 Distribution of the corticospinal tract (long pathway) and corticobulbar tract (short pathway). Actual representation, *left;* schematic, *right.*

interrelate motor activities of the cerebral cortex, cerebellum, and brain stem. The descending output of this system originates largely from the globus pallidus with synapses in course on the red nucleus and adjacent nuclei. The descending pathways terminate on motor (ventral horn) neurons within the spinal cord.

Generally the corticospinal tract *controls* precise, voluntary movements, and the basal ganglia, in conjunction with the cerebellum, *stabilize* motor movements. Lesions of the basal ganglia result in abnormal motor movements such as those seen in Parkinson's disease.

The basal ganglia may be defined in many ways. A strict anatomic definition of the basal ganglia is outlined as follows:

I. Corpus striatum
   A. Caudate nucleus
   B. Lentiform nucleus
      1. Putamen
      2. Globus pallidus
II. Claustrum
III. Amygdala

It could be argued that the claustrum and amygdala are not truly dimensions of the basal ganglia. Structures that are interconnected with the basal ganglia are (1) the red nucleus, (2) the thalamus, (3) the cerebral cortex, and (4) the reticular formation.

A simplified illustration of many of the interrelationships of the nuclei and tracts of the basal ganglia is presented in Figure 2-13. The pathways, shown in the form of neurons projecting to anatomic areas, give only general basal ganglia relationships and do not fully represent all pathways.

A lateral view of the left cerebral hemisphere, including the precentral and postcentral gyri, is represented in Figure 2-13, *A*. Neurons located in the frontal and parietal lobes and neurons close to the precentral and postcentral gyri project their axons to the striatum, that is, the caudate nucleus and the putamen. These axons traverse the corona radiata and the internal capsule. These projections from the cortex are transmitting motor information to the striatum. The caudate nucleus in part (Figure 2-13, *B*) integrates this information and projects to the putamen.

The neurons of the putamen distribute their axons within the putamen to the globus pallidus (which is subdivided into internal and external sections) and to the substantia nigra (Figure 2-13, *C*) through the striatonigral pathway. Most neurons within the putamen secrete gamma-aminobutyric acid (GABA) as their primary neurotransmitter and are referred to as GABA (gabanergic) neurons. Gamma-aminobutyric acid is an inhibitory neurotransmitter. The putamen also receives projections from dopamine-secreting neurons located within the substantia nigra via the nigrostriatal tract.

The globus pallidus sends a significant number of gabanergic axons to the subthalamic nucleus, the substantia nigra, and the red nucleus, as well as to nuclei of the dorsal thalamus (DeLong, 1989).

The subthalamic nucleus projects glutaminergic neurons (excitatory neurons) to the globus pallidus as well as to the putamen (not illustrated). The pallidal neurons whose axons pass to the red nucleus (Figure 2-13, *C*) stimulate two pathways (the rubrospinal and reticulospinal tracts), which are the primary pathways by which the basal ganglia ultimately influence the brain stem and spinal cord.

The rubrospinal tract (*rubro*, red) originates in the red nucleus and descends into the cervical spinal cord contralaterally (opposite side), where it terminates on ventral horn cells.

Information from the basal ganglia passes to the dorsal thalamus and then, by way of thalamocortical fibers, through the internal capsule and corona radiata, to terminate on premotor cortex, immediately anterior to the precentral gyrus. Although not illustrated in Figure 2-13, the motor cortex incorporates and utilizes this information when discharging through the corticospinal tract.

Within the basal ganglia there are three major feedback loops. The one already discussed involves a circuit of synapses from the frontoparietal cortex to the striatum; impulses then pass from the putamen to the globus pallidum, from the globus palli-

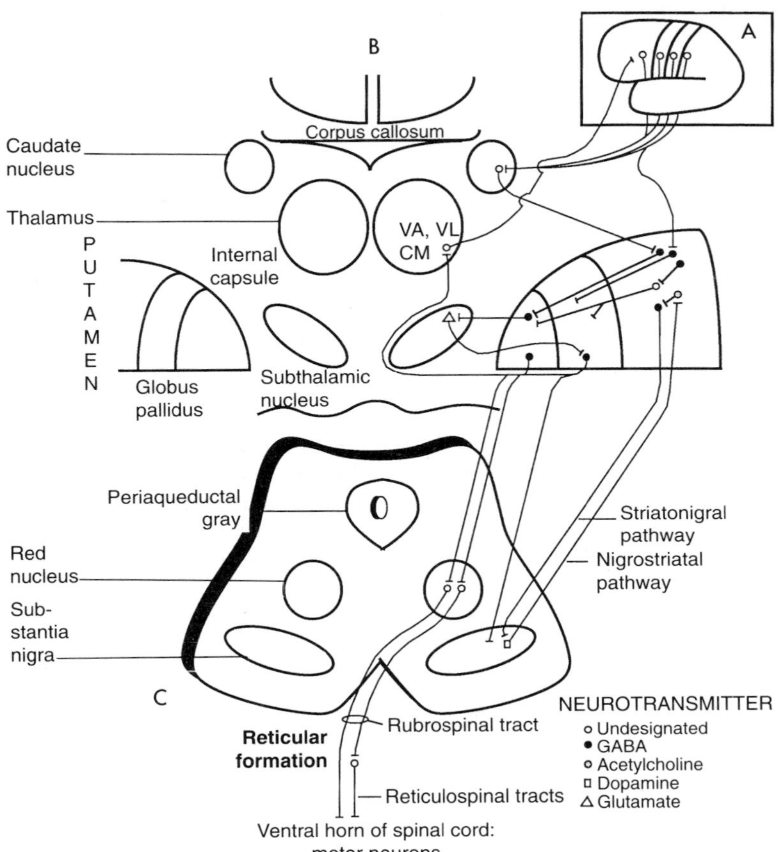

Figure 2-13 Basal ganglia system and its interconnections, including identified neurotransmitters. **A,** Left view of cerebral hemisphere. **B,** Coronal section of brain through corpus striatum. **C,** Midbrain. *VA,* Ventral anterior; *VL,* ventrolateral; and, *CM,* centromedian thalamic nuclei.

dum to the dorsal thalamus, and from the dorsal thalamus to the cortex. The second loop is from the globus pallidus to the subthalamic nucleus and then to the globus pallidus, and the third is from the putamen to the substantia nigra and then to the putamen. The latter circuit is of great interest to clinicians. The striatonigral pathway has already been mentioned as a gabanergic pathway passing from the putamen to the substantia nigra. These neurons synapse on dopaminergic neurons in the substantia nigra, which in turn sends axons to the putamen via the nigrostriatal pathway. The dopaminergic neurons are believed to synapse on acetylcholine (ACh) neurons intrinsic within the putamen. These ACh neurons then excite the previously mentioned putamen gabanergic neurons. The interaction of dopamine, ACh, and GABA and their relative concentrations are important in the control of movement disorders (Afifi and Bergman, 1986). Clinical neuropharmacologists and clinicians who treat problems within this system use drug therapy, brain implants, and psychosurgery.

LIMBIC LOBE

The limbic lobe (Figure 2-14) is the portion of the telencephalon that forms a border, or limbus, between the telencephalon and diencephalon. The limbic lobe frequently has been referred to as the rhinencephalon, or "nose-brain," because it is intimately involved with the perception and transmission of olfactory impulses. The so-called limbic lobe is not a separate anatomic division within the central nervous system but comprises structures that are found in the frontal lobe and pass through the parietal lobe, as well as structures found within the temporal lobe. The limbic lobe is concerned with the utilization of visceral functions for survival mechanisms and with the development of preferential visceral functions that are involved in eating and sexual activity. Structures most commonly included in the limbic lobe are (1) the olfactory nerves, (2) the olfactory bulbs and olfactory tracts, or striae, (3) the septum or parolfactory area of Broca, (4) the amygdala, (5) the parahippocampal gyrus, (6) its underlying hippocampal formation, (7) the major projection bundle from the hippocampus, the fimbria-fornix, and (8) the preoptic area. To understand the limbic lobe one must have some appreciation of its connections. Mitral cells in the olfactory bulbs that are receiving olfactory impulses from the nasal mucosa transmit these impulses along the olfactory striae. The medial olfactory tract or stria terminates largely in the parolfactory area of Broca. The impulses are relayed from the parolfactory area of Broca (the septum) to the hypothalamus by way of the medial forebrain bundle. It is well known and documented that the hypothalamus and the discharges from the hypothalamus are concerned with visceral responses to olfactory stimuli. Thus olfactory impulses, which ultimately reach the hypothalamus, influence the major discharge of two pathways from the hypothalamus, the dorsal longitudinal fasciculus and the hypothalamotegmentoreticular pathways. Both of these pathways descend through the brain stem to terminate on cranial nerve parasympathetic and motor nuclei concerned with visceral impulses, such as feeding. Hence there is a multisynaptic pathway by

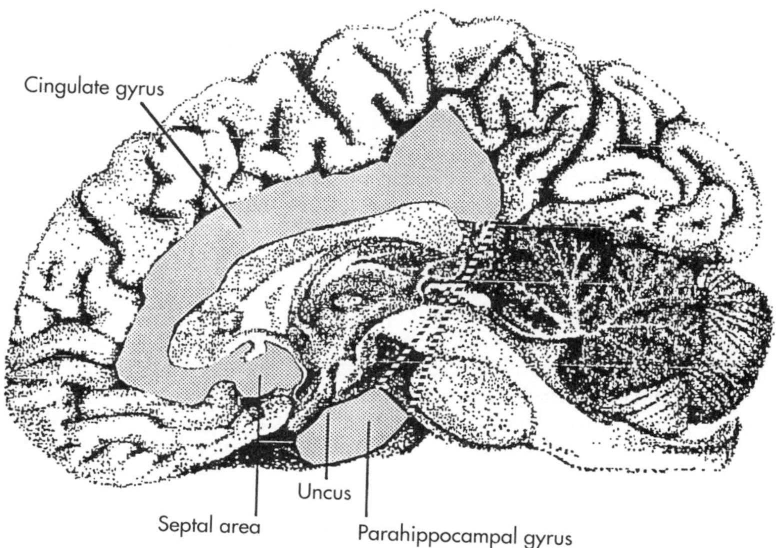

Figure 2-14 Limbic lobe as seen from a medial midsagittal view of the brain. (From Nolte J: *The human brain,* ed 3, St Louis, 1992, Mosby.)

which olfactory impulses may pass from the primary receptive areas within the telencephalon into the brain stem so that we might salivate in response to olfaction. Olfaction related to higher cortical functions is largely accomplished through the connections of the lateral olfactory tract. Olfactory impulses are transmitted along the lateral olfactory tract to terminate principally in the corticomedial amygdaloid nucleus, as well as in the prepyriform cortex. From the corticomedial amygdaloid nucleus there are interconnections with the basolateral amygdaloid nucleus. From the basal lateral amygdaloid nucleus these impulses are transmitted into the temporal lobe to the parahippocampal gyrus. The parahippocampal gyrus in turn projects these impulses to the underlying hippocampal formation, which, through the cornu ammonis, gives rise to the fimbria-fornix. The fimbria-fornix projects mainly to the mammillary bodies of the hypothalamus. The major projections from the mammillary bodies is through the mammillothalamic tract (bundle of Vicq d'Azyr), which terminates in the anterior nucleus of the dorsal thalamus; however, the mammillary bodies are also interconnected with other hypothalamic nuclei and thus may influence the discharge of the descending pathways previously mentioned. It must be remembered that the temporal lobe contains primary auditory cortex and auditory association cortex. The temporal lobe also receives long association bundles from the occipital lobe and from the parietal lobe. Thus the temporal lobe is stimulated by connections from many widely varying cortical areas. These impulses are transmitted to the hippocampal gyrus and to the hippocampal formation and take part in the stimulation of the fimbria-fornix.

Not only is the amygdala connected with the parahippocampal gyrus, but also there are direct projections from the amygdala into the hypothalamus by way of the ventral amygdalohypothalamic tract. Thus olfactory impulses that reach the amygdala may not only ultimately stimulate the various structures within the medial temporal lobe but also may influence the discharge of the hypothalamus through this pathway. It is often thought, and has been stated, that the amygdala is concerned with visceral impulses related to pleasurable and discriminatory activities. Bilateral lesions of the amygdala result in what is known as a Klüver-Bucy syndrome. The pure state is usually not seen in human's and was described originally in experimental studies performed on monkeys. Bilateral destruction of the medial temporal lobes, including the amygdala, results in an animal that is frequently placid. These animals have a tendency to examine everything in their environment by utilizing their oral cavities. They also may lose sexual discrimination, and their eating preferences are altered. Occasionally these animals (rather than being placid) are extremely aggressive and hostile; this behavior has sometimes been referred to as "sham" rage. Trauma in human beings may result in bilateral damage to the temporal lobes, and in such cases a combination of these symptoms is often seen. Herpes encephalitis, which has a predilection for the temporal lobes, may also result in a combination of these various symptoms.

One cannot discuss the connections of the medial temporal lobes and the hippocampus without considering those structures included in what has become known as Papez's circuit. This circuit includes a number of important interconnections between the temporal lobe, the hypothalamus, the cingulate gyrus, and its underlying long association bundle, the cingulum. Impulses, as stated previously, are transmitted from the hippocampal formation through the fimbria-fornix to the mammillary bodies. From the mammillary bodies impulses are projected to the anterior nucleus of the dorsal thalamus by way of the mammillothalamic tract. The anterior nucleus of the dorsal thalamus relays these impulses by way of anterior thalamic radiations, which pass through the anterior limb of the internal capsule, to the cingulate gyrus. The cingulate gyrus gives rise to the long association bundle, the cingulum, which then transmits impulses that pass along its length through the isthmus and ultimately into the temporal lobe, where it terminates in relation to the hippocampal gyrus. As stated previously, there are interconnections between the parahippocampal gyrus and the hippocampal formation. Because impulses may be transmitted along both directions through this circuit, it may be said to be a "two-way street." It is now known that bilateral lesions of Papez's circuit, particularly those involving the fornix, result in profound loss of recent memory. It is well documented that the removal of tumors from the third ventricle, which interrupts the fornix bilaterally, results in a patient who is no longer able to lay down new or recent memory. Bilateral lesions of the hippocampal formation have also been noted to have this profound result. Patients with these kinds of injuries may have intact long-term memory, but their ability to make new memories is frequently severely impaired. Thus it is thought that the integrity of Papez's circuit is vital for the ability to learn.

REFERENCES

Afifi AK, Bergman RA: *Basic neuroscience: a structural and functional approach*, ed 2, Baltimore, 1986, Urban & Schwarzenberg.

Barr ML, Kiernan JA: *The human nervous system: an anatomical viewpoint*, Philadelphia, 1988, JB Lippincott.

DeLong MR: Symposium. Basal ganglia: structure and function, *Soc Neuroscience* 15(1):952, 1989 (abstract).

ADDITIONAL READINGS

Berne RM, Levy MN: *Physiology*, ed 3, St Louis, 1992, Mosby.

Crill WE: The milieu of the central nervous system. In HD Patton et al, editors: *Textbook of physiology*, vol 1, Philadelphia, 1989, WB Saunders.

Doane BK, Livingston KF, editors: *The limbic system: functional organization and clinical disorders*, New York, 1983, Raven.

Franck JAE et al: The limbic system. In HD Patton et al, editors: *Textbook of physiology*, vol 1, Philadelphia, 1989, WB Saunders.

Isaacson RL: *The limbic system*, New York, 1982, Plenum.

Lindsley DF, Holmes JE: *Basic human neurophysiology*, New York, 1984, Elsevier.

Narabayashi H: Stereotaxic vim thalamotomy for treatment of tremor, *Eur Neurol* 29:29, 1989.

Neuwelt EA, editor: *Implications of the blood-brain barrier and its manipulation*, vol 2. *Clinical aspects*, New York, 1989, Plenum.

Nolte J: *The human brain: an introduction to its fundamental anatomy*, ed 3, St Louis, 1993, Mosby.

Papez JW: A proposed mechanism of emotion, *Arch Neurol Psychiatry* 38:725, 1937.

Rowland LP: Blood-brain barrier, cerebrospinal fluid, brain edema, and hydrocephalus. In Kandel ER, Schwartz JH: *Principles of neural science*, New York, 1985, Elsevier.

Squire LR: Mechanisms of memory, *Science* 232:1612, 1986.

CHAPTER 3

Review of Neurotransmitters

RICHARD A. SUGERMAN

Neurons are the basic subunit of the nervous system. They transmit information by sending action potentials, or waves of electrical depolarization, down their processes and on to other neurons. Most action potentials travel from one neuron to another by sending a chemical called a neurotransmitter across a minute space (or synapse), which separates these cells, to evoke the next action potential. It is in or around this space, or synapse, that many drugs have their site of action in the nervous system.

SYNAPTIC TRANSMISSION

Figure 3-1 depicts two neurons. The first neuron is the presynaptic neuron, and its axon is going to a dendrite of the second neuron, or postsynaptic neuron. The presynaptic membrane often has on its surface synaptic boutons, button- or bulb-shaped projections on the end of the axon, that are directly opposite the postsynaptic membrane. Synaptic boutons are about 1 μm in diameter and contain synaptic vesicles carrying neurotransmitters. An action potential arriving at a synaptic bouton (Figure 3-2) causes a change in the membrane potential of the bouton by opening calcium channels and allowing extracellular calcium (Ca^{++}) to enter the bouton. The increased intracellular calcium in the bouton triggers the vesicles to fuse with the bouton's cellular membrane and releases the transmitter into the synaptic cleft, a 20-nm space between the cells. The neurotransmitter then diffuses across the synaptic cleft to the postsynaptic membrane of the next neuron, where it binds only to specific receptors. For example, the neurotransmitter acetylcholine (ACh) binds only with the ACh receptors on the postsynaptic membrane of the next neuron. This binding allows sodium ions into and potassium ions out of opened channels. If enough ACh diffuses to the postsynaptic membrane (receptors), an action potential can be gener-

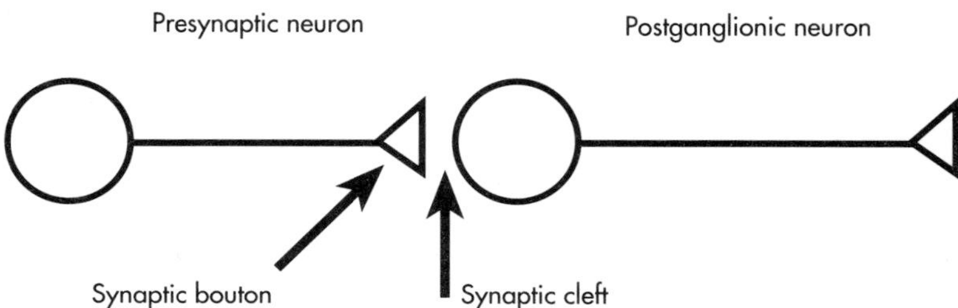

Figure 3-1 Two-neuron chain showing the presynaptic and postsynaptic neurons interconnected by a synapse. The synapse is composed of a synaptic bouton *(triangle)* that is on the presynaptic membrane, the synaptic cleft, and the postsynaptic membrane, which in this instance is the dendrite or cell body *(circle)* of the postsynaptic neuron.

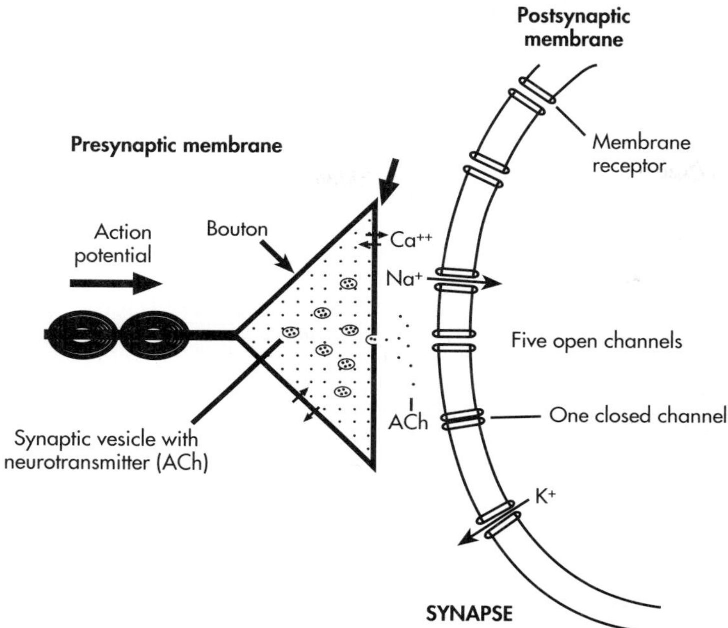

Figure 3-2 An action potential opens calcium ion channels and allows Ca^{++} to enter the presynaptic membrane (bouton). The Ca^{++} triggers the vesicles to fuse with the membrane and release the neurotransmitter (ACh) into the synaptic cleft. Two molecules of ACh then bind with an ACh receptor on the postsynaptic membrane of the target cell, which allows sodium (Na^+) influx and potassium (K^+) efflux through opened channels in the target cell membrane. The channels are normally closed, except when activated by the ACh-receptor complex.

ated by the postsynaptic neuron. Most neurotransmitters, after binding to the receptors, are quickly and actively "reuptaken" by the presynaptic boutons or surrounding glial cells. Acetylcholine is an exception to this general principle. It is broken down in the synaptic space by the enzyme acetylcholinesterase. The rapid degradation of ACh allows only a short burst of activity at the postsynaptic membrane.

Types of Synapses

At one time neuroscientists were aware of only a few types of synapses. The classic axon synapsed on the dendrites, somas (cell body), and axons—the axodendritic, axosomatic, and axoaxonic synapses, respectively. With the advent of the electron microscope scientists found somatosomatic and dentrodendritic synapses. In addition, electron micrography has allowed scientists to find reciprocal synapses between two neurons, for example, dendrodendritic (Shepard, 1983). These reciprocal synapses probably form minuscule local positive or negative feedback loops. Furthermore, many neurons receive input from more than 1000 other neurons. Thus the true complexity of the neuronal milieu begins to be appreciated.

MEMBRANE RECEPTORS

Receptors are cell membrane proteins that react to specific neurotransmitters. These proteins are depicted as hollow tubes that extend their openings between the extracellular and intracellular spaces. These openings are referred to as pores or channels. When a neurotransmitter binds with its specific receptor, a conformational change takes place that opens or closes the channel to the flow of specific ions, for example, sodium, potassium, and chloride. The ACh receptor molecule is a glycoprotein with a molecular weight of 268,000 and five separate polypeptides that extend into the extracellular space (Hille, 1989). The exposed polypeptides help in providing the specificity for the receptors.

Classically pharmacologists working with ACh have operationally defined ACh receptors as either nicotinic or muscarinic, depending on whether the alkaloid nicotine or muscarine has an excitatory (agonistic) effect at the synapse. For example, ACh receptors that are stimulated by nicotine are **nicotinic** and ACh receptors that are stimulated by muscarine are *muscarinic*. Acetylcholine receptors at the neuromuscular junction of skeletal muscle and in sympathetic ganglia are nicotinic, whereas ACh receptors found on effector organs such as glands, smooth muscle, and cardiac muscle are muscarinic. Therefore ACh has more than one type of receptor. In addition, the excitatory effects of ACh at the receptors can be blocked selectively by different agents or antagonists. For example, nicotinic receptors on skeletal muscle are selectively blocked by curare, whereas muscarinic receptors are blocked by atropine. Thus the presence of specific agonists and antagonists for the membrane receptors have enabled scientists to classify receptors for ACh and other neurotransmitters into more than one type. Scientists now know that there are many different types of receptors that are specific for individual neurotransmitters.

Mechanisms of Receptor Action

When a neurotransmitter binds with a receptor, ion channels are opened or closed, allowing specific ions to start or stop moving across the postsynaptic membrane and evoking local changes in the membrane potential. In neuron excitation, when a sufficient amount of neurotransmitter binds with a threshold-level number of receptors, an action potential takes place and travels along the entire length of the neuron. When the neurotransmitter-receptor complex results in direct change of the membrane potential, it is referred to as *first messenger transmission*. First messenger transmission requires only a few milliseconds to initiate its changes to the cell membrane. First messenger transmission also can initiate a series of intracellular reactions by triggering *secondary messenger transmission* that causes not only delayed ion channel opening or closing but also the regulation of many cell functions. These secondary messengers are cell membrane proteins that relay the "message" from the neurotransmitter-receptor complex to a chain of chemical reactions in the neuroplasm of the cell (Patton, 1989). Thus hormones and neurotransmitters can activate intracellular mechanisms to initiate cell division, protein synthesis, and the like. First messenger transmission can be viewed as evoking rapid, *direct* membrane changes, and secondary messenger transmission as a slower, *indirect* process with broad applications.

NEUROTRANSMISSION

Neuron Excitation and Inhibition

Neuron excitation of the postsynaptic membrane is due to the stimulation of the receptor by the neurotransmitter. This stimulation causes an influx of sodium ions into the neuron, which results in the depolarization of the postsynaptic membrane. Inhibition is due to an efflux of potassium ions or an influx of chloride ions, or both, that causes a hyperpolarization of the postsynaptic membrane. Neurotransmitters are sometimes classified as excitatory or inhibitory, *but the mechanism of action actually depends on the postsynaptic receptor*. Acetylcholine can be either excitatory or inhibitory, depending on the receptor that it activates.

Defining Neurotransmitters

The following specific criteria are used to define a chemical as a neurotransmitter:

1. The chemical must be found in the presynaptic boutons and must be released when the neuron is stimulated.
2. The chemical must somehow be inactivated after it is released. Two mechanisms of inactivation have been found. The most common is reuptake of the chemical by the presynaptic membrane, and the second is the degradation of the chemical by an extracellular enzyme.
3. If the chemical is applied exogenously at the postsynaptic membrane, the effect will be the same as when the presynaptic neuron is stimulated. The quantity of chemical applied must be in a reasonable concentration.
4. The chemical applied to the synapse must be affected in a manner similar to that of the normally occurring chemical.

ACTION AND SYNTHESIS OF NEUROTRANSMITTERS

Neurotransmitters have been divided into four major groups or systems: *cholinergics, monoamines, neuropeptides*, and *amino acids* (see Table 3-1). In this section neurotransmitters are classified by major group or system, and their sites of action, their modes of synthesis, and their mechanisms of action are discussed. Neurotransmitters occur in neurons and tracts in too many locations to discuss in detail; therefore only significant anatomic locations are mentioned.

Cholinergic System

The neurotransmitter in the cholinergic system is ACh (Mathews and Van Holde, 1990; Taylor and Brown, 1989). Acetylcholine is found in the peripheral nervous system (PNS) at the myoneural junction of skeletal muscle, in autonomic ganglia and at parasympathetic postganglionic-effector synapses, and in the central nervous system (CNS) within the spinal cord, basal ganglia, and cerebral cortex. Several pathways in the brain have been identified as ACh tracts. The basal nucleus of Meynert projects fibers to the cerebral cortex and has been implicated as a site of lesion in Alzheimer's disease. The septal area, an area rostral to the hypothalamus, sends ACh fibers to the hippocampus. Acetylcholine is synthesized by the union of acetylcoenzyme A (acetyl-CoA) and choline in the axonal boutons and stored in synaptic vesicles (Figure 3-3, *A*).

As stated earlier, ACh is released from the presynaptic membrane, crosses the synaptic cleft, and attaches to its receptor. Acetylcholinesterase in the synaptic cleft breaks down the ACh into its component molecules (Figure 3-3, *B*). Much of the choline in the bouton is obtained by reuptake from the synaptic cleft and is used subsequently for ACh synthesis. It was also stated earlier that ACh has two major categories of membrane receptors, nicotinic and muscarinic. Both nicotinic and muscarinic receptors can be further divided into subtypes, which are beyond the scope of this review. The nicotinic receptors are found at the postsynaptic membrane at the

Table 3-1 Classification of Neurotransmitters and Pathways

Neurotransmitter	Chemical transmitter	Location found	Major pathways
Cholinergic systems	ACh	Myoneural junctions, postganglionic neurons, autonomic ganglia, parasympathetic postganglionic neurons	Basal nucleus of Meynert to cerebral cortex, septal area (rostral to hypothalamus) to hippocampus
Monoamine systems	Catecholamines		
	Dopamine		Nigrostriatal
	Norepinephrine	Locus ceruleus	Locus ceruleus (in midbrain) to thalamus, cerebral cortex, cerebellum, and spinal cord; lateral midbrain to hypothalamus and basal forebrain
	Epinephrine		Central tegmental tract
	Serotonin	Raphe nuclei	Central brain stem nuclei up to forebrain and down to spinal cord
Neuropeptides	Enkephalins	Spinal cord, hypothalamus, midbrain, and the like	
	Endorphins	Spinal cord, hypothalamus, midbrain, and the like	
	Substance P	Spinal cord, hypothalamus, and many other places	
	Somatostatin, VIP, CCK, ACTH, neurotensin, angiotensin II, and others		
Amino acids	GABA	Most neurons indicating ubiquitous distribution	
	Glycine	Spinal cord, brain stem, and many other CNS areas	
	Glutamate	Widely distributed in the CNS	
	Asparate	Hippocampus, dorsal root ganglion	

ACh, Acetylcholine; *ACTH*, adrenocorticotropic hormone; *CCK*, cholecystokinin; *CNS*, central nervous system; *GABA*, gamma-aminobutyric acid; *VIP*, vasoactive intestinal polypeptide.

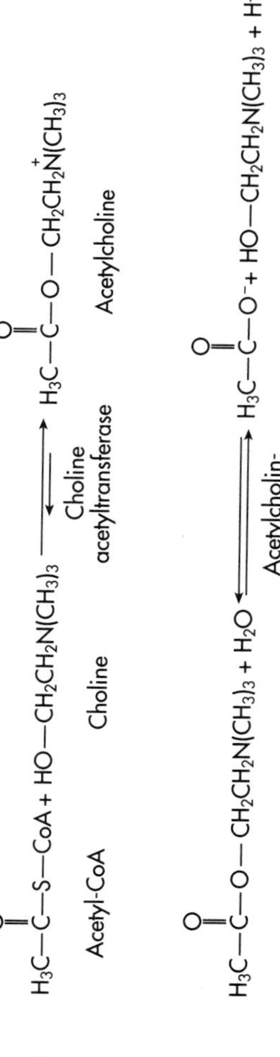

Figure 3-3 A, Synthesis of acetylcholine (ACh) and, **B,** its subsequent breakdown, facilitated by acetylcholinesterase.

myoneural junction and, rarely, in the CNS. The muscarinic receptors are located on sympathetic effector organs and in the CNS. Nicotinic receptors appear to be excitatory in function and utilize first messenger transmission. The muscarinic receptors trigger secondary messenger transmission and can affect the postsynaptic membrane in a number of ways, including membrane hyperpolarization.

Monoamine Systems

Neurotransmitters containing one amine group are called monamines (Mathews and Van Holde, 1990; Weiner and Molinoff, 1989). These include the catecholamines (dopamine, norepinephrine, and epinephrine), serotonin, and histamine. The term *adrenergic* refers to neurons activated by catecholamines, which are adrenalin-like substances also derived from the adrenal gland. The catecholamines are common neurotransmitters that are widely dispersed in the CNS and PNS. Dopamine neurons project from the substantia nigra to the putamen via the nigrostriatal pathway, a major pathway affected in Parkinson's disease. Additional dopamine sites are located in the caudate nucleus, amygdala, and temporal lobe. High concentrations of dopamine appear to be involved in schizophrenia. Norephinephrine cells in the locus ceruleus (in the midbrain) send their processes to the thalamus, cerebral cortex, cerebellum, and spinal cord. Norepinephrine is also the neurotransmitter of the sympathetic postganglionic neurons. Epinephrine (adrenalin) is found in neurons that run from the red nucleus to the medulla oblongata in the central tegmental tract. Serotonin is found in central midbrain nuclei and in neuronal processes up to the forebrain and down to the spinal cord. The catecholamines are all derived from tyrosine (Figure 3-4).

Tyrosine is found in the neurons, where it is converted to levodopa (L-dopa) and then to dopamine. Dopamine is then taken up into storage vesicles and converted to norepinephrine within these vesicles. There are six classes of catecholamine receptors (D1, D2, alpha 1, alpha 2, beta 1, and beta 2), and these receptors appear to influence ion channels by secondary messenger mechanisms. Many of these receptors affect the postsynaptic neurons by stimulating adenylate cyclase to convert adenosine

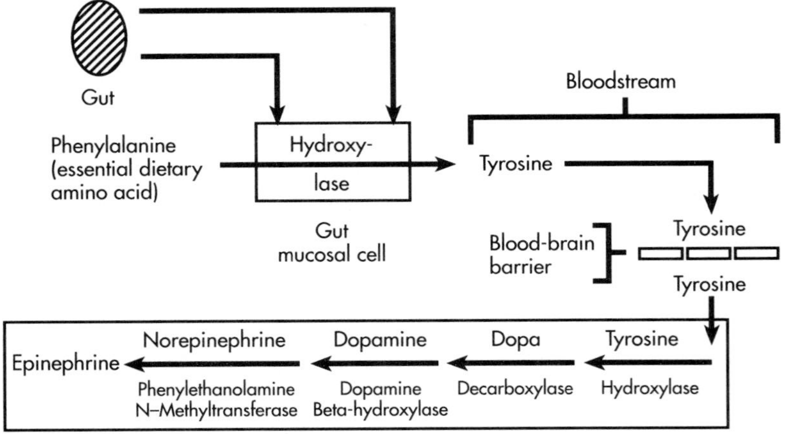

Figure 3-4 Normal synthesis of the catecholamines.

triphosphate (ATP) to cyclic adenosine monophosphate (AMP). Cyclic AMP is an important secondary messenger.

Serotonin (5-hydroxytryptamine) is derived from tryptophan within the CNS. Serotonin receptors have been described as activating secondary messenger transmission. Serotonin is involved in the spinal pain pathway, in facilitating motor activity, and possibly in modulation of human behavior. Both norepinephrine and serotonin have been implicated in depression.

Histamine is found in low quantities in the brain. Its precursor is histidine, which is the chemical that crosses the blood-brain barrier. Histamine neurons are located primarily in the hypothalamus, and their processes extend to many CNS areas. The receptors for histamine initiate secondary messenger transmission. Histamine is believed to be involved in such body functions as the regulation of biorhythms and thermoregulation and in neuroendocrine functions.

The monoamines can be excitatory or inhibitory transmitters, depending on the action mediated by their receptors. These receptors primarily give rise to secondary messenger transmission that can be slow-acting initially but have an extended duration of action. Therefore for a full understanding of the action of neurotransmitters one needs to understand the action of the specific receptors.

Neuropeptides

Neuropeptides are proteins that act as neurotransmitters or hormones. These are highly diverse proteins that have a common ability to excite or inhibit the activity of cell membranes. This discussion is limited to the neuropeptides that act as neurotransmitters in the CNS. Some of these proteins are released from their neurons in a manner similar to that of other transmitters. However, these neurotransmitters may enter either synaptic clefts or the bloodstream (pituitary hormones). Receptors on the postsynaptic membrane initiate secondary messenger transmission. Neuropeptides have been found to be released in conjunction with other neurotransmitters. For example, ACh and vasoactive intestinal polypeptide (VIP) have been shown to be released from cortical neurons at the same boutons (Detwiller and Crill, 1989). Therefore the principle that one neuron releases one neurotransmitter (Dale's principle) does not reflect current information. Theoretically, then, one might expect to find multiple transmitters from the same neuron working synergistically or antagonistically on the postsynaptic receptors. Hence the quantity and distribution of the receptors are of importance in the forming of neural circuits.

The synthesis of neuropeptides is hypothesized to be performed in one of two ways: by messenger ribonucleic acid (mRNA) or by enzymatic action. Large neuropeptides are proteins that originate from the interaction of mRNA with polyribosomes on the endoplasmic reticulum in the cell body. Since these proteins will be involved in secretory processes, they are transported to the golgi apparatus as prohormones, where they are packed in membranes and shipped by axonal transport to the cell processes for storage, degradation to the active molecule, and release (Holaday, 1985; Schwartz, 1985). Small neuropeptides can be synthesized by means of enzymatic action through the processes of glycolysis, citric acid cycle, and related mechanisms.

Opioids. In 1975 Hughes et al. discovered that the brain contained its own opioid system and that the system appeared to be involved with pain and pleasure. The receptors of this system are stimulated by endogenous opioid-like chemicals and morphine and can be blocked by naloxone, a narcotic antagonist. The chemicals are called endorphins. Endorphins are defined as endogenous molecules of the body that have an opioid-like action. The broad term *endorphin* encompasses a large group of diverse neuropeptides. In this section beta-endorphin and a smaller group of endorphins called enkephalins are discussed. These chemicals are widely distributed throughout the CNS.

Beta-endorphin, which contains 31 amino acids, is an excellent representative of the endorphin group. It has been found to be 48 times as potent as morphine. Beta-endorphin has been localized to the hypothalamus, with projecting processes to the midbrain and other CNS locations. It is synthesized from the prohormone proopiomelanocortin, which is broken down in vesicles into adrenocorticotropin, or adrenocorticotropic hormone (ACTH), beta-lipotropin, and a number of other active neuropeptides. Beta-lipotropin is further processed into beta-endorphin and another peptide. Under stress, beta-endorphin and ACTH are released simultaneously into the blood, which helps demonstrate the common prohormone origins (Kelly, 1985).

Enkephalins are specific endorphins. They are all pentapeptides. Enkephalins are widely distributed throughout the CNS in primarily small neurons that are locally active. The prohormones for enkephalins are proenkephalin and prodynorphin. The synthesis is similar to that of endorphin formation in that a number of neuropeptides are formed in the process of the cell dismantling the prohormones. The enkephalins have been implicated in such physiologic areas as pain perception, taste and olfaction, arousal, emotional behavior, vision and hearing, neurohormone secretion, motor coordination, and water balance (Dorsa, 1989; Holaday, 1985; Kutchai, 1993; Simon and Miller, 1989).

Substance P. Substance P was discovered in 1931 from the precipitate of horse brain. It is composed of a chain of 11 amino acids. The activity of substance P was shown at that time to be similar to that of ACh, but it was not blocked, as ACh is, by atropine. Substance P is found in great quantities in the ventral horn of the spinal cord and is widely distributed throughout the CNS. In the spinal cord it appears to be the neurotransmitter of the small-diameter, peripheral pain neurons (Dorsa, 1989).

Somatostatin. Somatostatin is produced inside the brain and in D cells of the pancreas. It is composed of a chain of 14 amino acids. One fourth of the brain somatostatin has been localized to the hypothalamus, and it is also found in the small-diameter, peripheral pain neurons with substance P. Somatostatin is both a hormone and a neurotransmitter. Somatostatin affects the postsynaptic membrane by hyperpolarizing (inhibiting) the membrane (Dorsa, 1989; Erulkar, 1989).

Other Neuropeptides

Vasoactive intestinal polypeptide (VIP)
Cholecystokinin (CCK)
Adrenocorticotropic hormone (ACTH)
Neurotensin
Angiotensin II

Amino Acid Transmitters

The amino acid transmitters are a special group of amino acids that are normally found in cells. They are formed, like many other amino acids, as products during the normal cellular processes of glycolysis and the citric acid cycle (Figure 3-5) (Mathews and Van Holde, 1990). These chemicals include gamma-aminobutyric acid (GABA), glycine, glutamate, and aspartate. Gamma-aminobutyric acid and glycine are well-

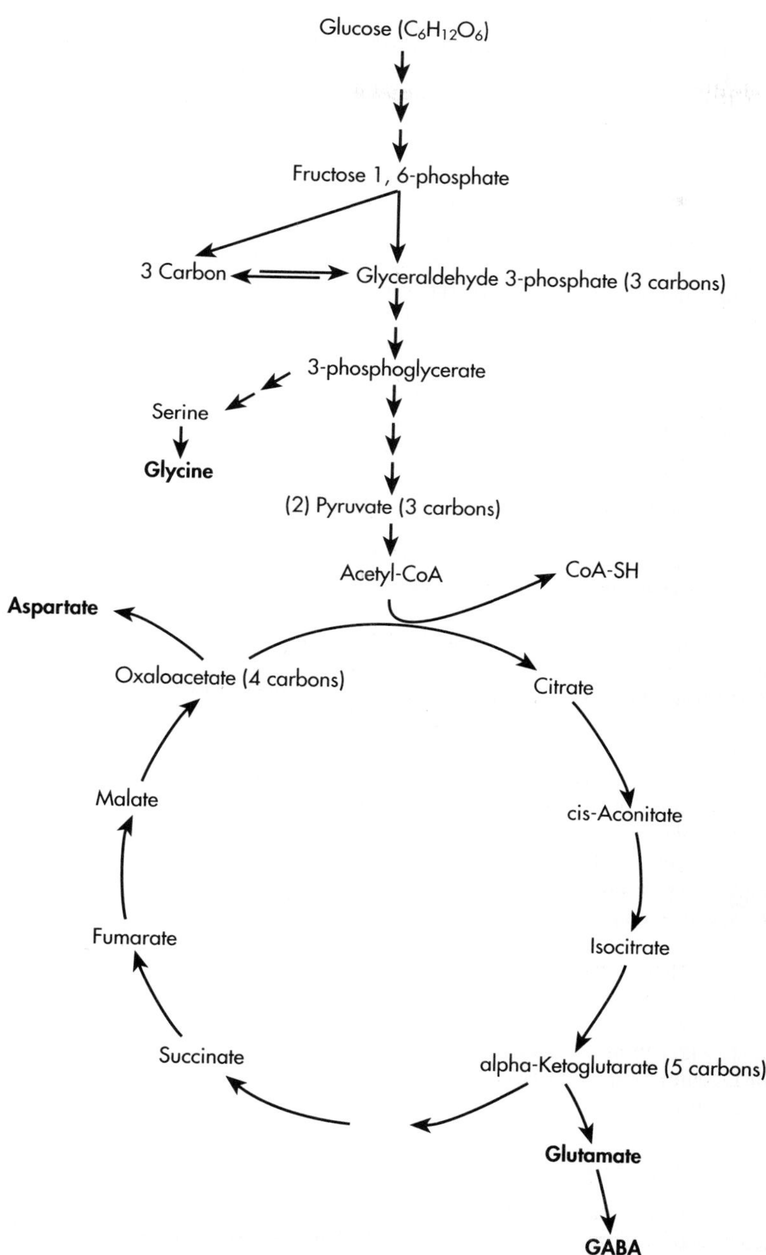

Figure 3-5 Reactions of glycolysis and the citric acid cycle and synthesis of glycine, aspartate, glutamate, and gamma-aminobutyric acid (GABA).

known inhibitory transmitters; glycine and aspartate are excitatory transmitters. These amino acid transmitters are widely distributed throughout the nervous system.

Gamma-aminobutyric acid receptors have been localized on all neurons that have been investigated (Detwiller and Crill, 1989), which indicates a ubiquitous distribution in the nervous system. Gamma-aminobutyric acid receptors are designated *A* and *B* (Gottlieb, 1988). Type A receptors function by first messenger transmission, whereas type B receptors utilize the indirect secondary messenger transmissions. Both receptors, when activated, result in an influx of chloride ions into the neuron, which causes hyperpolarization of the membrane potential, that is, inhibition. Glial cells, which form a dense network around neurons, have an affinity for GABA, and by removing it from the synaptic cleft, they prevent GABA buildup (Gottlieb, 1988; Crill, 1989). Gamma-aminobutyric acid is synthesized by the decarboxylation of glutamate (Figure 3-5) via alpha-ketoglutaric acid from the citric acid cycle.

Glycine has been localized in the cerebellum, brain stem, and spinal cord. Both glycine and GABA have been isolated from the two types of Renshaw cell, from interneurons, and in the spinal cord. The receptor for glycine utilizes the fast-acting first messenger transmission. The storage mechanism within the neuron for both glycine and GABA has not yet been determined. The mechanism for inhibition is the same as that described for GABA. Glycine is synthesized directly from serine, which is derived from glycolysis (Figure 3-5) (Detwiller and Crill, 1989; McGeer and McGeer, 1989).

Glutamate has been found in the cortex, hippocampus, cerebellum, and spinal cord. Two receptor types have been classified, N-methyl-D-aspartate (NMDA) and non-NMDA. Both receptors evoke first messenger transmission to cause depolarization of the membrane potential, that is, excitation. When glutamate loses an ammonium ion, glutamine is formed. Glutamine is readily diffusible into the blood and the cerebrospinal fluid. Therefore measuring the glutamine level in the cerebrospinal fluid provides an indicator of the ammonia concentration in the brain. High ammonia concentrations in the brain can lead to coma (McGeer and McGeer, 1989).

Aspartate is found in the hippocampus and the dorsal root ganglion. Its activity is similar to glutamate. Asparate is synthesized (Figure 3-5) directly from oxaloacetic acid, again a primary chemical in the citric acid cycle. It should be mentioned that it is difficult to distinguish between glutamate and asparate by means of current technology.

NEUROTRANSMITTERS AND NEUROCHEMISTRY OF BEHAVIOR

It is important to recognize that all neurotransmitters and pathways have multiple functions. Only a few are discussed in this review. Further, more than one neurotransmitter may be released at any synapse. When this occurs the synergistic effect or a differential effect may take place. Finally, receptors act to select which transmitter will activate or inhibit the neuron. The following section discusses some of these neurotransmitters with respect to the neurochemistry of behavior. Additionally, the functional neuroanatomic pathways rising from the reticular formation (see Chapter 2) are known to be involved in the integration, modulation, and regulation of several neurotransmitter systems, for example, acetylcholine, norepinephrine, serotonin, and dopamine. Our basic understanding of these systems is useful when considering the actions and effect of pharmacologic agents. Moreover, current neurophysiologic studies, postmortem studies, and molecular genetics studies are seeking to further clarify the role of these systems in the behavioral neurobiology of pharmacologic agents.

In this chapter neurochemical systems have already been characterized with respect to their neurochemical transmission and communication between presynaptic and postsynaptic receptors. Additionally, the potential for transmission at the postsynaptic receptor site through ion channels and the influence of second messenger systems have been discussed. Also, projections arising from the reticular formation, including the locus ceruleus, dopaminergic tracts such as the arcuate nucleus, and serotonergic tracts, including raphe nuclei, have been presented in Table 3-1 and are important in the understanding of the proposed effects of psychotropic drugs.

The neurochemistry of many behaviors and mechanisms of several classes of psychotropic agents may be best understood through an appreciation of the interaction among the neuroanatomic structures and the interplay of the neurochemical systems, especially the case of certain pharmacologic compounds that have been discovered or developed along these conceptual frameworks. For example, the initial observations further leading to the neurochemical explanations of many behaviors were stimulated in the 1950s by Labrec, a French anesthesiologist, who was trying to invent a cocktail to relieve anxiety and stress associated with surgical procedures. In Labrec's work with a chemist to invent a new antihistamine, chlorpromazine was identified as the active ingredient of his cocktail. The cocktail was then given to schizophrenic and psychotic patients in a French asylum and shown not only to calm the patients but also to reduce the other symptoms, that is, hallucinosis, paranoia, and agitation, in these patients. This experiment resulted in the dramatic changes discussed in Chapter 1 and many historical advances; in addition, it led to the neurochemical studies of chlorpromazine and other chemicals, which were believed to be possibly useful in clinical practice.

Chlorpromazine, from the phenothiazine class or family, was found to be similar in structure to dopamine, especially in its ring structure and tailed nitrogen. The molecule was found to fit or interact with the dopamine receptor and to act as a dopamine antagonist, preventing transmission of dopamine impulses believed responsible for schizophrenic and other psychotic symptoms. It was observed that a concentration of approximately 600 mg per day was necessary for the desired clinical effect, probably because of its relatively low affinity for the dopamine receptors. Other drugs in the phenothiazine family found later included triflupromazine, trifluoperazine, fluphenazine, and others that were much more potent, had a higher affinity for the receptor, and were much more likely to be clinically effective at lower doses. Two such drugs were haloperidol and thiothixene. These agents are discussed fully in Chapter 4.

Further study of the phenothiazine family of agents resulted in further delineation of the dopaminergic tracts. The mesolimbic and mesofrontal tracts were identified as the main ones responsible for schizophrenic behavior. The nigrostriatal tract was involved in symptoms that were identified with Parkinson's disease. It was also noted that these tracts communicated with the retina. Thus when chlorpromazine is administered to a patient, it interacts with dopamine receptors in the terminal portion of the striatum and can result in extrapyramidal symptoms that mimic Parkinson's disease. These symptoms are referred to as pseudoparkinsonian symptoms and include dyskinetic movement, dystonia, and other frank parkinsonian symptoms. The development of tardive dyskinesia, which is discussed in detail in Chapter 4, as well as other undesired effects, results from the "upregulating" of dopamine receptors, particularly D_2 receptors.

As with the discovery of antipsychotic agents, the antidepressant drugs were discovered rather serendipitously. After the success of treating tuberculosis with isonicotinic acid was established, pharmaceutical companies began seeking to create similar compounds. This research resulted in the development of iproniazid, which was placed in clinical trials. After tuberculous patients had been taking this drug for 3 to

4 months, their moods were found to be significantly improved but the tuberculosis was not. Iproniazid, which acts as a monoamine oxidase (MAO) enzyme inhibitor, had many effects on neurotransmitters, including the potentiation of norepinephrine and serotonin, neurotransmitters thought to play a key role in depression. Because it took 3 to 4 months to see these effects, these drugs did not have significant abuse potential and this class of drug (MAO inhibitors) was later developed as a conventional antidepressant (see Chapter 5). Another pharmaceutical company attempted to develop alternative forms of chlorpromazine and developed a compound called mipradine. When they tested this drug, they found that it was also successful in the treatment of depression. This compound was the predecessor to the tricyclic antidepressants and was later noted to block the reuptake of various biogenic amines.

The discovery of the MAO inhibitors and tricyclic antidepressants resulted in further consideration of depression as an illness in which both mood and behavior were affected and induced by neurochemical changes, which resulted in the biogenic amine theory of depression. Subsequent hypotheses included the serotonin hypothesis, which was developed after it was found that the concentrations of specific serotonin metabolites (5-hydroxyindoleacetic acid [5-HIAA]) in the cerebral spinal fluid of depressed patients was biomodally distributed. This simply means that one group had normal levels of 5-HIAA, and the other had low 5-HIAA levels. This finding indicated that low serotonin synthesis and turnover was occurring in one subgroup of depressed patients. Since the vast majority of serotonin is produced in the central nervous system by the raphe nuclei that supply the limbic system and frontal cortical system, this distribution made serotonin a likely suspect in the cause of depressive illness. Tricyclic antidepressants prevented the reuptake of this neurochemical from the synapse by the presynaptic terminal, which in turn increased the relative amount of serotonin in the synapse and corrected the relative deficiency. The initial result was a greater-than-normal response because of the supersensitivity of the serotonin receptor site. In short, these receptor sites were hungry for serotonin and these pharmacologic agents, the MAO inhibitors and the tricyclic antidepressants, enabled those receptors to have an increased supply.

Subsequently the norepinephrine hypothesis of depression was developed. The major nuclei of the norepinephrine production are found within the locus ceruleus. This structure, the virtual command-and-control center of norepinephrine, sends projections to the limbic system and cortex in a manner similar to that of serotonin. Norepinephrine was also deemed to be important in certain depressive syndromes, particularly when a decrement of norepinephrine production was occurring. It was proposed that certain agents, in particular, tricyclic antidepressants, acted with norepinephrine as they did with serotonin. That is, they blocked the reuptake of norepinephrine at the presynaptic terminal and supersensitized the postsynaptic membrane. Thus a greater synaptic supply of norepinephrine was available.

The action of the tricyclic antidepressants were observed to show a lag time of approximately 2 to 5 weeks before any effects of treatment were seen. It was further learned that the amount of neurotransmitter in the synapse increased *immediately* because of the block of the reuptake by the presynaptic terminal. However, the changes in the sensitivity of the postsynaptic receptors occurred *over time*. This seems to be the critical step in how this class of agents has its clinical effect. Furthermore, effects at differential receptor sites are now thought to be critical to the clinical efficacy of these and other antidepressant compounds, including novel agents such as bupropion and newer agents such as the serotonin selective reuptake inhibitors.

Many other agents that affect neurotransmitter systems outlined in this chapter are discussed in chapters specific to disorders. For example, generalized anxiety disorder that occurs in patients with persistent, severe, and disabling anxiety involves the GABA–benzodiazepine chloride system. Psychostimulants such as amphetamines and methylphenidate (Ritalin) may cause brief periods of euphoria but are more commonly used to treat the dreaded attention deficit hyperactivity disorder. These drugs increase the amount of synaptic dopamine, suggesting that this disorder may be caused by too little dopamine. It has also been noted that when psychostimulants are given to schizophrenic patients, a significant worsening of their condition occurs.

Other connections between neurotransmitter systems and identified psychiatric disorders include the role of ACh and other cholinergic systems in memory processes. The degeneration of cholinergic neurons of the basal nucleus of Meynert into the hippocampus is one of the many features found in Alzheimer's disease. Endorphins and enkephalins are known to be important in pain perception. Cholecystokinin and neurotensin may also be important in schizophrenia. Somatostatin may be found to be deficient in Alzheimer's disease. These neurochemical systems, as they are being explored, have certainly furthered our understanding of the biology of behavior, including the cause and course of many significant neuropsychiatric syndromes.

A final discussion of neurochemistry and the neurotransmitter systems as they relate to psychotropic agents might include current genetic and postmortem studies. For example, there is known to be a significant increase in D_2 receptors in the CNS in schizophrenics, and in patients with Alzheimer's disease, plaques and tangles may disrupt neurotransmitter systems. The core symptoms of both schizophrenia and Alzheimer's disease, as well as a host of psychiatric complications, are thought to be caused by these neurochemical deviations from normal.

The introduction of computerized tomography (CT), magnetic resonance imaging (MRI), and other imaging techniques, including single photon emission computerized tomography and positron emission spectroscopy, may also be useful in examining structural and functional defects in individuals who have major psychiatric syndromes. These technologies have also been useful, through the use of radioisotopes, in the study of the influence of pharmacologic agents on certain receptor sites and structures. These technologies allow us to view the inside of the brain, including the ventricular system, receptors sites, and brain tissues. Positron emission spectroscopy scanning with the use of radioisotopes, which are taken up readily into the cells, may also enable the evaluation and assessment of metabolic disturbances and the relative value of pharmacologic agents in correcting these defects. For example, obsessive compulsive disorder is known to be characterized by the hypermetabolism of the striatum and frontal cortex. Drugs such as clomipramine (Anafranil) are known to correct this functional defect.

Molecular genetics, which allows the identification of certain disorders based on specific chromosomal defects, may be useful in developing certain genetic pharmacologic and chemical agents that can serve to correct these defects. This could certainly open up further development of chemical treatments for psychiatric disorders. Identifying the gene, cloning it, getting the DNA to express its protein product, and figuring out how the protein affects behavior, may ultimately correct abnormal function. This is indeed an interesting time in the field of neurochemistry of behavior and is largely accountable for the National Institutes of Health deeming the 1990s "the decade of the brain."

REFERENCES

Crill WE: The milieu of the central nervous system. In Patton HD et al, editors: *Textbook of physiology*, vol 1, Philadelphia, 1989, WB Saunders.

Detwiller PB, Crill WE: Synaptic transmission. In Patton HD et al, editors: *Textbook of physiology*, vol 1, Philadelphia, 1989, WB Saunders.

Dorsa DM: Neuropeptides as neurotransmitters. In Patton HD et al, editors: *Textbook of physiology*, vol 2, Philadelphia, 1989, WB Saunders.

Erulkar SD: Chemically mediated synaptic transmission: an overview. In Siegel GJ et al, editors: *Basic neurochemistry*, New York, 1989, Raven.

Gottlieb DI: GABAergic neurons, *Scientific American* 258:82, 1988.

Hille B: Neuromuscular transmission. In Patton HD et al, editors: *Textbook of physiology*, vol 1, Philadelphia, 1989, WB Saunders.

Holaday JW: *Endogenous opioids and their receptors: current concepts*, Kalamazoo, Mich, 1985, Upjohn.

Hughes H et al: Identification of two related pentapeptides from the brain with potent opiate agonist activity, *Nature* 258:577, 1975.

Kelly DD: Central representation of pain and analgesia. In Kandel ER, Schwartz JH, editors: *Principles of neural science*, New York, 1985, Elsevier.

Kutchai HC: Cellular physiology. In Berne RM, Levy MN, editors: *Physiology*, ed 3, St Louis, 1993, Mosby.

Mathews CK, Van Holde KE: *Biochemistry*, Redwood City, Calif, 1990, Benjamin-Cummings.

McGeer PL, McGeer EG: Amino acid neurotransmitters. In Siegel GJ et al, editors: *Basic neurochemistry*, New York, 1989, Raven.

Patton HD: The autonomic nervous system. In Patton HD et al, editors: *Textbook of physiology*, vol 1, Philadelphia, 1989, WB Saunders.

Schwartz JH: Chemical messengers: small molecules and peptides. In Kandel ER, Schwartz JH, editors: *Principles of neural science*, New York, 1985, Elsevier.

Shepard GM: *Neurobiology*, New York, 1983, Oxford University.

Simon EJ, Miller JB: Opioid peptides and opioid receptors. In Siegel GJ et al, editors: *Basic neurochemistry*, New York, 1989, Raven.

Taylor P, Brown JH: Acetylcholine. In Siegel GJ et al, editors: *Basic neurochemistry*, New York 1989, Raven.

Weiner N, Molinoff PB: Catecholamines. In Siegel GJ et al, editors: *Basic neurochemistry*, New York, 1989, Raven.

UNIT II

Drugs Used in the Treatment of Mental Disorders

CHAPTER 4

Schizophrenia and Other Psychoses

HISTORICAL CONSIDERATIONS

Schizophrenia is the diagnostic category defined by the *Diagnostic and Statistical Manual of Mental Disorders (Third Edition-Revised [DSM-III-R])* criteria (American Psychiatric Association, 1987) that describes a psychiatric disorder characterized by psychosocial withdrawal and disturbances in thought, motor behavior, and interpersonal functioning. The *DSM-III-R* criteria are depicted in the box on pp. 43-44. Individuals with schizophrenia may appear dull and colorless, dependent and apathetic, emotionally isolative, or agitated and threatening; these and other characteristic symptoms determine which subtype is assigned, that is, paranoid, catatonic, disorganized, undifferentiated, or residual. The cost in human suffering is incalculable: it is known that about 1% of the population meets conventional criteria for schizophrenia. Economic costs are estimated in the tens of billions of dollars each year.

Morel was the first to assign a name to the psychiatric symptoms described in the preceding paragraph. In 1856, while treating an adolescent boy, he used the phrase *démence précoce* (precocious senility) to describe the group of observed symptoms. Kahlbaum (in 1868) and Hecker (in 1870) added to the lexicon with their diagnostic categories, *catatonia* and *hebephrenia*, respectively. Kraepelin added the term *paranoia* and engaged in a rigorous study of a variety of disorders that we now recognize as schizophrenia. He noted the symptomatic commonalities among these mental disorders, *catatonia, hebephrenia*, and *paranoia*, and in 1896 attached the label *dementia praecox*. Kraepelin (1919) believed schizophrenia was the result of neuropathologic disturbance and also made an effort to distinguish between cases with florid symptoms and those characterized by persistent losses or deficits. He envisioned a progressive deteriorating course for the latter group, which resulted in a more disabling degree of mental impairment with little hope of recovery (Andreasen et al., 1990). Kraepelin described the fundamental deficit in schizophrenia as "annihilation of the will" (Lewine, 1990).

Bleuler (1950) in the early 1900s actually coined the term *schizophrenia* in a book subtitled *The Group of Schizophrenias*. Bleuler observed that schizophrenia did not always follow a course of deterioration, so dementia was thought to be an inappropriate term, nor did schizophrenia always begin early in life, so praecox was also an inappropriate term. Bleuler broadened Kraepelin's concept by focusing on symptoms rather than clinical outcomes. Kraepelin, for instance, on finding an individual who "recovered," believed that the individual had never actually had schizophrenia. On the basis of Bleuler's wider grouping, pessimism eased and some clinicians began to see improvements in their patients. Bleuler, largely influenced by Freud and other psychodynamic theorists, explored psychologic explanations for schizophrenia, yet he never abandoned the biologic theories of Kraepelin. In recent years a resurgence of interest in biologic research has resulted in renewed respect for Kraepelin's work. In

DSM-III-R Diagnostic Criteria for Schizophrenia

A. Presence of characteristic psychotic symptoms in the active phase: either (1), (2), or (3) for at least one week (unless the symptoms are successfully treated):
   1. Two of the following:
      a. Delusions
      b. Prominent hallucinations (throughout the day for several days or several times a week for several weeks, each hallucinatory experience not being limited to a few brief moments).
      c. Incoherence or marked loosening of associations.
      d. Catatonic behavior.
      e. Flat or grossly inappropriate affect.
   2. Bizarre delusions (i.e., involving a phenomenon that the person's culture would regard as totally implausible, e.g., thought broadcasting, being controlled by a dead person).
   3. Prominent hallucinations [as defined in 1.b above] of a voice with content having no apparent relation to depression or elation, or a voice keeping up a running commentary on the person's behavior or thoughts, or two or more voices conversing with each other.

B. During the course of the disturbance, functioning in such areas as work, social relations, and self-care is markedly below the highest level achieved before onset of disturbance (or, when the onset is in childhood or adolescence, failure to achieve expected level of social development).

C. Schizoaffective disorder and mood disorder with psychotic features have been ruled out, i.e., if a major depressive or manic syndrome has ever been present during an active phase of the disturbance, the total duration of all episodes of a mood syndrome has been brief relative to the total duration of the active and residual phases of the disturbance.

D. Continuous signs of the disturbance for at least six months. The six-month period must include an active phase (or at least one week or less if symptoms have been successfully treated) during which there were psychotic symptoms characteristic of schizophrenia (symptoms in A), with or without a prodromal or residual phase, as defined below.
   Prodromal phase: A clear deterioration in functioning before the active phase of the disturbance that is not due to a disturbance in mood or to a psychoactive substance use disorder and that involves at least two of the symptoms listed below.
   Residual phase: Following the active phase of the disturbance, persistence of at least two of the symptoms noted below, these not being due to a disturbance in mood or to a psychoactive substance use disorder.
   Prodromal or Residual Symptoms:
   1. Marked social isolation or withdrawal
   2. Marked impairment in role functioning as wage-earner, student, or homemaker

From American Psychiatric Association: *Diagnostic and statistical manual of mental disorders, third edition, revised,* Washington, DC, 1987, The Association.

Continued.

DSM-III-R Diagnostic Criteria for Schizophrenia—cont'd

3. Markedly peculiar behavior (e.g., collecting garbage, talking to self in public, hoarding food)
4. Marked impairment in personal hygiene and grooming
5. Blunted or inappropriate affect
6. Digressive, vague, overelaborate, or circumstantial speech, or poverty of speech, or poverty of content of speech
7. Odd beliefs or magical thinking, influencing behavior and inconsistent with cultural norms, e.g., superstitiousness, belief in clairvoyance, telepathy, "sixth sense," "others can feel my feelings," overvalued ideas, ideas of reference
8. Unusual perceptual experiences, e.g., recurrent illusions, sensing the presence of a force or person not actually present
9. Marked lack of initiative, interests, or energy

Examples: Six months of prodromal symptoms with one week of symptoms from A; no prodromal symptoms with six months of symptoms from A; no prodromal symptoms with one week of symptoms from A and six months of residual symptoms.

E. It cannot be established that an organic factor initiated and maintained the disturbance.

F. If there is a history of autistic disorder, the additional diagnosis of schizophrenia is made only if prominent delusions or hallucinations are also present.

contrast, the introduction of the *Diagnostic and Statistical Manual of Mental Disorders, Third Edition (DSM-III)* in 1980 resulted in the view that Bleuler's contributions, albeit significant, had "softened the diagnostic criteria" and obscured the deteriorating course of the illness. This "softening" possibly led to overdiagnosis, particularly in blacks and lower socioeconomic groups (American Psychiatric Association, 1980; Jones and Gray, 1986).

DSM-III-R TERMINOLOGY AND CRITERIA

Since the inception of schizophrenia as a diagnostic entity, attempts have been made to divide it into homogeneous subtypes (Kendler, Gruenberg, and Tsuany, 1988). Early attempts at identifying homogeneous groups resulted in the subtypes catatonia, hebephrenia, and paranoia. Bleuler later added *simple* schizophrenia to the nomenclature. This early thinking is still reflected in the current official diagnostic classification system (see the box on pp. 43-44).

The most useful subtyping approach is derived from Kraepelin's earlier work and is now advocated by biologically oriented diagnosticians. Andreason and Olsen (1982), Andreason et al. (1990), Crow (1980), and others have developed two subtypes, positive and negative schizophrenia, based on well-designed research. Positive or type 1 schizophrenia has a different constellation of symptoms than does negative or type 2 schizophrenia. Type 1 is positive in the sense that symptoms are an embellishment of normal cognition and perception: the symptoms are "additional." Posi-

Table 4-1 Comparison of Positive Schizophrenia (Type 1) and Negative Schizophrenia (Type 2)

Positive schizophrenia (type 1)	Negative schizophrenia (type 2)
Positive symptoms	Negative symptoms
Hyperdopaminergic process	Nondopaminergic process
Normal brain structure	Structural changes, i.e., increased ventricular-brain ratios, decreased cerebral blood flow
Good response to treatment	Poor response to treatment

tive symptoms are believed to be caused by a subcortical dopaminergic process (too much dopamine) affecting cortical areas. Type 2 is labeled negative because symptoms are essentially an absence of what should be, that is, lack of affect, lack of energy, and so forth. Type 2 is thought to be nondopaminergic and to be caused by cortical structural changes, (e.g., cerebral atrophy) not unlike those in Alzheimer's disease. Neurobiologic disturbances consistently reported in the literature include decreased cerebral blood flow, particularly in frontal areas, and increased ventricular-brain ratios. The basic differences between type 1 and type 2 are listed in Table 4-1.

According to biologic theory, antipsychotic drugs, drugs that effectively block dopamine receptors, are likely to be more beneficial for individuals with positive schizophrenia; quite possibly, since negative schizophrenia is more related to a structural defect and not as specifically related to disturbances in dopamine function, the use of dopamine-blocking drugs or antipsychotics are relatively less effective and their continuous administration more controversial (Johnson, 1990). Accordingly, the more flagrant the psychotic symptoms characteristic of positive schizophrenia, the greater the likelihood of a positive response to an antipsychotic drug.

ANTIPSYCHOTIC DRUGS

Antipsychotic drugs are used to treat the symptoms of psychosis and various other manifestations of mental illness. These drugs are particularly important in the prevention of relapse, but rates of compliance are low. Table 4-2 presents a comparative description of these drugs. Chronic mental illness, specifically, schizophrenia accompanied by symptoms of florid psychosis, and acute agitation in mania or in other psychotic or motor-disturbed patients are the major targets of these compounds (Harris, 1981; Overall et al., 1989). Other uses are acknowledged and discussed briefly in this chapter.

History

In the late 1940s a pharmaceutical company developed a cold remedy that caused mild sedation, potentiated the effects of analgesics, and calmed anxious surgical patients. Further studies led to the discovery of a derivative, chlorpromazine, that effectively reduced psychotic symptoms in psychiatrically disturbed patients.

Antipsychotic drug use in public hospitals began in about 1954. Before the introduction and acceptance of chlorpromazine and the related drugs eventually manufactured, hundreds of thousands of patients with severe psychiatric disturbances were

Table 4-2 Antipsychotic Drugs

Antipsychotic agent	Approximate equivalent oral dose (mg)*	Adult daily dosage range (mg)	Sedation	Extrapyramidal symptoms	Anticholinergic effects	Orthostatic hypotension	Concentration (ng/ml)	Relative market share % (rank)‡
Phenothiazines								
Aliphatic phenothiazines								
Chlorpromazine (Thorazine)	100	30-800	+++	++	++	+++	30-500	12.0% (3)
Promazine (Sparine)	200	40-1200	++	++	+++	++		0.7% (10)
Trifluopromazine (Vesprin)	25	60-150	+++	++	+++	++		0.5% (14)
Piperidine phenothiazines								
Mesoridazine (Serentil)	50	30-400	+++	+	+++	++		1.5% (9)
Thioridazine (Mellaril)	100	150-800	+++	+	+++	+++		31.2% (1)
Piperazine phenothiazines								
Fluphenazine (Prolixin, Permitil)	2	0.5-40	+	+++	+	+	0.13-2.8	5.6% (6)
Perphenazine (Trilafon)	10	12-64	+	+++	+	+	0.8-1.2	4.2% (7)

Trifluoperazine (Stelazine)	5	2-40	+	+++	+	+		8.7% (4)
Butyrophenone								
Haloperidol (Haldol)	2	1-15	+	+++	+	+	5-20	24.2% (2)
Thioxanthenes								
Chlorprothixene (Taractan)	100	75-600	+++	++	++	++		0.5% (12)
Thiothixene (Navane)	4	8-30	+	+++	+	+	2-57	8.2% (5)
Dibenzoxazepine								
Loxapine (Loxitane)	15	20-250	++	+++	+	++		1.9% (8)
Dihydroindolone								
Molindone (Moban)	10	15-225	+	+++	+	+		0.6% (11)
Dibenzodiazepine								
Clozapine (Clozaril)	50	300-900	+++	+	+++	+++	>350†	Too new

Adapted from Olin BR, editor: *Drug facts and comparisons*, Philadelphia, 1990, JB Lippincott.
*Many clinicians believe that for most schizophrenic patients the effective dosage should be at or above 400 mg/day of chlorpromazine or its equivalent. (From Beresford TP, Hall RCW: *Psychiatr Med* 8[4]:1, 1990.)
†Perry JP et al found that 64% of treatment-resistant schizophrenic patients improved. (From Perry JP et al: *Am J Psychiatry* 148[2]:236, 1991.)
‡Wysowski DK, Baum C: Antipsychotic drug use in the United States: 1976-1985, *Arch Gen Psychiatry* 46:929, 1989.
Incidence of side effects: +++ = high; ++ = moderate; + = low.

hospitalized under sometimes poor conditions. Psychosocial isolation, physical restraint, and occasional treatment with aggressive measures, for example, psychosurgery or lobotomy, were employed. These treatments rarely restored the patient to a state that enabled productive social or occupational functioning, and affected individuals often were unable to interact reasonably with others.

Although some of the hopes and expectations for antipsychotic drugs have not been realized, these drugs have had a dramatic impact on psychiatric care and therapeutic outlook. Their use in the psychiatric community has resulted in more early and effective treatments; many of the ineffective or restrictive treatments have been abandoned, and the number of long-term hospitalizations has declined from more than half a million patients in 1955, before the widespread use of antipsychotic drugs, to about 120,000 in the mid-1980s. In short, most patients who previously would have been hospitalized are now living and functioning well socially and occupationally largely because of the efficacy of antipsychotic drug treatment. However, the vast homeless population includes many previously hospitalized, mentally ill persons; thus psychopharmacologic treatment alone is not enough and is ideally combined with other social, behavioral, and psychotherapeutic approaches.

The drugs discussed in this chapter are generally called antipsychotic agents, but they have also been referred to as major tranquilizers, ataractics (i.e., drugs that produce calmness or serenity), or neuroleptics, since they can also produce neurologic symptoms (Keltner, 1989).

Classification Systems

Antipsychotic drugs are generally classified in two ways. The first and most accurate classification system is based on chemical and structural class. These drugs have diverse chemical properties, although they all effectively reduce various psychiatric symptoms. Drug differences are mainly attributed to a drug's potential for sedation and other side effects. For instance, because of chemical class differences the type, intensity, and frequency of side effects vary among individual antipsychotic drugs. Also, when a drug is "not working," a switch to a drug of a different class is often considered.

A second means of classifying antipsychotic drugs is based on potency. This system is admittedly less "scientific" than classification by means of chemical class but has gathered support because of its clinical utility. Essentially, some drugs are required in much higher doses to achieve clinical results similar to those of other drugs. For example, about 100 mg of chlorpromazine (Thorazine) is required to achieve the same clinical effect as 2 mg of haloperidol (Haldol). Drugs that are one to four times as potent as chlorpromazine are designated as low potency, and those 20 or more times as potent, as high potency (Gomez and Gomez, 1990). Accordingly, chlorpromazine is referred to as a low-potency antipsychotic drug and haloperidol as a high-potency one. In clinical practice it appears that low-potency antipsychotic drugs produce more frequent and intense anticholinergic side effects and are more likely to produce orthostatic symptoms; in contrast, high-potency antipsychotic drugs are more likely to produce more frequent and intense extrapyramidal side effects (EPSEs).

Neurochemical Theory of Schizophrenia

Although various theories of schizophrenia exist and are vigorously debated, the neurochemical theory affords the best explanation for the effectiveness of antipsychotic agents. The neurochemical theory states that schizophrenia and psychotic symptoms, for example, hallucinations and delusions, are caused by increased levels of dopamine in the limbic system of the brain. Since antipsychotic drugs are dopamine blockers, it follows that their effectiveness can be attributed to this dopamine-blocking activity. Furthermore, this theory of schizophrenia is supported by clinical observations and clinical research, which demonstrate that high doses of levodopa and amphetamines can produce schizophrenic symptoms.

Pharmacologic Effects (Therapeutic Effects)

Chlorpromazine and the other antipsychotic drugs are used primarily to treat psychiatric disorders, specifically, schizophrenia and other mental illness associated with psychotic or motor disturbances. Well-designed clinical research has produced impressive evidence *for* their effectiveness. Not all patients respond, but many who do have the potential to live their lives unencumbered by the oppressive symptoms of psychosis. Psychosis is a phenomenon of brain activity. Therefore a drug that affects psychosis acts primarily in the central nervous system (CNS). Tolerance to an antipsychotic effect is uncommon. Peripheral nervous system (PNS) effects are discussed in the section on side effects (undesired effects). Chlorpromazine, a phenothiazine and the prototype antipsychotic agent is discussed extensively, and a more condensed discussion of the other drugs is included.

Central nervous system effects. Central nervous system effects include sedation, emotional quieting, and psychomotor slowing; thus at one time these drugs were generally referred to as major tranquilizers. This emotional quieting enables the patient to take advantage of other forms of therapeutic intervention, for example, the therapeutic relationship and the therapeutic milieu.

Other CNS effects include a sedating quality that decreases insomnia and sleep disturbances frequently observed in persons with psychoses. Whether the sedating effect itself or the "freeing" from disturbing thoughts, or a combination of the two, enhances sleep is not precisely known. Not all antipsychotic drugs are equally sedating. High-potency drugs are less sedating than are the low-potency drugs. For example, haloperidol and fluphenazine (Prolixin, Permitil) are not generally sedating yet are quite effective. Thus the effectiveness of antipsychotic agents results from more than "just" their tranquilizing qualities.

Psychiatric Symptoms Modified by Antipsychotic Drugs

Antipsychotic drugs are prescribed because other people note a patient's behavior to be disturbed (objective symptoms) or because the individual is experiencing psychotic symptoms (subjective symptoms) and seeks relief. As previously discussed, antipsychotic drugs are more effective in treating the positive symptoms of schizophrenia (Table 4-1). Positive symptoms include hallucinations, delusions, and to some extent the acute motor and thought disturbances. Negative symptoms are less responsive to antipsychotic drug therapy, including symptoms that develop insidiously such as flat or restricted affect, verbal paucity or laconic speech, and a lack of drive or volitional, goal-directed activity. Improvement in objective and subjective symptoms or in positive and negative signs of schizophrenia is the yardstick by which progress is gauged. Psychotic symptoms associated with other disorders, for example, mania, depression, organic mental syndromes, or disorders of cognitive impairment, may also respond well to antipsychotic drugs.

Perceptual disturbances. As a general rule the more bizarre the behavior associated with psychosis, the more likely that an antipsychotic drug will be found beneficial. Hallucinations and illusions usually diminish or remit with the use of these drugs. Even when symptoms are not fully eradicated, antipsychotic drugs may enable the individual to understand that hallucinations and illusions are, indeed, not real or can be tolerated without influencing behavior.

Thought disturbances. The use of antipsychotic drugs may also improve reasoning and decrease ambivalence and delusions or suspiciousness. Since disturbed reasoning, ambivalence, and delusional thinking may produce frustration and behavioral consequences, an antipsychotic agent can free the patient from these symptoms while improving the ability to communicate and cooperate with others.

Motor disturbances. Individuals with schizophrenia and other psychotic disorders are frequently found to be hyperactive or agitated because of internal turmoil and, perhaps, because of the disturbed neurobiology. Antipsychotic drugs may slow or normalize psychomotor activity. Low-potency drugs such as chlorpromazine are inherently sedating, and this effect may be particularly useful for agitated and combative persons.

Altered consciousness. Mental confusion found among psychotic and schizophrenic patients is possibly due to the anxiety and disturbed processing of thought associated with psychosis. Some mental health professionals have promulgated that these symptoms are among the most disabling. Antipsychotic drugs may be effective in decreasing disturbances of thought and in clearing mental confusion.

Interpersonal disturbances. Schizophrenic patients often have a history of asociality and withdrawal and may have few if any close personal relationships, including inconsistent relationships with family members. An individual with schizophrenia typically may invest little in his appearance and is not especially aware of his behavior. Introspection and self-focused speech combine to produce ineffective communication patterns, which reinforce isolation. These behaviors may also offend other people or result in social dysfunction. The individual with schizophrenia may have little to give to society and may be seen as socially unfit. Antipsychotic drugs together with other forms of therapy may enable the patient to become less self-focused and to divert his or her attention away from self to others. The socially damaging introspectiveness may simply be due to the considerable energy expended to maintain some degree of equilibrium in the face of psychologic turmoil. This pattern may parallel the regression and lack of attention given to appearance or behavior when an individual is ill. For the psychotically disturbed individual, antipsychotic drugs can often reduce the inner turmoil, freeing psychic energy for more effective interpersonal relationships and for the establishment and maintenance of a therapeutic relationship.

Affective disturbance. Affective symptoms alone are not treated with antipsychotic drugs, but flat affect, inappropriate affect, or lability of affect seen in schizophrenia may respond to antipsychotic drug therapy.

Other Uses and Effects

The site of neuronal control of nausea and vomiting is the chemoreceptor trigger zone, which is well supplied by dopaminergic receptors. When these receptors are stimulated with dopamine, nausea and vomiting occur. Because antipsychotic drugs block dopamine, most phenothiazines are effective antiemetics. Prochlorperazine (Compazine) is prescribed primarily for its antiemetic qualities. Chlorpromazine also is used to prevent nausea and vomiting during surgery, for intractable hiccups, and as adjunctive therapy for tetanus. Antipsychotic drugs also block PNS muscarinic acetylcholine receptors and alpha-adrenergic receptors, which are responsible for some of the side effects discussed later.

Pharmacokinetics

Chlorpromazine enters the CNS rapidly. A tranqulizing effect occurs within 60 minutes of an oral dose and within 10 minutes of an intramuscular dose. However, the actual antipsychotic effect may not be realized for several weeks or months. Chlorpromazine accumulates in fatty tissue and is released slowly from these sites. Traces of metabolites of this drug are found in the urine months after therapy has stopped, which may explain why patients who abruptly stop their medication continue to experience an antipsychotic effect for a time, that is, the chlorpromazine continues to be released from fatty storage sites after use is discontinued. This slow release from fatty stores may also account for noncompliance, since the patient who stops taking this medication does not experience an immediate return of symptoms.

Because most of the chlorpromazine (95% to 98%) binds tightly to plasma proteins, the proportion that crosses the blood-brain barrier may be negligible, that is, only a fraction of the drug ingested accounts for its effect. Interestingly, chlorpromazine might have an increased effect in an elderly individual, who may have decreased protein-binding capabilities.

Chlorpromazine is metabolized in the liver and has a half-life of 10-30 hours. Impaired hepatic function extends its half-life and therefore its effect.

Although many individual antipsychotic drugs are available, no one drug is more effective than another. Some patients, however, show a differential and individual response: one patient may respond best to chlorpromazine and another to haloperidol. Therefore the choice of antipsychotic drug is usually based on the physician's preference and experience, the likelihood, for example, on the basis of the patient's previous response to a certain drug, that a certain drug will be helpful, and an educated guess about the potential for a particular agent to produce unwanted side effects. Because the nurse has prolonged contact with inpatients and periodic contact with outpatients, few psychiatric professionals have a better opportunity to assess both desired and undesired responses that affect the selection of the best drug for a particular patient. Additionally, since nearly half of all orders for antipsychotic medications are written as needed, the nurse may have added reason to evaluate the response to these drugs (Blair, 1990).

Most antipsychotic drugs are available in oral and parenteral forms (see Table 4-3). Oral administration is the preferred route for a variety of reasons, not the least of which is that the patient prefers this route. Tablets, however, have consistently created a problem because they may be "cheeked." "Cheeking" occurs when an individual places the tablet to one side of the mouth and pretends to swallow it. Moreover, an estimated 46% of patients, both inpatients and outpatients, take less of their medications than prescribed (Blair, 1990). Noncompliance is perhaps the single most important cause of symptom exacerbation, relapse, and rehospitalization. Psychiatric patients may not comply with medical regimen for several reasons, including the stigma of illness or the sick role, paranoid fears of poisoning, or unpleasant reactions or side effects (see the box on p. 52). Many inpatient units use liquid forms of antipsychotic and other psychotropic drugs to reduce noncompliant tendencies. However, liquids or concentrates may have an unpleasant taste and should be diluted. Two

Table 4-3 Parenteral Antipsychotic Drug Use

Drug	Parenteral administration (intramuscular)
For acute agitation*	
Chlorpromazine (Thorazine)	Initially 25 mg, repeated in 1 hour as needed; switch to oral dose as soon as possible
Haloperidol (Haldol)	Initially 2-5 mg, repeated every 1-8 hours as needed
For long-term maintenance or noncompliant behavior	
Fluphenazine decanoate (Prolixin decanoate)†	Initially 12.5-25 mg, repeated every 2-4 weeks
Haloperidol decanoate (Haldol decanoate)†	Initially 10 to 15 times the oral dose of haloperidol; usually maintenance dosage of 50-100 mg every 4 weeks

*See Chapter 9 for a complete review.
†Long-acting antipsychotics.

Issues in Antipsychotic Therapy

Relapse

There is a general consensus that about one-third of all schizophrenic patients will relapse over a two year period, even when taking prescribed levels of antipsychotic drugs. Johnson* suggests that antipsychotic medication be continued for at least 12 months after remission. Among all schizophrenic patients relapse rates are expected to be as high as 50% in the first year and 20% in the second year after hospitalization.†

Noncompliance

Van Putten‡ in a much quoted paper stated that 24% to 63% of outpatients and 15% to 33% of inpatients do not take the prescribed amounts of antipsychotic drugs. In general, extrapyramidal side effects and, specifically, akathisia were the primary cause of noncompliant behavior. Interestingly, in a study by Lund and Frank,† the authors found that psychiatric nurses believe noncompliance to be an educational issue, whereas the patients themselves give many reasons for noncompliant behavior.

*Johnson DAW: *Drugs* 39(4):481, 1990.
†Lund VE, Frank DI: *J Psychosoc Nurs* 29(7):6, 1991.
‡Van Putten T: *Arch Gen Psychiatry* 31:67, 1974.

other issues related to "cheeking" and noncompliance are decompensation and hoarding.

For severely disturbed patients, chlorpromazine 25 mg three times a day is a usual starting dosage and is typically increased every 1 or 2 days by 20 to 50 mg, up to a daily dose of 400 mg. Daily dose may range from 30 to 800 mg.

Another form of administration is the parenteral route. Parenteral drugs are usually employed to treat acutely disturbed patients or those who represent significant compliance risks. Both haloperidol and fluphenazine are available in long-acting injectable forms that require injection as seldom as once per month. These depot compounds are particularly beneficial in community outpatient clinics. Middlemiss and Beeber (1989) have described a Z-track injection technique used to decrease skin irritation in these cases. Other antipsychotics available in parenteral form and used on an acute, short-term basis include the following:

Chlorprothixene (Taractan)
Loxapine (Loxitane)
Mesoridazine (Serentil)
Perphenazine (Trilafon)
Thiothixene (Navane)
Trifluoperazine (Stelazine)

When a patient is not responding to an antipsychotic drug, a reassessment of the patient is necessary. Three principles guide assessment of the patient's response and raise the possibility of a change of drug. These principles are listed in the box below.

Side Effects

The antipsychotic drugs produce numerous side effects because of PNS and CNS actions (see the box on pp. 54-55). Side effects due to PNS autonomic blocking (that is, anticholinergic and antiadrenergic) actions are more likely to be caused by low-potency forms such as chlorpromazine (Richelson, 1984). Extrapyramidal symptoms in the CNS are more likely to be caused by high-potency drugs such as haloperidol.

Patient Responses Suggesting a Possible Drug Change

1. Is the patient able and willing to comply with the original drug therapy as ordered? The potential therapeutic value cannot be established if the patient is noncompliant.
2. Has the drug currently being prescribed been given a fair trial with respect to dosage and time interval? Daily therapy at an effective dose for 3 to 6 weeks (or more) may be needed before a drug's effectiveness can be ascertained. The emphasis on short hospital stays may make evaluation of a response more difficult.
3. If a change of medication is indicated, is the new agent from a different chemical class (or subclass of the phenothiazines) so that the patient benefits from any inherent differences between classes? Drugs within a class or subclass act similarly and may offer no therapeutic advantage; for example, fluphenazine and trifluoperazine are both high-potency piperazine phenothiazines.

Side Effects of Antipsychotic Drugs and Appropriate Clinical Interventions

Peripheral nervous system effects

Constipation

Encourage high dietary fiber and increased water intake; give laxatives as ordered.

Dry mouth

Advise patient to take sips of water frequently; provide sugarless hard candies, sugarless gum, and mouth rinses.

Nasal congestion

Give over-the-counter nasal decongestant if approved by physician.

Blurred vision

Advise patient to avoid potentially dangerous tasks. Reassure patient that normal vision typically returns in a few weeks, when tolerance to this side effect develops. Pilocarpine eyedrops can be used on a short-term basis.

Mydriasis

Advise patient to report eye pain immediately.

Photophobia

Advise patient to wear sunglasses outdoors.

Hypotension or orthostatic hypotension

Ask patient to get out of bed or chair slowly. He or she should sit on the side of the bed for 1 full minute while dangling feet, then slowly rise. If hypotension is a problem, measure blood pressure before each dose is given. Observe to see whether a change to another antipsychotic agent is indicated.

Tachycardia

Tachycardia is usually a reflex response to hypotension. When intervention for hypotension (previously described) is effective, reflex tachycardia usually decreases. With *clozapine,* hold the dose, if pulse rate is greater than 140 pulsations per minute.[†]

Urinary retention

Encourage frequent voiding and voiding whenever the urge is present. Catheterize for residual fluids. Ask patient to monitor urine output and report output to nurse. Older men with benign prostatic hypertrophy are particularly susceptible to urinary retention.

Urinary hesitation

Provide privacy, run water in the sink, or run warm water over the perineum.

Sedation

Help patient get up early and get the day started.

Weight gain

Help patient order an appropriate diet; diet pills should not be taken.

Agranulocytosis

A high incidence of agranulocytosis (1% to 2%) is associated with *clozapine.* White blood cell count (WBC) should be performed weekly. When baseline WBC is less than 3500 cells/mm^3, treatment should not be initiated. After treatment begins, a WBC of less than 3000 cells/mm^3 and a granulocyte count of less than 1500 cells/mm^3 indicate treatment interruption to monitor for infection. If no signs of infection are present, treatment can resume. If WBC is less than 2000 cells/mm^3 and granulocyte count is less

Side Effects of Antipsychotic Drugs and Appropriate Clinical Interventions—cont'd

than 1000 cells/mm^3, stop therapy and do not rechallenge the patient. If infection develops, antibiotics should be prescribed.

Central nervous system effects

Akathisia

Be patient and reassure patient who is "jittery" that you understand the need to move and that appropriate drug interventions can help differentiate akathisia and agitation. Since akathisia is the chief cause of noncompliance with antipsychotic regimens, switching to a different class of antipsychotic drug may be necessary to achieve compliance.

Dystonias

If a severe reaction such as oculogyric crisis or torticollis occurs, give antiparkinson drug (e.g., benztropine mesylate [Cogentin]) or antihistamine (e.g., diphenhydramine [Benadryl]) immediately, as needed, and offer reassurance. More than likely an order for intramuscular administration will not have been written, so call the physician at once to obtain the order. For less severe dystonias, notify the physician when an order for an antiparkinson drug is warranted.

Drug-induced parkinsonism

Assess for the three major parkinsonism symptoms, tremors, rigidity, and bradykinesia, and report to physician. Antiparkinson drugs will probably be indicated.

Tardive dyskinesia

Assess for signs by using the abnormal inventory movement scale. Drug holidays may help prevent tardive dyskinesia. Since antipsychotic drugs may mask tardive dyskinesia, their use should be reviewed. Anticholinergic agents will worsen tardive dyskinesia, so question their indiscriminate prophylactic use. However, young men taking large doses of high-potency antipsychotic drugs (e.g., haloperidol) are one group in which prophylactic use of antiparkinson drugs may be more prudent than not using them.*

Neuroleptic malignant syndrome

Be alert for this potentially fatal side effect. *Routinely* take temperatures and encourage adequate water intake among all patients on a regimen of antipsychotic drugs, and *routinely* assess for rigidity, tremor, and the like.

Seizures

Seizures occur in approximately 1% of patients receiving antipsychotic drug treatment. *Clozapine* causes an even higher rate, up to 5% of patients taking 600 to 900 mg/day. For dosages of clozapine greater than 600 mg/day a normal EEG should be performed. If a seizure occurs, it may be necessary to discontinue clozapine. See Chapter 7 for appropriate antiepileptic therapy.

*American Psychiatric Association Task Force on Tardive Dyskinesia: *Am J Psychiatry* 137:1163, 1980.

†Jaretz, Flowers, and Millsap: *Perspect Psychiatr Care* 28:19, 1992.

Peripheral nervous system effects. Anticholinergic PNS effects—dry mouth, blurred vision, and photophobia—are common and often can be managed with non-drug interventions. Mydriasis can cause an increase in intraocular pressure, which can aggravate glaucoma. Other relatively common anticholinergic effects are constipation and urinary hesitance. Patients with a history of glaucoma or prostatic hypertrophy are not ordinarily placed on regimens of these drugs. Tachycardia is another PNS effect, and patients with cardiovascular disease should be carefully evaluated before these drugs are prescribed. Sudden death related to arrhythmias and decreased cardiac output has been reported with antipsychotic drugs. Thioridazine (Mellaril) has been implicated in more cases of sudden death than has any other antipsychotic drug (Mehtonen et al., 1991).

Hypotension is the major antiadrenergic effect of antipsychotic drugs. Hypotension often occurs when the individual stands or changes position suddenly (orthostatic hypotension). Orthostatic symptoms occur most often in elderly persons (Gomez and Gomez, 1990). Thus precautions against falls must be instituted. Additionally, hypotension may cause a reflex tachycardia that can in turn cause general cardiovascular inefficiency. Thus low-potency antipsychotic drugs are usually not prescribed for individuals with severe hypotension, heart failure, or a history of arrhythmias.

Central nervous system extrapyramidal side effects. In up to 75% of patients receiving antipsychotic medications EPSEs develop (Blair, 1990). Abnormal involuntary movement disorders develop because of a drug-induced imbalance between two major neurotransmitters, dopamine and acetylcholine (ACh), in portions of the brain. This imbalance seems to be caused more readily by high-potency antipsychotic drugs, for example, haloperidol. Extrapyramidal side effects may be characterized as akathisia, dystonias, dyskinesias, akinesias, and drug-induced parkinsonism. Neuroleptic malignant syndrome and tardive dyskinesia (TD), a late-appearing dyskinesia, also may result from dopamine depletion and are the most serious side effects and (in the case of TD) the least treatable. Guidelines for minimizing EPSEs are listed in the box on p. 57.

Akathisia. "Akathisia is an EPSE that results from antipsychotic medication and is by far the most dramatic; akathisia may also be the most dangerous . . .," according to Dauner and Blair (1990). Akathisia, literally "the inability to sit" (Blair and Dauner, 1992), is an unpleasant subjective and objective response to antipsychotic drugs. Perhaps the most common EPSE (about 50% of all EPSEs), akathisia probably accounts for more noncompliant behavior than do the other side effects. Some clinicians believe that a majority of patients receiving antipsychotic drugs have akathisia. Akathisia was first described in 1911, long before antipsychotic drugs were available, suggesting that other variables may contribute to its occurrence. *Subjectively* the patient often feels jittery or uneasy. He or she may report a lot of "nervous energy." *Objectively* the patient is restless and cannot sit still, even during group activities, and assaultive behavior can result. Planasky and Johnston (1971) found that 79% of suicidal schizophrenic patients had akathisia. Restlessness and verbal reflections of subjective anguish can be misinterpreted as a worsening of the psychotic process. *If additional antipsychotic medication is given (i.e., a dose "as needed") because of this misinterpretation, the patient will suffer much more.* Akathisia may respond to anticholinergic drugs (see chapter 14) such as trihexyphenidyl but can be resistant to this intervention. Benzodiazepines may also be useful. However, Keepers and Casey (1986) pointed out that other approaches, including waiting for tolerance to develop and decreasing the dosage of the antipsychotic agent, may be the best approach to the treatment of akathisia.

Dystonias. Dystonic reactions may cause rigidity in muscles that control posture,

Guidelines for Minimizing EPSEs

1. Antipsychotic drugs are used for approved indications, that is, they are not used, for example, to treat anxiety.
2. The dose for certain patients is limited. Elderly persons, for instance, are especially susceptible to hypotension and tardive dyskinesia.
3. As with all drugs, but especially because of a dose-EPSE relationship, the lowest effective dose of an antipsychotic drug is given. Since these drugs are metabolized primarily in the liver, persons with reduced liver function as a result of old age or liver disease should be given lower doses than normal.
4. Drug holidays, brief periods when the patient is taken off a regimen of drugs, can decrease side effects without jeopardizing the therapeutic value of the drug.
5. After 1 year of continuous antipsychotic drug therapy the patient is gradually weaned from the drug. This taper allows the treatment team or clinician to evaluate the current need for the drug and also permits the detection of an emerging tardive dyskinesia.

gait, or ocular movement. Remington et al. (1990) in a small prospective study (N = 41) found that 67% of the schizophrenic patients taking parenteral haloperidol became dystonic. In oculogyric crisis the eyes roll back, a frightening experience. Torticollis, another dystonic reaction, is a contracted state of the cervical muscles, producing torsion on the neck. A laryngeal-pharyngeal dystonia, which is associated with gagging, cyanosis, respiratory distress, and asphyxia (particularly in young men), is life threatening. All these conditions respond to intramuscular anticholinergic antiparkinsonism drugs or may respond to intramuscular or intravenous diphenhydramine (see Chapter 14).

Akinesia. Akinesia refers to an absence of movement. More often a state of bradykinesia, or a slowing of movement, exists. Movement is difficult to initiate and maintain. The patient lacks spontaneity in movement and speech. Paradoxically these same symptoms (for different reasons) are common in schizophrenia, the focus of treatment. Historically it has not been uncommon for nurses to mistake bizarre postures caused by EPSEs for exacerbation of schizophrenic symptoms. The dilemma is real. If a manifestation of schizophrenia is occurring, more medication may be indicated; if the condition is an EPSE, more medication will worsen the symptoms.

Drug-induced parkinsonism. Antipsychotic drugs can produce the constellation of symptoms peculiar to parkinsonism: tremors, rigidity, and bradykinesia are possible consequences of antipsychotic drug therapy. Antipsychotic drugs can intensify existing "naturally occurring" parkinsonism, so antipsychotics are avoided if at all possible for persons with this condition.

Dyskinesias and tardive dyskinesia. *Dyskinesia* refers to abnormal involuntary skeletal muscle movements, which usually produce a jerky motion. Treatment with any antipsychotic drug involves the risk of tardive dyskinesia, which is a serious side effect. The term *tardive* means "late-appearing." Typically TD appears after months or years of drug usage; however, TD can appear sooner. Although EPSEs, much like parkinsonism, are caused by a dopamine deficiency, TD theoretically is caused by hypersensitivity to dopamine (and, possibly, cholinergic deficit). In a sense TD is the pharmacologic opposite of the EPSEs (Lieberman et al., 1988). Therefore, although anticholinergic antiparkinsonism drugs (e.g., trihexyphenidyl and benztropine) are beneficial for the other EPSEs, they may worsen TD and thus exacerbate it. Tardive dyskinesia is thought to affect about 15% to 25% of the patients who receive antipsychotic drug treatment; however, current research (Yassa et al., 1990) suggests even higher levels (34%) of this illness.

Tardive dyskinesia usually affects the muscles of the mouth and face. Signs of tardive dyskinesia include lip smacking, grinding of the teeth, rolling or protrusion of the tongue, tics, and diaphragmatic movements, which may impair breathing. These involuntary movements are generally coordinated, fluctuate in severity, and disappear during sleep. Patients with TD are three times as likely to have an impaired gag reflex. Tardive dyskinesia is most often severe in young men and most common in women over 70 years of age (Appleton, 1988).

Because TD is considered irreversible (except in the early stages, when it is more appropriately termed "withdrawal dyskinesia"), a physician should be notified and the patient or family, or both, educated when TD is suspected. The abnormal involuntary movement scale (AIMS) provides a mechanism for assessing TD. The dopamine agonist bromocriptine (Parlodel) and reserpine have been used to treat this side effect, as has clonazepam and vitamin E (which apparently works by neutralizing free radicals). However, no highly effective treatment approach has yet been established.

Neuroleptic malignant syndrome. A final side effect or adverse event worthy of discussion is the neuroleptic malignant syndrome (NMS), an underdiagnosed adverse response to antipsychotic drugs (Keltner and McIntyre, 1985). Neuroleptic malignant syndrome may occur in as many as 1% (some research estimates run as high as 2.4%) of patients receiving antipyschotic drugs; of this number from 14% to 30% may die (Hooper, Herren, and Goldwasser, 1989). Neuroleptic malignant syndrome is most often associated with high-potency antipsychotic drugs, especially when prescribed with a large loading dose. Deng, Chen, and Phillips (1990) in a large prospective study (9700 inpatients) found fluphenazine decanoate (Prolixin decanoate), when used without an antiparkinson agent, to be a major risk factor. However, NMS is not related to toxic drug levels and may occur after only a few doses. Neuroleptic malignant syndrome shares some symptoms with the EPSEs. Hyperthermia, muscular rigidity, tremors, impaired ventilation, muteness, altered consciousness, and autonomic hyperactivity are observed. Perhaps the cardinal symptom is high body temperature. Temperatures as high as 42.2° C (108° F) have been reported. Historically risk factors associated with NMS have been young adulthood, male sex, nonschizophrenic illness, and high-potency drugs. Pharmacologic treatment has included the use of bromocriptine, dantrolene (Dantrium), and amantadine (Symmetrel) (see Chapter 14).

Other side effects. Other side effects that may occur in association with antipsychotic drugs include hyperglycemia, jaundice, blood dyscrasias, susceptibility to hyperthermia, blue-gray skin rash, sun-sensitive skin (sunburn), nasal congestion, wheezing, galactorrhea (seepage from breast), gynecomastia (enlarged breast in either sex), impaired ejaculation, and amenorrhea. A CNS effect that is not an extrapyramidal symptom is memory loss. Since the cholinergic system is implicated in memory and learning, anticholinergic antiparkinsonism drugs and low-potency antipsychotic drugs could play a role in this cognitive symptom. A new antipsychotic, clozapine (Clozaril), causes agranulocytosis in 1% of the persons who take it (Barrett, Ormiston, and Molyneux, 1990). Thirty-five percent of those in whom agranulocytosis developed in 1986 died. Clozapine is discussed at end of this chapter.

Implications

Individual profiles for each antipsychotic can be found in Part Two of this book.

Therapeutic versus toxic levels. Overdoses of antipsychotic drugs may be fatal but are less likely with the high-potency agents. Symptoms of overdose include severe CNS depression (somnolence to coma), hypotension, and EPSEs. Restlessness or agitation, convulsions (antipsychotic drugs lower the seizure threshold), hyperthermia, increased anticholinergic symptoms, and arrhythmias are other indicators of an overdose. Treatment is mostly supportive: gastric lavage to empty the stomach, amphetamine for severe CNS depression (although a risk of seizure is incurred), and antiparkinson drugs for severe EPSEs. Norepinephrine can be used for severe hypotension. *Epinephrine aggravates hypotension.*

Use in pregnancy. Although the risks to the fetus are statistically low, exposure to antipsychotic drugs during the first trimester is still to be avoided. During the remainder of the pregnancy the lowest possible dose is desirable. If possible, antipsychotic drugs should be discontinued to reduce the risk of transient neonatal toxicity (Cohen, 1989).

Side effects. Peripheral nervous system anticholinergic and antiadrenergic effects of antipsychotic drugs are troublesome but are not always as serious or as disturbing to the patient as the CNS EPSEs. Nurses are often the first psychiatric professionals to observe side effects. There are several specific interventions the nurse can provide to ameliorate the side effect or to prevent serious consequences (see the box on pp. 54-55).

Interactions. Antipsychotic drugs compromise and are compromised by many other drugs (Watsky and Salzman, 1991). Since these drug-drug interactions can be serious, it is important, first, to know potential offending agents and, second, to advise the family and patient accordingly. Central nervous system depressants such as alcohol, antihistamines, antianxiety drugs, antidepressants, barbiturates, meperidine, and morphine have additive effects that can cause profound CNS depression. The clinician should review prescriptions for the possible inadvertent combination of these and the antipsychotic drugs and should advise the patient to avoid both alcohol and certain over-the-counter medications.

Since antacids decrease absorption of antipsychotic drugs, administer these agents 1 to 2 hours after an oral antipsychotic drug has been given.

Be aware of other drugs that interact adversely with the antipsychotic drugs (see the box on pp. 60-61).

Patient education. Patient education is an important dimension of the care of patients who are taking antipsychotic drugs. Use discretion in selecting the content of education sessions, since the patient may have a tendency to become anxious about potential side effects. Focus on symptoms that can be seen or felt. Some patient education issues have been discussed throughout this chapter. Those recommendations not previously mentioned include the following:

- Avoid hot tubs, hot showers, and hot tub baths, since hypotension may occur and may cause falls.
- Avoid abrupt drug withdrawal, thereby reducing the risk of EPSEs.
- Use sunscreen to prevent sunburn.
- Adhere to the drug regimen as prescribed: noncompliance is the primary cause of symptom exacerbation.

Adverse Interactions of Antipsychotics with Other Drugs

Amoxapine, fluoxetine
Increased EPSEs

Amphetamines
Decrease antipsychotic effect

Anticholinergic antiparkinson drugs
Increased anticholinergic effect; delayed onset of the effects of oral doses of antipsychotics; potential increased risk of hyperthermia

Barbiturates, nonbarbiturate hypnotics
All cause respiratory depression and increase sedation; all decrease antipsychotic serum levels; hypotension

Benzodiazepines
Increased sedation; respiratory depression with lorazepam and loxapine

Beta-adrenergic blocking agents (propranolol)
Effect of either or both drugs increased

Cimetidine
Chlorpromazine absorption decreased; increased sedation with chlorpromazine

Diazoxide
Can cause severe hyperglycemia

Dopaminergic antiparkinson drugs (e.g., bromocriptine)
Antagonize the antipsychotic effect

Guanethidine
Control of hypertension is decreased

Insulin, oral hypoglycemics
Control of diabetes is weakened

L-dopa
Decreased antiparkinsonian effect of L-dopa; may exacerbate psychosis

Lithium
Decreases antipsychotic effect; may cause neurotoxicity when combined with haloperidol; lithium toxicity may be masked by antiemetic effect of antipsychotic drugs; increases EPSEs

Narcotics
Hypotension with chlorpromazine and meperidine; increased sedation; hypotension augmented; respiratory depression augmented

Adverse Interactions of Antipsychotics with Other Drugs—cont'd

Phenytoin
May increase phenytoin toxicity; decreased antipsychotic blood serum levels

Trazodone
Additive hypotension with phenothiazines

Tricyclics
Possible ventricular arrhythmias with thioridazine; possible increased blood serum levels of both; hypotension; sedation; anticholinergic effect; increased risk of seizures.

Pay attention to and communicate symptoms of sore throat, malaise, fever, or bleeding: such signs and symptoms may indicate the emergence of a blood dyscrasia.

Adopt appropriate dress in hot weather, and increase fluid intake to avoid heat stroke.

Chemical Class and Structure of Specific Drugs

True therapeutic differences among antipsychotic agents have not been substantiated (with the possible exception of clozapine). Any differences between individual drugs are those of sedation and side effects as forementioned (Johnson, 1990) (see Table 4-2 for a review of these drug effects).

Phenothiazines. The phenothiazines are divided into three subclasses, aliphatics, piperidines, and piperazines.

Aliphatics: chlorpromazine, promazine, and triflupromazine. The aliphatics are more sedative and more likely than other phenothiazines to produce orthostatic hypotension. Chlorpromazine has been described previously in detail. The other two drugs, *promazine* (Sparine) and *trifluopromazine* (Vesprin), are seldom ordered.

Piperidines: thioridazine and mesoridazine. Piperidines have a lower risk of EPSEs, but important concerns about eye toxicity exists. Thioridazine is almost as old as chlorpromazine and is the largest-selling antipsychotic in the United States (Wysowski and Baum, 1989). It is frequently ordered, and many patients respond or tolerate it. Thioridazine is sometimes prescribed for the short-term treatment of depression accompanied by anxiety in adult patients and for agitation, anxiety, depressed mood, tension, sleep disturbances, fears, and other symptoms in geriatric patients. In children with severe behavioral problems marked by combativeness, thioridazine has been therapeutic. In a regimen of thioridazine the maximum daily dose is 800 mg; with higher doses the risk of pigmentary retinopathy or retinitis pigmentosa occurs. Mesoridazine is not prescribed as often as thioridazine but has the advantage of being available as an injectable and is more easily metabolized. Mesoridazine is sometimes preferred in alcohol abusers or other persons with liver disease. Elderly persons are exquisitely sensitive to mesoridazine-induced hypotension.

Piperazines: fluphenazine, trifluoperazine, and perphenazine. Piperazines are moderately sedative; they seldom cause orthostatic hypotension but do cause significant levels of EPSE. The two most often prescribed piperazines are fluphenazine and trifluoperazine. Fluphenazine, a high-potency antipsychotic, is available in a long-acting or depot form. Fluphenazine decanoate (Prolixin decanoate), the long-acting form, is beneficial for patients who do not comply with a daily oral medication regimen. An injection can be given every 2 to 4 weeks. Fluphenazine hydrochloride has a "regular" duration and is available in tablet, concentrate, and "regular-acting" parenteral forms. There are restrictions for diluting the concentrate: it should not be mixed with tea, apple juice, or caffeine (e.g., coffee and colas).

Trifluoperazine is prescribed relatively often. It is available in tablets and concentrate and for parenteral use and is indicated for excessive anxiety, tension, and agitation, as well as for psychotic manifestations.

Perphenazine is often used with antidepressants for patients who are both psychotic and depressed. It can be given separately or is available in a fixed-dose combination with amitriptyline (Elavil). The fixed-dose combination of perphenazine and amitriptyline is Triavil.

Butyrophenone: haloperidol. Haloperidol is in the butyrophenone chemical class of antipsychotic drugs. It is a high-potency drug (2 mg of haloperidol is equivalent to 100 mg of chlorpromazine) and tends to cause EPSEs but has fewer anticholinergic side effects than do the low-potency agents. Haloperidol is the most frequently prescribed high-potency antipsychotic and is used extensively in the elderly (because of fewer anticholinergic effects) and in pediatric psychiatry. Haloperidol is also used for Gilles de la Tourette's syndrome, which is characterized by facial grimaces, tics, purposeless movements of the upper body, shoulder, and arms, coprolalia (frequent extreme profanity), and echolalia (repetition of words spoken to patient). Whereas dosages of up to 100 mg per day have been given for psychosis, Rifkin et al. (1991) found that smaller dosages of more than 10 mg per day had no additional benefit.

Haloperidol decanoate is a long-acting depot form and can be given every 2 to 4 weeks (or with longer intervals). This preparation is particularly beneficial for patients with compliance difficulties.

Thioxanthenes: chlorprothixene and thiothixene. Chlorprothixene and thiothixene have different potencies. Chlorprothixene is similar to chlorpromazine or the aliphatic phenothiazines in potency. Thiothixene is 20 times as potent as chlorpromazine, or more like the piperazine phenothiazines. Thiothixene is prescribed relatively often. Thiothixene exhibits weak anticholinergic properties but relatively powerful EPSEs.

Dibenzoxazepine: loxapine. Loxapine is available in capsule, concentrate, and parenteral forms. The concentrate is unpleasant and should be diluted with orange or grapefruit juice shortly before administration. Specific EPSEs have been reported frequently (in approximately 20% of patients), particularly during the first few days of treatment. Specific EPSEs include akathisia and parkinsonism symptoms: tremors, rigidity, sialorrhea, and masked facies. As with other agents, reduction of the loxapine and the administration of an antiparkinson drug usually controls these manifestations.

Dihydroindolone: molindone. Molindone (Moban) is about 10 times as potent as chlorpromazine and is used exclusively for the treatment of psychosis. Some studies indicate that molindone may be the ideal antipsychotic because it has fewer overall side effects than the other antipsychotic drugs. Available only for oral administration, molindone has several unique properties; for example, it provokes heavy menstruation in previously amenorrheal women and contains calcium ions that can interfere with the absorption of tetracycline antibiotics or phenytoin (Dilantin).

Dibenzodiazepine: clozapine. Clozapine *(Clozaril),* manufactured by Sandoz, Inc. (Hanover, New Jersey), is the first new antipsychotic agent to be introduced in the United States in 20 years. Although it was first introduced in 1960, it has taken three decades to be marketed in the United States (Safferman et al., 1991). Clozapine is a dibenzodiazepine derivative and has pharmacologic features unique among antipsychotic drugs. It has an affinity for limbic rather than striatal neurons. This affinity probably explains the relative lack of EPSEs associated with clozapine. Clozapine binds with dopamine receptors, as do other antipsychotic drugs, thus limiting the effects of dopamine in the brain. Clozapine's primary importance is that patients resistant to other antipsychotics have responded to its use (Meltzer, 1989). Approximately 10% to 20% of schizophrenic patients are not responsive to traditional antipsychotics, and another 20% to 30% who are initially responsive to antipsychotics other than clozapine relapse within 1 year. Some studies suggest that as many as 64% of treatment-resistant schizophrenic patients show a favorable response to clozapine (Perry et al., 1991). "One of the pluses of the development of clozapine is that for the first time professions . . . are accepting the importance of biologically based therapy," according to Lawson (1992).

Sandoz, Inc. (1992) estimates that there are 200,000 suitable candidates for clozapine (Salzman, 1990). Although clozapine has been used for some time in Europe and China for the treatment of schizophrenia, clozapine was not approved in the United States until 1990, largely because of the seriousness of the side effect, agranulocytosis. Agranulocytosis is a sudden and severe drop in the number of white blood cells that leads to death, which is usually caused by overwhelming infection. The period of maximum risk is 4 to 18 weeks (Safferman et al., 1991). A study made in 1986 revealed that in about 1% to 2% of the patients who take clozapine, agranulocytosis develops and that of these, 35% die. However, recent information from the manufacturer indicates that since the introduction of the Clozaril Patient Management System or other similar monitoring formats, seven clozapine-related deaths have been reported as of October, 1992 (Sandoz, Inc., Hanover, New Jersey).

Clinical implications. Until the advent of clozapine all antipsychotic drugs were considered equally effective. Some drugs helped some people more than other drugs, but one could not say, for instance, that haloperidol was superior to chlorpromazine. Clozapine is the first drug for which an improved rate of response is suggested. However, because of the high risk of bone marrow suppression or bone marrow failure and death, certain precautions must be observed by the clinician and patient. Although clinicians agree that clozapine treatment succeeds where treatment with other neuroleptics fails, its efficacy for purely negative symptoms is unknown (Safferman et al., 1991).

Frequent monitoring of white blood cells and platelets. When white blood cells and platelets are monitored frequently, impending bone marrow failure can be detected early, thus greatly reducing the risk associated with infection.

Prominent side effects. Sedation, hypersalivation, dizziness, tachycardia, hypotension, and constipation are the most frequent side effects of clozapine treatment. Hypersalivation (sialorrhea), by some anecdotal accounts, affects most patients taking clozapine and can be extremely embarrassing (Jaretz, Flowers, and Millsap, 1992).

Weekly distribution. Clozapine should be distributed to the patient once a week to ensure that monitoring standards are followed.

Clinical criteria. Pelonero and Elliot (1990) have outlined the following guidelines for the selection of patients who could benefit from clozapine:

1. Treatment-resistant schizophrenia or severe, persistent tardive dyskinesia, or both are present.
2. No medical contraindication (such as blood dyscrasia, epilepsy, or hepatic or renal disease) is present.
3. Patient has the ability to give informed consent.
4. Patient has the ability to comply with the treatment regimen, including the Clozaril Patient Management System.

A public and professional outcry concerning the Clorazil Patient Management System caused the manufacturer to provide a mechanism for other patient management systems. In the original Clorazil Patient Management System patients did not receive clozapine through a pharmacy; instead, they received weekly home visits from a nurse or a technologist. Each week a blood sample was drawn and tested for agranulocytosis. Patients received only a 1-week supply of clozapine. Because dispensing clozapine was so labor- and technology-intensive, the drug was expensive, costing about $9000 per year, or about $25 per day (Griffith, 1990). In comparison the cost of azidothymidine (AZT), the drug used in the treatment of acquired immunodeficiency syndrome (AIDS), is about $8000 per year. Thus few state departments of mental health could afford to purchase clozapine. For instance, in California the state department of mental health prohibited the prescribing of clozapine unless the family or patient would pay for it (Bergmann, 1990). In fairness to the manufacturer, this expensive system succeeded in reducing the number of incidents of agranulocytosis.

In May 1991, physicians and pharmacists were allowed to monitor clozapine patients according to locally developed systems. These systems must include a weekly WBC; no more than 1 week's supply of clozapine is given to each patient, and patients taken off a regimen of clozapine must be monitored for a minimum of 4 weeks. The new systems have reduced the cost of clozapine to $4160 per year.

REMARKS

The dopamine hypothesis of schizophrenia states that schizophrenia is caused by excessive levels of dopamine in the brain. Antipsychotic drugs block dopamine receptors, which accounts for the ability of these drugs to effectively "combat" the excessive level of dopamine. Antipsychotic drugs are most accurately classified according to chemical structure; however, a classification system based on potency seems to offer clinical utility. Antipsychotics sedate, quiet emotions, and slow psychomotor agitation while alleviating major symptoms of schizophrenia and psychoses (i.e., alteration in perception, thoughts, consciousness, affect, and the like).

Antipsychotic drugs produce three major side effects, anticholinergic side effects, extrapyramidal side effects (EPSEs), and to a lesser extent, hypotension. For the most part anticholinergic side effects are annoying, whereas EPSEs and severe hypotension with orthostasis are often serious. Low-potency antipsychotics (such as chlorpromazine) tend to produce anticholinergic side effects and hypotension, whereas high-potency antipsychotics (such as haloperidol) produce EPSEs.

Overdoses of antipsychotics, especially the high-potency agents, are seldom fatal, but drug interactions with other CNS depressants such as alcohol can be serious. All health care professional with direct responsibilities for patient care should be alert for signs and symptoms of EPSEs, including tardive dyskinesia and neuroleptic malignant syndrome.

REFERENCES

American Psychiatric Association: *Diagnostic and statistical manual of mental disorders, third edition,* Washington, DC, 1980, The Association.

American Psychiatric Association: *Diagnostic and statistical manual of mental disorders, third edition-revised,* Washington DC, 1987, The Association.

Andreasen NL, Olsen S: Negative vs positive schizophrenia, *Arch Gen Psychiatry* 39:789, 1982.

Andreasen NL, et al: Positive and negative symptoms in schizophrenia: a critical reappraisal, *Arch Gen Psychiatry* 47:615, 1990.

Appleton WS: *Practical and clinical psychopharmacology,* Baltimore, 1988, Williams & Wilkins.

Barrett N, Ormiston S, Molyneux V: Clozapine: a new drug for schizophrenia, *J Psychosoc Nurs* 28:24, 1990.

Bergmann GT: Clozapine: will states ration care? *State Health Reports* 57:1, 1990.

Blair DT: Risk management for extrapyramidal symptoms, *Quality Review Bulletin, J Quality Assurance* 17:116, 1990.

Blair DT, Dauner A: Dangerous consequences: neuroleptic-induced tardive akathisia, *J Psychosoc Nurs* 30(3):41, 1992.

Bleuler E: *Dementia praecox or the group of schizophrenias.* Translated by Zinkin J, New York, 1950, International Universities Press.

Cohen LS: *Psychopharmacology: psychotropic drug use in pregnancy, Hosp Community Psychiatry* 40:566, 1989.

Crow TJ: Molecular pathology of schizophrenia: more than one disease, *Br Med J* 280:66, 1980.

Dauner A, Blair DT: Akathisia: when treatment creates a problem, *J Psychosoc Nurs* 28(10):13, 1990.

Deng MA, Chen GQ, Phillips MR: Neuroleptic malignant syndrome in 12 of 9,792 Chinese inpatients exposed to neuroleptics: a prospective study, *Am J Psychiatry* 147:1149, 1990.

Gomez GE, Gomez EA: The special concerns of neuroleptic use in the elderly, *J Psychosoc Nurs* 28:7, 1990.

Griffith EEH: Clozapine: problems for the public sector, *Hosp Community Psychiatry* 41:837, 1990.

Harris E: Antipsychotic medication, *Am J Nurs* 81:1316, 1981.

Hooper JF, Herren CK, Goldwasser H: Neuroleptic malignant syndrome, *J Psychosoc Nurs* 27:13, 1989.

Jaretz N, Flowers E, Millsap L: Clozapine: nursing care considerations, *Perspect Psychiatr Care* 28:19, 1992.

Johnson DAW: Pharmacological treatment of patients with schizophrenia: past and present problems and potential future therapy, *Drugs* 39(4):481, 1990.

Jones BE, Gray BA: Problems in diagnosing schizophrenia and affective disorders among blacks, *Hosp Community Psychiatry* 37:61, 1986.

Keepers GA, Casey DE: Clinical management of acute neuroleptic-induced extrapyramidal symptoms. In Masserman JH, editor: *Current psychiatric therapies,* New York, 1986, Grune & Stratton.

Keltner NL: Antipsychotic drugs. In Shlafer M, Marieb E, editors: *The nurse, pharmacology, and drug therapy,* Menlo Park, Calif, 1989, Addison-Wesley.

Keltner NL, McIntyre CW: Neuroleptic malignant syndrome, *J Neurosurg Nurs* 17:362, 1985.

Kendler KS, Gruenberg AM, Tsuany MT: A family study of the subtypes of schizophrenia, *Am J Psychiatry* 145:57, 1988.

Kraepelin E: *Dementia praecox and paraphrenia, with historical introduction (1919).* Translated by Barclay RM, New York, 1971, RE Krieger.

Lawson WB: Drugs versus other therapies, *Hosp Community Psychiatry* 43(1):84, 1992.

Lewine RRJ: A discriminate validity study of negative symptoms with a special focus on depression and antipsychotic medication: *Am J Psychiatry* 147:1463, 1990.

Lieberman J et al: Pharmacologic characterization of tardive dyskinesia, *J Clin Psychopharmacology* 8(4):254, 1988.

Lund VE, Frank DI: Helping the medicine go down, *J Psychosoc Nurs* 29(7):6, 1991.

Mehtonen et al: A survey of sudden death associated with the use of antipsychotic or antidepressant drugs: 49 cases in Finland, *Acta Psychiatrica Scandinavica* 84:58, 1991.

Meltzer HY: Duration of a clozapine trial in neuroleptic-resistant schizophrenia, *Arch Gen Psychiatry* 46:672, 1989.

Middlemiss MA, Beeber ZS: Depot antipsychotics, *J Psychosoc Nurs* 27:36, 1989.

Overall JE et al: Justifying neuroleptic drug treatment, *Hosp Community Psychiatry* 40:749, 1989.

Pelonero AL, Elliot RL: Ethical and clinical considerations in selecting patients who will receive clozapine, *Hosp Community Psychiatry* 41:878, 1990.

Perry PJ et al: Clozapine and norclozapine plasma concentrations and clinical response of treatment refractory schizophrenic patients, *Am J Psychiatry* 148(2):231, 1991.

Planasky K, Johnston R: The occurrence and characteristics of suicidal preoccupation and acts in schizophrenia, *Acta Psychiatr Scand* 47:473, 1971.

Remington GJ et al: Prevalence of neuroleptic-induced dystonia in mania and schizophrenia, *Am J Psychiatry* 147:1231, 1990.

Richelson E: Neuroleptic affinities for human brain receptors and their use in predicting adverse effects, *J Clin Psychiatry* 45:331, 1984.

Rifkin A et al: Dosage of haloperidol for schizophrenia, *Arch Gen Psychiatry* 48:166, 1991.

Safferman A et al: Update on the clinical efficacy and side effects of clozapine, *Schizophr Bull* 17(2):247, 1991.

Salzman C: Notes from a state mental health director's meeting on clozapine, *Hosp Community Psychiatry* 41:838, 1990.

Sandoz, Inc.: Clozaril systems data, *Treatment Trends* 1:2, 1992.

Watsky EJ, Salzman C: Psychotropic drug interactions, *Hosp Community Psychiatry* 42(3):247, 1991.

Wysowski DK, Baum C: Antipsychotic drug use in the United States: 1976-1985, *Arch Gen Psychiatry* 46:929, 1989.

Yassa R et al: Factors in the development of severe forms of tardive dyskinesia, *Am J Psychiatry* 147:1156, 1990.

CHAPTER 5

Mood Disorders

HISTORICAL CONSIDERATIONS

Mood or affective disturbances are a part of the normal human condition and can become evident as a symptom, a syndrome, or a specific diagnostic disorder. *Descriptions of depression* have been noted since ancient times and were first recorded by Hippocrates (Lewis, 1967). The term *melancholia* is attributed to him and was thought to result from the influence of black bile and phlegm on the brain, which darkened the spirit and led to melancholia. *Descriptions of bipolar disorder* can be traced to early in the second century, when Aretaeus of Cappadocia recognized association between melancholia and mania.

Although references to melancholia can be found in the historical record from ancient times, it was not until the end of the 1800s that another major contribution to our understanding was developed. In 1896 Kraepelin made this contribution to psychiatry by separating the functional psychoses into two groups, dementia praecox and manic-depressive psychosis. Subsequently patients with chronic depression were included in this group (Kraepelin, 1921; Winokur, 1972). Freud in 1917 published *Mourning and Melancholia*, which described his theories of depression (Freud, 1957). He noted that depression and grief had in common the process of mourning, that is, the response to the loss of a love object. He further observed that although grief was a healthy response, it differed from melancholia in that the latter involved intense expression of ambivalent, hostile feelings formerly associated with the object.

The controversy concerning endogenous (biologic) versus reactive depressions (reactions to life events) undoubtedly arose as a result of the differing viewpoints of Kraepelinians and Freudians. A large part of the existing literature assumes that the two basic forms of depression do indeed exist. However, clinical observations in the last decade indicate that primary mood disorders are more appropriately divided into bipolar and unipolar forms (American Psychiatric Association, 1987). Other mood or affective spectrum disorders have been identified and subclassified as minor forms of mood disturbances (Goodwin and Guze, 1984).

SCOPE OF THE PROBLEM

Estimates of the prevalence of mood disturbances depend on the sample of the population studied and on the definition of the illness. Lifetime incidences as high as 18% for major depression have been reported. The Epidemiological Catchment Area (ECA) studies, sponsored by the National Institutes of Mental Health, found much lower lifetime incidences of 6.7%, 3.7%, and 5.7% for New Haven, Connecticut; Baltimore; and St. Louis, respectively (Myers et al., 1985). The prevalence of bipolar disorder has been investigated primarily through treatment cases because it occurs infrequently. The ECA studies revealed a 6-month incidence ranging from 0.4% to 0.8% for men and from 0.4% to 0.9% for women.

Women are at greater risk than men for major depression, and the patient age at onset is usually the late twenties. No differences are found among races in its distribution. Differences among social classes and familial differences have been shown; depression is most common in lower socioeconomic groups and most likely to emerge in individuals with a positive family history of depression (American Psychiatric Association, 1987). Negative events are often identified as precipitators or as having occurred before the onset of a depressive disorder.

The occurrence of bipolar disorder is equal between men and women and among races; the patient age at onset is typically the early twenties (American Psychiatric Association, 1987). This disorder is most common in higher socioeconomic groups and in religious communities, for example, Old Order Amish. Family history is particularly important insofar as genetic contributors are present, and often a positive family history is found among affected individuals. The relative effect of life events on the onset of an episode is currently unknown.

Primary mood disorders are the psychiatric problem for which patients are most frequently admitted to hospitals and to many psychiatric clinics. Depression is also a common reason for psychiatric consultation; secondary depressions are frequently found among elderly and medically ill individuals who are referred for consultation. Depression may be induced by drugs, foods, or substances of abuse (see Chapter 12).

Criteria for a Major Depressive Episode

1. There is a 2-week period of maladaptive functioning (i.e., a clear change from previous functioning) in which five of the following symptoms are present and in which one of the symptoms is either depressed mood or loss of interest or pleasure.
   a. Depressed mood
   b. Inability to experience pleasure or markedly diminished interest in pleasurable activities
   c. Appetite disturbance (more than 5% change in body weight within 1 month)
   d. Sleep disturbance
   e. Psychomotor disturbance
   f. Fatigue or loss of energy
   g. Feelings of worthlessness or excessive or inappropriate guilt
   h. Diminished ability to concentrate or indecisiveness
   i. Recurrent thoughts of death or suicidal ideations
2. At no time during the disturbance have there been delusions or hallucinations for as long as 2 weeks in the absence of prominent mood symptoms. (If there have been, think "schizoaffective disorder.")
3. There is no evidence of an organic etiology or other major mental disorder.

The episode is designated as mild, moderate, severe (with or without psychotic features), in remission (full or partial), chronic, melancholic, or seasonal based on the number, severity, duration, and/or pattern of the depressive episode(s).

Adapted from American Psychiatric Association: *Diagnostic and statistical manual of mental disorders, third edition-revised,* Washington, DC, 1987, The Association.

DIAGNOSTIC CONSIDERATIONS

Diagnostic criteria for major depression and mania (bipolar disorder) are presented in the boxes on pp. 68 and 69. Those for adjustment disorder and dysthymic disorder are depicted in the boxes on p. 70. Residual categories exist for individuals who do not meet complete criteria. It is recognized that a mood disturbance may be related to adjustment problems, may be a component of another major psychiatric disorder, or may be associated with a seasonal pattern (American Psychiatric Association, 1987). Some individuals with depression may meet conventional criteria for melancholia, the most severe form of depression. Melancholia is characterized by agitation, somatic or nihilistic delusions, loss of pleasure in all or almost all activities, excessive anhedonia, increased depression in the morning, early morning awakening, and excessive or inappropriate guilt.

Major Depression

The chief complaint of patients with major depressive disorder is usually psychologic, that is, feelings of worthlessness or despair or ideas of self-harm. However, a significant portion of depressed individuals also complain of somatic disturbances combined with a dysphoric mood. They may describe themselves as having feelings of hopelessness, irritability, fearfulness, worry, or discouragement. Patients who somatize may have a tendency to minimize feelings of dysphoria and focus on insomnia

Criteria for Bipolar Disorder: Manic Episode

1. There is a distinct period of abnormally euphoric, expansive, or irritable mood, which is of sufficient severity to cause marked impairment in social or occupational functioning.
2. During the mood disturbance, at least three of the following are also present:
   a. Grandiosity
   b. Decreased need for sleep
   c. Hyperverbal or pressured speech
   d. Flight of ideas or racing thoughts
   e. Distractibility
   f. Increase in goal-directed activity or psychomotor agitation
   g. Excessive involvement in pleasurable activities that have a high potential for painful consequences
3. At no time during the disturbance have there been delusions or hallucinations for as long as 2 weeks in the absence of prominent mood symptoms.
4. There is no evidence of an organic etiology or other major mental disorder.

Designate as mild, moderate, severe (with or without psychotic features), or in remission (full or partial) based on the severity of the symptoms. If psychotic symptoms are present, designate as mood-congruent or mood-incongruent.

Adapted from American Psychiatric Association: *Diagnostic and statistical manual of mental disorders, third edition-revised,* Washington, DC, 1987, The Association.

Criteria for Adjustment Disorder*

1. The condition develops as a psychologic reaction to identifiable stressors or events.
2. The reaction clearly reflects a change in the individual's normal personality and can be distinguished as different from the person's usual style of functioning.
3. The psychologic reaction is maladaptive in that normal functioning (including social and occupational functioning) is grossly impaired or the reaction is in excess of what would normally be expected of others in similar circumstances.
4. The psychologic reaction is not an exacerbation of some other mental disorder.
5. The reaction begins within 3 months of the stressor(s) but resolves within 6 months of its onset.

Adapted from American Psychiatric Association: *Diagnostic and statistical manual of mental disorders, third edition-revised,* Washington, DC, 1987, The Association.
*May become evident primarily as anxiety, depression, or mixed features.

Criteria for Dysthymia*

1. There is a chronic, mildly depressed mood state that is generally present most of the day, on more days than not, and for a period of at least 2 years (1 year in children and adolescents).
2. There is never a 2-month period when there are no depressive symptoms.
3. The depression is associated with at least two of the following:
   a. Vegetative symptoms
      Sleep disturbance
      Appetite disturbance
      Decreased energy or fatigue
   b. Cognitive symptoms
      Low self-esteem
      Feeling of hopelessness
      Poor concentration or difficulty making decisions
4. There is no unequivocal evidence of a major depressive episode during the *first 2 years* of the disturbance or of any other major mental disorder *during the course* of the illness.
5. There is no evidence of an organic cause.

Adapted from American Psychiatric Association: *Diagnostic and statistical manual of mental disorders, third edition-revised,* Washington, DC, 1987, The Association.
*May become evident primarily as anxiety, depression, or mixed features.

and anorexia, the so-called vegetative disturbances (Ford, 1983; Stone and Folks, in press). Agitation may be so overwhelming in some depressed individuals that other symptoms of mood disturbance go unnoticed. In contrast, other patients may have prominent motor retardation to the point that they become mute or even catatonic. Psychotic symptoms, for example, suspiciousness and perceptual disturbances, may complicate a depressive episode. Delusions or hallucinations or both may or may not be congruent with the mood disturbance per se. Depressed patients may or may not be able to identify precipitating events that have contributed to the illness. In fact, some of the "precipitators" actually may have occurred *after* the onset of depressive symptoms. For instance, a failed marriage may be either the cause of or the result of depression.

A variety of biologic correlates are known concomitants of depression, such as reduction in slow-wave sleep, shortened rapid eye movement (REM) latency, and increased REM density. Neuroendocrine disturbances, for example, alterations in the response to dexamethasone, may also be present, but a discussion of these is beyond the scope of this book. It has been suggested that these biologic correlates might be used to determine when an antidepressant treatment should be discontinued (Greden et al., 1980).

Bipolar Disorder

The cardinal features of mania are euphoria, hyperactivity, and disturbances of thinking, that is, flight of ideas and pressured speech (see the box on p. 69). Many bipolar patients are primarily irritable. Elderly manic patients may have mixtures of manic and depressive symptoms. Psychotic symptoms, especially, persecutory and grandiose delusions, hallucinations, or ideas of reference, also complicate mania.

Suicide and Other Risks

There is a clear association between depression and suicide; in fact, 50% to 70% of those who commit suicide are found retrospectively to have had symptoms characteristic of depression. Of those who are depressed it is suggested that approximately 15% eventually die by suicide (Guze and Robins, 1970). Disregarding suicide, patients with primary mood disturbance still show an increased mortality when compared by age and sex to members of the general population (Kerr, Schapira, and Roth, 1969). Alcoholism and poor judgement are other risks of primary affective disorders, especially among manic patients. The postpartum period is significant also, especially in women with bipolar disorder, who are likely to have episodes of depression or mania during the postpartum period.

Diagnostic Dilemmas

Depressed patients may show impairment in concentration and short-term but not long-term memory (Sternberg, Jarvik, 1976). Sometimes the memory impairment associated with depression mimics dementia. This condition is referred to as pseudodementia (see Table 5-1). The differential diagnosis between primary mood disturbance and grief can be difficult (see Table 5-2). Differential diagnosis includes anxiety disorders, hypochondriasis or other somatoform disorders, and other major psychiatric syndromes such as schizophrenia and organic mental syndromes. Syndromes in which a mood disturbance is secondarily induced as a side effect of certain drugs or as a complication of various medical problems are also prominent (see the boxes on pp. 73 and 74).

Table 5-1 Comparison of Dementia and Depression

Feature	Dementia	Depression
Onset	Insidious, indeterminate	Rapid, abrupt
Symptom duration	Longer	Shorter
Mood	Variable	Depressed
Cognitive deficits	Consistent	Inconsistent
Mental status assessment	Wrong answer	Refuses to attempt answer
Neurologic deficit	Aphasia, apraxia, agnosia	None

Table 5-2 Comparison of Grief and Depression

Grief	Depression
Guilt/self-reproach	Guilt/self-reproach
Somatic symptoms	Somatic symptoms
Duration of 6 months or less	Greater than 6 months' duration
Remains functional	Becomes debilitated
Usually not suicidal	Possibly suicidal

TREATMENT CONSIDERATIONS

Depression

The management of depression ideally combines an indicated drug treatment together with other interventions. Insight-oriented psychotherapy, for example, may involve examinations of motives and feelings; cognitive psychotherapy may focus on defects in the individual's perception of self, the environment, or future outlook. Other forms of psychotherapy, including interpersonal, behavioral, group, and marital therapy, may contribute significantly to patient outcome. Studies have repeatedly shown that psychotherapy is more efficacious than nontreatment and that the combination of psychotherapy and antidepressant medication is more efficacious than either drug treatment alone or no treatment (Roundsville, Klerman, and Weissman, 1981). Some patients do not wish to receive drug treatment, and many patients cannot tolerate the side effects of antidepressant medication. Still others may not wish to enter into any form of psychotherapy, and these patients, of course, should not be denied treatment with antidepressants (Weissman, 1979).

No definitive data suggest that patients will recover as a result of one type of treatment rather than another or that an individual with a particular subtype of depression will benefit from drugs or psychotherapy, or a combination of the two. However, the best approach to the management of major depressive illness is often drug treatment or electroconvulsive therapy (ECT), or both. Choosing the most suitable antidepressant medication for a particular patient remains more of an art than a science (Goodwin and Guze, 1984). It is not yet clear how antidepressant medication shortens depressive episodes, and electroconvulsive therapy may be the most effective treatment available for depression, especially major depression (see Chapter 11)

Medical Illnesses Commonly Associated with Depression

Central nervous system disorders
Alzheimer's disease (senile and presenile)
Amyotrophic lateralizing sclerosis
Brain tumor (especially, nondominant lobe)
Cerebrovascular accident (stroke)
Chronic subdural hematoma
Multiple sclerosis
Normal-pressure hydrocephalus
Parkinson's disease
Subarachnoid hemorrhage

Infections
Acquired immunodeficiency syndrome
Hepatitis
Infectious mononucleosis
Influenza
Syphilis
Tuberculosis
Viral pneumonia
Encephalitis

Collagen vascular disease
Polymyalgia rheumatica
Rheumatoid arthritis
Systemic lupus erythematosus
Temporal arteritis

Neoplastic disorders
Carcinoma of head of pancreas
Chronic myelogenous leukemia
Lymphoma
Other malignant diseases
Small-cell carcinoma of lung

Toxic-metabolic disturbances and endocrinopathies
Addison's disease
Apathetic hyperthyroidism
Cushing's disease
Diabetes mellitus
Electrolyte disorders
Hypothyroidism
Hypoglycemia
Metal intoxication
Parathyroid disorders
Uremia

Others
Chronic fatigue syndrome
Chronic obstructive pulmonary disease

Adapted from Ford CV, Folks DG: *Southern Med J* 78(4):397, 1985.

Drugs and Toxins that May Induce Depression

Analgesics
Phenacetin
Pentazocine

Antibiotics
Aminoglycosides
Chloramphenicol
Sulfonamides

Anticonvulsants
Carbamazepine (rare)
Clonazepam
Phenytoin
Phenobarbital
Primidone
Succinimide

Antihypertensives
α-Methyldopa
Calcium channel blockers (possibly)
Clonidine
Hydralazine (possibly)
Propranolol
Reserpine

Antiinflammatory agents
Corticosteorids
Indomethacin

Cardiovascular agents
Digitalis
Disopyramide
Procainamide

Psychotropic and central nervous system agents
Aliphatic phenothiazines
Amphetamines
Appetite suppressants
  Fenfluramine
  Phenmetrazine
Barbiturates
Benzodiazepines
High-potency neuroleptics*

Miscellaneous
Baclofen
Choline
Cimetidine
Disulfiram
Phenylephrine
Physostigmine

Antituberculosis agents
Ethambutol
Isoniazid

Antineoplastic agents
Asparaginase
Corticosteorids
Nonsteroidal antiinflammatory drugs
Phenylbutazone

Antiparkinsonian agents
Amantadine
Levodopa
Cycloserine
Vinblastine sulfate

Adapted from Ford CV, Folks DG: *Southern Med J* 78(4):397, 1985.
*May cause akinesia as a form of secondary depression (see Chapter 4).

(Kalinowsky and Hippius, 1969). Generally ECT is no more dangerous than treatment with drugs.

Bipolar Disorder

Mania may be effectively treated with antipsychotics, lithium or alternative agents, or ECT. Of these methods ECT is probably the least effective. Lithium is the drug of choice, but antipsychotic agents may be particularly useful in active or agitated manic patients. The usefulness of lithium or other alternative agents such as carbamazepine or valproate may be limited to the treatment of acute mania. Growing evidence suggests that these drugs, particularly carbamazepine, may reduce morbidity, that is, they may prevent depression as well as mania (Angst et al., 1970; Mendels, Secunda, and Dyson, 1972; Keltner and Folks, 1991).

Other Mood Disorders

The use of drugs to treat other mood disturbances depends largely on the "target" symptoms that are present. The identification of target symptoms and a rationale for treatment are considered carefully before the institution of therapy. Patients with dysthymic disorder, adjustment disorder with depressed mood, cyclothymia, or other mood disturbances may derive great benefit from drug treatment. Substantial data to support this conventional wisdom does not exist, and it remains the subject of further studies.

ANTIDEPRESSANTS

Historical Considerations

The introduction of pharmacologic agents with antidepressant action in the 1950s revolutionized our thinking about the causes, pathogenic mechanisms, and management of depressive illness. As a consequence, many patients with depressive illness were able to function normally and lead productive lives. Electroconvulsive therapy, developed in the 1930s, remains an effective and safe modality for treatment of depressions that fail to respond to pharmacotherapy and is discussed in Chapter 11.

Before the 1950s and after the initial development of ECT, amphetamines for the treatment of psychomotor retardation and barbiturates for the treatment of agitation were used in patients with depression. Although amphetamines and barbiturates are still used in the initial treatment of depression in medically ill, abulic, or demented patients, there is little reason to use these drugs in most cases of depression. Moreover, the use of amphetamines in persons with severe depression is not indicated and may actually worsen any associated agitation or psychosis, or both (see Chapter 13).

The antidepressant actions of the monoamine oxidase inhibitors (MAOIs) were discovered serendipitously in the 1950s; these were the first drugs to have a true mood-elevating effect. Clinical pharmacologists also began to observe and correlate changes in brain chemistry with changes in mood and behavior, which led to a better understanding of some of the mechanisms of action of these drugs and the biologic contributors to psychiatric illness (Goodman and Charney, 1985). Subsequently in the 1960s the now dominant class of tricyclic antidepressant compounds (TCAs) were introduced for the treatment of depression. The TCAs first developed were actually an outgrowth of attempts to find antipsychotic drugs that were chemically related to the phenothiazines and more effective. The tricyclics remain the mainstay of pharmacologic treatment of depressive illness, although many new agents are now being developed and introduced. Depending on molecular configuration, some of these new agents are more correctly identified as bicyclic or tetracyclic. To reduce repetition, an encompassing classification, "heterocyclic," has been developed to embrace "bicyclic, tricyclic, and tetracyclic" antidepressants. Although these categories are not identical, it is common for all to be referred to as tricyclic antidepressants, or TCAs, in the literature. Figure 5-1 shows the chemical structures of current available heterocyclic antidepressants. Tables 5-3 and 5-4 show the reuptake antagonism, half-life, and the relative effects resulting from cholinergic, histaminergic, alpha-adrenergic, and dopaminergic blockade (discussed in the section on side effects).

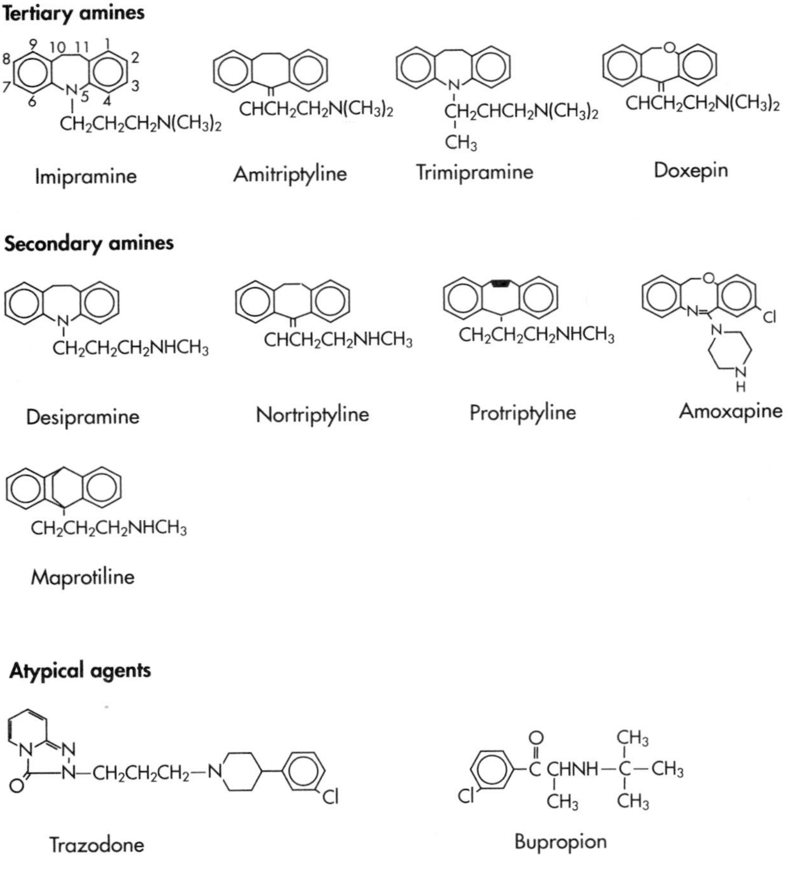

Tertiary amines

$CH_2CH_2CH_2N(CH_3)_2$
Imipramine

$CHCH_2CH_2N(CH_3)_2$
Amitriptyline

$CH_2CHCH_2N(CH_3)_2$, CH_3
Trimipramine

$CHCH_2CH_2N(CH_3)_2$
Doxepin

Secondary amines

$CH_2CH_2CH_2NHCH_3$
Desipramine

$CHCH_2CH_2NHCH_3$
Nortriptyline

$CH_2CH_2CH_2NHCH_3$
Protriptyline

Amoxapine

$CH_2CH_2CH_2NHCH_3$
Maprotiline

Atypical agents

$N{-}CH_2CH_2CH_2{-}N$
Trazodone

$C\ CHNH{-}C{-}CH_3$, CH_3, CH_3, CH_3
Bupropion

Figure 5-1 Chemical structures of antidepressants.

All the antidepressant agents depicted in Tables 5-3 and 5-4 are effective in alleviating the symptoms of depressive illness. Melancholia, including sadness and hopelessness as well as vegetative, somatic, and motor symptoms, is responsive to drug treatment. The abilities to reengage in social, occupational, and relationship functioning and to recapture quality of life are among the many benefits that may be derived from antidepressant therapy. Patients generally experience an improvement in energy level, a decrease in fatigue and psychomotor symptoms, and the disappearance of suicidal thoughts (Bernstein, 1988).

Neurochemical Theory of Effectiveness

Although a number of theories concerning the cause of depression have been promulgated, the efficacy of antidepressants is best understood from a neurochemical and neurobiologic perspective. The biogenic amine theory of depression essentially implies that an imbalance or a relative deficiency exists of certain neurotransmitters or biogenic amines, for example, serotonin and norepinephrine. Specifically, deficien-

Table 5-3 Pharmacologic Properties of Antidepressants

Drug	Usual daily adult dosage range (mg)	Therapeutic plasma levels (ng/ml)	Neurotransmitter effect*	
			Serotonin	Norepinephrine
Heterocyclics				
Amitriptyline (Elavil, Endep)	S 25 tid-qid M 40-100 hs	110-250	4x	2x
Amoxapine (Asendin)	S 50 bid or tid M 100-300 hs	200-500	2x	3x
Clomipramine (Anafranil)	S 25 qd M 100-150 hs	150-300	4x	2x or 3x
Desipramine (Norpramin, Pertofrane)	S 100-200/day M 100-200 hs	125-300	2x	4x
Doxepin (Adapin, Sinequan)	S 75/day M 75-150 hs	100-200	2x	x
Imipramine (Tofranil)	S 75-100/day M 50-150 hs	200-350	4x	2x
Maprotiline (Ludiomil)	S 25 tid M 75-150/day	200-300	0/x	3x
Nortriptyline (Aventyl, Pamelor)	S 25 tid-qid M 50-100/day	50-150	3x	2x
Nonheterocyclics				
Bupropion (Wellbutrin)	S 100 bid M 100 tid	—	+/0	+/0
Fluoxetine (Prozac)	S 20 in AM M 10-40/day (AM and noon)	—	5x	x
Sertraline (Zoloft)	S 50/day M 50-200/day	—	5x	0
Trazodone (Desyrel)	S 50 tid M 150-400/day	800-1600	3x	0

Adapted from Olin BR, editor: *Drug facts and comparisons,* Philadelphia, 1990, JB Lippincott.
S, to start; *M,* maintenance*; *x,* relative intensity of effect; *0,* none; —, unknown.
*Based on manufacturer information.

cies of these substances result in a neurochemical imbalance. Perhaps alterations exist in the functioning of the receptor site or the secondary messenger systems that modulate the activity of the receptor site postsynaptically (hence the term "neuromodulator").

Psychopharmacologic treatment (Figure 5-2) is based on the restoration of normal levels of neurotransmitter systems (1) by *TCAs* blocking neurotransmitter uptake in the nerve ending, (2) by inhibiting neurotransmitter breakdown (*MAOIs*), or (3) possibly by reducing the stimulation at the site of the receptor, specifically, of beta-adrenergic receptors, through norepinephrine pathways (both *TCAs* and *MAOIs*). Whether the amine-potentiating actions of antidepressants are either necessary or sufficient to account for the clinical actions of antidepressants remains uncertain. Thus considerable risk is taken in the process of simply developing new antidepressants by

Table 5-4 Receptor Blockade and Nontherapeutic Effects of Antidepressants

	Potential side effects caused by receptor blockage (scale of 0-4)				
	Cholinergic (muscarinic)	**Histaminergic**	**α_1-adrenergic**	**α_2-adrenergic**	**Dopaminergic**
	Blurred vision; dry mouth; sinus tachycardia; constipation; urinary retention; memory dysfunction	**Sedation drowsiness; weight gain; hypotension; potentiation of central nervous system depressants**	**Postural hypotension; dizziness; reflex tachycardia; additive with antihypertensive prazosin**	**Block antihypertensive effects of clonidine, quanabenz, and methyldopa; priapism**	**Extrapyramidal movement disorders; endocrine changes (prolactin elevation)**
Antidepressant					
Heterocyclics					
Amitriptyline (Elavil, Endep)	+3	+3	+4	+2	+1
Amoxapine (Asendin)	+/0	+2	+3	+1	+2
Clomipramine (Anafranil)	+2	+2	+3	+1	+1
Desipramine (Norpramin, Pertofrane)	+1	+1	+2	+/0	+1
Doxepin (Adapin, Sinequan)	+2	+4	+4	+2	+1

Imipramine (Tofranil)	+2	+2	+3	+1	+1
Maprotiline (Ludiomil)	+/0	+3	+3	+/0	+1
Nortriptyline (Aventyl, Pamelor)	+1	+1	+3	+1	+1
Nonheterocyclics					
Bupropion (Wellbutrin)	0	+/0	+/0	0	?
Fluoxetine (Prozac)	+/0	+/0	+/0	+/0	+1
Sertraline (Zoloft)	+/0	+/0	+/0	+/0	+1
Trazodone (Desyrel)	0	+1	+3	+2	+1
Reference agent	(Atropine [belladonna alkaloid]) +4	(Diphenhydramine [Benadryl]) +2	(Phentolamine [Regitine]) +4	(Phentolamine [Regitine]) +3	(Haloperidol [Haldol]) +4

Modified from Richelson E: *McClean Hosp J* 13:67, 1988.

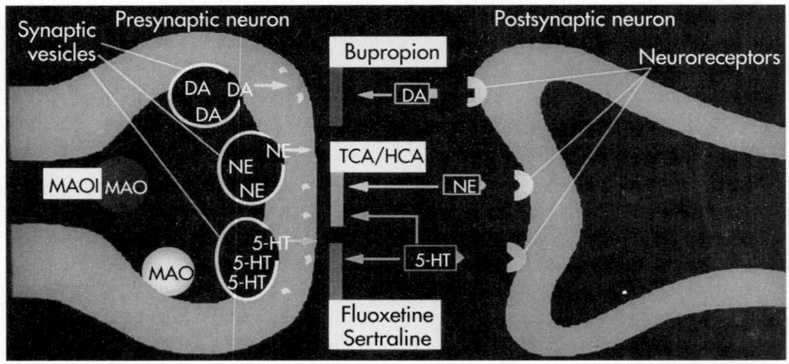

Figure 5-2 Mechanism of action of antidepressant agents. *DA,* Dopamine; *NE,* norepinephrine; *5-HT,* serotonin. (From Dista Products Co., Indianapolis, Ind.)

screening for a chemical compound's ability to inhibit the uptake of norepinephrine or serotonin or to otherwise alter neurochemical transmission. Nonetheless, this type of circular reasoning is tempting in view of the apparent association of these drugs' effects and the clinical response (Baldesserini, 1985).

Two new agents, fluoxetine (Prozac) and sertraline (Zoloft), are classified as selective serotonin reuptake inhibitors and seem to have great promise for patients with depression. Another new agent, clomipramine (Anafranil), possesses selective beneficial effects in the treatment of obsessive-compulsive disorder by blocking the reuptake of both norepinephrine and serotonin. Furthermore, some effective antidepressants neither block the uptake of monoamines nor inhibit monoamine oxidase but probably exert subtle influences on neuronal processes; trazodone and bupropion are good examples of these drugs. Thus it would seem that antidepressants with similar actions on neurotransmitters may be selectively beneficial for dissimilar disorders and that antidepressants with dissimilar actions on neurotransmitters may be selectively beneficial for similar disorders. These differences raise doubts about the biogenic amine theories of depression.

Although the influence of monoamines is the most studied neurochemical aspect of mood disorders, other important receptor interactions are also useful in predicting clinical side effects and potential toxic effects (Tables 5-3 and 5-4). These effects account for both therapeutic and nontherapeutic actions of antidepressants. Their variable effects in blocking the reuptake of norepinephrine and serotonin, and other effects, undoubtedly account for some of the variability in side-effect profiles.

TRICYCLIC, HETEROCYCLIC, AND NON-MAOI ANTIDEPRESSANTS

Pharmacokinetics

The tricyclic, heterocyclic, and non-MAOI antidepressant agents are well absorbed from the gastrointestinal tract and are usually given orally. Imipramine and amitriptyline are available in parenteral forms. Antidepressant compounds are metabolized in the liver, and some metabolites have active antidepressant effects and are marketed as such. For example, desipramine is a metabolite of imipramine; nortriptyline is a metabolite of amitriptyline.

Peak plasma concentrations of antidepressants are generally reached in 3 to 4 hours. Tricyclic, heterocyclic, and other antidepressant compounds are water soluble and are highly bound to plasma proteins. Their effects are due to a small fraction of free drug; thus even a small increase in free drug is potentially significant. Individuals with diminished liver function, with decreased plasma proteins, and with decreased total body water are at special risk for elevated serum levels. Antidepressant compounds are also relatively lipophilic but are avidly bound to tissue and plasma proteins, which makes it virtually impossible to remove the heterocyclic agents by hemodialysis, adding to the danger of acute overdoses.

The ratio of parent tricyclic compound to the active secondary amine products varies markedly among patients by as much as 50 fold (Baldesserini, 1985). After a fixed dose of antidepressant drug the plasma levels of active agents may vary by 10 to 20 fold among individuals. Assays of antidepressant compounds may not be reliable, but such measurements do help to confirm patient compliance with medication regimens and may be useful in the evaluation of unexpected or untoward clinical outcomes.

Tolerance to many of the side effects of heterocyclic and other antidepressant compounds, for example, sedation and the autonomic effects, is usual. Occasional symptoms suggestive of physical dependence have been reported, especially after a discontinuation, and a withdrawal syndrome consisting of malaise, chills, coryza, and muscle ache has been described. Therefore gradual withdrawal is considered a reasonable and standard practice. These compounds are eliminated similarly to the elimination of antipsychotic compounds.

The individual and structural characteristics and pharmacologic properties of the antidepressant medications are shown in Figures 5-1 and 5-2 and in Tables 5-3 and 5-4. A discussion of the side effects or undesirable effects may begin with the tricyclic antidepressants, comparing these agents with newer drugs and the MAOIs.

Side Effects

Patients for whom TCAs are prescribed have both peripheral and central nervous system side effects (see the box on p. 82).

Peripheral nervous system effects. Peripheral nervous system side effects include anticholinergic effects on the peripheral autonomic nervous system, which often affect patient tolerance and may also affect compliance; these side effects include dry mouth and visual disturbances, including blurred vision, tearing, and photosensitivity resulting from mydriasis. These symptoms are more annoying than dangerous; however, the narrow mydriatic action of the tricyclics can precipitate an acute attack of glaucoma. Moreover, TCAs should not be prescribed for individuals with narrow-angle glaucoma. Other anticholinergic side effects include slowing of the gastrointestinal tract that leads to constipation and slowing of bladder function, which can lead to hesitancy or urinary retention. Elderly individuals are most susceptible to these side effects (see Chapter 17).

Anticholinergic effects on the cardiovascular system are common enough to warrant some consideration. Tachycardia, reflex tachycardia, and arrhythmias can lead to myocardial infarction or heart block, or both. Essentially the potential reduction in cardiac conduction time is of greater concern than is the potential for inducing arrhythmias except in patients who have a preexisting arrhythmia or bundle branch block. The tricyclic antidepressants possess a quinidine-like effect and may actually prove to be beneficial for patients with arrhythmia. In any event, patients with a history of cardiac problems should be carefully evaluated and closely monitored when receiving treatment with a tricyclic antidepressant. More recently the secondary

Side Effects and Nursing Interventions for Tricyclic Antidepressants

Peripheral nervous system effects

Dry mouth

Advise frequent sips of water, hard candies, sugarless gum.

Mydriasis

Advise wearing of sunglasses outdoors.

Diminished lacrimation

Suggest artificial tears.

Blurred vision

Caution about driving and potential for falls. The patient should remove objects in the house that might be tripped over (e.g., throw rugs and small tables).

Eye pain

Advise patient to report eye pain immediately, since it may indicate an acute glaucoma attack. All elderly persons should be screened for glaucoma before treatment with TCAs is initiated.

Urinary hesitancy or retention

Monitor fluid intake. Patient should be told to avoid putting off urinating. Running water or pouring water over the perineum can stimulate urination. Catheterization may be needed.

Constipation

Monitor fluid and food intake. Urge patient to heed the urge to defecate. A high-fiber diet and large amounts of water (2500 to 3000 ml per day) are helpful.

Anhidrosis

Decreased sweating can lead to increased body temperature. Adequate fluid intake, appropriate clothing, and sensible exercise should be stressed.

Cardiovascular effects

Tricyclic antidepressants are contraindicated during the recovery phase of myocardial infarction.

Orthostatic hypotension

Advise patient to assume sitting position on side of bed, to wait and dangle feet for 1 full minute, then to rise slowly. Patients should not stand in one position too long and should avoid hot showers and tub baths. Elderly patients may require assistance at these times.

Central nervous system effects

Sedation

Caution patient about driving.

Delirium or mania

Discontinue the drug and call the physician.

Suicidal patients

Observe patients closely, since TCAs may increase energy for suicide.

amine TCA, nortriptyline, has gained some favor in the treatment of persons with cardiac conditions because of its ability to be monitored by means of serum level determinations and because of its relatively favorable profile with respect to the potential for causing orthostasis and other hemodynamic instabilities. Newer agents, including fluoxetine, sertraline, and buproprion, are much less likely to result in cardiovascular side effects. However, these agents have not been used or studied to the extent that the TCAs have been.

Central nervous system effects. A number of CNS effects have been reported with the TCAs. Sedation is common but sometimes represents a "fringe therapeutic benefit," since insomnia frequently accompanies depression. Less pleasant CNS effects include confusion, disorientation, delusions, agitation, hallucination, and lowering of the seizure threshold. These neuropsychiatric side effects are probably due to CNS anticholinergic effects and may be found in as many as 5% to 15% of patients (Meador-Woodruff, 1990). These CNS effects are more likely to occur when serum TCA levels are elevated. Other potential CNS effects include anxiety, insomnia, nightmare, ataxia, and tremors. Some patients report nightmares so terrifying that they avoid sleep even though they are sleep deprived.

Implications

Therapeutic versus toxic levels. Tricyclic antidepressants do not produce euphoria and are nonaddictive, so their potential for abuse is minimal. However, overdose of these agents is a real issue: TCA overdose accounts for 25% to 50% of all hospital admissions for overdose (Harsch and Holt, 1988). The difference is slight between a therapeutic dose and a health-impairing or lethal dose. As little as 10 to 30 times the daily dose can be fatal. TCA serum levels should be monitored, and since many clinicians do not attempt to memorize all acceptable therapeutic plasma values, the information in Table 5-5 should be kept available. Toxic blood levels may result in sedation, ataxia, agitation, stupor, coma, respiratory depression, and convulsions. Exaggeration of side effects previously mentioned can also occur. Cardiovascular reac-

Table 5-5 Tricyclic Antidepressant Blood Levels

Drug	Range (ng/ml)	Relationship
Imipramine and desipramine (combined levels)	150-250	Linear
Desipramine	150-250 100-155	Linear; plateau above 250 ng/ml; ?therapeutic window
Amitriptyline and nortriptyline (combined levels)	100-250 130-220	Linear; ?therapeutic window
Nortriptyline	50-140	Curvilinear; therapeutic window
Protriptyline	80-240	Linear; ?therapeutic window
Doxepin and desmethyldoxepin	120-250	Linear; ?therapeutic window
Maprotiline	150-250	Linear

Clinical application of TCA blood level monitoring (1) is not necessary in routine treatment with imipramine and amitriptyline, for which a linear relationship exists; (2) is useful in elderly patients who achieve higher levels with standard doses; (3) is useful in nonresponders who may not be taking medication properly; and (4) is necessary in titrating dosage of tricyclic drugs such as nortriptyline, for which a curvillinear therapeutic window exists. There are inadequate data to reliably correlate plasma drug concentration with therapeutic response for amoxapine, trimipramine, and trazodone.

tions can occur suddenly and cause acute heart failure. On the other hand, cardiovascular reactions can be delayed, that is, they can occur after recovery from depression. For these reasons all TCA overdoses should be considered serious, and the patient should be admitted to a hospital for monitoring. However, some studies suggest that imipramine also has antiarrhythmic properties. Imipramine's arrhythmic and antiarrhythmic properties underscore the need for more knowledge about TCAs.

TCAs have a paradoxic effect. Although they are effective antidepressants, they also have the ability to energize suicidal patients. Apparently, as TCAs begin to exert their antidepressant effect, patients who otherwise might be "too depressed" to act on suicidal thoughts slowly begin to accrue the energy to act in self-destructive ways. Because of the potential lethality of TCAs it is not uncommon for outpatients to be restricted to a 7-day supply when suicide is a risk. Inpatients should be watched for hoarding. Interventions for TCA overdose are given in the box below.

Use in pregnancy. Depressive symptoms such as loss of appetite can interfere with fetal development by preventing adequate fetal weight gain. During pregnancy, TCAs with low anticholinergic effects (such as nortriptyline and desipramine) are preferred to those with high anticholinergic effects. The TCAs must be tapered off before delivery to avoid transient perinatal toxicity (Cohen, 1989).

Side effects. TCAs, as noted previously, cause many CNS and peripheral nervous system side effects. Although some are simply annoying, others are significant, even dangerous, and warrant clinical attention. A common CNS effect is sedation. Sedation can be beneficial for depressed patients who have insomnia, and a drug such as amitriptyline (Elavil) can be ordered, to take advantage of its sedating properties. In other situations, such as when a patient must continue to work, sedation can present an array of problems from dozing off at work to impairment of driving. Protriptyline (Vivactil) can be ordered for patients who experience unacceptable sedation. This one side effect underscores the need for individual consideration when prescribing TCAs. The box on page 82 reviews interventions.

Interactions. Several serious drug interactions occur with TCAs. These interactions can be categorized as CNS depression, cardiovascular and hypertensive interactions, and additive anticholinergic effects.

Interventions for TCA Overdose

Monitor blood pressure, heart rate and rhythm, and respirations.
Maintain patent airway.
Monitor cardiovascular system with electrocardiogram.
Induce vomiting or gastric lavage with activated charcoal to prevent further drug absorption (for up to 24 hours).
Sodium bicarbonate (hypertonic, 1 *M*) IV has been used effectively to treat cardiac arrythmias and hypotension. If cardiac arrythmias do not respond, lidocaine or phenytoin may be used. If hypotension does not respond, fluid expansion and vasopressors (e.g., dopamine) may be required.

Modified from Keltner NL. In Shlafer M, Marieb E, editors: *The nurse, pharmacology, and drug therapy*, Redwood City, Calif, 1989, Addison-Wesley.

Central nervous system depression. When taken with drugs such as the antipsychotics, benzodiazepines, sedatives, antiepileptics, alcohol, and some antihypertensives (e.g., beta-blockers, clonidine, and reserpine), TCAs can increase CNS depression.

Cardiovascular and hypertensive effects. Cardiovascular arrhythmias or hypertension can occur when sympathomimetic drugs that increase norepinephrine levels in the synaptic cleft are given with TCAs. Interactants to avoid include norepinephrine, dopamine, ephedrine, and phenylpropanolamine. The latter drug is a major component of over-the-counter weight-loss stimulants. Monoamine oxidase inhibitors, another class of antidepressants, must also be avoided for similar reasons. The MAOI-TCA combination, although perhaps not as lethal as once thought, can cause a severe reaction, including high fever, seizures, and a fatal hypertensive crisis. Since MAOIs are not typically prescribed unless TCAs fail, care should be taken when switching the TCA-resistant patient to MAOIs. The *Physicians Desk Reference* (1992) recommends a minimum of 14 days between the time TCAs are discontinued and MAOIs are given. TCAs block the release of several antihypertensives from presynaptic cells, thus contributing to the failure of antihypertensives to control hypertension.

Additive anticholinergic effects. An "atropine-poisoning" effect can occur when TCAs are mixed with other anticholinergic drugs. Especially troublesome drugs include antipsychotic drugs, atropine, scopolamine, anticholinergic-antiparkinsonism drugs, and antihistamines. Elderly persons are at special risk for this interaction, and all the central and peripheral anticholinergic effects mentioned in the side effects section can be intensified.

Patient education. Besides the teaching related to side effects, the following areas of education are worth discussing with the patient and his or her family:

A "lag period" of 2 to 4 weeks occurs before full therapeutic effects are experienced.

Certain interactants must be avoided, including over-the-counter products (see the section on interactions).

Abrupt discontinuation of TCAs can cause nausea, headache, and malaise.

Eye pain must be reported immediately.

SPECIFIC TRICYCLIC ANTIDEPRESSANTS

Tricyclic antidepressants are usually divided into tertiary and secondary amine TCAs (based on their structure). *Imipramine* (Tofranil) is the oldest of the TCAs. Imipramine has relatively high anticholinergic and sedative effects. However, none of the newer antidepressant agents has proven to be more effective. Imipramine pamolate (Tofranil PM) is available in a single bedtime dose for adults. *Amitriptyline* (Elavil and Endep) preferentially potentiates serotonin and exerts the greatest anticholinergic and antianxiety effects among the tertiary amine TCAs. Amitriptyline is sedating and is often prescribed to be taken at bedtime to enhance sleep. Amitriptyline is also available in a parenteral form and in a fixed-dose combination with the antipsychotic drug perphenazine (Triavil). *Amoxapine* (Asendin) is a relatively recent drug but not specifically a tricyclic antidepressant. It is a metabolite of the antipsychotic drug loxapine and also blocks dopamine receptors. Amoxapine potentiates norepinephrine preferentially and, perhaps because of its neuroleptic effects, has a faster rate of onset of action than other antidepressants. However, extrapyramidal and other side effects often noted with the antipsychotic agents have been reported with amoxapine and are no doubt related to the dopamine blocking properties.

Doxepin (Sinequan) is a widely used TCA that potentiates serotonin preferentially.

Doxepin is sedating, has significant anticholinergic activity, and is often touted as a drug that effectively enhances sleep and reduces anxiety. Doxepin has often been recognized as a compound well tolerated among cardiac patients; however, there is no substantial evidence to show that doxepin is superior to other tertiary (or secondary amine) TCAs.

Trimipramine (Surmontil) is a TCA that theoretically potentiates serotonin; however, this effect has not been clearly established. Trimipramine, like the other tertiary amine TCAs, is quite sedating and has moderate anticholinergic effects.

Secondary amine TCAs are represented by *desipramine* (Norpramin and Pertofrane), a widely used TCA that potentiates norepinephrine preferentially. Desipramine is a naturally occurring metabolite of imipramine, and many clinicians have noted its utility in depressed elderly patients sensitive to anticholinergic effects and in elderly individuals with open angle glaucoma or prostatic hypertrophy, because of its low incidence of anticholinergic effects. This drug is also considered less sedating than other tricyclics and therefore is sometimes referred to as an "activating" antidepressant agent.

Nortriptyline (Aventyl and Pamelor) is a TCA often preferred because it has a lower potential for sedating and anticholinergic effects than other TCAs. It is a natural metabolite of amimitriptyline, and because of the reliability of its measured serum levels, it is often used in patients for whom toxicity or compliance is an issue.

Protriptyline (Vivactil) is different from other TCAs in that it is quite stimulating. Protriptyline may produce a greater incidence of tachycardia and cardiovascular problems than other tricyclics and certainly has a high potential for anticholinergic side effects. Because some depressed patients have hypersomnia rather than insomnia, protriptyline may enable these individuals to reduce their amount of sleep.

Maprotiline (Ludiomil) is a new antidepressant that is not a tricyclic but a tetracyclic. It potentiates norepinephrine, has a relatively mild potential for anticholinergic effects, and is sedating. Its *neurochemical effects* are similar to those of desipramine. Dosage increases are generally made more slowly than with the tertiary amine TCAs because this drug is almost twice as potent.

In addition to amoxapine and maprotiline, *trazodone* (Desyrel) is the other heterocyclic that was introduced after the TCAs were. Trazodone potentiates serotonin and is prescribed often because of its virtual lack of anticholinergic effects and low potential for cardiac effects. An exception is the report of ventricular arrhythmia occurring in patients with preexisting cardiac conditions. Trazodone's absorption is increased by 20% when it is taken with a meal, an unusual reaction. Another unusual adverse reaction to this drug is priapism, that is, prolonged penile erection. Emergency or surgical intervention has been required in a small percentage of affected men. If priapism occurs, the patient should stop the medication and seek medical advice.

RECENTLY DEVELOPED AGENTS

Among the newer agents *bupropion* (Wellbutrin), *fluoxetine* (Prozac), and *sertraline* (Zoloft) have been introduced. Fluoxetine and, more recently, sertraline represent the subgroup of antidepressant agents now referred to as selective serotonin reuptake inhibitors (SSRIs) (Figure 5-3). Fluoxetine, which preferentially and selectively potentiates serotonin, has a half-life of 7 to 9 days and may be given once per day or less often to a schedule of 3 times per week. This drug should generally be taken before noon because of its ability to result in insomnia or contribute to sleep disturbance. However, in selected individuals the drug may have no potential for causing activation and, in fact, may paradoxically result in sedation. Fluoxetine may cause a rash or

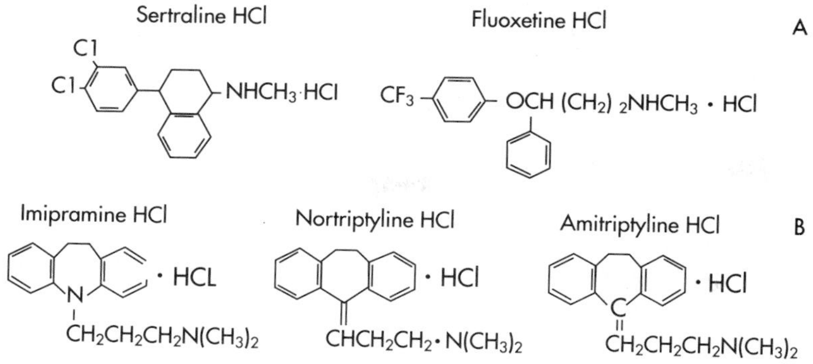

A

Sertraline HCl

Cl, Cl, $NHCH_3 \cdot HCl$

Fluoxetine HCl

CF_3, $OCH\ (CH_2)_2NHCH_3 \cdot HCl$

B

Imipramine HCl

N, $\cdot$ HCL, $CH_2CH_2CH_2N(CH_3)_2$

Nortriptyline HCl

$\cdot$ HCl, $CHCH_2CH_2 \cdot N(CH_3)_2$

Amitriptyline HCl

C, $\cdot$ HCl, $CH_2CH_2CH_2N(CH_3)_2$

Figure 5-3 The chemical structures of the SSRIs, **A,** sertraline and fluoxetine, differ from each other. In contrast, TCAs, **B,** have chemical structures that are similar to one another.

cause weight loss in anorectic patients. However, the risk is minimal. Because of its long half-life, this drug not only has the potential to interact with MAOIs but also may do so for as long as 4 to 6 weeks after its discontinuation. Therefore, the use of MAOIs for that interval of time after discontinuation or concomitantly is strictly forbidden.

Fluoxetine is widely used and prescribed, possibly because of its utility and favorable side effect profile; however, the drug's cost, about $1.50 per tablet (Monroe, 1990), may limit its use. Despite much controversy about fluoxetine's ability to disrupt sleep and contribute to the risk of suicide, there are few substantial data to warrant any actions beyond monitoring for these potential adverse events.

Sertraline, another SSRI, has similar effects and a similar side effect profile to those of fluoxetine; however, it may have the advantages of reduced half-life and reduced cost (Table 5-3).

Bupropion is a recently introduced agent that is neither a TCA nor an MAOI. Clinical tests indicate that orthostatic hypotension, cardiovascular conduction problems, anticholinergic effects, daytime sedation, and other typical effects of tricyclics are not seen with this compound. However, this drug is also "activating," and agitation is sometimes produced. Buproprion is contraindicated in patients with seizure disorders or in patients for whom prior diagnosis of bulimia or anorexia may exist. Bupropion, as with the other antidepressants, should not be given in combination with the MAOIs because of the potential for drug interaction and hypertensive crisis.

Other antidepressants currently under investigation include fluvoximine, paroxetine, geprirone, and nefazadone. The discussion of these agents is beyond the scope of this text. However, their mechanisms of action and chemical classes vary and are somewhat unique, suggesting the possibility for future continued progress in the development of antidepressant agents.

Implications

Therapeutic versus toxic levels. The SSRIs are new agents, and their toxicity levels are still being determined. Only three deaths resulting from fluoxetine overdose have been reported (Dista Products Co., Indianapolis, Indiana, 1992), and none has been reported for sertraline overdose, which occurs at a dose of approximately

750 to 2100 mg (Roerig, New York, New York, 1992). Two of the deaths attributed to fluoxetine overdose involved other drugs. A 3000-mg dose of fluoxetine alone has been survived.

Nausea and vomiting are the primary symptoms of fluoxetine overdose. Other symptoms include agitation, restlessness, hypomania, and CNS hyperstimulation. Sertraline overdose manifests as intensification of adverse responses previously noted.

Treatment for overdose includes supportive care such as airway maintenance and adequate oxygenation and ventilation. Activated charcoal with sorbitol is thought to be more effective than lavage or emetic for the treatment of sertraline overdose. Monitoring of vital signs and supportive nursing care as indicated are consistent with conservative management practices.

Use in pregnancy. Both fluoxetine and sertraline are classified as Food and Drug Administration (FDA) pregnancy category B (see Appendix). Their teratogenic effects are unknown; caution is advised. Fluoxetine is known to be excreted in breast milk of nursing mothers; it is unclear whether sertraline is excreted. Again, given the concerns surrounding pregnancy and nursing mothers, these drugs should be given only when benefits to the mother outweigh potential harm to the baby.

Side effects. During clinical trials of both fluoxetine and sertraline, 15% of patients discontinued treatment because of adverse responses to these drugs. Prominent effects were nervousness, anxiety, and insomnia. When tolerance to these effects does not develop, discontinuance remains an option.

Other common effects include dry mouth, general gastrointestinal tract complaints, headaches, and dizziness. Interventions noted previously for dry mouth, nausea, diarrhea, constipation, headaches, and dizziness are also appropriate for SSRIs. Male sexual dysfunction, primarily, ejaculatory delay, seems to be prominent in patients receiving sertraline (15.5%) and less prominent in patients taking fluoxetine (1.9%); a number of men stopped taking sertraline because of this side effect.

Interactions. Fluoxetine should not be combined with MAOIs, tryptophan, or other antidepressants. Fluoxetine can interact with MAOIs for as long as 4 to 6 weeks after discontinuation. Combining fluoxetine with lithium leads to both increased and decreased lithium serum levels. Fluoxetine also prolongs the half-life of diazepam, and presumably this combination could cause CNS depression. Sertraline also prolongs the half-life of diazepam but has unclear effects on lithium. When combining lithium with either, drug lithium serum levels should be monitored. Selective serotonin reuptake inhibitors should be used cautiously with other CNS-active drugs. Selective serotonin reuptake inhibitors are highly bound to plasma proteins, and combining these drugs with another tightly bound drug could cause a displacement in one or the other and the occurrence of potential adverse effects.

Patient education. Patients and their families should be instructed as follows concerning SSRIs:

Although it is not clear that combining alcohol or over-the-counter medications with SSRIs is harmful, the patient should be cautioned against doing so and encouraged to discuss such decisions with the physician or nurse.

When sedation results from taking these drugs, driving or operating hazardous machinery should be avoided.

Pregnancy or breast-feeding should be discussed with the primary health care provider, since the harmful effects of SSRIs during these developmental stages are not clear.

MONOAMINE OXIDASE INHIBITORS

Monoamine oxidase inhibitors, another class of antidepressants, are usually administered to hospitalized patients or to outpatients who may be closely monitored and are compliant. These drugs are almost always prescribed after TCAs or other agents have been tried and have failed. An argument can be made that MAOIs are particularly effective in treating atypical depression, for example, depression characterized by hypersomnia and neurotic compulsions such as excessive eating, or in treating certain types of anxiety syndromes, for example, panic associated with depression. The second-class status afforded the MAOIs is generally related to their potential for serious adverse reactions. Although many expert clinicians think the fear of MAOIs is unwarranted, the reluctance to use them seems to be the norm (Folks, 1982).

As a general rule the MAOIs can be divided into hydrazines and nonhydrazines (see Table 5-6). These drugs block monoamine oxidase, the major enzyme involved in the metabolic decomposition and thus the inactivation of norepinephrine, serotonin, and dopamine. The increased level of these neurotransmitters in the peripheral and the central nervous systems can be dramatic. According to the biogenic amine theory of depression, depressed individuals have a deficiency of these neurotransmitters. MAOIs help achieve the "normal" amount of neurotransmitters by slowing the deactivation of these enzymes. This mechanism is in contrast to mechanisms of TCAs and other agents, which achieve the "normal" level or restore the relative deficiency by preventing the reuptake of amines or by directly affecting the postsynaptic receptor (Figure 5-2). Generally a period of 10 days to 4 weeks is required for the antidepressant effects of the MAOIs to occur but, as with the tricyclic antidepressants, the physiologic action, that is, the inhibition of monoamine oxidase, occurs immediately. This phenomenon suggests that factors other than low level of specific neurotransmitters are involved in the pathogenesis of depression.

Pharmacokinetics

Monoamine oxidase inhibitors are well absorbed from the gastrointestinal tract and are given orally. They are metabolized in the liver, and metabolites are excreted in the urine. They have long half-lives. Table 5-6 gives usual doses for these drugs.

Side Effects

Monoamine oxidase inhibitors induce central nervous system, cardiovascular, and anticholinergic side effects.

Table 5-6 Monoamine Oxidase Inhibitors

Drug	Usual daily dose (mg)
Isocarboxazid (Marplan)	S = 30/d M = 10-20/d
Phenelzine (Nardil) Most sedating; preferred MAOI	S = 15 tid, then increase to 60-90/d M = 15/d
Tranylcypromine (Parnate)	S = 30 mg/d, may increase to 60 mg/d M = 10, 1-2 times per day

S, Start; *M*, maintenance; *MAOI*, monoamine oxidase inhibitor.

Peripheral nervous system effects. In the peripheral nervous system the slow release of norepinephrine causes decreased heart rate, decreased vasoconstriction, and hypotension. Monoamine oxidase inhibitors also inhibit monoamine oxidase in the liver, which may lead to elevated levels of other drugs that are normally metabolized in the liver by a monoamine oxidase.

Hypotension is the most common nontherapeutic effect. Interestingly, pargyline (Eutonyl) is an MAOI that is not used as an antidepressant but rather is indicated for use as an antihypertensive agent. The slowdown in the release of norepinephrine is the presumed mechanism of action. Unlike the effect of tricyclic antidepressants, a reflex tachycardia does not occur, because of the slowed release of norepinephrine experienced by the adrenergic system, and the heart rate does not reflexively speed up. Thus hypotension combined with the failure of compensatory increased heart rate may lead to heart failure in predisposed individuals. Monoamine oxidase inhibitors may also cause anticholinergic effects such as dry mouth, blurred vision, urinary hesitancy, and constipation, although constipation occurs to a lesser extent than observed with the tertiary amine TCAs. Hepatic and hematologic dysfunctions may rarely occur and are potentially serious. Blood cell counts and liver function tests should be obtained before therapy begins; symptoms indicating bone marrow suppression or liver dysfunction should be investigated.

Central nervous system effects. Because MAOIs increase the availability of biogenic amines in the brain, CNS hyperstimulation may also occur, causing agitation, acute anxiety, restlessness, insomnia, and euphoria. Full schizophrenic episodes may

Food-Drug Interactions with MAOIs

Sympathomimetic drugs should not be combined with MAOIs.

Thramine-containing foods must not be ingested by the patient who is taking MAOIs.

MAOIs are contraindicated as follows:

- In the patient with a history of stroke or cardiovascular disease
- In the patient with a pheochromocytoma, a tumor that secretes pressor substance
- In the patient undergoing elective surgery (because of the hypotensive potential of combined MAOIs and anesthesia)

MAOIs should not be given in combination with the following:

- Other MAOIs
- TCAs
- Meperidine (Demerol)

Hypertensive crisis is a major concern. If it occurs, the nurse should respond as follows:

- Discontinue MAOIs and contact the physician
- Know that therapy to reduce the blood pressure is warranted, and know that phentolamine (Regitine) 5 mg intravenously is the appropriate drug
- Manage fever by external cooling
- Institute supportive nursing care as indicated

Adapted from Keltner NL. In M Shlafer M, Marieb E, editors: *The nurse, pharmacology, and drug therapy*, Redwood City, Calif, 1989, Addison-Wesley.

also develop in individuals with quiescent schizophrenia as a response to MAOIs. Hypomania (less than full mania) is also a common effect.

Specific Interactions

Monoamine oxidase inhibitors have a number of serious interactions. Potentially lethal interactions may occur with both drugs and foods (see the boxes on pp. 90 and 91 and Table 5-7). Drug and food interactions should be considered, particularly with compounds potentially causing hypertension, anticholinergic effects, or sympathomimetic effects. Sympathomimetic drugs are classified as direct acting, indirect acting, and mixed acting, that is, having both direct and indirect properties. Indirect-acting and mixed-acting sympathomimetics may cause serious and sometimes fatal hypertension. Direct-acting sympathomimetics act by adding new norepinephrine to the body, whereas indirect agents release existing epinephrine or norepinephrine from the neuron. Since MAOIs increase the amount of stored norepinephrine in the peripheral nervous system, the potential for these indirect or mixed-acting sympathomimetics to release relatively large amounts of norepinephrine makes the avoidance of these interacting drugs crucial. Even small amounts may trigger a hypertensive crisis. Typical indirect-acting and mixed-acting sympathomimetics include amphetamines cocaine, methylphenidate, dopamine, metfenturomine, and ephedrine. Over-the-counter weight-loss and stimulant products such as phenylephrine, phenylpropanolamine, and pseudoephedrine, which are mixed or indirect-acting sympathomimetics, should be avoided altogether. Direct-acting sympathomimetics, that is, norepinephrine, epinephrine, and isopropeterenol, theoretically should not trigger the release of

Tyramine-rich Foods to Avoid While Taking MAOIs

Alcoholic beverages
Beer and ale
Chianti and sherry wine

Dairy products
Cheese: cheddar, blue, brie, and mozzarella
Sour cream
Yogurt

Fruits and vegetables
Avocados
Bananas
Fava beans
Canned figs

Meats
Bologna
Chicken liver

Fish, dried
Liver
Meat tenderizer
Pickled herring

Salami
Sausage

Other foods
Caffeinated coffee, colas, and tea (large amounts)
Chocolate
Licorice
Soy sauce
Yeast

Adapted from Keltner NL. In Shlafer M, Marieb E, editors: *The nurse, pharmacology, and drug therapy*, Redwood City, Calif, 1989, Addison-Wesley.

Table 5-7 Drugs to Avoid While Taking MAOIs

Drugs	Interaction
Anticholinergic drugs	Compound anticholinergic response
Anesthetics (general)	Deepen CNS depression
Antihypertensives (diuretics, β-blockers, hydralazine)	
CNS depressants	Intensify CNS depression
Guanethidine, methyldopa, reserpine	Produce severe hypertension
Sympathomimetics (mixed and indirect-acting)	Precipitate hypertensive crisis, cardiac stimulation, arrhythmias, cerebrovascular hemorrhage
Amphetamines, methylphenidate, dopamine, phenylpropanolamine (in many over-the-counter hayfever, cold diet medications)	
Sympathomimetics (direct-acting)	Same as for mixed and indirect-acting sympathomimetics but theoretically should not produce as severe a reaction
Epinephrine, norepinephrine, isoproterenol	
	Less likely to cause problems
Tricyclic antidepressants	Same as for epinephrine, norepinephrine, isoproterenol

Adapted from Keltner NL. In Shlafer M, Marieb E, editors: *The nurse, pharmacology, and drug therapy*, Redwood City, Calif, 1989, Addison-Wesley.

existing norepinephrine. As previously noted, MAOIs should not be given in combination with TCAs except in unusually refractory cases of depression, in hospitalized patients, or in patients who are closely monitored.

The initial symptoms of hypertensive crisis are palpitation, tightness in the chest, stiff neck, and a throbbing, radiating headache. Extremely high blood pressure with elevation of heart rate is common. Cardiovascular consequences have included myocardia infarctions, cerebral hemorrhage, myocardial ischemias, and arrhythmias; diaphoresis and pupillary dilation are also prominent signs.

Anticholinergic effects may be present to a greater extent when other anticholinergic drugs are given in concert with the MAOIs. Typical anticholinergic side effects are similar to those for the TCAs.

Since MAOIs inhibit monoamine oxidase in the liver, some drugs, particularly central nervous system depressants, are not metabolized there; with these drugs, serum levels may be achieved more rapidly and may be high enough to seriously depress the central nervous system. Meperidine (Demerol) is specifically contraindicated; a marked potentiation of this drug can occur.

Hypotensive drugs are also potentiated by the MAOIs; hence these are relatively contraindicated. Food-drug interactions center around the amino acid tyramine, a precursor to dopamine, norepinephrine, and epinephrine. Tyramine is found in many foods commonly consumed in a North American diet; in fact, all high-protein foods that have undergone protein breakdowns by means of aging, fermentation, pickling, or smoking should be avoided. Hypotension and hypertensive crisis can develop from these food-drug combinations by the mechanism previously discussed.

Implications

Therapeutic versus toxic levels. As with the TCAs, with the MAOIs an intensification of the effects already discussed may occur with overdosage. A lethal dose of MAOIs may be achieved at only 6 to 10 times the usual daily dose (Table 5-6). Careful monitoring when medications are being ingested should occur. As noted with the antipsychotic agents, cheeking and hoarding of these drugs could be disastrous and these possibilities should be considered in individuals at risk. When an MAOI overdose is suspected, the following should be performed:

1. Emesis and gastric lavage, which are particularly helpful if performed early
2. Monitoring of vital signs
3. External cooling, which is particularly warranted when high fever occurs
4. Standard treatment of hypotension

Use in pregnancy. Monoamine oxidase inhibitors should be given during pregnancy only when anticipated benefit justifies the potential risk to the fetus and should be avoided altogether in the first trimester.

Side effects. Several important side effects associated with MAOIs and appropriate interventions are listed in the box below.

Interactions. As previously discussed, drug-MAOI and food-MAOI interactions are significant. General guidelines for these interactions include the following. (1) *Sympathomimetic* drugs should not be combined with MAOIs. (2) *Tyramine-containing* foods should not be ingested by the patient taking MAOIs. (3) Do not give MAOIs in combination with another MAOI or with a TCA except in unusually refractory patients and then under close supervision. (4) Avoid MAOIs in combination with

Side Effects and Nursing Interventions for MAOIs

Central nervous system hyperstimulation
Reassure the patient. Assess for developing psychosis, hypomania, or seizures. When symptoms warrant, withhold the drug and notify the physician.

Hypotension
Monitor blood pressure frequently, and intervene to prevent falls and injuries; having patient lie down may help return blood pressure to normal.

Anticholinergic effects
See the section on TCA side effects for appropriate nursing interventions.

Hepatic and hematologic dysfunction
Blood cell counts and liver function tests should be performed. When dysfunction is apparent, MAOI should be discontinued.

Adapted from Keltner NL. In Shlafer M, Marieb E, editors: *The nurse, pharmacology, and drug therapy*, Redwood City, Calif, 1989, Addison-Wesley.

meperidine (Demerol). (5) If a hypertensive crisis is suspected, the following measures should be instituted:

Discontinue the MAOI.

Have phentolamine (Regitine) available. Phentolamine 5 mg intravenously reduces blood pressure.

Manage fever by external cooling.

Provide supportive care as indicated.

Patient education. Because combining MAOIs with a variety of interactants is a serious matter, it is important to be consistent in teaching both the patient and his or her family about these drugs (see Table 5-7). Although in current thinking these interactions are not regarded quite as pessimistically as they were by the clinicians of a few years ago, appropriate education remains appropriate. Teaching includes the following general points:

A "lag time" of 10 days to 4 weeks occurs before a full therapeutic effect is experienced.

Driving should be avoided if sedation is pronounced.

The patient should inform all medication prescribers when he or she is taking MAOIs.

High tyramine-containing foods should be avoided.

Headaches, palpitations, and stiff neck should be reported immediately.

SPECIFIC MONOAMINE OXIDASE INHIBITORS

Three MAOIs are used in the treatment of depression. *Isocarboxazid* (Marplan) is considered the mildest MAOI; a clinical response may not be noticed for 4 weeks or longer after therapy is initiated. *Phenelzine* (Nardil) has been found to be the most effective in depressed individuals who are characterized as atypical on clinical examination. Phenelzine is considered the most effective MAOI and is the most sedative. A clinical response is generally experienced or begins to be experienced in about 4 weeks. *Tranylcypromine* (Parnate) seems to be the most effective MAOI for treatment of severe or endogenous depression. A clinical effect may be experienced rapidly, in about 10 days, more quickly than with the other MAOIs. Tranylcypromine is the most stimulating MAOI. As mentioned previously, pargyline is not used as an antidepressant.

TREATMENT ISSUES AND CAVEATS

Initial treatment with an antidepressant medication is often administered in doses divided throughout the day. The patient can gradually accommodate unwanted side effects, and there is opportunity to titrate the dosage upward until the desired clinical effect is achieved. Once an optimal dose is achieved or a therapeutic response experienced, the patient who is tolerating the medication satisfactorily may be given a single dose of tricyclic or heterocyclic agents with equal therapeutic efficacy. The only exception may be trazodone, with its short half-life. A single bedtime dose may not be desirable in elderly patients or in patients sensitive to the anticholinergic effects of the antidepressant, who may tolerate the drug better when the dose is divided throughout the day (Bernstein, 1988). Patients may benefit from a similarly divided dosage scheduled to alleviate anxiety without the need to add an anxiolytic medication to the regimen. Coadministration of antianxiety or antipsychotic agents may sometimes be necessary while awaiting the therapeutic response of an antidepressant (Robertson and Trimble, 1982; Folks, 1990). In the event that a benzodiazepine is used concurrently, short-to-intermediate half-life agents are the best choice, for example, oxazepam (see Chapter 6).

For patients with paranoid ideation and delusional thinking, concomitant treatment with the institution of a potent antipsychotic agent, for example, haloperidol, is preferable (see Chapter 4). Low-potency agents are unlikely to be useful and particularly should be avoided, since they can induce postural hypertension and undoubtedly add to the anticholinergic effects in those patients who are receiving TCAs. Amoxapine has been found to be effective in treating psychotic depression without the need for simultaneous administration of a neuroleptic drug (Anton, Hitri, and Diamond, 1986).

Two common problems with antidepressant medications are the prescription of inadequate doses and the discontinuation of drug treatment before the patient has recovered from the immediate depressive symptoms. Prophylaxis, and therefore guarding against recurrence of the depression, can more likely be achieved if these two problems are avoided (Prien and Kupfer, 1986).

Another continuing problem in achieving a prompt, satisfactory response to antidepressant drugs is the inability to predict which patient will respond optimally to which type or class of antidepressant agent. Several reports have employed the use of stimulant drugs, that is, dextroamphetamine or methylphenidate, as predictors of antidepressant responsiveness (Goff and Jenike, 1986). Most commonly methylphenidate 5 to 20 mg, as a single or divided dose, is prescribed. Patients who experience a prompt mood improvement after stimulant drug administration are often responsive to a noradrenergic antidepressant such as desipramine (Sabelli, Fawcett, and Javaid, 1983). Patients who experience a dysphoric response to the stimulant test may, generally speaking, not respond well to noradrenergic antidepressants but more often are observed to achieve a favorable therapeutic response to "serotonergic" drugs, for example, amitriptyline (Van Kammen and Murphy, 1978).

Tricyclics had been widely used as antidepressant agents for many years before plasma level monitoring became available. Thus the routine measurement of plasma concentration is generally not necessary for effective therapy. However, if the patient fails to respond and is, indeed, taking the medication, it is generally appropriate to increase the dose and evaluate the response. Most evidence supports a linear relationship between plasma concentration and therapeutic response, although a therapeutic window for nortriptyline and, possibly, desipramine has been suggested in the literature (Bernstein, 1988). Table 5-5 suggests some generally accepted ranges of plasma levels (Risch, Janowsky, Hyey, 1981). Patients of any age who fail to respond to standard tricyclics may benefit from the measurement of plasma tricyclic concentrations, since many patients fail to take their medication or are noncompliant. Monitoring the plasma TCA level may help to point out to the noncompliant patient the reason for nonresponse and give added emphasis to restructuring of a therapeutic relationship. Inadequate data exist to support reliable statements regarding the correlation of therapeutic response and plasma levels for recently developed agents such as amoxapine, trimipramine, trazodone, fluoxetine, sertraline, and bupropion.

Patients who do not respond easily or quickly to antidepressant medication may not do so because of inadequate dosage or duration of treatment. However, treatment-resistant depression does exist. Once measurements of plasma concentrations and assessment of patient compliance is complete, consideration of an alternate agent or adjuncts should be considered. Some nonpsychotic depressed patients have a more favorable response when a low-dose neuroleptic is added to the antidepressant regimen (Stern and Mendels, 1981).

Premature discontinuation of antidepressant medication is a common cause for relapse in depressed patients (Prien and Kupfer, 1986). Although a 4-month course of medication may be appropriate with the first episode of depression, it is more reasonable to plan for a 6- to 12-month course followed by cautious tapering, particularly in an individual with a previous episode or a positive family history. As previously discussed, antidepressant medication should not be withdrawn abruptly and the dosage should be tapered, preferably over several weeks. Depressed individuals with recurrent episodes of depression, even in the absence of mania, may also benefit from maintenance doses of lithium alone or lithium in conjunction with an appropriately chosen medication, in addition to the use of antidepressant drugs.

ANTIMANIC AND MOOD-STABILIZING DRUGS

LITHIUM

Lithium, a naturally occurring element, is not much different from sodium. The differences, however, are significant enough to make lithium useful in the treatment of bipolar mood disorder. Lithium was discovered in 1817 by Arfwedson, who named it after the Greek word for stone. Lithium was touted as a cure for epilepsy, gout, and other problems. In the 1940s lithium was used as a salt substitute for cardiac patients in the United States. However, it was removed from the market after some of these individuals died of toxic effects of lithium.

John Cade, an Australian physician, employed lithium urate in his investigation of toxicity of urea in guinea pigs and found that the animals developed extreme lethargy while remaining fully conscious. Cade had been involved in this work in relationship to his search for a toxin in the urine of manic patients. He then employed lithium salts experimentally in an attempt to produce sedation in manic patients; he also used lithium preparations in persons with epilepsy because of the apparent anticonvulsant action of the preparations (Cade, 1949).

Before Cade's application of lithium in psychiatric patients, Henderson and Gillespie (1944) noted that the waters from certain wells appeared to have special efficacy in the treatment of mental illness. The use of lithium in the treatment of mental illness in psychiatric patients, beginning with this remarkable early work of Cade, spread to England and Denmark, throughout Europe, and eventually to the United States, which became the last country to authorize the therapeutic use of lithium.

Although precisely how lithium achieves its normalizing effects in mania is not known, the lithium ion substitutes for the sodium ion, thereby compromising the ability of neurons to release, activate, or respond to neurotransmitters. Although indicated only for the treatment of mania and for maintenance in patients with a history of mania, lithium treatment of a variety of other psychiatric illnesses has been noted throughout the world. These other uses of lithium remain controversial, despite an expanding literature supporting a therapeutic efficacy broader than simply the treatment and prophylaxis of mania (Jefferson et al., 1987).

Pharmacokinetics

Lithium is well absorbed from the gastrointestinal tract and is normally given in oral tablets, capsules, or concentrates. Peak blood serum levels are reached in 1 to 4 hours. More than 95% of the amount ingested is excreted by the kidneys; that is, it is not metabolized. The plasma half-life is approximately 24 hours. Renal insufficiency or disease lengthens the half-life, necessitating reduction in dosage. Absorption and excretion of lithium are closely linked to those of sodium. When dietary sodium intake increases, serum levels of lithium are likely to drop, since lithium is excreted more rapidly. Conversely, when sodium in the diet decreases or when sodium is lost in ways other than through the kidney, that is, sweating or diarrhea, lithium serum levels increase. Since a therapeutic serum level of lithium is not much lower than a toxic serum level, such considerations are significant. Diet and activity levels should not change abruptly.

Lithium is manufactured primarily in 300-mg capsules or tablets (lithium carbonate). A 450-mg sustained-release capsule is available. Lithium is effective in as many as 80% of cases; however, it takes 1 to 2 weeks to achieve a clinical response. Lithium dosage is based on both the clinical response and lithium serum levels. The typical dosage for acute mania is 600 mg 3 times per day, usually producing a serum level of 1.0 to 1.5 mEq/L. Desirable serum levels for maintenance are 0.6 to 1.2 mEq/L, which can be maintained on an average dose of 900 to 1200 mg per day. Lithium serum levels over 1.5 mEq/L are usually toxic.

The use of L-triiodothyronine (T_3) at a dose of 25 to 50 μg in conjunction with a conventional antidepressant may also enhance the speed or magnitude of response to an antidepressant. In most instances, T_3 may be discontinued within several weeks of achieving the desired response and the patient continues to do well. Measurements of thyroid function are generally found to be normal before the initiation of this type of adjunctive therapy (Goodwin et al., 1982).

Although there is not total agreement as to the antidepressant efficacy of lithium carbonate, some studies have indicated its beneficial effect in patients with depressed mood (Ortiz, Dabbagh, and Gershon, 1984). Lithium carbonate in conjunction with TCAs or MAOIs may be quite useful in many patients who have not responded to adequate trials of antidepressants. Controlled studies have confirmed the ability of lithium to augment a therapeutic response (Heninger, Charney, and Sternberg, 1983; Price, Charney, and Heninger, 1985). Carbamazepine may also improve depressed mood when used alone or in combination with a heterocyclic or an MAOI-type antidepressant (Folks, 1982). A patient who has not responded to an adequate trial of antidepressant may benefit.

Treatment-resistant patients may also benefit from MAOI–heterocyclic antidepressant combinations, particularly in severely refractory cases. The incidence and severity of adverse drug reactions and proper monitoring of this combined regimen are not dissimilar to those for patients receiving any one of the antidepressant drugs singly (Bernstein, 1988). Although there is general agreement about the safety of combined heterocyclic antidepressant–MAOI therapy, data are less substantial regarding the efficacy.

A patient whose depression fails to respond to pharmacologic treatment should undoubtedly receive a course of ECT, after which the patient's condition should be stabilized with an appropriate prophylactic regimen consisting of an antidepressant, an MAOI, or lithium, or a combination of these. In some cases the combined lithium-antidepressant drug therapy provides the most effective prophylaxis against recurrent depression.

The efficacy of lithium in the treatment of acute mania has been well documented (Jefferson et al., 1987). In addition to the monitoring of lithium serum levels and other values in patients taking lithium in the acute phase of manic illness, lithium requires a cooperative patient who will take daily oral medication, whereas neuroleptic drugs may also be given orally or intramuscularly as required. Perhaps the major disadvantage of lithium in the treatment of acute mania is that improvement is slow and gradual. It may take up to 3 weeks to adequately control manic symptoms. Thus haloperidol or other antipsychotic agents may be used alone or in combination, with dramatic and rapid impact in controlling behavior in manic patients. Although low-potency agents such as chlorpromazine or thioridazine may produce considerable sedation, these drugs do little to alter qualitatively the underlying manic symptoms (Shopsin et al., 1975). As previously noted, the optimal therapeutic lithium serum level in the treatment of acute manic or it prophylaxis is generally quoted to be at 0.6 to 1.2 mEq/L.

Lithium serum levels ideally should be measured approximately 12 hours, plus or minus 2 hours, after administration of the last dose of lithium (Jefferson et al., 1987). Clinical observations and well-documented compliance should coincide with this practice.

Considerable evidence supports the beneficial effect of lithium and the prophylaxis of recurrent depression in persons with bipolar illness. Lithium may also be beneficial in the treatment of recurrent depression in patients who do not have a manic component to the mood disorder (Quitkin et al., 1976). Perhaps the most interesting and important application of lithium in depression is its apparent ability, as previously noted, to facilitate a therapeutic response to a conventional antidepressant (Nelson and Majore, 1986).

Side Effects

Lithium, an ion interchangeable with sodium, has a variety of physiologic and pathophysiologic actions in various organ systems. Thus it is important to ascertain whether the patient is in good health, has any medical contraindications to lithium, and has sufficient renal function to clear the ion adequately so that lithium intoxication may be prevented (Jefferson et al., 1987). Determination of serum creatine or blood urea nitrogen level should be obtained. For patients on a low-salt diet or a diuretic regimen, electrolyte values should also be determined. A baseline electrocardiogram (ECG) is necessary, since lithium often produces repolarization (ST segment and T wave) changes in the ECG and about 20% of patients taking lithium have a T-wave flattening or inversion at therapeutic blood levels, which are not indicative of underlying heart disease (Jefferson et al., 1987; Bucht et al., 1984). Patients who have lithium intoxication may show a variety of cardiovascular abnormalities, including arrhythmia, conduction disturbance, and hypotension (Mitchell and MacKenzie, 1982). Since lithium may be associated with the development of a euthyroid goiter, hyperthyroidism with or without thyroid gland enlargement or abnormalities in serum determinations of thyroid function warrant baseline measurements of thyroid function. Also, because lithium administration is frequently associated with weight gain partially related to fluid retention and to increased caloric intake, the patient should be considered at risk for this nontherapeutic effect.

Lithium frequently produces benign reversible leukocytosis; white blood cell counts of 12,000-15,000 cells/mm^3 are frequently seen during therapy. This condition does not indicate any hematologic disease and does not require discontinuation of lithium (Jefferson et al., 1987).

Because lithium is a simple ion whose entry into the body is governed by the same physiologic mechanisms as sodium, lithium reaches virtually all bodily tissues. Lithium's side effects, however, are linked primarily to serum blood levels. Blood levels greater than 1.5 mEq/L can be toxic, and generally levels above 2.0 mEq/L induce toxic signs and symptoms. Common side effects include nausea, dry mouth, diarrhea, and thirst. Drowsiness, mild hand tremor, polyuria, weight gain, a bloated feeling, sleeplessness, and headaches are other relatively common side effects.

A lithium tremor tends to be irregular in rhythm and amplitude, affecting the fingers. Jerky motions of the flexion and extension of fingers are also commonly associated with lithium therapy (Tyrer, Lee, and Trotter, 1981). These tremors often disappear spontaneously when the dose is held constant for the first 2 to 3 weeks of lithium treatment. Sometimes reducing the dose of lithium or advising the patient to take smaller dosages several times throughout the day alleviates this unwanted effect.

However, when the tremor is persistent and severe enough to cause inconvenience to the patient in daily activities, propanalol, metaprolol, and nadolol, beta-adrenergic blocking agents, are highly effective in controlling the tremor (Zubenko, Cohen, and Lipinski, 1984). The use of slow-release lithium preparations may reduce the severity of lithium tremor by reducing serum blood level peaks.

Side effects unrelated to serum levels include weight gain, a metallic taste, headache, edema of the hands and ankles, and pruritus. Lithium, even in therapeutic levels, can affect thyroid gland function. In some patients thyroid hormone therapy may be required. Lithium may also impair the mental or physical capabilities required for driving.

Polyuria and polydipsia develop in many patients taking lithium. These symptoms are generally benign and are not indicative of renal or metabolic disease. Of patients studied and reported in the literature who have renal changes in association with therapeutic doses of lithium, none has been reported to have renal failure (Bernstein, 1988). To prevent kidney damage, lithium should not be prescribed unless there is both a reasonable clinical indication of its necessity and the likelihood that it will provide a useful therapeutic benefit. It may add somewhat to the safety of long-term lithium management and provide reassurance to the patient and the clinician to measure urine osmolality once or twice yearly, after a 12-hour period of fasting. This practice is, of course, in addition to periodic determinations of lithium serum levels, which should be monitored.

During lithium treatment patients who have edema of the ankle or lower legs generally do so in the context of normal renal, cardiovascular, and hepatic function. This edema may disappear spontaneously or may respond favorably to spironolactone 50 mg two times a day, a specific aldosterone inhibitor that perhaps attempts to normalize tubular reabsorption of sodium, which has some role in the edema formation (Demers and Heninger, 1970). Additionally, patients who have edema may also respond favorably to an intermittent dose of a thiazide diuretic, for example, hydrochlorothiazide 50 mg daily or every other day. If administered on a regular basis, hydrochlorothiazide should be prescribed in association with the monitoring of serum potassium and supplemental oral potassium levels as indicated, as with any patient receiving a thiazide diuretic and lithium simultaneously.

Although weight gain is common in patients taking lithium and may in part be due to the fluid retention described previously, variable changes in glucose metabolism may be an important mechanism in weight gain (Jefferson et al., 1987). Patients should be educated about this possibility and taught to maintain adequate fluid and salt intake during the course of any rapid weight loss. Moreover, it is often appropriate to measure lithium serum concentration more frequently in those who may be on a weight-reducing diet.

Lithium therapy may be associated with the development of goiter in the presence of normal thyroid function tests and a euthyroid state. This condition is usually associated with an increased thyroid-stimulating hormone level and an enlargement of the thyroid gland as it is attempting to maintain the euthyroid state. Hypothyroidism may also be induced by lithium treatment. This occurrence does not indicate that the dosage needs to changed or the medication discontinued; however, proper evaluation and replacement therapy with an appropriate thyroid hormone regimen may be necessary in conjunction with lithium treatment (Myers et al., 1985).

Dermatologic reactions may occur with lithium (Folks and Kinney, 1991). Acne may worsen, and lithium has also been reported to exacerbate psoriasis. Occasionally a maculopapular rash with or without puritis may emerge during the course of lithium treatment. Hair loss may also occur and may be limited to the scalp or may affect other body regions.

Many patients taking lithium have gastrointestinal tract complaints, most commonly upper gastric burning sensations and persistent indigestion. Taking lithium at mealtime or with a snack often alleviates these symptoms. Mild diarrhea is also occasionally associated with conventional therapeutic doses and serum levels of lithium but is more apt to occur in the presence of excessive lithium serum concentration. A major risk is posed by vomiting, which contributes to dehydration and in turn may worsen any lithium intoxication. Patients who have nausea, vomiting, or other flulike symptoms during lithium therapy should be advised to discontinue lithium and maintain adequate fluid intake for a short time.

Lithium intoxication is a common problem; when it is suspected, the drug should be discontinued and blood samples sent for determinations of lithium serum concentration and serum creatinine and electrolyte levels. Specific interventions include adequate hydration, antiemetics as necessary, and monitoring of serum levels of electrolytes, lithium, and creatinine, which in turn can guide the rate and nature of fluid replacement. An ECG should also be obtained, since the possibility of cardiac arrhythmia is always present. A patient with lithium intoxication may also have a variety of central nervous system effects, including confusion, stupor, and the potential for seizure (Sansone and Zeigler, 1985; Himmelhoch et al., 1980).

Implications

Therapeutic versus toxic levels. Therapeutic lithium serum levels are 0.6 to 1.2 mEq/L. At serum levels above 1.5 mEq/L adverse reactions can occur. Typically the higher the serum levels, the more severe the reaction. Mild to moderate toxic reactions occur at levels of 1.5 to 2.5 mEq/L, and moderate to severe reactions at 2.0 to 2.5 mEq/L. Diarrhea, vomiting, drowsiness, muscular weakness, and lack of coordination can be early signs of lithium intoxication. At higher levels ataxia, giddiness, tinnitus, blurred vision, and large output of dilute urine may be seen. At serum levels above 3 mEq/L multiple organs and organ systems may be involved, leading to coma and death (Sugarman, 1984). Serum levels as high as 10 mEq/L have been survived. Serum levels should be monitored and should not be allowed to exceed 2 mEq/L.

There is no antidote for lithium poisoning. When supportive intervention is available, discontinuing the drug may be enough. In the treatment of acute overdose, gastric lavage has been used successfully. Parenteral normal saline solution infused over 6 hours (1-2 L) may provide enough volume to prevent hypovolemia and restore blood pressure and enough sodium to counteract lithium's ill effects, enhancing renal excretion for serum levels below 2.5 mEq/L. Forced diuresis may be necessary for patients with lithium poisoning, and mannitol may be used. Acetazolamide, which alkalinizes the urine, may also be given to increase lithium excretion in case of an acute overdose. In some severe cases hemodialysis has been found to be helpful.

Use in pregnancy. Cessation of lithium during pregnancy is suggested because of its relationship to Ebstein's anomaly and other teratogenic effects in the first trimester. If antimania treatment is essential during this time, treatment with thioridazine or, perhaps, carbamazepine or valproate may be beneficial. These drugs, when used instead of lithium, also carry unknown risks when prescribed in the second and third trimesters. Doses should be reduced as much as 50% before the delivery because of the potential for neonatal intoxication resulting from high maternal serum levels of lithium (Cohen, 1989).

Side effects. Because lithium has a narrow therapeutic index, lithium serum levels should be determined frequently. Levels are determined daily in some acute treatment units. Once the patient's condition is stabilized, monthly serum level determinations are usually adequate. Blood is usually drawn before administration of the first dose of lithium in the morning (usually 8 to 12 hours after the last dose). However, do not rely on laboratory tests alone: continue to evaluate the patient.

Interactions. Familiarity with the drugs that can elevate lithium serum levels is essential. Diuretics, with the exception of acetazolamide, increase sodium excretion, thereby elevating serum lithium levels. Indomethacin and, possibly, other nonsteroidal antiinflammatory agents increase serum levels of lithium by reducing renal elimination. Switching to a low-salt diet also elevates lithium serum levels.

Some drugs decrease serum lithium levels and pose problems of inadequate treat-

Patient Guidelines for Taking Lithium

To achieve a therapeutic effect and prevent toxic effects of lithium, patients taking lithium should be advised of the following:

1. Lithium must be taken on a regular basis, preferably at the same time daily. If a patient is taking lithium, for example, on a three-times-daily schedule and forgets a dose, he or she should wait until the next scheduled time to take the lithium but should not take twice the amount at that time, since lithium intoxication could occur.
2. When lithium treatment is initiated, mild side effects such as a fine hand tremor, increased thirst and urination, nausea, anorexia, and diarrhea or constipation may develop. Most of the mild side effects are transient and do not represent toxic effects of lithium. Also, in some patients who are taking lithium some foods such as celery and butter have an unappealing taste.
3. Serious side effects of lithium that necessitate its discontinuance include vomiting, extreme hand tremor, sedation, muscle weakness, and vertigo. If any of these occur, the prescribing physician should be notified immediately.
4. Lithium and sodium compete for elimination from the body through the kidneys. An increase in salt intake increases lithium elimination, and a decrease in salt intake decreases lithium elimination. Thus it is important that the patient maintain a balanced diet and salt intake. If the patient wishes to alter his or her diet, he or she should first consult with the prescribing physician.
5. Various situations can require an adjustment in the amount of lithium administered to a patient, for example, the addition of a new medication to the patient's drug regimen, a new diet, or an illness with fever or excessive sweating.
6. Blood should be drawn in the morning for determination of lithium levels, approximately 8 to 14 hours after the last dose was taken.

Adapted from Keltner NL. In Shlafer M, Marieb E, editors: *The nurse, pharmacology, and drug therapy,* Redwood City, Calif, 1989, Addison-Wesley.

ment and symptom exacerbation. This decrease may occur in one of two ways, by increasing lithium excretion or by decreasing lithium absorption. Drugs that increase lithium excretion include acetazolamide, caffeine, and alcohol.

Lithium and antipsychotic drugs are frequently combined. Antipsychotics are prescribed with lithium because lithium's clinical response time is delayed to 1 to 2 weeks. Antipsychotic agents are prescribed to produce an immediate neuroleptic or antipsychotic effect (see Chapter 9). A potential problem with this combination that has not previously been mentioned is that the antiemetic properties of the antipsychotic agent can potentially mask the early signs of lithium intoxication, that is, nausea and vomiting. Moreover, there are some concerns that the specific combination of lithium and haloperidol has a greater-than-normal potential for neurotoxicity. This possibility, however, seems to be primarily a matter of drug interaction and should be a concern with any combination of lithium and an antipsychotic agent. Lithium also prolongs the paralyzing effect of some neuromuscular blocking agents that may be given before surgery or used during ECT. Appropriate measures should be taken in these cases.

Patient education. The patient and family alike must be familiar with the nontherapeutic effects of lithium and the symptoms of minor and major toxic effects (see the box on p. 101). Side effects associated with lithium should be reviewed, and in individuals of child-bearing age appropriate measures should be taken to avoid conception during lithium treatment because of its definitive ability to harm the fetus. Avoidance of driving until the patient is stabilized on a regimen of lithium is a reasonable expectation. The interventions outlined in the box below should also be considered in applicable cases.

ALTERNATIVE ANTIMANIC AND MOOD-STABILIZING DRUGS

Lithium is highly effective, generally safe, and produces a tolerable level of side effects in the great majority of patients. However, when lithium is not tolerated or when response does not occur, alternative agents may be required. The alternative

Nursing Interventions for Patients Taking Lithium

Prepare the patient for expected side effects in a nonanxious manner.

Discuss which side effects should subside (nausea, dry mouth, diarrhea, thirst, mild hand tremor, weight gain, bloatedness, insomnia, and lightheadedness).

Identify the side effects that require immediate notification of the physician (e.g., vomiting, severe tremor, sedation, muscle weakness, and vertigo).

Suggest taking lithium with meals to reduce nausea.

Suggest drinking 10 to 12 8-oz (240 ml) glasses of water per day to reduce thirst and maintain normal fluid balance.

Advise patient to elevate feet to relieve ankle edema.

Advise patient to maintain a consistent dietary sodium intake but to increase sodium if there is a major increase in perspiration.

Adapted from Keltner NL. In Shlafer M, Marieb E, editors: *The nurse, pharmacology, and drug therapy*, Redwood City, Calif, 1989, Addison-Wesley.

antimanic and mood-stabilizing drugs discussed here are compounds that are currently marketed for treatment of other conditions and are not at this writing approved by the FDA for the treatment of mood disorders. However, the literature is replete with many alternative pharmacologic approaches.

Carbamazepine (Tegretol) is perhaps the best alternative treatment for manic episodes when lithium is ineffective, contraindicated, or not tolerated (Table 5-8). As noted previously, carbamazepine may also be used in individuals at great risk during pregnancy. Although an effective antiepileptic drug, carbamazepine is chemically related to the tricyclic antidepressants. Patients with rapid-cycling manic depressive episodes may respond especially well to carbamazepine, and at times carbamazepine may be given in combination with lithium (Folks et al., 1982). Although the mechanism of the antimanic action of carbamazepine is unknown, early work focused on its ability to inhibit kindling (Post et al., 1982; Folks et al., 1982).

Although plasma concentrations of carbamazepine correlate to its anticonvulsant effect, the relationship of blood level to antimanic activity is less clear (Jefferson et al., 1987). Certainly, levels of 8-12 μg/ml should be achieved, when response does not occur at lower levels, before concluding whether the drug is ineffective (Ballenger, Post, and Bunney, 1982).

Nausea, anorexia, and occasional vomiting may occur with carbamazepine, particularly when the drug is administered on an empty stomach or when relatively high doses are used. Sedation and drowsiness are other common side effects, which may be minimized by lowering initial doses and by slower titrating. Indeed, the sedative effect of carbamazepine may be useful in managing insomnia and agitation in some patients with mood disturbances (see Chapter 9).

The most serious and rare side effect of carbamazepine is its potential to produce agranulocytosis (Jefferson et al., 1987; Folks et al., 1982). Mild to moderate leukopenia, anemia, and thrombocytopenia may also occur. Complete blood cell counts and examination of the blood smear should be performed weekly during the first month of therapy and may be performed at progressively longer intervals during the course of treatment. Complete blood cell counts and other appropriate laboratory tests in patients receiving maintenance therapy with carbamazepine should be moni-

Table 5-8 Comparison of Side Effects Profiles for Lithium and Carbamazepine

Lithium* (0.7-1.2 mEq/L)	Frequency (%)	Carbamazepine† (5-12 μg/ml)
Memory disturbances‡	—	?
Thirst and polyuria	50-70	—
Tremor	30-50	—
Weight gain‡	10-30	?
Diarrhea	10-20	—
Hypothyroidism	5-10	Essentially absent
Psoriasis	1	—
	—	Blood dyscrasias
	—	Hepatitis
	—	Dizziness and ataxia
	—	Water intoxication

*Vestergaard P, Shou M: *Pharmacopsychiatry* 17:199, 1984.
†Post RM et al: *J Clin Psychopharmacol* 4:178, 1984.
‡Reasons for noncompliance. (From Jamison KR, Akisal HS: *Psychiatr Clin North Am* 6:175, 1983.)

tored every 3 to 4 months during the continuation of treatment. For patients who benefit greatly, periodic monitoring of those with mild leukopenia, anemia, or thrombocytopenia may be acceptable and tolerated. In addition to its antimanic effect, carbamazepine has been shown to possess antidepressant actions when employed alone or in conjunction with other antidepressant drugs (Post et al., 1986).

Toxic effects of carbamazepine, as well as drowsiness, may occur with coadministration of erythromycin; neurotoxic effects may result from the ability of this antibiotic to inhibit carbamazepine metabolism. When given alone or in combination with other antiepileptic drugs, for example, phenobarbital, carbamazepine may induce its own metabolism through microsomal induction. Carbamazepine may also increase serum lithium concentration and decrease serum neuroleptic concentration. Neurotoxic effects may occur when carbamazepine is combined with calcium channel blockers or angiotensin in converting enzyme inhibitors (Bernstein, 1988).

Another anticonvulsant, *valporic acid* (Depakene), has been used occasionally and is becoming accepted as an alternative treatment for mania (Emrich, Dose, and Von Zerssen, 1985; McElroy, Keck, and Pope, 1987). Current studies are underway to assess the ability of this drug to be used alone for the treatment or the prophylaxis of mania, or both. A number of clinical reports have noted the use of sodium valporate in conjunction with lithium, neuroleptics, carbamazepine, or other drugs, which may also contribute to the successful treatment of many patients who are nonresponders to lithium. Complete blood cell counts and liver function tests should be monitored periodically during treatment with sodium valporate.

Clonazepam (Klonopin) has been suggested as a treatment or an adjunct for the treatment of mania and has been shown to have an acute effect in manic patients (Chouinard, Young, and Annable, 1983) (see Chapter 9). This drug may also reduce the need for doses of haloperidol or other neuroleptic agents; except for considerable drowsiness, minimal adverse effects are seen in patients receiving clonazepam doses of 2 to 16 mg per day (Chouinard, Young, and Annable, 1983; Victor et al., 1984; Chouinard, 1985).

Perhaps more important than the previously described use, clonazepam may be used as a maintenance drug in the treatment of bipolar affective disorder in conjunction with lithium or carbamazepine in patients who have previously required combined lithium-neuroleptic maintenance regimens. Clonazepam is also useful in patients for whom neuroleptic drugs cannot be employed, such as patients with Parkinson's disease. Similarly, *lorazepam* (Ativan) may be employed in lieu of neuroleptic drugs in conjunction with lithium. Lorazepam is perhaps the only benzodiazepine that has potential use and is reliable when administered intramuscularly (or intravenously). Lorazepam may also minimize the acute extrapyramidal side effects of high-potency antipsychotic drugs in the treatment of acute psychosis (see Chapter 9).

Several investigators have discussed the use of calcium channel blockers, specifically, verapamil, to exert a clinically significant antimanic effect (Pollack, Rosenbaum, and Hyman, 1987). Further investigation of the psychotropic effects of this drug is needed. A recent study has shown no improvement in manic symptoms (Barton and Gitlin, 1987). Moreover, there have been reports of patients receiving calcium channel blockers, including verapamil, diltiazem, and nifedipine, in whom symptoms of depression or dysphoria emerged as a possible side effect (Bernstein, 1988).

REFERENCES

American Psychiatric Association: *Diagnostic and statistical manual of mental disorders, third edition-revised*, Washington, DC, 1987, The Association.

Angst J et al: Lithium prophylaxis in recurrent affective disorders, *Br J Psychiatry* 116:604, 1970.

Anton RF, Hitri A, Diamond BI: Amoxapine treatment of psychotic depression: dose effect and dopamine blockage, *J Clin Psychiatry (Monogr Ser)* 4:32, 1986.

Ballenger JC, Post RM, Bunney WE: Carbamazepine in manic-depressive illness: a new treatment, *Am J Psychiatry* 139:115, 1982.

Baldesserini RJ: *Chemotherapy in psychiatry,* Cambridge, Mass, 1985, Harvard University.

Barton BM, Gitlin MJ: Verapamil in treatment-resistant mania: an open trial, *J Clin Psychopharmacol* 7:101, 1987.

Bernstein JG: *Drug therapy in psychiatry,* ed 2, Litton, Mass, 1988, PSG.

Bernstein JG, Hackett TP, Cassem NH, editors: *Massachusetts General Hospital handbook of general hospital psychiatry,* ed 2, Littleton, Mass, 1987, PSG.

Bucht G et al: ECG changes during lithium therapy: a prospective study, *Acta Med Scand* 216:101, 1984.

Cade JFJ: Lithium salts in the treatment of psychotic excitement, *Med J Aust* 2:349, 1949.

Chouinard G: Antimanic effects of clonazepam, *Psychosomatics* 26(suppl):7, 1985.

Chouinard G, Young SN, Annable L: Antimanic effects of clonazepam, *Biol Psychiatry* 18:451, 1983.

Cohen LS: Psychotropic drug use in pregnancy, *Hosp Community Psychiatry* 40:566, 1989.

Demers R, Heninger G: Pretibial edema and sodium retention during lithium carbonate treatment, *JAMA* 214:1845, 1970.

Dista Products Company: Prozac advertisement, *Hosp Community Psychiatry* 43(3):213, 1992.

Emrich HM, Dose M, Von Zerssen D: The use of sodium valproate, carbamazepine and oxcarbazepine in patients with affective disorders, *J Affective Disord* 8:243, 1985.

Folks DG: Clinical approaches to anxiety in the medically ill elderly, *Drug Ther Suppl* p 72, August 1990.

Folks DG, Kinney FC: Dermatology. In Stoudemire A, Fogel BS, editors: *Medical psychiatric practice,* vol 1, Washington, DC, 1991, American.

Folks DG et al: Carbamazepine treatment of selected affectively disordered inpatients, *Am J Psychiatry* 139:115, 1982.

Ford CV: *The somatizing disorders: illness as a way of life,* New York, 1983, Elsevier Biomedical.

Ford CV, Folks DG: Psychiatric disorders in geriatric medical/surgical patients. II. Review of clinical experience in consultation, *Southern Med J* 78(4):397, 1985.

Freud S: Mourning and melancholia. In *The complete psychological works of sigmund freud,* London, 1957, Hogarth.

Goff DC, Jenike MA: Treatment-resistant depression in the elderly, *J Am Geriatr Soc* 34:63, 1986.

Goodman WK, Charney DS: Therapeutic applications and mechanisms of action of monoamine oxidase inhibitor and heterocyclic antidepressant drugs, *J Clin Psychiatry* 46(10, sec 2):6, 1985.

Goodwin DW, Guze SB: *Psychiatric diagnosis,* New York, 1984, Oxford University.

Goodwin FK et al: Potentiation of antidepressant effects by L-triiodothyronine in tricyclic non-responders, *Am J Psychiatry* 139:34, 1982.

Greden JF et al: Normalization of dexamethasone suppression test: a laboratory index of recovery from endogenous depression, *Biol Psychiatry* 15:449, 1980.

Guze SB, Robins E: Suicide and primary affective disorders, *Br J Psychiatry* 117:437, 1970.

Harsch HH, Holt RE: Use of antidepressants in attempted suicide, *Hosp Community Psychiatry* 39:990, 1988.

Henderson DK, Gillespie RD: *Textbook of psychiatry,* ed 6, Oxford, 1944, Oxford University.

Heninger GR, Charney DS, Sternberg DE: Lithium carbonate augmentation of antidepressant treatment: an effective prescription for treatment-refractory depression, *Arch Gen Psychiatry* 40:1335, 1983.

Himmelhoch JM et al: Age, dementia dyskinesias, and lithium response, *Am J Psychiatry* 137:941, 1980.

Jefferson JW et al: *Lithium encyclopedia for clinical practice,* Washington, DC, 1987, American Psychiatric Association.

Kalinowsky LB, Hippius H: *Pharmacological, convulsive and other somatic treatments in psychiatry,* New York, 1969, Grune & Stratton.

Keltner NL: Drugs for treatment of depression and mania. In Shlafer M, Marieb E, editors: *The nurse, pharmacology, and drug therapy,* Menlo Park, Calif, 1989, Addison-Wesley.

Keltner NL, Folks DG: Alternatives to lithium in the treatment of bipolar disorder, *Perspect Psychiatr Care* 27(2):36, 1991.

Kerr TA, Schapira K, Roth M: The relationship between premature death and affective disorders, *Br J Psychiatry* 115:1277, 1969.

Kraepelin E: *Manic depressive insanity and paranoia*, Edinburgh, 1921, ES Livingstone.

Lewis A: Melancholia: a historical review. In *The state of psychiatry: essays and addresses*, New York, 1967, Science House.

McElroy SL, Keck PE, Pope HG Jr: Sodium valproate: its use in primary psychiatric disorders, *J Clin Psychopharmacol* 7:16, 1987.

Meador-Woodruff JH: Psychiatric side effects of tricyclic antidepressants, *Hosp Community Psychiatry* 41:84, 1990.

Mendels J, Secunda SK, Dyson WL: The controlled study of the antidepressant effects of lithium carbonate, *Arch Gen Psychiatry* 26:154, 1972.

Mitchell JE, MacKenzie TB: Cardiac effects of lithium therapy in man: a review, *J Clin Psychiatry* 43:47, 1982.

Monroe LR: New weapons in the assault on depression, *Los Angeles Times*, Jan 2, 1990.

Myers DH et al: A prospective study of the effects of lithium on thyroid function and on the prevalence of antithyroid antibodies, *Psychol Med* 15:55, 1985.

Nelson JC, Majore CM: Lithium augmentation in psychotic depression refractory to combined drug treatment, *Am J Psychiatry* 143:363, 1986.

Ortiz A, Dabbagh M, Gershon S: Lithium: clinical use, toxicology, and mode of action. In Bernstein JG, editor: *Clinical psychopharmacology*, ed 2, Boston, 1984 John Wright–PSG.

Physicians' desk reference, New Jersey, 1992, Medical Economics Data.

Pollack MH, Rosenbaum JF, Hyman SE: Calcium channel blockers in psychiatry, *Psychosomatics* 28:356, 1987.

Post RM et al: Kindling and carbamazepine in affective illness, *J Nerv Ment Dis* 170:717, 1982.

Post RM et al: Antidepressant effects of carbamazepine, *Am J Psychiatry* 143:29, 1986.

Price LH, Charney DS, Heninger GR: Efficacy of lithium-tranylcypromine treatment in refractory depression, *Am J Psychiatry* 142:619, 1985.

Prien RF, Kupfer DJ: Continuation of drug therapy for major depressive episodes: how long should it be maintained? *Am J Psychiatry* 143:18, 1986.

Quitkin F et al: Prophylaxis in unipolar affective disorder, *Am J Psychiatry* 133:1091, 1976.

Risch SC, Janowsky DS, Hyey LY: Plasma levels of tricyclic antidepressants and clinical efficacy. In Enna SJ, Malick JB, Richelson E, editors: *Antidepressants: neurochemical, behavioral, and clinical perspectives*, New York, 1981, Raven.

Robertson MM, Trimble MR: Major tranquilizers used as antidepressants, *J Affective Disord* 4:173, 1982.

Roerig: Zoloft advertisement, *Hosp Community Psychiatry* 43(3):216a, 1992.

Roundsville BJ, Klerman GL, Weissman MM: Do psychotherapy and pharmacotherapy for depression conflict? *Arch Gen Psychiatry* 38:24, 1981.

Sabelli HC, Fawcett J, Javaid JI: The methylphenidate test for differentiating desipramine-responsive from nortriptyline-responsive depression, *Am J Psychiatry* 140:212, 1983.

Sansone MEG, Ziegler DK: Lithium toxicity: a review of neurologic complications, *Clin Neuropharmacol* 8:242, 1985.

Shopsin B et al: Psychoactive drugs in mania, *Arch Gen Psychiatry* 32:34, 1975.

Stern SI, Mendels J: Drug combinations in the treatment of refractory depression: a review, *J Clin Psychiatry* 42:368, 1981.

Sternberg DE, Jarvik ME: Memory functions in depression, *Arch Gen Psychiatry* 33:219, 1976.

Stone T, Folks DG: Somatization in the elderly, In RCW Hall, editor, *Psychiatric medicine* (in press).

Sugarman JR: Management of lithium intoxication, *Fam Pract* 18:347, 1984.

Tyrer P, Lee I, Trotter C: Physiological characteristics of tremor after chronic lithium therapy, *Br J Psychiatry* 139:59, 1981.

Van Kammen DP, Murphy DL: Prediction of imipramine antidepressant response by a one-day *d*-amphetamine trial, *Am J Psychiatry* 135:1179, 1978.

Victor BS et al: Use of clonazepam in mania and schizoaffective disorders, *Am J Psychiatry* 141:111, 1984.

Weissman MM: The psychological treatment of depression, *Arch Gen Psychiatry* 36:1261, 1979.
Winokur G: Types of depressive illness, *Br J Psychiatry* 120:265, 1972.
Zubenko GS, Cohen BM, Lipinski JF: Comparison of metroprolol and propranolol in the treatment of lithium tremor, *Psychiatry Res* 11:163, 1984.

CHAPTER 6

Anxiety Disorders

HISTORICAL CONSIDERATIONS

Anxiety and insomnia (see Chapter 7) are among the most common symptoms for which drug therapy is prescribed (Folks, 1990). Anxiety may occur in association with a variety of medical or psychiatric illnesses. The onset, course, and symptoms associated with anxiety syndromes vary significantly. Anxiety may occur suddenly with or without a precipitating cause or may develop in a rather subtle course. Anxiety may be associated with a clearly definable stress or stressors or may accompany problems within the family or psychosocial constellation. Anxiety may also occur when manifest symptoms are primarily somatic, may be secondarily associated with a significant medical or surgical problem, or may even be induced by medication or dietary substances.

Regardless of the course or circumstances surrounding the onset, anxiety that is disabling with respect to daily activities, social or occupational functioning, or relationship functioning requires intervention. Intervention, of course, should always be preceded by adequate assessment so that underlying emotional, family, biologic, or others factors that may respond to a specific intervention are further appreciated. As with depression, the use of anxiolytic medications are ideally combined with psychotherapeutic approaches, behavioral therapy techniques, or other adjunctive interventions that promote compliance and increase the likelihood of both an initial and a sustained response.

Drugs historically used to treat anxiety, referred to as antianxiety or anxiolytic agents, include those listed in the box below. Clearly alcohol is the oldest known agent to be used both medically and nonmedically. Alcohol is still the most frequently *self-prescribed* treatment for anxiety. The development of anxiolytic compounds has improved safety and efficacy, yet the dangers of dependency and the complications associated with anxiolytic treatment persist. The risks and adverse effects of alcohol have been documented in sources as old as the first book of the Old Testament, which declares that Noah "drank of the wine, was drunken and uncovered within his tent."

Historical and Contemporary Anxiolytic Drugs

Alcohol	Antihistamines
Opiates	Beta-blockers
Belladonna	Benzodiazepines
Barbiturates	Monoamine oxidase inhibitors
Meprobamate	Cyclic antidepressants
Phenothiazines	Buspirone

After the widespread use of alcohol through the ages as a sedative and an anxiolytic medicine a variety of other compounds, presumably safer and more effective, were developed (Table 6-1). Many of these historical compounds were neither safe nor effective in long-term treatment. For example, in the early 1900s the bromo seltzers were proclaimed efficacious but bromide dependency became a significant problem, and these products were withdrawn from the market (Harvey, 1985). Subsequently the barbiturates were developed and were seen as another potentially safe class of drugs; again their development was followed by the recognition of adverse effects, including seizures and the potential for addiction, dependence, and withdrawal symptoms. These compounds, as well as the opiates and tincture of belladonna, were indeed fraught with problems.

Perhaps the first major advance after the development of barbiturates was the development of meprobamate in the mid-1950s. This drug was initially heralded as an effective and addiction-free agent that did not possess the disadvantages of the barbiturates. However, with widespread initial use of meprobamate a number of individ-

Table 6-1 Historical Anxiolytics

Agent	Trade name	Comments
Alcohols, aldehydes, and propanediols		
Ethanol	Generic	Not recommended*
Ethchlorvynol	Placidyl	Not recommended*
Chloral hydrate	Generic	1-2 gm for sleep
Paraldehyde	Generic	Not recommended*
Meprobamate	Equanil, Miltown, generic	Not recommended*
Tybamate	Tybatran, Solacen, generic	Not recommended*
Barbiturates		
Amobarbital	Amytal, generic	100-800 mg/hr, intravenously in diagnosis, or parenterally for emergency sedation
Methohexital	Brevital	10 mg/5 sec intravenously for ECT only
Pentobarbital	Nembutal, generic	Can be used for withdrawal in most sedative addictions†‡
Phenobarbital	Luminal, generic	30-90 mg/day†‡
Secobarbital	Seconal, generic	Not recommended†
Structural relatives of barbiturates (nonbarbiturates)		
Glutethimide	Doriden	Not recommended*
Methyprylon	Noludar	Not recommended*
Methaqualone	Quaalude, Sopor, generic	Not recommended*
Antihistamines		
Diphenhydramine	Benadryl	25-50 mg parenterally for dystonia
Hydroxyzine	Atarax, Vistaril	Not recommended*
Promethazine	Phenergan, generic	Not recommended*

Modified from Baldessarini RJ: *Chemotherapy in psychiatry*, Cambridge, Mass, 1985, Harvard University.

*These agents are not recommended for routine use.

†Short-acting barbiturates are prescribed for sleep because of their low cost; phenobarbital is inexpensive and not often abused.

‡Pentobarbital and phenobarbital are used to treat addiction to and dependence on the sedative-hypnotic class of drugs.

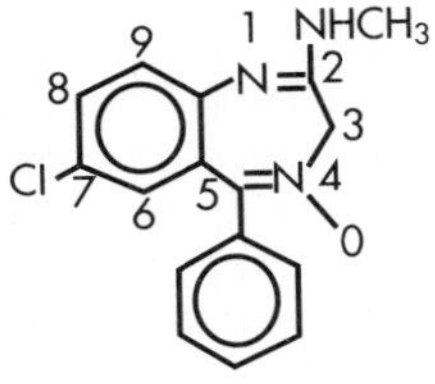

Chlordiazapoxide

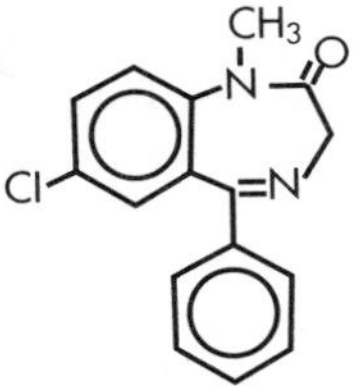

Diazapam

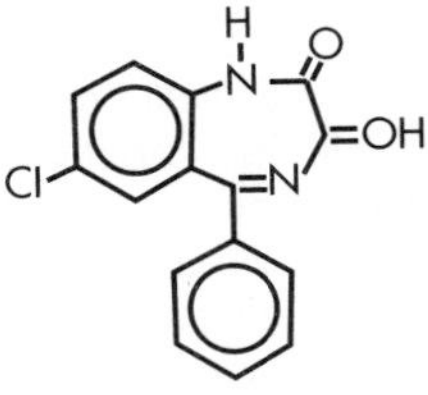

Oxazepam

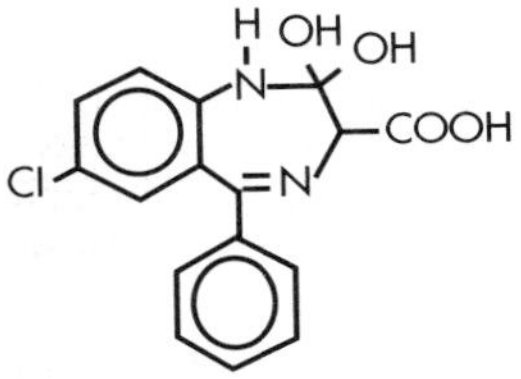

Clorazepate

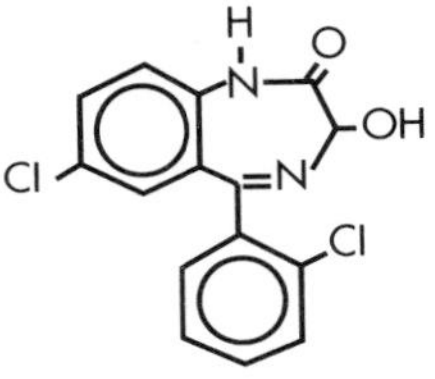

Lorazepam

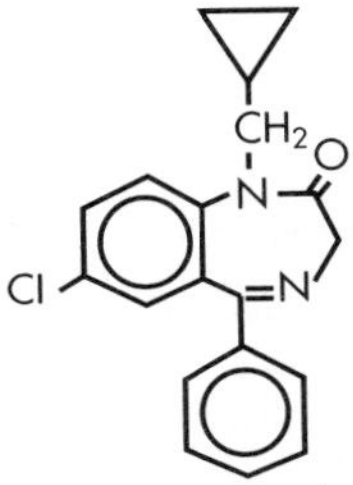

Prazepam

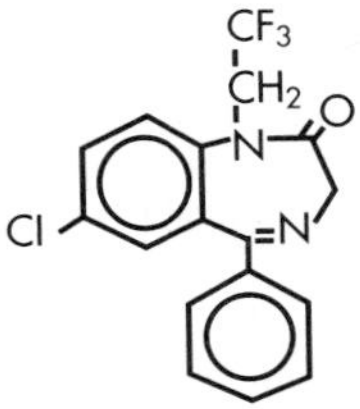

Halazepam

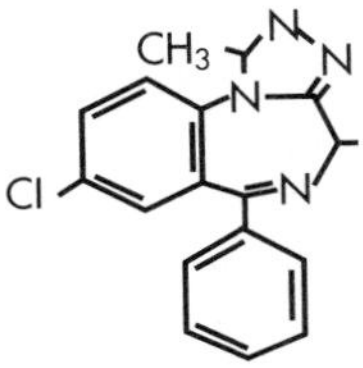

Alprazolam

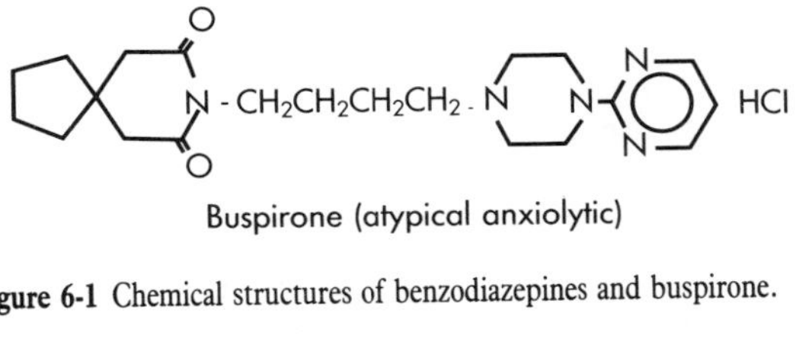

Buspirone (atypical anxiolytic)

Figure 6-1 Chemical structures of benzodiazepines and buspirone.

uals using the drug over an extended period began to have problems. Symptoms of addiction and withdrawal and grand mal seizures were observed and were similar to those associated with the barbiturates.

After meprobamate the first benzodiazepine, chlordiazepoxide (Librium), appeared on the scene in the 1960s (Figure 6-1). Again, this drug was introduced with the promise of efficacy and safety and a specific lack of risk for addiction, dependency, and withdrawal. As greater experience was gained, however, this compound and related compounds such as diazepam were associated with drug withdrawal symptoms similar to those seen with meprobamate and the barbiturates.

In 1986 buspirone, a structurally unique nonbenzodiazepine antianxiety drug, was introduced; this drug appears not to have the tolerance, dependency, or withdrawal symptoms associated with its predecessors (Figure 6-1). Compounds currently being investigated within this class and others hold promise that indeed anxiolytic compounds will someday be available without some of the adverse effects that have been so typical of the sedative-hypnotic class of the anxiolytics.

DIAGNOSTIC CONSIDERATIONS

The clinical picture of anxiety suggests that a variety of symptomatic presentations exists. Anxiety may represent a symptom, a syndrome, or a disorder or may simply be part of another underlying psychiatric disorder, for example, depression. Therefore a uniform clinical approach to the diagnosis and treatment of anxiety does not exist. Anxiety may be conceptualized in a variety of ways. For example, in the early psychoanalytic period anxiety was described as either signal anxiety, separation anxiety, or castration anxiety. Moreover, the current nomenclature suggests that anxiety may be experienced in anticipation of an unpleasant or stressful experience *(anticipatory anxiety)*, may be experienced as a component of a phobia in which excessive anxiety or apprehension is associated with a specific external situation or object, or may be quite severe and discrete, as with panic anxiety, in which severe episodes exist and may occur without an apparent external cause. Obsessive-compulsive disorder has emerged as a specific type or subtype of anxiety in which intrusive thoughts and compulsive rituals result in social, occupational, and relationship dysfunction. Other more generalized or *mixed syndromes* include mixed anxiety-depression and *posttraumatic stress disorder* (PTSD), in which symptoms follow a psychologically distressing event such as fear, terror, or helplessness. *Generalized anxiety* may be present when the essential features are associated with unrealistic or excessive anxiety and worry focused on two or more life circumstances. In this chapter the treatment approach to generalized and syndromal forms of anxiety and specific interventions that are currently applied to anxiety are discussed, as well as panic disorder, phobic disorders, and obsessive-compulsive disorder. Symptoms of anxiety may be generally described as psychologic, behavioral, or somatic (see the boxes on p. 112).

Anticipatory Anxiety

Anticipatory anxiety is a relatively common pathologic state and is generally less incapacitating than other forms of anxiety. Anxiety as an emotion most often does not require pharmacologic intervention, although the intermittent use of drugs such as benzodiazepines may be necessary when precipitating stress or situational factors are disabling.

Psychologic Symptoms of Anxiety

Anxious
Apprehensive
Fearful
Feeling of dread
Irritable
Frustrated
Intolerant
Nervous
Overconcerned
Sensitive to Shame
Worried

From Rosenbaum JF, Pollack MH. In Hackett TP, Cassem NH, editors: *Massachusetts General Hospital handbook of general hospital psychiatry*, ed 2, Littleton, Mass, 1987, PSG.

Behavioral Symptoms of Anxiety

Amotivational
Compulsive
Distractable
Frightened
Judgement impairment
Panicky
Phobic
Preoccupied
Reactive
Repetitive motor acts
Rigid
Threatened
Wound up

From Rosenbaum JF, Pollack MH. In Hackett TP, Cassem NH, editors: *Massachusetts General Hospital handbook of general hospital psychiatry*, ed 2, Littleton, Mass, 1987, PSG.

Somatic Signs and Symptoms of Anxiety

Anorexia
Backache
"Butterflies" in stomach
Chest discomfort
Diaphoresis
Diarrhea
Dizziness
Dyspnea
Dry mouth
Faintness
Fatigue
Flushing
Headache
Hyperventilation
Light-headedness
Muscle tension
Nausea
Pallor
Palpitations
Paresthesia
Sexual dysfunction
Shortness of breath
Stomach pain
Sweating
Tachycardia
Tremulousness
Urinary frequency
Vomiting

From Rossenbaum JF, Pollack MH. In Hackett TP, Cassem NH, editors: *Massachusetts General Hospital handbook of general hospital psychiatry*, ed 2, Littleton, Mass, 1987, PSG.

Posttraumatic Stress Disorder

In contrast to anticipatory anxiety, posttraumatic stress disorder (PTSD) generally follows exposure to a catastrophic event.

Posttraumatic stress disorder is characterized by anxiety that is *persistently experienced* in one of the following ways:

Recurrent or intrusive distressing recollections of the event

Recurrent distressing dreams of the event, or other sleep disturbances

Sudden acting or feeling as if the traumatic event were recurring, that is, flashback episodes, hallucinations, or illusions

Intense psychologic distress upon exposure to events that symbolize or reassemble an aspect of the trauma, including an anniversary reaction (Bernstein, 1987)

The current criteria of the *Diagnostic and Statistical Manual of Mental Disorders, Third Edition-Revised (DSM-III-R)* for PTSD is indicated in the box on pp. 114-115. Patients have persistent symptoms of arousal. They may experience sleep difficulties, personality changes, irritability, or outbursts of anger. Also common are concentration difficulties, hypervigilance, exaggeration of the startle response, and physiologic reactivity on exposure to events that resemble the traumatic event (American Psychiatric Association, 1987).

Mixed Anxiety-Depression

Especially noteworthy in primary care and ambulatory outpatient facilities are individuals who manifest mixed symptoms of anxiety and depression. These individuals often do not meet conventional diagnostic criteria for a mood or anxiety disorder but nonetheless come to medical attention with a mixed picture of mood and anxiety symptoms in an aggregate that appears to cause clinically significant impairment or distress, or both, and deserves recognition as a mental disorder (American Psychiatric Association, 1991). This subthreshold disorder may be particularly important in the selection of a pharmacologic agent. This syndrome may also be a most promising subject of further research. Specific symptoms of anxiety as target symptoms for treatment with newly developed pharmacologic agents have been considered as worthwhile areas of study (Table 6-2).

Generalized Anxiety

As stated previously, generalized anxiety disorder is manifested by unrealistic or excessive anxiety and worry about two or more life circumstances, for example, misfor-

Table 6-2 Mixed Symptoms of Anxiety-Depression

Symptom	Example
Affective	Dysphoria
Motor	Fears, worry, agitation, restlessness
Somatic	Insomnia, appetite disturbance, loss of libido, neuromuscular symptoms, cardiorespiratory symptoms, gastrointestinal tract symptoms
Psychologic	Concentration difficulty, memory complaints, indecisiveness, guilt, suicide*

*Suicide, although more likely to occur with depression, may also be likely to occur with anxiety, especially panic or obsessional anxiety.

Diagnostic Criteria for 309.89 Posttraumatic Stress Disorder

A. The person has experienced an event that is outside the range of usual human experience and that would be markedly distressing to almost anyone, e.g., serious threat to one's life or physical integrity; serious threat or harm to one's children, spouse, or other close relatives and friends; sudden destruction of one's home or community; or seeing another person who has recently been, or is being, seriously injured or killed as the result of an accident or physical violence.

B. The traumatic event is persistently reexperienced in at least one of the following ways:
   (1) Recurrent and intrusive distressing recollections of the event (in young children, repetitive play in which themes or aspects of the trauma are expressed)
   (2) Recurrent distressing dreams of the event
   (3) Sudden acting or feeling as if the traumatic event were recurring (includes a sense of reliving the experience, illusions, hallucinations, and dissociative [flashback] episodes, even those that occur upon awakening or when intoxicated)
   (4) Intense psychological distress at exposure to events that symbolize or resemble an aspect of the traumatic event, including anniversaries of the trauma

C. Persistent avoidance of stimuli associated with the trauma or numbing of general responsiveness (not present before the trauma), as indicated by at least three of the following:
   (1) Efforts to avoid thoughts or feelings associated with the trauma
   (2) Efforts to avoid activities or situations that arouse recollections of the trauma
   (3) Inability to recall an important aspect of the trauma (psychogenic amnesia)
   (4) Markedly diminished interest in significant activities (in young children, loss of recently acquired developmental skills such as toilet training or language skills)
   (5) Feeling of detachment or estrangement from others
   (6) Restricted range of affect, e.g., unable to have loving feelings
   (7) Sense of a foreshortened future, e.g., does not expect to have a career, marriage, or children or a long life

D. Persistent symptoms of increased arousal (not present before the trauma), as indicated by at least two of the follow:
   (1) Difficulty falling or staying asleep
   (2) Irritability or outbursts of anger
   (3) Difficulty concentrating
   (4) Hypervigilance
   (5) Exaggerated startle response

From American Psychiatric Association: *Diagnostic and statistical manual of mental disorders, third edition-revised*, Washington, DC, 1987, The Association.

Diagnostic Criteria for 309.89 Posttraumatic Stress Disorder—cont'd

(6) Physiologic reactivity upon exposure to events that symbolize or resemble an aspect of the traumatic event (e.g., a woman who was raped in an elevator breaks out in a sweat when entering any elevator)

E. Duration of the disturbance (symptoms B, C, and D) of at least 1 month. ***Specify delayed onset*** if the onset of symptoms was at least 6 months after the trauma.

tune occurring to one's child or worry about finances, which persists for 6 months or longer (American Psychiatric Association, 1987). Diagnostic criteria are listed in the box on p. 116. The symptoms of generalized anxiety may vary and are distinct from the types of anxiety associated with mood or psychotic disorders. Patients with generalized anxiety have a variety of autonomic or somatic signs and symptoms. Symptoms generally include psychologic and physical complaints that disturb concentration, result in irritability or sleep disturbance, and, if they persist, result in "chronic" anxiety. Essentially the anxiety and worry are excessive. The worry is pervasive and uncontrollable. The person finds it difficult to focus his or her attention on the tasks at hand because worry and energies are directed toward seeking relief.

Nonpsychiatric Anxiety

Anxiety may be present as a result of a nonpsychiatric medical condition, that is, an organic anxiety disorder, or may be induced by specific substances. It is often difficult to determine whether the anxiety exists primarily or secondarily; despite the presence of an organic disorder or substance use disorder, anxiety often becomes or needs to be a focus of treatment (Table 6-3; see the box on p. 117).

TREATMENT

The treatment approach to anxiety (as noted for depression in Chapter 5) ideally should combine pharmacotherapy, psychotherapy, and behavioral techniques in the context of medical and physiologic management. Adjunctive interventions, including the use of physical therapists, activity therapists, nutritionists, and so forth may also be essential to the therapeutic process. Despite the popularity of the sedative-hypnotic class of agents and, more specifically, the benzodiazepines, these drugs are too often prescribed in a universal or cavalier fashion. Providing the patient with quick relief may serve to alleviate distress but also may diminish the patient's awareness of what is actually happening within his or her body or environment. This diminished level of consciousness may interfere with the patient's ability to adapt, adjust his or her life-style, or improve coping behaviors.

A haphazard pharmacologic approach may also simply serve as a substitute for the time required to assist an anxious or unhappy individual to discover and modify the sources of his or her psychic pain. Of course, investigations for new methods of treating anxiety, including novel agents that may be nontranquilizing or may enhance the

Diagnostic Criteria for 300.02 Generalized Anxiety Disorder

A. Unrealistic or excessive anxiety and worry (apprehensive expectation) about two or more life circumstances, e.g., worry about possible misfortune to one's child (who is in no danger) and worry about finances (for no good reason), for a period of 6 months or longer, during which the person has been bothered more days than not by these concerns. In children and adolescents, this may take the form of anxiety and worry about academic, athletic, and social performance.

B. If another Axis I disorder is present, the focus of the anxiety and worry in *A* is unrelated to it, e.g., the anxiety or worry is not about having a panic attack (as in panic disorder), being embarrassed in public (as in social phobia), being contaminated (as in obsessive-compulsive disorder), or gaining weight (as in anorexia nervosa).

C. The disturbance does not occur only during the course of a mood disorder or a psychotic disorder.

D. At least 6 of the following 18 symptoms are often present when anxious (do not include symptoms present only during panic attacks):

Motor tension

(1) Trembling, twitching, or feeling shaky
(2) Muscle tension, aches, or soreness
(3) Restlessness
(4) Easy fatigability

Autonomic hyperactivity

(5) Shortness of breath or smothering sensations
(6) Palpitations or accelerated heart rate (tachycardia)
(7) Sweating, or cold clammy hands
(8) Dry mouth
(9) Dizziness or light-headedness
(10) Nausea, diarrhea, or other abdominal distress
(11) Flushes (not flashes) or chills
(12) Frequent urination
(13) Trouble swallowing or "lump in throat"

Vigilance and scanning

(14) Feeling keyed up or on edge
(15) Exaggerated startle response
(16) Difficulty concentrating or "mind going blank" because of anxiety
(17) Trouble falling or staying asleep
(18) Irritability

E. It cannot be established that an organic factor initiated and maintained the disturbance, e.g., hyperthyroidism or caffeine intoxication.

From American Psychiatric Association: *Diagnostic and statistical manual of mental disorders, third edition-revised*, Washington, DC, 1987, The Association.

Table 6-3 Drug-Induced Anxiety*

Drug	Example
Stimulants	Caffeine
Anorectics	Fenfluramine
Analgesics	Salicylates
Anticholinergics	Diphenhydramine
Hallucinogens	Cannabis
Sympathomimetics	Ephedrine
Neuroleptics (akathisia)	Haloperidol
Diuretics	Acetazolamide

*Anxiety may emerge acutely or with long-term treatment.

Organic Causes of Anxiety

Cardiovascular disorders
Arrhythmias, especially paroxysmal
Atrial tachycardia
Angina pectoris
Mitral valve prolapse
Orthostatic hypotension
Myocardial infarction

Endocrine disorders
Hyperthyroidism
Hypothyroidism
Pheochromocytoma
Hypoglycemia
Carcinoid syndrome
Hypoparathyroidism
Insulinoma
Cushing's syndrome
Acute intermittent porphyria

Respiratory disorders
Chronic obstructive respiratory disease
Hypoxia resulting from any cause
Pulmonary embolism
Asthma

Neurologic disorders
Aura of migraine
Early dementia
Cerebral neoplasia
Delirium
Partial complex seizures
Demyelinating disease
Vestibular disturbance
Postconcussive syndrome
Withdrawal from sedative-hypnotics, caffeine, or nicotine

From Rosenbaum JF, Pollack MH. In Hackett TP, Cassem NH, editors: *Massachusetts General Hospital handbook of general hospital psychiatry*, ed 2, Littleton, Mass, 1987, PSG.

processes of improved coping and life-style adjustment are underway. Perhaps buspirone (Buspar) represents the first of a new generation of anxiolytic compounds that fall conceptually within this subtype of nonbenzodiazepine anxiolytics.

Of the anxiolytics that are most effective and are frequently recommended for the treatment of anxiety, perhaps the benzodiazepines, buspirone, and certain conventional antidepressant agents are the most efficacious agents available. These agents are later discussed in detail. Additionally, beta blockers may also represent a class of drug that is useful in the treatment of somatic anxiety, since an anxious patient may feel uncomfortable and nervous and may have prominent physical signs and symptoms (see the box on p. 112). In fact, severe anxiety is usually accompanied by a variety of somatic or autonomic nervous system manifestations, including dry mouth, tachycardia, palpitations, irregular heart rhythm, dizziness, diarrhea, abdominal pain, headache, and other neuromuscular symptoms. These physiologic, somatic, and autonomic manifestations may be present in each of the various types of anxiety that have been discussed previously. These symptoms are less likely to be fully responsive to benzodiazepines or other conventional anxiolytic compounds. However, beta-adrenergic blocking drugs, for example, propranolol, metoprolol, and atenolol, may dramatically inhibit these physiologic manifestations of anxiety when administered alone or in conjunction with modest doses of an anxiolytic compound (Noyes et al., 1984). This ability to inhibit physiologic anxiety has made beta blockers a popular "stage fright" antidote.

Patients with anxiety symptoms require assessment and ideally are assigned a specific diagnosis. This diagnosis helps identify those individuals who may have a specific anxiety subtype (discussed later in this chapter) for which a monoamine oxidase inhibitor (MAOI), tricyclic antidepressant (TCA), selective serotonin reuptake inhibitor (SSRI), or other novel compound is more effective than the generalized approach of the prolonged benzodiazepine administration. The practitioner should also consider whether the patient might benefit from a nonbenzodiazepine and nonsedative hypnotic agent such as buspirone. Although buspirone appears to have no specific antipanic or antiphobic effects, it may be effective and useful in patients with generalized syndromes or mixed anxiety-depression (Rakel, 1990). The Food and Drug Administration has recently approved buspirone use for anxiety with dysphoric mood.

ANXIOLYTICS

BENZODIAZEPINES

Despite the lengthy history of the use of barbiturates and extensive experience with benzodiazepines and a variety of other sedative-class medications, the mechanisms of actions of anxiolytics are not fully understood. Among anxiolytics the benzodiazepines have dominated recent clinical practice and are emphasized in the following discussion. The structures of most of the readily available agents are shown in Figure 6-1. The clinical characteristics and pharmacologic doses of these agents are provided in Table 6-4. Compounds used frequently before 1964 that are still used include several barbiturates and related agents, compounds that share structural and pharmacologic properties with alcohol, and the sedative antihistamines, diphenhydramine (Benadryl) and hydroxyzine (Vistaril) (Table 6-1). Most of these agents are used infrequently and are not recommended because of their inferior effects or their potentially dangerous pharmacologic and toxicologic properties.

Pharmacologic Effect

Many benzodiazepine agents used for the treatment of anxiety are also useful in the induction of sleep and exert a general depressing effect on the central nervous system (CNS) that is dose related (see Chapter 8). Benzodiazepines compete for gamma aminobutyric acid (GABA) receptors in the brain and for specific benzodiazepine receptors responsible for the selective actions of these drugs on neuronal pathways throughout the CNS. The anxiolytic potency of the various benzodiazepines correlates with their affinity for benzodiazepine receptors.

Gamma aminobutyric acid increases the affinity of benzodiazepines for their specific receptor sites; it is a naturally occurring inhibitory neurotransmitter. Benzodiazepines increase the frequency with which anion channels open in response to GABA (Enna, 1984). The relationship of GABA to specific anxiolytic effects of benzodiazepines is not definitively proven; however, the gabaminergic action of benzodiazepines may at least partially account for their anticonvulsant and muscle relaxant effects. There is also evidence that benzodiazepines may decrease norepinephrine and serotonin turnover rates. This mechanism may partially account for the antianxiety and hypnotic effects of the benzodiazepines.

The structural and pharmacologic properties of buspirone are unrelated to those of the benzodiazepines (Figure 6-1). Busiprone is not a CNS depressant, nor does it produce significant sedation; yet it alleviates many symptoms of generalized anxiety. Because this drug does not cross-react with the benzodiazepines, it theoretically does not protect against benzodiazepine withdrawal symptoms; it does not appear to produce tolerance or dependency. Its utility in the treatment of substance abuse is discussed in a later chapter. A comparison of buspirone and the benzodiazepine, diazepam, and the antipsychotic, haloperidol, is presented in Table 6-5. An expanded discussion of buspirone appears later in the chapter.

Pharmacokinetics

Benzodiazepines differ from one another in pharmacokinetic profile and metabolism. Diazepam (Valium) is a rapidly absorbed benzodiazepine, reaching peak plasma levels in less than half an hour after oral administration; clorazepate (Tranxene) is also rapidly absorbed. Intravenously administered diazepam has an almost immediate effect, but with the possible exception of lorazepam (Ativan), diazepam and other benzodiazepines are absorbed unpredictably when injected intramuscularly. Benzodiazepines that have high potency and are rapid acting may perhaps be the most likely to be abused or to induce intoxication. However, most benzodiazepines are absorbed at an intermediate rate, with peak plasma levels appearing between 1 and 3 hours after administration. The relative rates of absorption, the approximate half-life, the presence of active metabolites, and usual daily doses of benzodiazepines and busiprone are summarized in Table 6-4.

Benzodiazepines are lipophilic and highly bound to plasma membranes, 85% to 90%. Pharmacokinetics of benzodiazepines are often complex, since many of these agents have active metabolites that dominate the course of their activities. Agents with slowly eliminated active metabolites have prolonged clinical actions and an elimination half-life from plasma in excess of 2 days (long-acting benzodiazepines). Plasma levels twice the level considered effective and safe may be associated with undesirable degrees of sedation or may result in toxicity. Thus long-acting benzodiazepines should be given in two to four single daily doses that are small. Shorter-acting agents are best given in two to four small portions as well, particularly for the treatment of daytime anxiety, in which a minimal risk of oversedation is desirable.

Lorazepam, oxazepam (Serax), and, possibly, alprazolam (Xanax) are exceptional benzodiazepines in that they have virtually no important pharmacologically active metabolites. However, all three agents ultimately rely on conjugation with glucuronic acid to form inactive metabolites. Because of the heavy reliance on hepatic mechanisms, benzodiazepines should be used cautiously in patients with liver disease, whose ability to eliminate these agents may be reduced significantly. Oxazepam, lorazepam, and, possibly, alprazolam may represent the safest benzodiazepine agents for patients with inefficient hepatic functioning.

Table 6-4 Pharmacologic Doses and Clinical Characteristics of Benzodiazepines and Buspirone

Nonproprietary name	Trade name	Usual daily dose (mg)[a]	Extreme daily dose (mg)	Rapidity of absorption[b]	Half-life (hr)[c]	Metabolites[d]
Anxiolytic benzodiazepines						
Alprazolam	Xanax	0.75-4	0.5-10	+++	12	Minor
Chlordiazepoxide	Libritabs	15-60	10-100	+++	18	Yes
Chlordiazepoxide hydrochloride[e]	Librium, A-poxide	15-60	10-100	+++	18	Yes
	SK-lygen	50-100 (IV per dose)	300 (IV)			
Clorazepate dipotassium[f]	Tranxene	30	7.5-90	++++	100	Yes
Diazepam[f,g]	Valium	4-40; 2-20 (IV per dose)	2-60	+++++	60	Yes
Halazepam	Paxipam	60-160	20-160	+++	14	Yes
Lorazepam[g]	Ativan	2-4; 2-4 (IM or IV per dose)	1-10	+++	15	No
Oxazepam	Serax	30-60	10-120	++	8	No

Prazepam	Centrax	20-40	5-60	+	100	Yes
Anticonvulsant benzodiazepine						
Clonazepam[h]	Klonopin	1.5-10	0.5-20	++	34	Yes
Anxiolytic nonbenzodiazepine						
Buspirone[i]	Buspar	15-40	10-60	Not applicable	7	Minor

Modified from Baldessarini RJ: *Chemotherapy in psychiatry*, Cambridge, Mass, 1985, Harvard University.

a. The daily doses are given as total milligrams per day, assuming doses are divided into two to four portions per day.

b. Ranked from 5+ (fastest: diazepam, <1 hour) to 1+ (slowest: prazepam, about 6 hours).

c. Elimination half-life is an estimated average, including active metabolites.

d. Most include desmethylated products, notably the long-acting nordiazepam; alprazolam has some active desmethylated and hydroxylated products that do not greatly prolong elimination.

e. Chlordiazepoxide is also available in combination with clidinium bromide (Librax and Clipoxide) or amitriptyline (Limbitrol).

f. Clorazepate dipotassium is also available as slow-release tablets (Tranxene-sd) containing either 11.25 or 22.5 mg to be taken once daily. Diazepam is also available as slow-release capsules (Valrelease) containing 15 mg.

g. Parenteral preparations are available only for chlordiazepoxide hydrochloride, diazepam, and lorazepam; intramuscular administration is not advisable, except with lorazepam (which is also very active sublingually); for details concerning intravenous use, see the manufacturer's instructions.

h. Clonazepam, while used primarily as an anticonvulsant for petit mal epilepsy and other non-grand mal seizure disorders, has been reported to have antimanic and antipanic activity as well.

i. Buspirone should be given in 2 to 4 daily divided doses with food or snack.

Table 6-5 Comparative Properties of Buspirone in Humans

Property	Diazepam	Haloperidol	Buspirone
Anxiolytic	++	0	++
Antipsychotic	0	++	0
Extrapyramidal	0	++	0
Sedation	++	+	+−
Muscle relaxant	++	0	0
Physical dependence	+	0	0
Anticonvulsant	++	-	0

From Neppe VM: *Innovative psychopharmacotherapy*, New York, 1989, Raven.
++ = Marked effect; + = mild effect; 0 = no effect; - = mild effect against; +-= dubious effect.

Side Effects

The most commonly encountered nontherapeutic side effects of the benzodiazepines are sedation with drowsiness, decreased mental acuity, and some decrease in coordination, occupational efficiency, and productivity with increased risk of accidents. Combining the drugs with alcohol increases these risks.

Autonomic side effects, anticholinergic side effects, and extrapyramidal side effects are rarely encountered. Liver damage, blood dyscrasia, and other end-organ toxic effects are also rare. Benzodiazepines are frequently associated with dysphoria, irritability, agitation, or otherwise "disinhibited" behavior. These reactions seem to be more characteristic of benzodiazepines than of barbiturates or meprobamate (Baldessarini, 1985). Some nonspecific side effects of benzodiazepines, including weight gain, skin reactions, headaches, impairment of sexual function, and menstrual irregularity, have been described in the literature. However, it is often difficult to determine whether these are symptoms or side effects of anxiety. Additionally, when doses are temporarily discontinued or dosage reduction occurs rapidly, it is sometimes difficult to determine whether the patient is having a resurfacing of anxiety symptoms or a mild withdrawal reaction.

Perhaps the most serious unwarranted effect of the benzodiazepines and other sedative hypnotics is their relative tendency to produce tolerance, physiologic dependence, and psychologic habituation. Tolerance can contribute to innocent self-medication and dose escalation. Further, these drugs, because of their ability to produce euphoria or intoxication, may have street value. The probability of becoming physiologically dependent or of developing tolerance depends largely on the daily dose and the duration of use. Physical dependence on the benzodiazepines chlordiazepoxide and diazepam has been studied extensively; however, the greatest risks of tolerance and dependence may be more significant with the new, shorter-acting benzodiazepines, especially those of high potency, that is, alprazolam and lorazepam.

Implications

Therapeutic versus toxic levels. Therapeutic levels of benzodiazepines have a comfortable margin of safety in comparison with those of other sedatives. However, overdoses equivalent to approximately twice a monthly supply, or even less, when taken with alcohol, have led to death. Moreover, the use of long-acting benzodiazepines, as well as the use of intravenous diazepam to control seizures or cardiac arrhythmias, is occasionally complicated by respiratory depression, apnea, ventricular arrhythmias, or even cardiac arrest. Most deliberate overdoses seem to involve more than one agent; typically alcohol is involved. Thus it is difficult to assess or determine what supply of benzodiazepines would be considered safely dispensed. The continued use of benzodiazepines for longer than several weeks should be applied in the context of the critical appraisal of risks and benefits in individual cases.

Use in pregnancy. The safety of sedative tranquilizer use in pregnancy is not established. There is inconclusive evidence that benzodiazepines may be teratogenic, causing cleft lip and palate in the first trimester. The level of risk involved is probably below the overall level of risk for birth defects, and in general the risk of toxic effects of benzodiazepines is low.

Side effects. The most common side effects of benzodiazepines are related to mental alertness. The patient should be cautioned about driving or operating hazardous machinery. Tolerance to most side effects quickly develops. Blood pressure of inpatients should be monitored routinely, and a drop in pressure of 20 mm Hg (systolic) on standing warrants withholding the drug and notifying the prescriber.

Interactions. Benzodiazepines tend to have "minimal true" pharmacokinetic interactions with most other drugs, with the possible exception of the MAOIs, which potentiate the sedating effects of the benzodiazepines. Unlike phenobarbital, the benzodiazepines have relatively minor ability to induce their own hepatic metabolism. Also, in contrast to the barbiturates, benzodiazepines have less potential for tolerance building and dose escalating. In other words, in contrast to the barbiturates and most traditionally prescribed sedatives, to obtain a sustained antianxiety or hypnotic effect, steadily increasing doses of benzodiazepines are not usually required. However, a degree of tolerance to the sedating effects and habituation can develop. Marked withdrawal symptoms are usually indicative of prolonged use at high doses.

Recently developed benzodiazepines of high potency and relatively short duration of action may present an increased risk of habituation and minor symptoms of withdrawal, warranting the slow tapering of doses of these agents. Such risks are lessened or at least delayed with the use of long-acting benzodiazepines.

Interactions between benzodiazepines and other agents occur. Phenytoin and digitalis preparations, when combined with the benzodiazepines, can result in increased plasma levels via hepatic metabolic interactions. Antacids and agents with anticholinergic activity, especially clorazepate, chlordiazepoxide, and diazepam, may decrease the absorption of benzodiazepines. Alcohol (and the MAOIs) may increase the intoxication potential. Disulfiram and cimetidine, but apparently not other H_2-receptor blockers, increase the plasma levels of long-acting benzodiazepines like chlordiazepoxide but not short-acting benzodiazepines, particularly those metabolized exclusively by conjugation, that is, oxazepam and lorazepam. In addition, the interaction between benzodiazepines and food may produce a differential effect on absorption. These effects may include an initial decrease in absorption, followed by a gradual increase, particularly with diazepam (Baldessarini, 1985).

Patient education. Benzodiazepines have a great potential for abuse. Consequently it is important to teach the patient and his or her family about these drugs. The nurse or physician should instruct the patient and the family as follows:

Benzodiazepines are not used in response to the minor stresses of everyday life.
Over-the-counter drugs may potentiate the actions of benzodiazepines.
Driving should be avoided until tolerance develops.

Alcohol and other CNS depressants potentiate the effects of benzodiazepines.
Hypersensitivity to one benzodiazepine may mean hypersensitivity to another.
Benzodiazepine use should not be discontinued abruptly.

Clinical implications and treatment issues. Diazepam and, possibly, other benzodiazepines have been known to result in disinhibition, a phenomenon characterized by increasing agitation leading to violence or terror (Hall, 1981). This loss of behavioral control sometimes associated with explosive or violent behavior may occur during the course of benzodiazepine treatment. Some evidence suggests that oxazepam is least likely to have a disinhibiting effect (Gardos et al., 1968).

Alprazolam and triazolam (discussed in Chapter 8) are structurally unique among the benzodiazepines with a triazolo ring bearing a somewhat similar configuration to the TCAs (see Figure 6-1). Thus it is not surprising that studies have shown the specific antidepressant and antipanic effects of alprazolam (Feighner et al., 1983; Liebowitz et al., 1986). Loss of behavioral control may emerge in patients receiving alprazolam and may be connected with the antidepressant action or may simply parallel the disinhibiting effect of other benzodiazepines (Bernstein, 1987). Moreover, alprazolam has recently gained Food and Drug Administration approval for use in the treatment of panic disorder (discussed later in this chapter). Not surprisingly, alprazolam has been reported to induce mania. By contrast, clonazepam, differing somewhat in structure and having only partial agonist effects, may actually have an antimanic effect (Goodman and Charney, 1987).

Benzodiazepines have well-known amnestic properties. This phenomenon has been observed during the treatment of patients and in various studies assessing the anesthetic use of benzodiazepines. Diazepam, for example, selectively impairs anterograde episodic memory and attention while sparing access to information in long-term memory (Liebowitz et al., 1987; Kumar et al., 1987). Amnestic properties of triazolam are discussed in Chapter 8.

The use of benzodiazepines in a manner conducive to the development of addiction is of great concern to patients and clinicians alike. In patients who have used these drugs excessively or at high doses treatment should not be discontinued suddenly. Obviously the same applies to patients who are taking other hypnotic agents such as barbiturates, meprobamate, chloral hydrate, and others. Occasionally barbiturates, for example, phenobarbital, are used in the alleviation of anxiety. This use may be particularly important in psychotic patients who are receiving optimal doses of antipsychotic medication but in whom persistent agitation occurs. Meprobamate has also been cautiously employed to provide sedation, improving both anxiety and insomnia, in nonpsychotic individuals. Obviously, recognizing the potential risks of dependency associated with the long-term use of these agents and the benzodiazepines is important. In chronically anxious patients who need prolonged drug therapy, other agents are worthy of consideration, for example, buspirone.

Patients with discrete panic attacks, phobic anxiety, or obsessive-compulsive disorder (OCD) may benefit from different classes of drugs, that is, a TCA or an MAOI (discussed later). Heterocyclic antidepressants that have significant sedating effects may have some advantage in the management of the treatment of anxiety. Antipsychotic and neuroleptic drugs have also been both recommended and condemned in the treatment of chronic anxiety. Obviously those with strongly sedating properties are preferable, for example, thioridazine, at a regimen in the range of 10 to 50 mg, one to four times per day. Of course, the choice of these agents in the treatment of chronic anxiety avoids the risks of drug dependency. However, concern about the potential development of tardive dyskinesia is well established. With the development of new-generation anxiolytics, that is, buspirone, the use of antipsychotics and neuroleptics should be avoided, or these agents should be prescribed in the context of a risks-versus-benefits approach.

A variety of sedating antihistamines have been used for the management of anxiety (and insomnia) (Carruthers et al., 1978). These compounds exert some anticholinergic and other nontherapeutic effects. Hydroxyzine, diphenhydramine, and promethazine are examples. Recently hydroxyzine, a moderately sedating nonphenothiazine antihistamine, has, perhaps, been the most popularly used, in a regimen of 10 to 25 mg, one to four times daily. However, these drugs primarily exert antianxiety effects through the process of sedation and are not recommended.

BUSPIRONE

Buspirone (Buspar), which belongs to a new chemical subgroup, the azapirones, is the first in a class of pure anxioselective agents (Figure 6-2). Differing substantially in both clinical and pharmacologic characteristics from the benzodiazepines, buspirone does not cause the sedation, hypnosis, anticonvulsant effects, and muscle relaxant effects of the benzodiazepines; 3 to 6 weeks are required for buspirone to achieve maximal therapeutic effects as an anxiolytic. Consequently, improvement in target symptoms, such as decreased agitation, improved concentration, and improved function, should be sought during its first week of administration. On chemical analysis the mechanism of buspirone anxiolytic effect is uncertain but probably relates to its partial agonist effects at the serotonin 1A receptor. At high doses intrinsic dopaminergic activity occurs hypothetically at cerebral, cortical, and midbrain levels. However, the drug primarily has its effect on presynaptic dopamine, with no significant neuroendocrine effects or consequential antipsychotic effects.

The anxiolytic action of buspirone may also be due in part to an active metabolite, 1-2 pyrimidinyl piperazine (1PP). This compound is particularly useful in the treatment of anxiety or mixed anxiety-depression because it poses few of the disadvan-

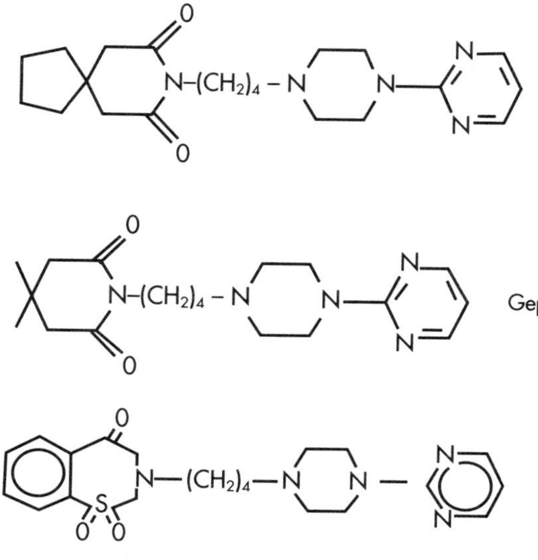

Figure 6-2 Structures of the prototype azapirones. (Only buspirone is currently marketed.)

tages associated with benzodiazepines, such as physical or psychologic dependence, and does not significantly interact with other compounds, with the exception of the MAOIs and haloperidol. Anxiety control is distinguished from sedative and euphoric actions of older anxiolytic drugs. In particular, symptoms of worry, apprehension, irritability, difficulty in concentrating, and cognitive difficulties, as well as the inability to cope, are the focus of treatment. Patients on regimens of buspirone frequently become less fearful, have fewer somatic symptoms, and are more interpersonally responsible than before treatment.

Pharmacokinetics

Buspirone is extensively metabolized, and after the first pass as little as about 1% becomes bioavailable. The main metabolite 1PP is also present and reaches relatively higher concentrations in the brain than does the parent compound buspirone itself. However, 1PP has only 1% to 20% of the potency of buspirone (Riblett et al., 1982). The distribution half-life of 1PP is four times longer than that of buspirone: the distribution half-life of buspirone is short and difficult to fully establish. Food increases its bioavailability by decreasing first-pass metabolism, and buspirone is rapidly and completely absorbed and widely distributed to all tissues. The drug is excreted almost exclusively as metabolites. Because of the large amount of hepatic metabolism of this lipid-soluble compound, one would expect this drug to antagonize effectively the cytochrome P450 enzyme system in the liver (Gammans, Mayol, and LaBudde, 1986).

Target symptoms in response to buspirone may begin to improve within days of initiation of an adequate dose, with the full effect at 3 to 6 weeks. The average daily dose is 20 to 30 mg given in divided doses, with a range of 15 to 60 mg per day. Buspirone may be particularly effective in mixed anxiety-depression or when cognitive and interpersonal problems exists (Rickels et al., 1982; Feighner, Merideth, and Hendrickson, 1983).

Implications

Therapeutic versus toxic levels. The most remarkable aspect of buspirone is its safety. There have been no reports of deaths resulting from the overdosage of buspirone when it is taken alone. Early studies in which doses of up to 2400 mg per day were used in patients with schizophrenia revealed no major untoward side effects.

Use in pregnancy. Buspirone can be administered with most medications; however, there are no data regarding the use of the drug during pregnancy. A comparison of the properties of buspirone, diazepam, and haloperidol in humans is given in Table 6-5.

Side effects. Common side effects associated with buspirone include headache, dizziness, light-headedness, and nausea, each of which can occur in 3% to 12% of patients (Domantay and Napoliello, 1989). These side effects can be treated as symptoms when they occur. In comparison with the benzodiazepines, with buspirone sedation seldom occurs; objective measures of motor impairment are far more common with the benzodiazepines, and the addictive effects seen when benzodiazepines are combined with alcohol are not observed with buspirone (Shuckit, 1984). Nonetheless, precautions against falls or driving are important, should a sedative response occur.

Interactions. As previously mentioned, drug interactions with buspirone are not observed; however haloperidol does interact with buspirone in as much as serum levels of haloperidol increase. Cimetidine has been reported to increase the 1PP metabolite by 30% (Gammans, Mayol, and LaBudde, 1986; Domantay and Napoliello, 1989). Interaction with MAOIs, resulting in a hypertensive reaction, has also been reported (Bristol-Myers Squibb, 1991).

Patient education. Buspirone has little potential for abuse; however, issues of safety and effective usage should be considered when this agent is discussed with the patient. Patients should be taught the following:

To avoid alcohol use, and to inform the prescriber about prescriptive and nonprescriptive drugs he or she is taking.

To discuss pregnancy and breast-feeding with the prescriber.

To avoid driving or operating hazardous machinery, if buspirone causes drowsiness, light-headedness, or dizziness.

Implications. An important clinical implication is that buspirone cannot be substituted immediately for benzodiazepines, that is, their pharmacologic characteristics are dissimilar, and in clinical practice buspirone takes many weeks to become fully therapeutic. Hence benzodiazepines must be gradually tapered while buspirone therapy is being initiated. Higher than usual doses of buspirone may be necessary for positive responses in patients who are not benzodiazepine naive (Kranzler, 1989). The common complaint of insomnia, which may be present in patients with mixed anxiety-depression, may be appropriately treated with trazodone, trimipramine, chloral hydrate, or other sedating compounds. Given the entirely different clinical and pharmacologic profiles of buspirone and benzodiazepines, buspirone and newly developed agents in this class require a shift of thinking with respect to anxiolytics (Neppe, 1989).

Because of the serotonergic effects and selectivity of buspirone, the potential for its use in the treatment of panic disorders, as previously noted, aggression (discussed in Chapter 9), and the affective spectrum disorders is noteworthy. Thus buspirone is effective in patients with mixed anxiety-depression but is as potent as diazepam for the control of psychic anxiety. Somatic anxiety may also be indirectly affected (Neppe, 1989).

The anxioselectivity of buspirone, without antipsychotic effects, extrapyramidal side effects, and the like, implies that it cannot induce tardive dyskinesia, despite its dopamine-related effects. Indeed its serotonin-modulating effects, its intrinsic dopaminergic activity, and its presynaptic action may help to alleviate tardive dyskinesia in patients with chronic psychosis on long-term regimens of neuroleptics (Neppe, 1989). Buspirone causes little sedation, is safe, and has no dependence-inducing properties. These features should diminish social stigma, but as a psychotropic agent it remains an unscheduled prescription drug. In contrast to the benzodiazepines, which impair cognitive and motor functioning and may compromise concentration, motivation, and functioning, buspirone acts on pathologic rather than normal anxiety while the patient is retaining concentration, motivation, and adequate functioning. The therapeutic relationship is critical to the successful implementation of buspirone treatment. As forementioned, a shift in thinking must be considered with buspirone in terms of patient education and compliance (Neppe, 1989).

SPECIFIC ANXIETY DISORDERS AND MIXED SYNDROMES

A number of specific anxiety disorders outlined earlier in this chapter have been identified as distinct entities; these disorders appear to be individualized expressions of related biochemical and physiologic disturbances of brain function. These include panic, obsessive-compulsive disorder (OCD), phobias, posttraumatic stress disorder (PTSD), and perhaps other syndromes that represent subthreshold syndromes or fall within the spectrum of affective disorders. Patients with panic, phobias, OCD, or other similar conditions have been viewed in the past as having unresolved psychologic conflicts; this point-of-view is clearly no longer tenable.

PANIC DISORDER

Patients with panic disorder have discrete episodes of intense fear, discomfort, or anxiety that may vary considerably in frequency and severity. During an attack pa-

Diagnostic Criteria for Panic Disorders

A. At some time during the disturbance, one or more panic attacks (discrete periods of intense fear or discomfort) have occurred that were (1) unexpected, i.e., did not occur immediately before or on exposure to a situation that almost always caused anxiety, and (2) not triggered by situations in which the person was the focus of others' attention.

B. Either four attacks, as defined in criterion A, have occurred within a four-week period, or one or more attacks have been followed by a period of at least a month of persistent fear of having another attack.

C. At least four of the following symptoms developed during at least one of the attacks:

(1) Shortness of breath (dyspnea) or smothering sensations
(2) Dizziness, unsteady feelings, or faintness
(3) Palpitations or accelerated heart rate (tachycardia)
(4) Trembling or shaking
(5) Sweating
(6) Choking
(7) Nausea or abdominal distress
(8) Depersonalization or derealization
(9) Numbness or tingling sensations (paresthesias)
(10) Flushes (hot flashes) or chills
(11) Chest pain or discomfort
(12) Fear of dying
(13) Fear of going crazy or doing something uncontrolled*Note:* Attacks involving four or more symptoms are panic attacks; attacks involving fewer than four symptoms are limited symptom attacks.

D. During at least some of attacks, at least four of the C symptoms developed suddenly and increased in intensity within 10 minutes of the beginning of the first C symptom noticed in the attack.

E. It cannot be established that an organic factor initiated and maintained the disturbance, e.g., amphetamine or caffeine intoxication, or hyperthyroidism.

Note: Mitral valve prolapse may be an associated condition, but does not preclude a diagnosis of panic disorder.

From *American Psychiatric Association: Diagnostic and statistical manual of mental disorders, third edition-revised,* Washington, DC, 1987, The Association.

tients most commonly complain of shortness of breath, dizziness, palpitations, and sweating, as noted in the *DSM-III-R* criteria presented in the box on p. 128. During a panic attack patients may have a sense of impending doom, a fear of "going crazy," and a profound loss of control. Sometimes these feelings are accompanied by feelings of depersonalization and derealization. Panic may be complicated by anticipatory anxiety, dependency, or more frequently, some degree of agoraphobia (see the box on p. 132).

The patient with panic must be reassured that this condition is not his or her fault and that, in fact, the condition exists as a biologic syndrome. The pharmacologic treatment alternatives for panic disorder are often best combined with other approaches, including behavioral techniques, psychotherapeutic intervention, and an attempt to identify any medical or physiologic contributors. Supportive psychotherapy along with pharmacotherapy may be beneficial, particularly with an emphasis on patient education about the disorder. Caffeine and other contributors to attacks can be identified and discussed with the patient (Charney, Heninger, and Breier, 1984).

Currently the biologic component of panic disorder is hypothesized to be increased sensitivity to augmented noradrenergic function with an impaired presynaptic noradrenergic regulation (Charney, Heninger, and Breier, 1984). An association between the occurrence of mitral valve prolapse and panic disorder has also been made (Liberthson et al., 1986). A subset of patients with atypical panic disorder may show hostility, irritability, severe derealization, and social withdrawal (Edlund, Swann, and Clothier, 1987). These patients may or may not show clear evidence of partial complex seizure disorder but typically show temporal lobe abnormalities on electroencephalogram and may show a therapeutic response to carbamazepine and to the conventional treatments discussed in the following section.

Treatment

Three classes of drugs have proven therapeutically effective in the management of panic disorder. Each class has advantages and disadvantages in the therapeutic profile and in side effects. Two benzodiazepines, alprazolam and clonazepam, have similar disadvantages, namely, the potential to produce excessive drowsiness, tolerance, and physical dependence. Tricyclic and heterocyclic antidepressants may exert an antipanic effect but produce dry mouth, constipation, tachycardia, postural hypotension, and other possible side effects or adverse nontherapeutic effects. MAOIs require dietary restriction and avoidance of certain medications, as noted in Chapter 5. Furthermore, the MAOIs may also produce significant dizziness and postural hypotension. Nevertheless, compared with placebo in patients with panic disorder, with each of these classes of drugs considerable benefit can be derived. Variations in efficacy between one drug and another may be evident between individuals (Ballenger, 1986; Garakani, Zitran, and Klein, 1984; Herman, Rosenbaum, and Brotman, 1987; Sheehan, 1984; Sheehan, Ballenger, and Jacobson, 1980).

The treatment of panic disorder with a benzodiazepine, either alprazolam or clonazepam, may be quite effective or particularly likely to provide immediate relief. Clonazepam has been used for a number of years as an anticonvulsant or an antiepileptic drug adjunct but recently has been employed in the treatment of anxiety disorders (Spier et al., 1986). The side effects and risks of benzodiazepines in general have been discussed. Liver enzyme abnormalities have been reported during treatment with clonazepam, and periodic liver function tests should be considered when high doses or long duration of administration is employed. Alprazolam has recently received an FDA-approved indication for use in patients with panic in a much larger number of controlled studies. However, clonazepam is probably equal or superior to alprazolam in the treatment of panic disorder. Clonazepam, particularly with its longer half-life and slower clearance, may be less likely than alprazolam to result in a withdrawal syndrome upon abrupt discontinuation of the drug after several weeks of treatment. However, the longer half-life and slower clearance of clonazepam may produce a greater cumulative effect, which must be considered in each individual case (Herman, Rosenbaum, and Brotman, 1987).

Clonazepam is likely to be twice as potent as alprazolam and can therefore be administered in smaller daily doses and can be taken once or twice daily, as opposed to the regimen of three or four doses per day for alprazolam. The average antipanic dose of alprazolam is approximately 3 mg per day, but 6 to 8 mg per day may be required to achieve a favorable response. Clonazepam exerts its antipanic effect at a daily dose of approximately 1.5 mg, although patients may require up to 4 to 6 mg daily. With either drug a low dosage should be used initially, with gradual upward titration as tolerated by the patient and as required to achieve symptom control. Alprazolam treatment may be started at a dosage of 0.25 mg three times per day, titrating at 0.25-mg doses every 1 to 3 days. Clonazepam treatment may be started at a dosage of 0.25 mg twice per day, with dosage increments of 0.25 mg every 1 to 2 days as tolerated. Since these benzodiazepines may produce drowsiness and impair performance, patients whose dosage is being titrated should be advised against driving, operating machinery, and the like until a stable dosage is established, at which time the patient is free of significant impairment.

Patients with panic disorder who are receiving a benzodiazepine and who either do not achieve the desired therapeutic response or do not wish to remain on a benzodiazepine regimen may have therapy initiated with another pharmacologic agent. Since tricyclic and heterocyclic antidepressants may lower seizure thresholds and seizures may occur in association with benzodiazepine withdrawal, it is especially important not to make an abrupt switch from a benzodiazepine to a TCA but rather to gradually titrate the benzodiazepine dosage downward as a tricyclic or heterocyclic agent is titrated upward (Fyer et al., 1987). Imipramine and, to a lesser extent, desipramine have been commonly used in the treatment of panic in the United States. Other heterocyclic antidepressants, including amitriptyline and trazodone, have also been reported to have antipanic effects (Mavissakalian et al., 1987; Ballenger, 1986). The dosages generally employed for tricyclic and heterocyclic agents in the treatment of panic are comparable to those used in the management of depressive illness (see Chapter 5). However, a low dosage should be initiated with careful titration, since a paradoxic effect may be observed in some individuals (Klein et al., 1980).

Clinical studies and extensive experience support the use of MAOIs in the treatment of panic. Phenelzine, isocarboxazide, and tranylcypromine have all been used effectively in the management of panic (Sheehan, 1984). Phenelzine is preferred, since it is a hydrazine compound and has less propensity to produce hepatic dysfunction than does isocarboxazide. The nonhydrazine compound, tranylcypromine, does not represent a hepatotoxic risk and is equally effective. In the treatment of panic with MAOIs, heterocyclics, tricyclics, and benzodiazepines alike, 1 to 3 weeks of pharmacotherapy are often required before significant reduction of panic symptoms is achieved.

When MAOIs are employed, it is extremely important that the patient be provided education regarding the dietary and medication restrictions, as previously discussed (see Chapter 5). Patients should receive this education in a nonthreatening and nonfrightening way, since many potential candidates will be terrified of the restrictions and cautions. Nonetheless, patients should be advised to go to the nearest hospital emergency department for evaluation and treatment if they experience a hypertensive reaction. Patients must also be advised and warned about headache, dizziness, and other symptoms that may be secondary to postural hypotension produced by the MAOIs. The patient's ability to monitor blood pressure at home may also be helpful during the course of treatment or when the possibility of elevated blood pressure may become a concern. It is, of course, important to measure each patient's blood pressure before initiating treatment with an MAOI and to monitor the blood pressure and pulse rate. A drop of 10 to 20 mm Hg in systolic pressure may occur in half to two thirds of patients receiving MAOIs (Davidson and Turnbull, 1986). In some cases, moderately severe symptomatic postural hypotension may be counteracted by increased salt intake. The cautious administration of the salt-retaining steroid fluorocortisone in low dosages of 0.05 to 0.1 mg once or twice daily may also be a useful technique.

PHOBIC DISORDERS

Phobic disorders have become more prominent with the increasing ability to provide treatment. The two most common phobic disorders seen in adult psychiatry are agoraphobia, which may occur in association with panic attacks, and social phobia. *Agoraphobia* comes to medical attention as a fear of being in places or situations from which escape may be difficult or embarrassing or places where help may not be readily available. Agoraphobic patients are often frightened to be away from their homes and may remain in the home, avoiding occupational, social, and relationship interactions. Some agoraphobic patients have elaborate schemes such that they leave their homes only in company with a significant other. Many agoraphobic patients attempt to participate in normal life situations and endure intense anxiety during the process. However, the majority of severely agoraphobic patients are unable to travel on public transportation and experience great difficulty in stores, theaters, or other public places. The diagnostic criteria for agoraphobia are shown in the box on p. 132.

Agoraphobic patients with or without panic attacks may benefit from pharmacologic intervention. These patients, like patients with obsessive-compulsive disorder, which is discussed later, may also have depression as a comorbid disorder.

The pharmacologic responsiveness of panic, agoraphobia, and depression, as well as obsessive-compulsive disorder (OCD), suggests that there may be some common denominators in these disorders with respect to underlying neurochemical disturbances. As discussed with panic disorder, patients with agoraphobia or social phobia may be significantly helped by behavioral techniques, including exposure and other types of interventions. These are particularly effective when combined with pharmacologic intervention (Mavissakalian and Michelson, 1986). In most instances, optimizing the medical and physiologic status of the patient enhances responsivity to pharmacologic intervention and may also be combined with psychotherapeutic interventions, including supportive or cognitive therapy.

Treatment

Pharmacologic approach to agoraphobia has generally included the use of benzodiazepines, heterocyclic antidepressants, and MAOIs. As with panic, alprazolam at relatively high doses, between 3 and 6 mg per day, may be effective. Imipramine alone or in combination with behavioral techniques has been reported to be highly beneficial in the treatment of agoraphobia (Mavissakalian and Perel, 1985).

Whereas patients with panic may be responsive to low doses of TCAs or may require higher doses, patients with agoraphobia may also respond to low doses but for the most part conventional doses of tricyclic or heterocyclic drugs are required, that

Diagnostic Criteria for Agoraphobia

Agoraphobia: Fear of being in places or situations from which escape might be difficult (or embarrassing) or in which help might not be available in the event of a panic attack. (Includes cases in which persistent avoidance behavior originated during an active phase of panic disorder, even if the person does not attribute the avoidance behavior to fear of having a panic attack.) As a result of this fear, the person either restricts travel or needs a companion when away from home, or else endures agoraphobic situations despite intense anxiety. Common agoraphobic situations include being outside the home alone, being in a crowd or standing in a line, being on a bridge, and traveling in a bus, train, or car.

Specify current severity of agoraphobic avoidance:

Mild: Some avoidance (or endurance with distress), but relatively normal life-style, e.g., travels unaccompanied when necessary, such as to work or to shop; otherwise avoids traveling alone.

Moderate: Avoidance results in constricted life-style, e.g., the person is able to leave the house alone, but not to go more than a few miles unaccompanied.

Severe: Avoidance results in being nearly or completely housebound or unable to leave the house unaccompanied.

In partial remission: No current agoraphobic avoidance, but some agoraphobic avoidance during the past 6 months.

In full remission: No current agoraphobic avoidance and none during the past 6 months.

Specify current severity of panic attacks:

Mild: During the past month, either all attacks have been limited symptom attacks (i.e., fewer than four symptoms), or there has been no more than one panic attack.

Moderate: During the past month attacks have been intermediate between "mild" and "severe."

Severe: During the past month, there have been at least eight panic attacks.

In partial remission: The condition has been intermediate between "In Full Remission" and "Mild."

In full remission: During the past six months, there have been no panic or limited symptom attacks.

From American Psychiatric Association: *Diagnostic and statistical manual of mental disorders, third edition-revised,* Washington, DC, 1987, The Association.

is, between 150 and 200 mg per day. Other heterocyclic antidepressants, including clomipramine, amitriptyline, and trazodone, are particularly effective in patients with agoraphobia but not as extensively studied as imipramine (Sheehan, 1984; Gloger et al., 1981).

MAOIs, particularly phenelzine, have demonstrated their utility in effective treatment of agoraphobia (Phol, Berchou, and Rainey, 1982). Bernstein (1987) suggested that MAOIs in agoraphobic patients may produce greater relief of symptoms than do other anxiolytics; however, the disadvantages of dietary and medication restrictions and the potential for postural hypotension must be considered carefully in each case.

Social phobia is a fairly common and limiting disorder characterized by persistent fear of situations in which one is exposed to the scrutiny of others; the patient with social phobia may be responsive to pharmacologic interventions with benzodiazepines such as alprazolam, used alone or in combination with beta-blocking drugs. Generally, establishing an effective pharmacologic regimen and response should precede any encouragement or effort to return the patient to normal function in all spheres of life. Many patients are responsive to beta-blocking agents such as propranolol in dosages of 10 to 20 mg three to four times a day, metaprolol in dosages of 25 to 50 mg twice daily, or atenolol in dosages of 50 to 100 mg once daily (Liebowitz et al., 1987; Gorman et al., 1985). Beta blockers may also be used in conjunction with alprazolam at low doses. Obviously, a careful history and assessment of blood pressure, pulse rate, heart, and lungs should precede the use of beta-adrenergic blocking agents. The histories of congestive heart failure, cardiac arrhythmia, and chronic obstructive pulmonary disease with asthma do pose a contraindication to treatment with beta-adrenergic blocking drugs.

Several studies have documented the therapeutic efficacy of MAOIs, primarily phenelzine, in the treatment of social phobia (Liebowitz et al., 1985). Treatment of social phobia with MAOIs should be used in conventional antidepressant doses, as previously discussed. Buspirone, which has demonstrated efficacy in the treatment of generalized anxiety and mixed anxiety-depression, is largely free of sedating or dependency-producing effects. However, buspirone has not been documented to be particularly effective in either panic, agoraphobia, or social phobia (Olajide and Lader, 1987). Nonetheless, this compound may be particularly useful in the treatment of anticipatory anxiety or may be useful when the patient is being provided with behavioral therapy techniques, such as exposure or desensitization.

OBSESSIVE-COMPULSIVE DISORDER

Individuals with OCD may experience both obsessions and compulsions, and either may occur individually. Current criteria as defined by *DSM-III-R* are listed in the box on page 134. In patients with OCD these symptoms worsen when coexisting symptoms of depression develop. As previously mentioned, the effect of antidepressant drugs in the treatment of OCD lends further support to the possibility that this condition shares some common neurochemical or neurobiologic disturbance with depression. In general, obsessions represent recurrent and persistent ideas, thoughts, impulses, or images that are experienced as intrusive or senseless.

Treatment

Both TCAs and MAOIs have proven to be the most effective therapeutic agents in the treatment of OCD. More recently buspirone has emerged as an alternative treatment (Mavissakalian, 1985; Jenike, Armentano, and Baer, 1987; Pato, 1990). Alprazolam may also be useful in the treatment of this condition (Tesar and Jenike, 1984). However, benzodiazepines may significantly exacerbate the symptoms of OCD while as the patient is feeling uncomfortable with sedation and other side effects; patients with coexisting symptoms of depression are much more likely to benefit from the use of an antidepressant or an MAOI. Neuroleptic medications may be useful for the treatment of hallucinations. Lithium may be occasionally found to be therapeutic either alone or as an adjunct. Conventional antidepressants remain the preferred pharmacologic agents (Tesar and Jenike, 1984; Stern and Jenike, 1983; Pies, 1984).

Clomipramine (Anafranil) at a dose of approximately 100 to 150 mg per day or

Diagnostic Criteria for 300.30 Obsessive-Compulsive Disorder

A. Either obsessions or compulsions:

Obsessions: (1), (2), (3), and (4):

(1) Recurrent and persistent ideas, thoughts, impulses, or images that are experienced, at least initially, as intrusive and senseless, e.g., a parent's having repeated impulses to kill a loved child, a religious person's having recurrent blasphemous thoughts

(2) The person attempts to ignore or suppress such thoughts or impulses or to neutralize them with some other thought or action

(3) The person recognizes that the obsessions are the product of his or her own mind, not imposed from without (as in thought insertion)

(4) If another Axis I disorder is present, the content of the obsession is unrelated to it, e.g., the ideas, thoughts, impulses, or images are not about food in the presence of an eating disorder, about drugs in the presence of a psychoactive substance use disorder, or guilty thoughts in the presence of a major depression

Compulsions: (1), (2), and (3):

(1) Repetitive, purposeful, and intentional behaviors that are performed in response to an obsession, or according to certain rules or in a stereotyped fashion

(2) The behavior is designed to neutralize or to prevent discomfort or some dreaded event or situation; however, either the activity is not connected in a realistic way with what it is designed to neutralize or prevent, or it is clearly excessive

(3) The person recognizes that his or her behavior is excessive or unreasonable (this may not be true for young children; it may no longer be true for people whose obsessions have evolved into overvalued ideas)

B. The obsessions or compulsions cause marked distress, are time-consuming (take more than an hour a day), or significantly interfere with the person's normal routine, occupational functioning, or usual social activities or relationships with others.

From American Psychiatric Association: *Diagnostic and statistical manual of mental disorders, third edition-revised,* Washington, DC, 1987, The Association.

fluoxetine at a dose of approximately 40 to 80 mg per day is perhaps the best potent antiobsessional agent. Clomipramine is a relatively selective serotonin reuptake inhibitor. Fluoxetine is a potent SSRI. Sertraline and other SSRIs being developed may also be effective in treating OCD. Recent evidence suggests that buspirone has efficacy either alone or as an adjunct in the treatment of OCD (Pato, 1990). Imipramine has also been studied in a number of clinical trials involving OCD and may also be effective at a dose of 150 to 200 mg per day. Excessive tremors, sweating, and other manifestations of serotonergic action may result in intolerable side effects (Insel et al., 1983).

Clomipramine is not a pure serotonin reuptake inhibitor, and its active metabolite desmethylclomipramine, a potent inhibitor of norepinephrine, may also account for its clinical efficacy (Asberg, Thoren, and Bertilsson, 1982). Three other carefully controlled double-blind studies using clomipramine have indicated its preferential effectiveness in reducing obsessional symptoms (Montgomery, 1980; Ananth et al., 1979; Insel et al., 1983). The treatment effect of clomipramine may not be fully apparent until 5 to 10 weeks after treatment. Plasma level determinations may be helpful in avoiding doses that are too high or low, both of which seem to be connected to poor outcome (Asberg, Thoren, and Bertilsson, 1982). Combining clomipramine with behavioral exposure treatment is desirable, and treatment is generally prolonged over several years. With the exception of dental problems that result from the reduced production of saliva, which can be avoided by careful mouth hygiene, no serious long-term effects have been described with clomipramine. In any event, heterocyclics, with clomipramine being the drug of choice, are clearly indicated in a depressed patient with OCD and may continue to be the drugs of first choice, even in nondepressed obsessional patients.

There are no controlled studies using MAOIs in patients with OCD. However, many case reports have alluded to favorable response (Jenike, Baer, and Minichiello, 1986). Generally the MAOIs may be particularly effective in patients with OCD who have associated panic or severe anxiety.

Some patients with OCD are responsive to lithium and may in fact have an underlying cyclothymia or manic depressive illness (Stern and Jenike, 1983). Likewise, antipsychotic agents may be useful in patients with psychotic symptoms. However, anxiolytic agents, in particular, alprazolam, possibly in part because of its antidepressant effects, may be successful in some patients with mixed anxiety-depression. Furthermore, as suggested for panic, patients may also be responsive to alprazolam, since it acts as an anticonvulsant. However, as with lithium and antipsychotic agents, anxiolytics have not been extensively studied.

Electroconvulsive therapy is generally regarded as not useful in the treatment of OCD. Although a link between depression and OCD may be present, ECT has not been found to be effective and there are not reports of success in patients who have classic OCD with rituals and the like. Many patients with OCD have had psychosurgery when severe illness is present and multiple therapeutic approaches have failed. The results of surgical intervention are impressive. A discussion of this topic, however, is beyond the scope of this text.

POSTTRAUMATIC STRESS DISORDER

Although numerous articles have discussed the characteristics of PTSD, little has been written about the pharmacotherapy of this syndrome. Posttraumatic stress disorder has been associated primarily with combat experience but occurs in other situations in which individuals are exposed to overwhelming stress, such as rape, robbery, and disasters affecting themselves, their families, or others with whom they have close relationships.

Treatment

There is yet no significant experience with the potential utility of buspirone in the treatment of PTSD, but buspirone may prove to be beneficial in view of its lack of ability to cause disinhibition or dependence. Some similarities between PTSD and panic disorder suggest the possible utility of TCAs and MAOIs. These drugs have been shown to be effective in patients who are able to comply with medical regimen and abstain from alcohol use (Falcon et al., 1985; van der Kolk, 1983). Lithium has been found to be effective in some patients with PTSD. Beta-adrenergic blocking drugs may also blunt some of the autonomic symptoms or autonomic arousal that occurs. Carbamazepine may be useful in decreasing impulsivity (Bernstein, 1987).

MIXED ANXIETY-DEPRESSION

Primary-care patients and patients in outpatient mental health and cross-cultural settings do not often meet full syndromal criteria for a mood or anxiety disorder. Nonetheless, patients seek medical advice with a mixed picture of mood and anxiety disturbance. In aggregate these syndromes appear to cause functional impairment or distress, or both. Currently referred to as a subthreshold disorder, mixed anxiety-depression may emerge as a disorder in future diagnostic schemata. The diagnosis of mixed anxiety-depression may simply be applied for individuals in whom diagnostic criteria are not clearly identified either because of the setting or because of the brevity of the assessment.

Treatment

Mixed anxiety-depression disorders are generally responsive to anxiolytics, especially alprazolam or buspirone, or to sedating antidepressants, that is, imipramine. Alprazolam or other benzodiazepines are best reserved for cases in which anxiety is overriding or related to situational factors. The distinct disadvantages of the benzodiazepines, that is, the potential for sedation and impairment of cognition or motor functioning, together with the potential for addiction, dependence, and withdrawal, must be carefully considered.

REFERENCES

American Psychiatric Association: *Diagnostic and statistical manual of mental disorders, third edition-revised,* Washington, DC, 1987, The Association.

American Psychiatric Association: *Diagnostic and statistical manual of mental disorders, fourth edition, options book: work in progress,* Task Force on *DSM-IV,* Washington, DC, 1991, The Association.

Ananth J et al: Clomipramine therapy for obsessive-compulsive neurosis, *Am J Psychiatry* 136:700, 1979.

Asberg M, Thoren P, Bertilsson L: Psychopharmacologic treatment of obsessive-compulsive disorder: clomipramine treatment of obsessive disorder, biochemical and clinical aspects, *Psychopharmacol Bull* 18:13, 1982.

Baldessarini RJ: *Chemotherapy in psychiatry,* Cambridge, Mass, 1985, Harvard University.

Ballenger JC: Pharmacotherapy of the panic disorders, *J Clin Psychiatry* 47(suppl 6):27, 1986.

Bernstein JG: Lithium and other mood-stabilizing drugs. In Hackett TP, Cassem NH, editors: *Massachusetts General Hospital handbook of general hospital psychiatry,* ed 2, Littleton, Mass, 1987, PSG.

Bristol-Myers Squibb: Personal communication, 1991.

Carruthers SG et al: Correlation between plasma diphenhydramine level and sedative and antihistamine effects, *Clin Pharmacol Ther* 23:375, 1978.

Charney DS, Heninger GR, Breier A: Noradrenergic function in panic anxiety, *Arch Gen Psychiatry* 41:751, 1984.

Davidson J, Turnbull CD: The effects of isocarboxazid on blood pressure, *J Clin Psychopharmacol* 6:139, 1986.

Domantay AG, Napoliello MJ: Buspirone for elderly anxious patients, *Int Med Certif* 3:1, 1989.

Edlund MJ, Swann AC, Clothier J: Patients with panic attacks and abnormal EEG results, *Am J Psychiatry* 144:508, 1987.

Enna SJ: Role of gamma-aminobutyric acid in anxiety, *Psychopathology* 17:15, 1984.

Falcon S et al: Tricyclics: possible treatment for post-traumatic stress disorder, *J Clin Psychiatry* 46:385, 1985.

Feighner JP, Merideth CH, Hendrickson RM: A double-blind comparison of buspirone and diazepam in outpatients with generalized anxiety disorder, *J Clin Psychiatry* 43:102, 1982.

Feighner JP et al: Comparison of alprazolam, imipramine and placebo in the treatment of depression, *JAMA* 249:3057, 1983.

Folks DG: Clinical approaches to anxiety in the medically ill elderly, *Drug Ther Suppl* p 72, August 1990.

Fyer AS et al: Discontinuation of alprazolam treatment in panic patients, *Am J Psychiatry* 144:303, 1987.

Gammans RE, Mayol RF, LaBudde JA: Metabolism and disposition of buspirone, *Am J Med* 80(suppl 3B):41, 1986.

Garakani H, Zitran CM, Klein DF: Treatment of panic disorder with imipramine alone, *Am J Psychiatry* 141:446, 1984.

Gardos G et al: Differential actions of chlordiazepoxide and oxazepam on hostility, *Arch Gen Psychiatry* 18:757, 1968.

Gloger S et al: Treatment of spontaneous panic attacks with clomipramine, *Am J Psychiatry* 138:1215, 1981.

Goodman WK, Charney DS: A case of alprazolam, but not lorazepam, inducing manic symptoms, *J Clin Psychiatry* 48:117, 1987.

Gorman JM et al: Treatment of social phobia with atenolol, *J Clin Psychopharmacol* 5:298, 1985.

Hall RCW, Zisook S: Paradoxical reactions to benzodiazepines, *Br J Clin Pharmacol* 11:995, 1981.

Harvey SC: Hypnotics and sedatives. In Gilman AG, Goodman LS, Rall TW, editors: *The pharmacological basis of therapeutics*, ed 7, New York, 1985, Macmillan.

Herman JB, Rosenbaum JF, Brotman AW: The alprazolam-to-clonazepam switch for the treatment of panic disorder, *J Clin Psychopharmacol* 7:175, 1987.

Insel TR et al: Obsessive-compulsive disorder: a double-blind trial of clomipramine and clorgyline, *Arch Gen Psychiatry* 40:605, 1983.

Jenike MA, Armentano ME, Baer L: Disabling obsessive thoughts responsive to antidepressants, *J Clin Psychopharmacol* 7:33, 1987.

Jenike MA, Baer L, Minichiello WE: *Obsessive-compulsive disorders: theory and management*, St Louis, 1986, Mosby.

Klein DF et al: *Diagnosis and drug treatment of psychiatric disorders: adults and children*, ed 2, Baltimore, 1980, Williams & Wilkins.

Kranzler HR: Buspirone treatment of anxiety in a patient dependent on alprazolam, *J Clin Psychopharmacol* 9:153, 1989.

Kumar R et al: Anxiolytics and memory: a comparison of lorazepam and alprazolam, *J Clin Psychiatry* 48:158, 1987.

Liberthson R et al: The prevalence of mitral valve prolapse in patients with panic disorders, *Am J Psychiatry* 143:511, 1986.

Liebowitz MR et al: Social phobia, *Arch Gen Psychiatry* 42:729, 1985.

Liebowitz MR et al: Alprazolam in the treatment of panic disorders, *J Clin Psychopharmacol* 6:13, 1986.

Liebowitz MR et al: Pharmacotherapy of social phobia, *Psychosomatics* 28:305, 1987.

Mavissakalian M, Michelson L: Two-year follow-up of exposure and imipramine treatment of agoraphobia, *Am J Psychiatry* 143:1106, 1986.

Mavissakalian M, Perel J: Imipramine in the treatment of agoraphobia: dose-response relationships, *Am J Psychiatry* 142:1032, 1985.

Mavissakalian M et al: Tricyclic antidepressants in obsessive-compulsive disorder: antiobsessional or antidepressant agents? *Am J Psychiatry* 142:572, 1985.

Mavissakalian M et al: Trazodone in the treatment of panic disorder and agoraphobia with panic attacks, *Am J Psychiatry* 144:785, 1987

Montgomery SA: Clomipramine in obsessional neurosis: a placebo-controlled trial, *Pharmacol Med* 1:189, 1980.

Neppe VM: Buspirone: an auxioselective neuromodulator. In: VM Neppe, editor: *Innovative psychopharmacotherapy*, New York, 1989, Raven.

Noyes R et al: Diazepam and propranolol in panic disorder and agoraphobia, *Arch Gen Psychiatry* 41:387, 1984.

Olajide D, Lader M: A comparison of buspirone, diazepam, and placebo in patients with chronic anxiety states, *J Clin Psychopharmacol* 7:148, 1987.

Pato MT: Treatment of obsessive-compulsive disorder with serotonergic agents, *Drug Ther Suppl* p 122, August 1990.

Phol R, Berchou R, Rainey JM: Tricyclic antidepressants and monoamine oxidase inhibitors in the treatment of agoraphobia, *J Clin Psychopharmacol* 2:399, 1982.

Pies R: Distinguishing obsessional from psychotic phenomena, *J Clin Psychopharmacol* 4:345, 1984.

Rakel RE: Mixed anxiety-depression. *Drug Ther Supple* p 137, August 1990.

Riblett LA et al: Pharmacology and neurochemistry of buspirone, *J Clin Psychiatry* 43:11, 1982.

Rickels K et al: Buspirone and diazepam in anxiety: a controlled study, *J Clin Psychiatry* 43:81, 1982.

Sheehan DV: The treatment of panic and phobic disorders. In Bernstein JC, editor: *Clinical psychopharmacology,* ed 2, Boston, 1984, John Wright-PSG.

Sheehan DV, Ballenger J, Jacobson G: Treatment of endogenous anxiety with phobic, hysterical, and hypochondriacal symptoms, *Arch Gen Psychiatry* 37:51, 1980.

Schuckit MA: Clinical studies of buspirone, *Psychopathology* 17(suppl 3):61, 1984.

Spier S et al: Clonazepam in the treatment of panic disorder and agoraphobia, *J Clin Psychiatry* 47:238-242, 1986.

Stern TA, Jenike MA: Treatment of obsessive-compulsive disorder with lithium carbonate, *Psychosomatics* 24:671, 1983.

Tesar GE, Jenike MA: Alprazolam as treatment for a case of obsessive-compulsive disorders, *Am J Psychiatry* 141:689, 1984.

van der Kolk BA: Psychopharmacological issues in post-traumatic stress disorder, *Hosp Community Psychiatry* 34:683, 1983.

CHAPTER 7

Seizure Disorders

Drugs used to treat seizure disorders have been traditionally referred to as anticonvulsants. Current preferred usage is moving toward classifying these drugs as antiepileptics. Epilepsy is the most common seizure disorder, and according to McKenna, Kane, and Parrish (1985), about 7% of the patients diagnosed as having epilepsy have a persistent psychosis. When compared with the 1% to 4% range for psychosis found among patients with posttraumatic stress disorder (PTSD), (Boudewyns et al., 1991), this level of comorbidity is striking. When this level of disorder (7%) is compared with the morbidity rate for schizophrenia in the general population (about 1%), it appears that a relationship exists between epilepsy and psychosis (Trimble, 1991). Since seizure disorders among a psychiatric population are not uncommon, antiepileptic drug information is an important part of both the mental health and the primary care clinicians' resources.

EPILEPSY

Epilepsy is a condition in which abnormal electrical activity in the brain occurs. The abnormal electrical activity has varying effects, hence several distinguishable forms of epilepsy are recognizable. The incidence of epilepsy is thought to be between 0.5% and 2.0% of the population. Onset is most common during childhood or after 50 years of age; however, onset is not limited to these particular development stages. Epilepsies may be broadly categorized as either acquired (i.e., caused by brain injury, meningitis, acute alcohol withdrawal, anoxia, stroke, fevers, toxic substances, etc.) or idiopathic (cause unknown). The extent of genetic influence is not known, but even clinicians who are prone to look for environmental factors in other illnesses consent to genetic predisposition for epilepsy. Treatment is aimed at controlling seizure activity; for many individuals this entails a lifelong dependence on antiepileptic therapy.

Categories of Seizures

Epileptic seizures are grouped according to characteristic physical and neurologic signs (Table 7-1). Each subtype also has a characteristic electroencephalogram (EEG) pattern. Seizures are divided into the two broad categories, partial seizures and generalized seizures (Barry and Teixeira, 1985). The diagnosis of each of these seizure types can be refined to include several subtypes.

Partial seizures. Partial seizures are more common than generalized seizures, accounting for approximately 70% of all seizures in adults and 40% of all seizures in children. By definition partial seizures typically begin in a focal area. Abnormal brain activity can spread to other parts of that cerebral hemisphere or even to the other hemisphere (Delgado-Escueta, Treiman, and Walsh, 1983). Partial seizure subtypes

Table 7-1 Major Characteristics of Epileptic Seizures, Based on International Classification

Seizure type	Comments
Partial seizures (focal or local)	Most common seizure type (accounts for about 70% of adults and 40% of children with epilepsy); EEG changes initially are localized, may evolve into other seizure types
Simple partial seizures	Typically no loss of consciousness; motor symptoms (jacksonian); sensory symptoms (visual, auditory, gustatory, and hallucinations) and somatosensory symptoms (tingling); autonomic symptoms (pallor, sweating, vomiting, and flushing)
Complex partial seizures	Consciousness is impaired at onset of seizure or later, after onset of simple partial seizure
Partial seizures evolving to generalized tonic-clonic seizures	
Generalized seizures	Involve symmetric (both hemispheres) distribution of abnormal brain discharge; bilateral motor changes; consciousness may be totally impaired
Nonconvulsive seizures	
Absence seizures	Abrupt loss of consciousness, usually lasting <10 sec; usually begin in childhood, often stop spontaneously during teenage years; mild clonic component; atonic component: diminution of muscle tone; automatisms; autonomic components
Myoclonic seizures	Single or multiple jerks, typically lasting 3-10 sec; sudden, brief, shocklike contractions, generalized or confined
Atonic seizures	Sudden diminution of muscle tone ("drop attacks")
Convulsive seizures	
Clonic seizures	Occur mostly in childhood; generalized convulsive seizures lacking tonic component; characterized by clonic jerks; postictal phase typically short
Tonic seizures	Sustained contraction of large muscles; continuous tension of chest musculature impairs ventilation and causes pallor or more serious problems if prolonged
Tonic-clonic	Consciousness lost abruptly; series of muscle spasms lasting 3-5 min from onset to recovery; postictal state may last from a few minutes to about half an hour; often characterized by confusion, dizziness, sleepiness, and "glazed" look
Status epilepticus	Could apply to any prolonged or repetitive seizure, but best applied to repetitive or fused tonic-clonic seizures; a medical emergency requiring immediate drug intervention to prevent brain damage or death resulting from impaired ventilation; only seizure for which there is no contraindication to drug use
Unclassified epileptic seizures	Includes all seizures that cannot be classified, whether because of inadequate or incomplete criteria or characteristics

Modified from Commission on Classification and Terminology of the International League Against Epilepsy: *Epilepsia* 22:489, 1981.

include simple partial seizures, complex partial seizures, and partial seizures evolving to generalized tonic-clonic seizures.

Simple partial seizures. Simple partial seizures do not impair consciousness, and since electrical abnormality is localized, symptoms depend on the area affected. Motor symptoms include localized jerks, focal jerks that "march" to involve other muscle (sometimes referred to as jacksonian seizures), and speech involvement. Sensory symptoms (visual, auditory, gustatory, and hallucinations) and somatosensory symptoms (i.e., tingling) also develop. Autonomic symptoms such as pallor, sweating, vomiting, flushing, tachycardia, hypotension, and hypertension are distressing to patients.

Complex partial seizures. Complex partial seizures are also known as psychomotor or temporal lobe epilepsy. Consciousness is impaired, and violent behavior may be a major component of seizure activity. Complex partial seizures typically begin as a perceived aura. A number of cognitive, affective, perceptive, and psychomotor symptoms can occur. Deja vu, fear and anxiety, hallucinations, and automatic behaviors (automatism) are commonly present.

Generalized seizures. Generalized seizures involve a symmetric distribution of abnormal electrical activity in the brain. Generalized seizures include a number of nonconvulsive seizures that primarily cause unresponsiveness and amnesia and convulsive seizures that cause unconsciousness and major convulsions. Nonconvulsive seizures include absence seizures, myoclonic seizures, and atonic seizures. Major motor tonic-clonic seizures and status epilepticus are major types of convulsive seizure.

Absence seizures. Absence seizures are characterized by a sudden loss of responsiveness. Often the loss of consciousness is so brief (10 seconds) that those around the person are unaware of a change. A variant of absence seizure is the true petit mal seizure, which produces a distinct three-per-second spike-and-wave EEG patten. These seizures typically start in childhood and remit during the teenage years (Norman and Browne, 1981).

Convulsive seizures. Tonic-clonic convulsions (also called grand mal seizures) are characterized by intense, repetitive tonic-clonic contractions of the whole body. Abnormal brain activity is symmetric, with most brain pathways involved. Seizures may last only a few minutes, but prolonged seizure activity can result in brain hypoxia. A number of other physical consequences may result.

Status epilepticus is a seizure type in which tonic-clonic convulsions occur successively without intervals of restored consciousness or normal muscle movement. Brain damage can occur as a result of prolonged hypoxia. Status epilepticus is a medical emergency requiring immediate attention (Delgado-Escueta et al., 1982).

ANTIEPILEPTIC DRUGS

The straightforward goals for antiepileptic treatment are as follows: (1) Control seizure activity, (2) keep side effects that result from antiepileptic therapy to a minimum, and (3) attempt maintenance with a regimen of one drug (monotherapy), if possible. Five categories of antiepileptic drugs may be distinguished; when these are added to noncategorized drugs called "other antiepileptics," a substantial number of individual drugs are at the clinician's disposal. The five major categories are the hydantoins, the long-acting barbiturates, the succinimides, the oxazolidinediones, and the benzodiazepines. The "other antiepileptics" group includes promising drugs such as carbamazepine, valproic acid (Depakene), and rarely used anticonvulsants such as lidocaine. Some of the drugs have rather broad indications; others have limited application. For instance, phenacemide is used only for complex partial seizures and then only after the disorder has proven refractory to safer drugs. Antiepileptic drugs may also be categorized according to their presumed mechanisms of action.

Careful medical evaluation is needed before an antiepileptic is prescribed. Based on an evaluation that includes the analysis of the EEG, a specific seizure type may be identified and an antiepileptic drug selected. The choice of the antiepileptic drug is based on the following considerations:

Size of the patient
Expense of the drug
Allergic response to the drug, if any
Child-bearing potential
Tolerance of side effects

Table 7-2 Seizure Types Matched with Appropriate Antiepileptic Agents

Antiepileptic agents	Tonic-clonic	Absence (petit mal)	Simple partial (focal)	Complex partial (psychomotor)	Status epilepticus
Hydantoins					
Ethotoin	X	—	—	X	—
Mephenytoin	X(R)	—	X(R)	X(R)	—
Phenytoin	DOC	—	X	X	2
Barbiturates					
Mephobarbital	X	X	—	—	—
Metharbital	X	X	—	—	—
Phenobarbital	2	—	X	X	2,3
Primidone	2	—	X	X	—
Succinimides					
Ethosuximide		DOC			
Methosuximide		2			
Phensuximide		X(R)			
Benzodiazepines					
Clonazepam		2*	—	—	—
Diazepam		—	—	—	DOC
Other antiepileptics					
Acetazolamide	X	2	—	—	—
Carbamazepine	DOC	—	—	2	—
Lidocaine†	—	—	—	—	X(R)
Magnesium sulfate‡	—	—	—	—	—
Paraldehyde§	—	—	—	—	—
Phenacemide	—	—	—	X(R)	—
Trimethadione	—	X(R)	—	—	—
Valproic acid	DOC	DOC	—	X	—

DOC, Drug of choice; *2*, second-choice drug; *3*, third-choice drug; *(R)*, used when seizures are refractory to other drugs; *X*, may be used.
*Includes Lennox-Gestaut seizures.
†Used as a last choice for refractory status epilepticus.
‡Used for seizures related to magnesium deficiency.
§Used for seizures related to alcohol withdrawal.

General Rules for Using Antiepileptics

1. When possible (i.e., when there is not great urgency, as there is during status epilepticus), start with a low dose and gradually increase until a steady therapeutic blood level of the drug is reached. For example, an initial dose should be one fourth to one third the recommended therapeutic dose. This incremental approach is important with carbamazepine, valproic acid, and primidone and is less important with phenytoin and phenobarbital.
2. Give antiepileptics on time, to achieve a steady state and then to maintain the drug's therapeutic effect.*
3. Understand that drug dosage varies among individuals; accordingly each dosage must also be individualized.
4. Understand the patient's history, including baseline pretreatment laboratory test results.
5. When an antiepileptic is to be discontinued, do so gradually, to decrease the possibility of withdrawal-related seizures, i.e., status epilepticus.† Other caregivers should be made aware of the patient's drug regimen so that they may provide fully informed care of their own.
6. Monitor the patient's laboratory results, including serum drug levels, hematologic responses to drugs, and trough levels.‡ (Pellock, Willmore, 1991). Indications for drawing serum levels include therapeutic failure, noncompliance (may be as high as 50%), toxicity, and drug interactions. In general, serum drug level determinations are overused.
7. Attempt to use a single drug, if possible. Patients receiving combination therapy have twice as many adverse responses as patient's who receive one antiepileptic, i.e., monotherapy.

*From Woodward ES: *J Neurosurg Nurs* 14:166, 1982.
†From Callaghan N, Garrett A, Goggin T: *New Engl J Med* 318(15):942, 1988.
‡From Pellock JM, Willmore LJ: *Neurology* 41(7):961, 1991.

For example, more than one drug may control seizure activity but a preferred drug may be better tolerated. Since more than one seizure type may be present, determining whether a given drug might exacerbate a particular seizure pattern is a secondary consideration in selecting the correct antiepileptic. Table 7-2 matches seizure type with an appropriate antiepileptic agent. The box above gives guidelines for the use of antiepileptics.

In the following discussion a prototype drug from each of the five classes of antiepileptics will be highlighted, as well as significant drugs from the "other antiepileptics" group of drugs. Table 7-3 presents examples of antiepileptic drugs and their proposed mechanisms of action.

HYDANTOINS: PROTOTYPE DRUG, PHENYTOIN

Historically hydantoins have been considered the most effective antiepileptics. Hydantoins are particularly effective in the treatment of tonic-clonic and complex partial seizures. Phenytoin (Dilantin) is the most widely used hydantoin, but two other hy-

Table 7-3 Antiepileptic Drugs and Proposed Mechanisms of Action

Drug	Mechanism of action
Phenytoin	1
Carbamazepine	1
Phenobarbital	2
Primidone	1
Valproate	1,3
Ethosuximide	5
Benzodiazepines	6
Acetazolamide	6

Mechanisms of action

1. Modify Na^+, Ca^{++} conductances: Limit sustained high-frequency discharges
2. Prolong GABA-mediated synaptic inhibition: Depress neural activity preferentially in limbic brain
3. Depress neuronal activity; other mechanisms uncertain
4. Augment GABA-mediated synaptic inhibition i.e., Cl^- channel
5. Uncertain mechanisms
6. Carbonic anhydrase inhibitor

GABA, Gamma-aminobutyric acid.

dantoins, ethotoin and mephenytoin are available. Since hydantoins controlled seizures without causing sedation, it became apparent that central nervous system (CNS) depression was not a prerequisite for seizure control.

Pharmacologic Effects

The main site of action of hydantoins is in the motor cortex. Phenytoin inhibits the spread of abnormal brain electrical activity by normalizing abnormal fluxes of sodium across the nerve cell membrane during or after depolarization. This inhibition stabilizes a state of hyperexcitability. Hydantoins also decrease the activity of brain stem centers responsible for the tonic phase of grand mal seizures. Phenytoin also depresses cardiac electrical conduction, and this effect is used for therapeutic purposes in patients with arrhythmias.

Pharmacokinetics

Phenytoin is slowly absorbed from the gut after oral administration. The bioavailability can vary as much as 10% to 90% among the different brands of phenytoin. Peak serum levels are reached in 1.5 to 3 hours when the promptly absorbed form is used; the extended-acting form reaches peak levels in 4 to 12 hours. The therapeutic serum level is 10 to 20 μg/ml (Penry and Newmark, 1979). Four to 7 days of use is needed before a steady state is reached, because of the average half-life of 22 hours; however, the half-life is dose dependent and has little clinical importance. Phenytoin is seldom administered by intramuscular (IM) injection because it is stored in tissue and released slowly. Absorption can take up to 5 days, which necessitates a 50% dosage adjustment when switching between oral and intramuscular modes of administration. When switching from oral to intramuscular modes the dosage must be increased by 50%. When switching from intramuscular to oral routes, the dosage must be decreased

Table 7-4 Pharmacokinetic Comparison of Major Antiepileptics

Agent	Time to steady state (days)	Therapeutic serum levels (μg/ml)	Toxic blood level (μg/ml)	Half-life (hr)	Protein-bound (%)
Hydantoin					
Phenytoin	7-10	10-20	>20	7-42†	87-93
Barbiturates					
Phenobarbital	16-21	15-40	>40	80 (before increased hepatic metabolism rate is induced)	40-60
Primidone*	1-5	5-12	>12	3-12	0-50
Succinimide					
Ethosuximide	5-10	40-100	>100	30-60 (adult); 30 (child)	0
Benzodiazepines					
Clonazepam	3-7	20-80 nanograms	>80 nanograms	18-50	80
Other antiepileptics					
Valproic acid	2-4	50-100	>100	6-16	90
Carbamazepine	2-4	4-12	>12	12-17	76

*When primidone is administered, phenobarbital levels must also be measured. With therapeutic primidone doses, phenobarbital levels should be 10-30 μg/ml.
†Half-life increases as serum level increases.

by 50%. Table 7-4 compares the pharmacokinetics of the major antiepileptics.

Phenytoin is metabolized in the liver and excreted in the urine. A small amount (1% to 5%) is excreted unchanged. High serum levels can occur at "normal" doses when the patient has impaired liver function or congenital deficiencies in enzymes that break down phenytoin or when the patient is taking other drugs that interfere with phenytoin metabolism. Obviously, if the health care provider does not understand the difference in oral and parenteral forms of the drug, overdosing or underdosing can occur. Plasma protein binding is 87% to 93%. Table 7-5 summarizes dosages for antiepileptic agents.

Oral administration. Phenytoin is available for oral administration in tablets, capsules, and suspensions and in pediatric and extended-acting forms. The extended-acting form is the only one available for once-per-day dosage. Oral therapy in adults usually begins with a dosage of 100 mg three times per day. However, a loading dose of 1 g (given over 4 hours) can be given to hospitalized patients with good hepatic functioning. If a person remains seizure free on the 100-mg three-times-per-day regimen, extended-acting capsules may replace the former approach. An apparent advantage of once-a-day dosage is increased compliance; however, a forgotten dose

Text continued on p. 150.

Table 7-5 Dosage for Selected Antiepileptics

Drug and clinical indication	Dosage
Hydantoins	
Phenytoin (Dilantin)	
Tonic-clonic and complex partial seizures	*Oral:* Adults: 100-200 mg tid or qid; Dilantin Kapseals (extended form) can be given once daily. Children: 4-8 mg/kg/day; children > 6 yr may require minimum adult dose (300 mg/day).
Status epilepticus	*IV:* Adults: Give loading dose of 10-15 mg/kg; IV rate should not exceed 50 mg/min (or, in elderly patients, 25 mg/min); initial dose should be followed by maintenance dose of 100 mg orally or IV q6-8h. Children: Give 15-20 mg/kg slowly (not more than 1-3 mg/kg/min).
Mephenytoin (Mesantoin)	
Tonic-clonic, simple, and complex partial seizures	*Oral:* Adults: 200-600 mg/day. Children: 100-400 mg/day.
Ethotoin (Peganone)	
Tonic-clonic and complex partial seizures	*Oral:* Adult: 2000-3000 mg/day given in four to six doses after eating. Children: 500-1000 mg/day given in four to six doses after eating.
Long-acting barbiturates	
Phenobarbital (Luminal)	
Tonic-clonic and simple and complex partial seizures	*Oral:* Adults: 50-100 mg bid or tid. Children: 3-5 mg/kg/day given hs or in three divided doses.
Status epilepticus	*IV:* Adults: 200-300 mg, repeating in 6 hours, if needed. Children: 15-20 mg/kg over 10-15 min; then 6 mg/kg every 20 min prn to maximum dose of 40 mg/kg in 24 hr.
Mephobarbital (Mebaral)	
Tonic-clonic and absence seizures	*Oral:* Adults: 400-600 mg/day. Children > 5 yr: 32-64 mg tid or qid. Children < 5 yr: 16-32 mg tid or qid.
Metharbital (Gemonil)	
Tonic-clonic, absence, myoclonic, and mixed seizures	*Oral:* Adults: Initially 100 mg one to three times per day; adjust upward to 600-800 mg/day, if needed. Children: Initially 5-15 mg/kg/day; adjust until seizures are controlled.

Primidone (Mysoline) Tonic-clonic, simple and complex partial seizures	*Oral:* Adults and children > 8 yr: Days 1 to 3, 100-125 mg hs; days 4 to 6, 100-125 mg bid; days 7 to 9, 100-125 mg tid; day 10, up to 250 mg tid or qid per day, if needed. Children < 8 yr: 50 mg hs at first, then gradually increase by Day 10 to 10-25 mg/kg/day in divided doses (125-250 mg tid), if needed.
Succinimides	
Ethosuximide (Zarontin) Absence seizures (petit mal)	*Oral:* Adults and children > 6 years: 500 mg/day at first, then increase by 250 mg/day every 4 to 7 days until seizures are satisfactorily controlled (40-100 μg/ml). Children 3-6 yr: 250 mg/day at first, then increase by 250 mg/day every 4 to 7 days. (20 mg/kg/day is typical optimal dose.)
Methsuximide (Celontin) Absence seizures (petit mal)	*Oral:* Adults: 300 mg/day at first, then weekly increases of 300 mg/day up to 1200 mg/day, if needed. Children: Same as for adults; however, increments are 150 mg.
Phensuximide (Milontin) Absence seizures (petit mal)	*Oral:* Adults and children: 500-1000 mg bid or tid; 1500 mg/day is average maintenance dose.
Oxazolidinediones	
Trimethadione (Tridione) Absence seizures (petit mal) refractory to other drugs	*Oral:* Adults: 900 mg/day at first, then increase by 300 mg/day every 7 days until seizures are controlled or until symptoms of toxic effects occur; maintenance dose usually 300-600 mg tid or qid; maximum dose is 2400 mg/day. Children: 300-900 mg/day in three or four divided doses.
Paramethadione (Paradione) Absence seizures (petit mal) refractory to other drugs.	*Oral:* Adults: 900 mg/day at first, then increase by 300 mg/day every 7 days until seizures are controlled or until symptoms of toxic effects occur; maintenance dose usually 300-600 mg tid or qid; maximum dose is 2400 mg/day. Children: 300-900 mg/day in three or four divided doses.

Continued.

Table 7-5 Dosage for Selected Antiepileptics—cont'd

Drug and clinical indication	Dosage
Benzodiazepines	
Diazepam (Valium)	
Status epilepticus	*IM or IV (preferred route):* Adults: 5-10 mg, repeat every 10-15 min, if needed, up to a total dose of 30 mg; *must be given slowly*. Children > 5 yr: 1 mg every 2-5 min, up to 10 mg, repeated in 2 to 4 hours prn. Children from 1 mo to 5 yr: 0.2 to 0.5 mg every 2-5 min, up to a total dose of 5 mg.
Clonazepam (Klonopin)	
Absence (petit mal), Lennox-Gastaut, and myoclonic seizures	*Oral:* Adults: 0.5 mg tid at first, then increase every 3 days by 0.5-1.0 mg until seizures are controlled; 20 mg/day is the maximum dose. Children < 10 yr: 0.01-0.03 mg/kg/day in divided doses at first, then increase by 0.25 to 0.5 mg every 3 days until seizures are controlled; usual dose is 0.1-0.2 mg/kg/day in three divided doses.
Clorazepate (Tranxene)	
Partial seizures (adjunctive)	*Oral:* Adults and children > 12 yr: up to 7.5 mg tid to start, then increase by no more than 7.5 mg every week: maximum dose is 90 mg/day. Children 9 to 12 yr: Up to 7.5 mg bid to start, then increase by no more than 7.5 mg every week; maximum dose is 60 mg/day.

Other antiepileptics	
Valproic acid (Depakene) Absence, tonic-clonic, complex partial, and myoclonic seizures	*Oral:* Adults and children: 15 mg/kg/day at first, then increase weekly by 5-10 mg/kg/day up to a maximum dose of 60 mg/kg/day in divided doses.
Carbamazepine (Tegretol) Tonic-clonic, complex partial, and mixed seizures	*Oral:* Adult and children >12 yr: 200 mg bid at first, then increase by 200 mg/day every 7 days, if needed; maintenance dose usually 800-1200 mg/day in divided doses; adult dose rarely exceeds 1200 mg/day. Children 12-15 yr should not receive more than 1000 mg/day. Children 6-12 years: 100 mg bid at first, then increase by 100 mg/day every 7 days, if needed; maintenance dose is usually 400-800 mg/day in divided doses; do not exceed 1000 mg/day.
Phenacemide (Phenurone) Complex partial seizures	*Oral:* Adults: 250-500 mg tid to start; maintenance dose is typically 2000 to 3000 mg/day. Children 5-10 yr: Half the adult dose at the same intervals as for adults.

could cause serum levels of phenytoin to plummet, thus risking breakthrough seizures.

In children doses usually start at 5 mg/kg per day. Maintenance doses range from 4 to 8 mg/kg per day. Children over 6 years of age sometimes require the minimum adult dosage (300 mg per day).

Parenteral administration. Intramuscular phenytoin is given to patients who cannot tolerate oral administration or when a risk of seizure is suspected during or soon after surgery. Intramuscular use is absolutely *not indicated* for status epilepticus because of the slow absorption of the route; thus careful attention to the appropriate dosage must be observed.

Intravenous (IV) use of phenytoin for status epilepticus is warranted in many situations; however, diazepam is a first-line drug for status epilepticus, whereas phenytoin remains a second-line therapeutic agent. Diazepam only aborts the seizure in progress and is not appropriate for continuous use as an antiepileptic. Close scrutiny of IV phenytoin is advised because of its narrow therapeutic index. Maintenance dosages of 100 mg every 6 to 8 hours to prevent breakthrough seizures are warranted. Children may be given 15 to 20 mg/kg but at a rate no faster than 1 to 3 mg/kg per minute.

Side Effects

The most common side effects of phenytoin are those involving the CNS, that is, sluggishness, ataxia, nystagmus, confusion, and slurred speech (Table 7-6). Dizziness, insomnia, nervousness, and fatigue less frequently occur. Phenytoin is considered the least sedating antiepileptic.

Peripheral side effects include those involving the blood, the gastrointestinal (GI) tract, connective tissue, and the skin. Hematologic effects such as leukopenia, agranulocytosis, megaloblastic anemia, and coagulation deficits in newborns have been reported. Nausea, vomiting, and constipation are the major GI tract effects. Gingival hyperplasia (overgrowth of gums down over the teeth) is a fairly common side effect of phenytoin use in children and in those who do not engage in good oral hygiene. Psychiatric patients and individuals with developmental disabilities seem to be susceptible to gingival hyperplasia. Other connective tissue problems include enlarged lips, coarsened facial features, and excessive growth of body hair (hypertrichosis). Skin reactions can range from the embarrassing, such as worsening of acne in a teenager, to the potentially fatal exfoliative dermatitis. Other skin reactions are a mild measlelike (morbilliform) rash and lupus erythematosus. Other adverse responses include hepatitis and liver damage, hyperglycemia, edema, chest pain, numbness and parasthesia, photophobia, pulmonary fibrosis, osteomalacia caused by enhanced vitamin D metabolism, and lymphadenopathy (as severe as Hodgkin's disease).

Central nervous system side effects are particularly debilitating for elderly patients because of the high susceptibility to falls and a tendency to misjudge situations (i.e., forgetting that a medication was taken and then ingesting an extra dose). Megaloblastic anemia can be countered with folic acid; however, excessive doses of folic acid can lower phenytoin serum levels to a subtherapeutic range. Discontinuance of phenytoin can reverse lymph node involvement.

Implications

Therapeutic versus toxic levels. The typical therapeutic dose of phenytoin ranges from 300 to 800 mg per day given in several doses or, if the extended-acting

Table 7-6 Side Effects and Adverse Reactions of Major Antiepileptics

Side effect or adverse reaction	Phenytoin	Pheno-barbital	Primidone	Ethosux-imide	Clonazepam	Valproic acid	Carba-mazepine
CNS effects	C	C	C	C	C		C
Transient alopecia	—	—	—	—	R	X	—
Coarsening of facial features	X	—	—	—	—	—	—
Gingival hyperplasia	C	—	—	X	—	—	—
Cardiovascular	—	—	—	—	X	—	X
Gastrointestinal tract	X	X	X	C	X	XM	X
Hepatic toxic effects	R	X	—	X	—	R	X
Coagulation defects in infants	X	X	—	—	—	—	—
Blood dyscrasias	X	R	R	X	X	R	R
Osteomalacia	X	R	—	—	—	—	—
Exfoliative dermatitis	R	R	—	—	—	—	—
Skin rash	C	X	X	X	X	R	—
Hypertrichosis	X	—	—	—	X	—	—
Sedation	X	C	X	X	C	—	C
Fever	X	—	—	—	—	—	X

C, Occurs commonly; *CNS*, central nervous system; *X*, occurs; *XM*, occurs but with mild symptoms; *R*, occurs rarely.

form is used, once per day. Toxic serum levels can occur at normal dosage levels for a variety of reasons (i.e., impaired liver function, enzyme deficiencies, or drug interactions). Therapeutic serum levels range from 10 to 20 μg/ml. A toxic level of phenytoin occurs at serum levels above 20 μg/ml. Symptoms can include far-lateral nystagmus, ataxia, dysarthria, tremor, slurred speech, and nausea and vomiting. Diminished mental capacity occurs at serum levels above 40 μg/ml. Serum levels above 50 μg/ml may cause seizures. At serum levels above 100 μg/ml the same symptoms are intensified and hypotension, circulatory and ventilatory failure, coma, and death can occur. The estimated lethal dose in an adult is 2 to 5 g. Death is caused by respiratory and circulatory failure.

Treatment for overdose and toxic effects are driven by the principle of reducing further drug absorption. Induced emesis, repeated gastric lavage and suctioning, and providing activated charcoal are interventions useful in interrupting phenytoin absorption. Since there is no known antidote, supportive measures for respiratory and circulatory systems should be employed. Hemodialysis may be useful, since phenytoin is not completely bound to plasma proteins.

Use in pregnancy. Phenytoin has been implicated in congenital defects, that is, cleft lip, cleft palate, and heart malformations (Dalessio, 1985). In addition, children of women taking phenytoin are susceptible to coagulation defects caused by lower levels of vitamin K–dependent clotting factors, which can lead to hemorrhage. Prophylactic administration of vitamin K (phytonadione) to the mother at 1 month before delivery and to the newborn at birth (about 1 mg) can prevent the development of this hematologic disorder. Hematologic studies should be routinely acquired. Breast-feeding is not appropriate for women taking phenytoin because this drug is excreted in breast milk.

Side effects. Central nervous system symptoms are most troublesome for elderly patients. These individuals should be observed closely to prevent falls or other problems associated with impaired judgement. Evaluation of mood, affect, and memory provide data from which interventions can be formulated.

Hematologic disorders can be minimized through careful assessment for fever, sore throat, malaise, or bruises (Keltner, 1989). The patient should be instructed to self-assess for these signs and to report them. A contraindication for phenytoin use is the presence of bone marrow depression or a blood dyscrasia.

Nausea, vomiting, and other gastrointestinal problems are reduced when phenytoin is given with meals. Gingival hyperplasia, coarsening of facial features, and other connective tissue consequences of phenytoin therapy can cause a loss of self-esteem because of disfigurement. Thorough oral hygiene can reduce the severity of gingival hyperplasia.

Since skin rashes can range from mild, measle like (morbilliform) conditions to serious skin disorders such as exfoliative dermatitis and lupus erythematosus, phenytoin should be discontinued when a rash appears. Finally, acne is a frequent adverse reaction to phenytoin among teenagers and young adults and its potential to lower self-esteem should not be underestimated by those responsible for care. If another antiepileptic will control seizures, a change from phenytoin is indicated.

Parenteral phenytoin can cause cardiovascular effects such as hypotension, circulatory collapse, depression of cardiac conductility, and cardiac arrest. Patients with a history of sinus bradycardia, sinoatrial or second- or third-degree atrioventricular block, or Adams-Stokes syndrome should not be given this drug. Monitoring the patient's blood pressure and respirations while giving phenytoin slowly IV (50 mg/min) reduces the likelihood of triggering a cardiovascular response.

Interactions. Many drugs interact with phenytoin. These interactions can be generally categorized as those that cause an increase or decrease in phenytoin serum levels, those that cause a decrease in the action of the interacting drug, and those interactants with unpredictable effects. Nonetheless, if phenytoin serum levels are closely monitored, multiple drug therapy is possible without serious consequences for the patient.

Drugs that increase phenytoin serum levels (potential toxic effects). Other drugs increase serum phenytoin by one of the following means: (1) inhibiting phenytoin metabolism or (2) displacing phenytoin from plasma protein binding sites, thereby leading to excessive levels of free (and active) phenytoin. Interactants that inhibit metabolism include acute alcohol ingestion, allopurinal, H_1-receptor blocking antihistamines, chlordiazepoxide, chlorpromazine and most antipsychotics, diazepam, disulfiram, estrogens, ethosuximide, halothane, isoniazid, methylphenidate, phenylbutazone, proclorperazine, tolbutamide, and valproic acid. Diazepam and ethosuximide are antiepileptics that might be prescribed along with phenytoin, so a downward adjustment in the dose of phenytoin should be made. Disulfiram, a major drug treatment for chronic alcoholism, necessitates a low starting dose of phenytoin, monitoring of serum levels of phenytoin, and careful assessment of the patient. Drinking alcohol when taking phenytoin leads to higher serum levels of phenytoin because alcohol successfully competes for liver enzymes. Valproic acid and salicylates increase phenytoin serum levels by displacing phenytoin from plasma protein binding sites.

Drugs that decrease phenytoin serum levels (potential seizure breakthrough). A number of drugs decrease the serum levels of phenytoin by means of the following distinct mechanisms: (1) increasing phenytoin metabolism or (2) decreasing its absorption. Barbiturates (including phenobarbital), theophylline, carbamazepine, chronic alcoholism (enzyme induction), molindone (an antipsychotic), and reserpine decrease phenytoin serum levels by increasing its breakdown in the liver. Folic acid, sometimes given prophylactically to prevent megaloblastic anemia, antacids, antineoplastics, and calcium gluconate interfere with phenytoin absorption.

Interactant effects that are decreased by phenytoin. The effects of corticosteroids, oral anticoagulants, oral contraceptives, quinidine, and vitamin D are all compromised by phenytoin. Dangers of these interactive patterns include decreased corticosteroid effect; increased blood clotting; pregnancy, spotting, and breakthrough bleeding; reduced antiarrhythmic action; and increased risk of osteomalacia. Assessment should address these issues. Increasing the level of estrogen in the contraceptive may improve efficacy, and instructing the patient to seek medical help should a pregnancy be expected is a prudent measure to ensure optimal benefit. Additionally, fluid retention lowers the seizure threshold; since retention occurs with the use of contraceptives, alternate birth control methods should be considered. Increasing quinidine dosage can maintain its antiarrhythmic quality, and encouraging more vitamin D in the diet can forestall skeletal problems.

Psychotropic drugs whose metabolism is enhanced by phenytoin include clonazepam, haloperidol, and methadone.

Interactants that behave unpredictably. Several drugs may either increase or decrease phenytoin serum levels. Two antiepileptics, phenobarbital and valproic acid, may cause phenytoin serum levels to rise or fall. Consequently, monitoring of laboratory data is important. Paradoxically phenytoin can have the same effect on these two drugs, that is, their effects may increase or decrease.

Finally, tricyclic antidepressants (TCAs), although not true interactants, can trigger seizures in some susceptible patients, necessitating phenytoin dosage adjustment.

Patient education. Patient teaching should focus on helping the patient maximize the therapeutic benefits of phenytoin while preventing or minimizing its serious side effects. The patient should be familiar with the desired action of the drug, the importance of taking the drug on time and as prescribed (maintaining therapeutic serum levels), the difference in efficacy between oral and parenteral routes, and the need to notify the clinician when certain side effects occur. Side effects that must be punctually reported include sore throat, fever, malaise, petechiae, and bruising. The other major significant issues in patient teaching are meticulous oral hygiene (brushing and flossing) to reduce gingival hyperplasia, warnings against driving when CNS symptoms such as dizziness or sedation occur, care when rising (to reduce the risk of falls), and avoiding prescription drugs that interact with phenytoin (make all other health care providers aware of phenytoin therapy) and consumption of alcohol. It is generally advisable for individuals taking antiepileptic drugs to wear a medical identification bracelet.

Young women should be made aware of the potential for congenital deficits should they become pregnant, and those desiring to become pregnant should first talk with their physician. Individuals who have gastrointestinal (GI) tract effects as a result of phenytoin use should be encouraged to take the drug with their meals, since doing so enhances absorption and decreases GI tract upset.

Patients should be advised not to abruptly discontinue phenytoin, because of the potential for status epilepticus. As little as a 10% change in daily dose can result in a 50% change in serum concentration.

Related Hydantoins

The two hydantoins other than phenytoin that are successfully used in the treatment of epilepsy are ethotoin (Peganone) and mephenytoin (Mesantoin). Ethotoin is indicated for the treatment of tonic-clonic and psychomotor seizures. It can be given alone or in conjunction with another antiepileptic. The initial adult daily dose is 1000 mg or less, given in four to six divided doses. As the patient adapts to ethotoin, a maintenance dose of 2 to 3 g per day is required. Adults rarely receive less than 2 g per day. Children initially receive a dose of up to 750 mg per day. Pediatric dosages are age dependent, but a typical maintenance dose is 500 mg to 1 g per day. Therapeutic serum levels of ethotoin are 15 to 50 μg/ml. Ethotoin is compatible with all antiepileptics except phenacemide (Phenurone). The combination of ethotoin and phenacemide has been reported to cause a paranoid syndrome. Ethotoin is *contraindicated* in patients with known hepatic abnormalities.

Mephenytoin is usually not prescribed unless other, safer antiepileptics have been attempted. In adults the usual initial dose is 50 to 100 mg per day. After 1 week the dosage is increased by 50 to 100 mg per day at weekly intervals. No dose is increased until it has been taken for 1 week. Maintenance adult doses are 200 to 600 mg per day. Children typically require a dose of 100 to 400 mg per day for seizure control.

LONG-ACTING BARBITURATES: PROTOTYPE DRUG, PHENOBARBITAL

Barbiturates are relatively old drugs, as noted in Chapter 6. Many individual drugs are available, but only long-acting barbiturates have antiepileptic potential. Only the antiepileptic qualities of barbiturates are discussed in this chapter. Phenobarbital (Luminal) is the prototype long-acting barbiturate. Mephobarbital (Mebaral), metharbital (Gemonil), and primidone (Mysoline) are related drugs.

Antiepileptic treatment is the only therapy for which long-term use of barbiturates is recognized. Although barbiturates have been used for nearly a century as sedatives, at subsedation doses a few have been found to possess antiepileptic qualities. All barbiturates have antiepileptic properties at high doses. It is phenobarbital's ability to inhibit seizures without inducing sedation that makes it and the related drugs beneficial.

Pharmacologic Effects

By altering ion movements across nerve membranes and inhibiting nerve transmission to the cerebral cortex, phenobarbital slows the response of nerves to seizure-causing stimuli and also slows the spread of abnormal electrical activity. The net effect is to raise the seizure threshold, that is, diminish the likelihood of a seizure. Oral phenobarbital is effective for the treatment of tonic-clonic seizures and simple and complex partial seizures (Table 7-2). Parenteral phenobarbital (IV) is used to stop status epilepticus when diazepam or phenytoin is ineffective or unavailable.

Pharmacokinetics

Phenobarbital is usually given orally, absorbed in varying degrees, and uniformly distributed to all tissues (Table 7-3). Onset of action after an oral dose varies from 20 to 60 minutes. Phenobarbital is metabolized in the liver by the hepatic microsomal enzyme system, but up to 50% of its molecules are excreted unchanged in the urine. Nonetheless, phenobarbital has a dramatic effect on the hepatic enzymes by increasing the synthesis of those enzymes (enzyme induction). The net effect is to expedite the metabolism of those drugs, including phenobarbital, that are metabolized by these liver enzymes. This mechanism produces tolerance to many effects and contributes to drug interactions. Tolerance to phenobarbital's antiepileptic activity and to its lethal effects is slight. Phenobarbital has the lowest lipid solubility and the longest duration of action of all barbiturates.

The therapeutic plasma level for phenobarbital is 15 to 40 μg/ml and takes 16 to 21 days to reach a steady state. It has a half-life of 80 hours (a range of 53 to 118 hours) initially, but that time is reduced after the aformentioned enzyme induction occurs. Phenobarbital is 40% to 50% bound to plasma proteins.

Oral phenobarbital is typically prescribed for adults, 50 to 100 mg, two or three times per day; children are given 3 to 5 mg/kg per day, in divided doses or a single dose (Table 7-5). Because of these low doses, physical dependence and withdrawal symptoms are seldom encountered. Phenobarbital is usually preferred over phenytoin for the treatment of seizures in children because it does not cause gingival hyperplasia or the various skin problems associated with phenytoin. Elderly patients may require a reduced dosage. Patients who have status epilepticus or other acute seizures (i.e., cholera, eclampsia, or meningitis) can be given IV phenobarbital. Typically adults are given 200 to 300 mg and the dose is repeated after 6 hours, if needed. Children can be given 15 to 20 mg/kg over 10 to 15 minutes, then 6 mg/kg every 20 minutes to a maximum dose of 40 mg/kg in 24 hours. Phenobarbital is not the first choice for these emergency situations (diazepam is) because the high doses needed to stop these seizures can cause CNS, respiratory, and cardiovascular depression.

Oral administration. Phenobarbital is available in a variety of oral forms: tablets, capsules, and elixirs. Long-term antiepileptic therapy is typically accomplished by means of oral phenobarbital use.

Parenteral administration. Parenteral usage is to be avoided unless oral administration is not feasible or a prompt antieptileptic response is needed. Parenteral phenobarbital is used for treatment of status epilepticus and other emergency convulsive states. Intramuscular phenobarbital should be injected into large muscles (gluteus maximus or vastus lateralis), where there is less risk of injecting into a peripheral nerve trunk or artery.

Intravenous injections are preferred over IM injections and are typically reserved for emergency situations in which timely action is important. A vein must always be used because interarterial injection can lead to a gangrenous condition caused by vessel spasm. The drugs must be injected slowly, at a rate no faster than 50 mg per minute. The onset of action after IV injection is about 5 minutes. Again, parenteral phenobarbital is not the drug of choice for the treatment of status epilepticus. Diazepam or phenytoin is given.

Side Effects

Central nervous system depression is the most common side effect of phenobarbital, that is, drowsiness, ataxia, and sedation (Table 7-6). However, because seizure control is a long-term if not a lifetime concern, many of the side effects associated with phenobarbital become tolerated by the patient. A history of porphyria (excessive hepatic formation of porphyrins) remains a contraindication to the use of phenobarbital because it induces the synthesis of porphyrins. Hypotension and respiratory depression are potential adverse responses to high oral doses or to rapid IV infusion.

Another major side effect of phenobarbital administration is the induction of hepatic microsomal enzymes. The effect of this induction phenomena is the increased rate of metabolism of phenobarbital and other drugs metabolized in the liver. This effect leads directly to the development of tolerance mentioned in the preceding paragraph.

Vitamin D metabolism is stimulated by phenobarbital. The same concerns reviewed during the discussion of phenytoin pertain to phenobarbital. Barbiturates can at low doses cause excitability in children and elderly individuals.

Implications

Therapeutic versus toxic levels. The therapeutic serum phenobarbital level is 15 to 40 μg/ml. Serum phenobarbital levels over 40 μg/ml may be toxic. Although toxic doses vary among individuals, usually 1 g orally of phenobarbital can cause serious toxic effects and ingesting 2 to 10 g can be lethal.

A tolerance to many barbiturate effects develops with chronic use, but a tolerance to the antiepileptic effects does not develop. Therefore, although an increased amount of barbiturate many be needed for sedation, an increase is not required for continued seizure control, nor does tolerance to lethal levels develop. At toxic levels respiratory and CNS depression, tachycardia, hypotension, hypothermia, and coma can occur. In cases of severe overdose, apnea, circulatory collapse, respiratory arrest, and death have been reported.

Treatment for overdose consists of maintenance of a patent airway and assistance with ventilation and oxygenation, if needed. Gastric lavage can be used to empty the stomach. Monitoring of vital signs and fluid balance is important. When renal function remains normal, forced diuresis and alkalinizing of the urine help eliminate the phenobarbital.

Use in pregnancy. Phenobarbital has been implicated in congenital defects (Dalessio, 1985). Withdrawal symptoms can occur in infants born to mothers who take barbiturates in their last trimester, and a coagulation defect in infants has been associated with maternal barbiturate use.

Side effects. Central nervous system effects such as drowsiness can impair driving and put the patient at risk in many situations. Should an older patient or a child have paradoxic excitement after taking phenobarbital, precautions to prevent injury should be instituted. Patient assessment data should include information about a history of porphyria. Resuscitation equipment should be readily available when IV phenobarbital is given.

Interactions. Drugs that depress the CNS are the chief interactants with phenobarbital, so the patient who requires phenobarbital in conjunction with another CNS depressant should be carefully observed by physicians and nurses. Interactants can be categorized into two groups, drugs that increase the effects of barbiturates and drugs whose effects are decreased by barbiturates.

Drugs that increase effects of barbiturates (toxic effects). Central nervous system depressants such as sedatives, hypnotics, anesthetics, antihistamines, antipsychotics, and alcohol enhance the depressant effects of barbiturates. Alcohol and barbiturates should never be combined. Alcohol can reduce the antiepileptic effect of phenobarbital and dramatically increase the level of CNS depression. Many deaths each year are attributed to the combination of barbiturates and alcohol.

Other antiepileptic agents also interact with phenobarbital. Since multiple-drug therapy is common in the treatment of seizure disorders, it is important to recognize potential problems and to develop protocols for evaluating them. Valproic acid, for example, interacts with phenobarbital through a mechanism referred to as selective metabolism. The hepatic microsomal enzyme system selectively metabolizes valproic acid, delaying the metabolism of phenobarbital. Phenobarbital serum levels may increase by 200%, clearly presenting a serious risk of toxic effects.

Drugs whose effects are decreased by phenobarbital. Many drugs are compromised by coadministration with phenobarbital. The induction of hepatic microsomal enzymes that more speedily metabolize these drugs is responsible for their shortened response in the body (Keltner, Schwecke, and Bostrom, 1991). Most notably reduced in effect are acetaminophen, digitoxin, oral anticoagulants, oral contraceptives, and TCAs. Although the effect of phenobarbital on phenytoin is not precisely known, it is thought that phenytoin metabolism is accelerated and consequently renders the drug less effective. The concurrent use of these two antiepileptics is common, so frequent monitoring of serum levels of both drugs is appropriate. Other drugs whose effects are decreased include griseofulvin, quinidine, doxycycline, and monoamine oxidose inhibitors.

Patient education. Patient teaching focuses primarily on health and safety. Patients should be warned to avoid driving or operating hazardous machinery and to avoid combining phenobarbital, alcohol, and other CNS depressants. Other teaching concerns include the reporting of side effects and adverse responses. Although hematologic side effects are uncommon, symptoms such as sore throat, fever, and bleeding should be reported so that the development of blood dyscrasias can be prevented.

Related Barbiturates

Three barbiturates other than phenobarbital are effective antiepileptics: mephobarbital, metharbital, and primidone.

Mephobarbital is used in the treatment of both tonic-clonic and absence epilepsy. It has two major advantages over phenobarbital. First, mephobarbital can be used in the treatment of absence seizure, whereas phenobarbital cannot. Second, mephobarbital causes less drowsiness and sedation in adults and less excitability in children than does phenobarbital. This second feature accounts for the predominate rationale for prescribing mephobarbital. Adults typically receive a dose of 400 to 600 mg per day. In children under 5 years of age a daily dosage of 16 to 32 mg three or four times per day is prescribed; children over 5 years of age are given a dosage of 32 to 64 mg three or four times per day. Dosages are started at the lower end of the range and gradually increased.

Mephobarbital is sometimes used in combination with phenobarbital. When so used, the daily dose of both should be about half of what it would be if each were given alone (i.e., 50 to 100 mg of phenobarbital and 200 to 300 mg of mephobarbital). Mephobarbital can also be given concurrently with phenytoin. In this combination, phenytoin daily dose should be reduced (i.e., to about 230 mg per day) but mephobarbital can be given at its full dose.

Metharbital is indicated for the treatment of tonic-clonic, absence, myoclonic, and mixed types of seizures. Its major metabolite is barbital, the longest-acting barbiturate. Metharbital is used as a replacement for phenobarbital primarily and is used adjunctively with other antiepileptic drugs. The usual adult starting dosage is 100 mg one to three times per day. Children can be started on a dose of 5 to 15 mg/kg per day. Both daily doses can be gradually increased as tolerance develops. Adults may require up to 800 mg per day to control seizures. Therapeutic doses of metharbital are somewhat more sedating than equivalent doses of phenobarbital.

Primidone is used alone or in conjunction with other antiepileptics to control tonic-clonic, simple partial, and complex partial seizures. Two metabolites of primidone, phenobarbital and phenylethylmalonamide, are responsible for the antiepileptic properties of primidone. When a barbiturate is indicated, primidone is not a first-line drug because it is responsible for consequential side effects, that is, ataxia, vertigo, GI tract upset, nystagmus, diplopia, impotence, and minor rashes. Emotional disturbances, including paranoid thinking and mood fluctuations, have also been reported in some patients. Some side effects such as ataxia and vertigo disappear after continued use. Adults and children are started on a regimen of primidone at modest doses (100 mg at bedtime and 50 mg at bedtime, respectively); then dosages are carefully elevated over the next 10 days to arrive at a therapeutic maintenance dose. (For details on dosages, see Table 7-5 and Psychotropic Drug Profiles.) Adults are never given more than 2 g per day. Bioequivalence among brands of primidone is not supported by clinical experience, so switching products is not recommended.

SUCCINIMIDES: PROTOTYPE DRUG, ETHOSUXIMIDE

The succinimides are the third group of antiepileptic drugs discussed here. They are chemically distinct from the hydantoins and the long-acting barbiturates. The contribution of the succinimides to the antiepileptic arsensal lies in their effectiveness in the treatment of absence seizures (Table 7-2). The prototype drug of the succinimides is ethosuximide (Zarontin). The two related antiepileptics are methsuximide (Celontin) and phensuximide (Milontin).

Pharmacologic Effects

Ethosuximide decreases absence seizures by depressing the motor cortex and raising the threshold of the CNS to convulsive stimuli. The three-cycles-per-second spike-and-wave EEG pattern associated with absence seizures is also effectively suppressed. Ethosuximide is not the first drug of choice for absence seizures in adults; valproic acid is. Nonetheless, ethosuximide remains an important drug and is much preferred over the oxazolidinediones (paramethadione and trimethadione), which may cause serious side effects.

Pharmacokinetics

Ethosuximide is readily absorbed in the GI tract, and peak serum levels are reached within 3 to 7 hours (Table 7-4). The therapeutic range of ethosuximide is 40 to 100 μg/ml. Ethosuximide, because of a long half-life of 60 hours in adults and 30 hours in children, can be given in once-per-day dosages. It is extensively metabolized to inactive metabolites and excreted in the urine.

Ethosuximide is available in oral forms (capsules and syrup). Adults and children over 6 years of age are initially given a dose of 500 mg per day, followed by gradual increases in dosage every 4 to 7 days until the therapeutic level is reached (Table 7-4). Younger children (3 to 6 years of age) are started on a dose of 250 mg per day, followed by the same incremental increases as noted for adult patients. No patient should receive more than 1.5 g per day because of the risk of side effects and toxic effects. Ethosuximide can be used adjunctively with other antiepileptic agents in patients with seizures other than absence seizures; however, because ethosuximide can increase the risk of tonic-clonic seizure breakthrough, higher doses of the concurrent antiepileptic may be required. Used alone, ethosuximide can increase the risk of tonic-clonic seizures in some patients.

Side Effects

The common complaint associated with ethosuximide is GI tract upset. Nausea, vomiting, cramps, diarrhea, and anorexia are common but can be reduced by taking the medication with meals (Table 7-6). Psychiatric and CNS symptoms (dizziness and drowsiness) can occur in some patients. Succinimides have been reported to cause abnormal hepatic and renal function in humans, so monitoring studies of these functions is consistent with good care. Giving ethosuximide to a patient with impaired liver functioning prolongs the already long half-life, increasing the risk of long-lasting toxic effects. Hematologic effects (infrequent but significant) and dermatologic effects occur in a few patients.

Implications

Therapeutic versus toxic levels. The therapeutic serum level of ethosuximide is 40 to 100 μg/ml. Toxic effects occur when the serum level is higher than 100 μg/ml. A state of overdose results in intensified GI tract, CNS, hematologic, and dermatologic side effects. Ataxia, lethargy, dizziness, and sedation are frequently the first signs of toxicity. The most severe reactions to overdose are myopia, vaginal bleeding, CNS depression, and systemic lupus erythematosus. Overdoses are treated symptomatically, and patient care is supportive.

Use in pregnancy. Although in general antiepileptic drugs are known to contribute to fetal abnormalities, ethosuximide seems to be a drug that can be given safely without the risk of significant defects in newborns. With appropriate monitoring, pregnant women have been able to take ethosuximide during pregnancy. This drug, as with most antiepileptics, is not recommended for use during lactation.

Side effects. Hepatic and renal studies should be performed before ethosuximide therapy is initiated. Thereafter, regularly scheduled testing is desirable so that deleterious effects to those organs can be evaluated or prevented. Since a few patients have had lethal blood dyscrasias, obtaining periodic blood cell counts is prudent. If the patient becomes depressed or aggressive, it may be necessary to withdraw ethosuximide.

Interactions. Ethosuximide does not interact in a significant way with any other drugs; however, excessive sedation could be a result of concurrent administration with a CNS depressant (i.e., alcohol). Antipsychotic and antidepressant drugs lower the seizure threshold and increase the risk of seizure development when taken during ethosuximide therapy.

Patient education. Patients who have any of the GI tract symptoms mentioned previously should be advised to take ethosuximide with food or milk. Because of the long half-life of ethosuximide and its once-a-day dosage pattern, patients who miss a day of medication should not take a "double dose" the next day. To do so could substantially raise the serum level of ethosuximide and in turn cause intensified side effects and toxic effects.

Patients taking ethosuximide should be advised to avoid alcohol and to refrain from abrupt discontinuance of this drug because to abruptly discontinue use increases the risk of seizures. Because ethosuximide can cause drowsiness, driving a car or operating hazardous machinery should be limited until the drug is well tolerated. Patients should report symptoms that indicate blood dyscrasias to the physician.

Related Succinimides

The two related succinimides are methsuximide and phensuximide. Methsuximide is as effective as ethosuximide in treating absence seizures; however, it is slightly more toxic. Methsuximide reaches peak serum levels within 4 hours and has a much shorter half-life than ethosuximide (2.6 to 4 hours). Drowsiness, ataxia, and dizziness are the most frequent side effects of methsuximide.

Methsuximide is a second-choice antiepileptic. Typically an effort is made to prescribe the lowest effective dose of methsuximide, to reduce the toxic effects. The optimal dose is determined by clinical trial; 300 mg per day is a reasonable initial dose. Dose changes are made no more frequently than once per week. The maximum dose is 1.2 g per day.

Phensuximide is thought to be slightly less effective than either ethosuximide or methsuximide. Peak serum levels are reached within 4 hours, and the half-life of phensuximide is about 4 hours. Significant genitourinary tract side effects not associated with the other succinimides have been reported to be caused by phensuximide, that is, urinary frequency, renal damage, and hematuria. Also, a harmless urinary effect is pinkish, red, or red-brown urine. Regardless of patient age, the total daily dose may vary from 1 to 3 g.

OXAZOLIDINEDIONES: PROTOTYPE DRUG, TRIMETHADIONE

The oxazolidinediones are antiepileptics normally used only when other drugs have proven ineffective. The oxazolidinediones cause serious side effects and have been proven to be tetragenic.

Pharmacologic Effects

Trimethadione (Tridione) was introduced in 1946 and was the first drug developed to treat absence seizures (Table 7-2). It is an effective drug agent, but because of its serious side effects, it is not a first-line antiepileptic. Although the exact nature of trimethadione's antiepileptic effect is not known, it is thought that antiepileptic properties may be associated with its ability to decrease synaptic stimulation to low-frequency impulses.

Pharmacokinetics

Trimethadione is rapidly absorbed from the GI tract. It is metabolized to an active metabolite, dimethadione, which is slowly excreted in the urine. Peak serum levels are reached within 30 to 60 minutes; the serum half-life of trimethadione is 12 to 24 hours, and that of its active metabolite is 6 to 13 days.

Adult maintenance dosage is 900 to 2400 mg per day in three to four equally divided doses (300 to 600 mg three to four times per day). Children are given 300 to 900 mg per day in three to four equally divided doses.

Side Effects

Trimethadione causes several serious side effects, and occasionally patients on a regimen of trimethadione have died. Prominent among the adverse responses are hepatic impairment, nephrosis, blood dyscrasias, exfoliative dermatitis, systemic lupus erythematosus, lymphadenopathy, and a myasthenia gravis–like syndrome.

Less serious side effects include drowsiness early in the course of therapy, dose-related photophobia and hemeralopia (day blindness), and GI tract symptoms such as nausea, vomiting, anorexia, and weight loss. Acneform rashes, although usually innocuous, can also be indicative of an early stage of fatal exfoliative dermatitis.

Implications

Therapeutic versus toxic levels. Therapeutic serum levels for trimethadione have not been established, but it is known that plasma levels of about 700 μg/ml control absence seizures. Toxic levels of trimethadione cause drowsiness, nausea, dizziness, ataxia, and visual disturbances. Large overdoses can cause coma. Treatment for overdose includes general supportive care, monitoring of vital signs, gastric evacuation by emesis or lavage, and urinary alkalinzation to increase dimethadione excretion.

Use in pregnancy. Trimethadione is teratogenic, and of the available antiepileptics it *poses the greatest risk to the fetus*. Only when all other antiepileptics have proven ineffective and when it has been established that the risk of nontreatment to the mother is substantial should trimethadione be prescribed.

Side effects. Because of the seriousness of some of the side effects of trimethadione, strict supervision of patients receiving trimethadione is required. If lymph node enlargement or other manifestations of lupus erythematosus occur, the drug should be withdrawn. Appearance of even mild or acneform rashes are suggestive of more serious skin disorders such as exfoliative dermatitis and warrant discontinuance of trimethadione. Even apparently benign rashes should be allowed to completely clear before the drug treatment is resumed. Jaundice or laboratory values consistent with hepatic dysfunction are cause for drug discontinuance. Patients with a history of hepatic problems ordinarily should not receive trimethadione. Since fatal nephrosis has occurred with oxazolidinediones, renal function should be monitored and should abnormalities (i.e., proteinuria) occur, these agents should be withdrawn. Since depression of blood cell count can occur, obtain a complete blood cell count before therapy begins and regularly thereafter. A marked depression of the blood cell count (neutrophil count of less than 2500 cells per mm^3) requires discontinuance.

Interactions. Valproic acid elevates the blood level of trimethadione and causes a number of symptoms related to mild toxic effects. Other significant interactions with the oxazolidinediones have not been reported.

Patient education. Patients should be taught the following:

To take oxazolidinediones with food, if GI tract problems occur

To avoid abrupt discontinuance of these drugs because of the possibility of withdrawal seizures

To avoid bright lights, if they have photophobia or hemeralopia

To be cautious when driving because of the potential for drowsiness
To notify caregivers when any of the preceding problems occur and when a sore throat, bleeding or bruising, a skin rash, or a pregnancy occurs

Related Oxazolidinedione

Paramethadione (Paradione) is related to trimethadione and is similar to that drug in most respects. Dosage for the treatment of absence seizures is the same for both drugs, with the caveat that the liquid form should be diluted before it is given to children, because of its high alcohol content.

BENZODIAZEPINES: PROTOTYPE DRUG, DIAZEPAM

The benzodiazepines, which are primarily prescribed for their antianxiety properties, are thoroughly reviewed in Chapter 6. However, three benzodiazepines are indicated in the treatment of seizure disorders. The antiepileptic qualities of benzodiazepines are briefly reviewed in this chapter.

Diazepam (Valium) is the prototype benzodiazepine and is the drug of choice for the treatment of status epilepticus (Table 7-2). Diazepam is effective about 95% of the time in controlling these life-threatening seizures. Diazepam is also used adjunctively in the treatment of other types of epilepsy.

A dose of 5 to 10 mg of diazepam given IV stops most seizures within 5 minutes. Since the serum levels fall rapidly, it may be necessary to repeat the dose to maintain a seizure-free state. Typically, repeated doses at 10- to 15-minute intervals may be required. No more than 30 mg of diazepam should be given to treat a single episode of status epilepticus. If a second episode of status epilepticus should occur, this protocol can be repeated within 2 to 4 hours. Because of residual metabolites of diazepam, caution should be used. All IV injections of diazepam must be administered slowly (no more than 5 mg per minute) to avoid thrombosis, phlebitis, and venous irritation. Children and infants have a significantly lower dosage restriction than do adults. Infants and young children (30 days to 5 years of age) should be given 0.2 to 0.5 mg every 2 to 5 minutes up to a maximum dose of 5 mg. Children (5 years of age and older) should be given 1 mg every 2 to 5 minutes up to a maximum dose of 10 mg.

Due to the short-lived effect of diazepam, a phenytoin infusion (18 mg/kg or less at a rate no faster than 50 mg/min) can be hung to follow the first dose of diazepam, thereby avoiding repeated doses of diazepam.

If diazepam is used exclusively (up to 30 mg) and seizures are refractory to treatment, an IV phenytoin drip can be provided. A phenobarbital drip (at 100 mg/min) is the next option but should not follow diazepam because of the synergistic effect of these drugs in depressing respirations. For seizures still not controlled, a paraldehyde infusion should be considered. As a final resort, anesthesia coupled with a neuromuscular blocker can be administered to stop refractory status epilepticus.

Although the discussion of diazepam as the drug of choice for status epilepticus is informative, the real-life task of starting an IV line in a patient with this type of seizure is no easy matter. Should starting the IV line become impossible, an alternative is to inject the drug into a large muscle or to give a diazepam enema. These routes of administration are not as effective but decrease the seizures over time.

Diazepam can be given orally as an adjunct to chronic treatment of convulsive disorders (10 mg four times a day) when the possibility of withdrawal seizures is likely.

Because diazepam has a wide therapeutic index, when it is given alone it is a safe drug. When mixed with other CNS depressants, however, diazepam can cause severe CNS depression. This fact is of slight clinical importance when diazepam is being used in the treatment of the life-threatening emergency, status epilepticus, but becomes more significant when the drug is used adjunctively for the treatment of other seizure forms. In either situation, support for ventilation and monitoring of blood pressure are critical precautions. Pharmacokinetics, side effects, and clinical implications for diazepam usage are discussed in Chapter 6.

Related Benzodiazepines

Two benzodiazepines other than diazepam are used for their antiepileptic effect. Clonazepam (Klonopin) is effective in the treatment of Lennox-Gastaut syndrome, a variant form of absence seizure, and akinetic and myoclonic seizures. It may also be effective in the treatment of absence seizures not responding to the succinimides. Approximately one third of the patients taking clonazepam have breakthrough seizures, indicating a development of tolerance to this drug. Dosage adjustment can restore drug effectiveness. Therapeutic serum levels for clonazepam are 20 to 80 ng/ml. Clonazepam and valproic acid used concurrently can stimulate absence status epilepticus (prolonged absence seizures).

Adults are prescribed an initial dosage of 0.5 mg three times per day. Incremental increases of 0.5 to 1 mg every three days are recommended until seizures are controlled or until side effects make further increases prohibitive. A maximum acceptable dose is 20 mg per day. Children and infants are initially prescribed 0.01 to 0.03 mg/kg per day, given in divided doses. Typical daily doses range from 0.1 to 0.2 mg/kg. Other dimensions of clonazepam use are discussed in Chapter 6.

The final benzodiazepine to be discussed within the context of seizure treatment is clorazepate (Tranxene). Clorazepate is used adjunctively for the treatment of partial seizures. Adults (and children 12 years of age and older) are given an initial dosage of 7.5 mg three times per day. Dosage is increased in 7.5-mg weekly increments, up to a maximum dose of 90 mg per day. More rapid incremental changes result in drowsiness. In children 9 to 12 years of age the initial dosage should be 7.5 mg twice per day, with incremental increases of 7.5 mg per week until effectiveness is established or until a maximum dose of 60 mg per day of clorazepate has been attempted. Children under 9 years of age should not be given this drug. Clorazepate's antianxiety effects and pharmacokinetic properties are discussed in Chapter 6.

OTHER ANTIEPILEPTICS

Several important antiepileptics do not lend themselves to convenient groupings. The most significant of these are valproic acid, carbamazapine, and a handful of rarely used drugs for which antiepileptic properties are secondary uses, that is, phenacemide, acetazolamide, lidocaine, magnesium sulfate, and paraldehyde. The most significant of these drugs are the two first mentioned, valproic acid and carbamazepine. Both of these drugs are now being appreciated for more than their antiepileptic properties. For instance, both are effective in the treatment of refractory bipolar illness (Keltner and Folks, 1991).

VALPROIC ACID AND DERIVATIVES

Valproic acid and its derivatives, sodium valproate and divalproex sodium, are frequently prescribed antiepileptics. Valproic acid is labeled for use in the treatment of absence seizures, but the literature suggests that it can be used effectively for tonic-clonic, myoclonic, and complex partial seizures as well (Table 7-2). Valproic acid is gaining acceptance as the most effective drug for the treatment of generalized seizures.

Pharmacologic Effects

Valproic acid apparently inhibits the spread of abnormal discharges through the brain. Although the precise nature of this action is not known, it is hypothesized that three mechanisms may be responsible: an increase in gamma-aminobutyric acid (GABA), an increased postsynaptic response to GABA, or an increase in the resting membrane potential.

Pharmacokinetics

Valproic acid is rapidly absorbed after oral ingestion, whether taken in capsule or syrup form. Peak serum levels occur in less than 4 hours. Concurrent food intake and use of the enteric coated form, divalproex sodium, slows absorption. Valproic acid is rapidly distributed in the body and is highly bound to serum proteins (Table 7-3). The therapeutic serum level is 50 to 100 μg/ml. Valproic acid is metabolized mostly in the liver and excreted in the urine. The serum half-life is relatively short, 6 to 16 hours. Children with immature livers and older patients with cirrhosis or acute hepatitis have prolonged half-lives (67 hours and 25 hours, respectively).

The usual starting dose of valproic acid for both adults and children is about 15 mg/kg per day (Table 7-4). This is a low dose, but it effectively reduces the incidence of bothersome side effects. Dosage then can be systematically raised at weekly intervals (increased by 5 to 10 mg/kg per day) to the daily maintenance level of 20 to 60 mg/kg. Because of the short half-life of valproic acid, a steady-state blood level can best be achieved by dividing this daily dose into 3 or 4 doses.

Side Effects

Valproic acid causes relatively few serious side effects (Table 7-6). This quality and its broad clinical utility are responsible for its growing acceptance as a major antiepileptic. Some GI tract symptoms are common during early therapy, but these disappear after continued usage. Also, prescription of the enteric coated form reduces GI tract discomfort. Almost 10% of the patients taking valproic acid gain weight. At therapeutic levels, only phenytoin causes less drowsiness than valproic acid.

Fatal hepatic failure has been associated with valproic acid and is most likely to occur in children under 2 years of age. Valproic acid is often given with other antiepileptics, which confounds efforts to know the true extent of hepatoxicity. Nonetheless, valproic acid and its derivatives are contraindicated in patients with liver disease and in children most at risk, those under 6 months of age.

Other adverse reactions can include emotional upset, some aleopecia, and musculoskeletal weakness.

Implications

Therapeutic versus toxic levels. Therapeutic serum levels of valproic acid are 50 to 100 μg/ml. At serum levels above 100 μg/ml CNS depression and coma develop. These events are most likely to result when valproic acid and phenobarbital are given concurrently. Restlessness and visual hallucinations are also symptoms of overdosage.

Since valproic acid is absorbed quickly, treatment is supportive unless it begins soon after the drug was ingested. If little time has elapsed, gastric lavage and forced emesis can reduce absorption and should be attempted. If absorption has occurred, support of respiratory and cardiovascular systems is most appropriate. Hemodialysis has been used. Naloxone (Narcan), the narcotic antagonist, may reverse the CNS depressant effects of valproic acid. However, since naloxone could also reverse antiepileptic effects, it should be used cautiously.

Use in pregnancy. Valproic acid is teratogenic and should not be used unless other antiepileptics have been found ineffective. The Centers for Disease Control estimate a risk of 1% to 2% for spina bifida in infants of mothers taking this drug. Only when the risk to the mother's health is otherwise so great that withholding valproic acid could be deemed irresponsible practice should this drug be prescribed. Concentrations of valproic acid in breast milk have been found to be 1% to 10% of the mother's serum level of the drug.

Side effects. Again, serious side effects of valproic acid are uncommon. Drowsiness typically disappears after usage. Hepatoxicity, although potentially fatal, can be averted by obtaining results of tests of hepatic function before treatment and by screening certain groups of patients, that is, infants and children under 2 years of age (especially, those under 6 months of age) and individuals with liver dysfunction. Gastrointestinal tract problems are alleviated by taking this drug with food.

Interactions. Valproic acid interacts with many drugs. It potentiates the actions of other CNS depressants such as alcohol and barbiturates by inhibiting hepatic metabolism of those agents. Some seizure disorders may be best treated with a combination of valproic acid and clonazepam; however, available evidence also indicates a potential increased risk of absence seizures. Sedation also increases with this combination.

Drugs that increase serum level of valproic acid. Chlorpromazine *increases* the half-life of valproic acid, as does aspirin. Since valproic acid inhibits platelet aggregation, use with aspirin and warfarin can cause prolonged bleeding and warrants close monitoring.

Drugs that decrease serum level of valproic acid. Valproic acid serum levels are *decreased* by the interactants carbamazepine and phenytoin.

Drug serum levels increased by valproic acid. Phenytoin serum levels are *increased* by valproic acid (as a result of protein-binding displacement), as are the plasma levels of phenobarbital (inhibition of hepatic metabolism) and ethosuximide. Phenobarbital serum levels are increased by as much as 200% when valproic acid is given concurrently; consequently, when given together, the dosage of phenobarbital should be reduced. A similar interaction may occur with the related long-acting barbiturates, mephobarbital, primidone, and possibly, metharbital. The anticoagulation effects of aspirin and warfarin are enhanced by valproic acid.

Patient education. Teach the patient the following:

To take valproic acid with food, if GI tract upset should occur

To swallow tablets or capsules whole to avoid irritation of mouth and throat

To take the drug at bedtime to minimize effects of drowsiness, and to be cautious when driving

To notify those monitoring for diabetes because valproic acid may give false-positive blood and urine ketone values.

Related Drugs

Valproate (Depakene syrup) is the sodium salt of valproic acid, as is the enteric coated divalproex sodium (Depakote), a compound that contains equal portions of valproic acid and valproate. Dosages are equivalent. Noticeable differences are the more rapid absorption when the syrup is used and delayed absorption with the enteric coated divalproex. Divalproex may reduce GI tract irritation.

CARBAMAZEPINE

Carbamazepine (Tegretol) is a major antiepileptic that is finding considerable use in new and interesting ways. It is related to the TCAs, and some patients taking this antiepileptic testify to improved mood (see Chapter 5). Although carbamazepine is an effective antiepileptic, some clinicians are reluctant to prescribe it because of its potential toxic effects.

Pharmacologic Effect

Although the exact mechanism of action is not known, carbamazepine is thought to reduce polysynaptic responses, thus preventing the spread of seizures. Carbamazepine is indicated for complex partial, tonic-clonic, or mixed seizures. It is not effective in controlling absence seizures. Other uses for carbamazepine include pain relief in persons with trigeminal neuralgia and restless legs syndrome, the treatment of psycotic illnesses, particularly, manic depressive psychosis, and posttraumatic stress disorder.

Pharmacokinetics

Carbamazepine is slowly and incompletely absorbed from the GI tract. Peak serum levels are reached within 5 hours after oral administration, and steady state is achieved within 2 to 4 days. Therapeutic serum levels are between 4 and 12 μg/ml. Carbamazepine is bound to serum proteins (76%). Carbamazepine is metabolized in the liver to an active metabolite. Initially the half-life in drug-naive patients ranges from 25 to 65 hours, but after sustained dosage the half-life is reduced to 12 to 17 hours. Urinary (72%) and fecal (28%) excretions are the sources of carbamazepine elimination.

Adults and children over 12 years of age are given initial dosages of 200 mg twice per day (see Table 7-5). Maintenance doses are typically in the range of 800 to 1200 mg per day for adults and 400 to 800 mg for children 6 to 12 years of age.

Side Effects

The most serious side effects of carbamazepine are hematologic reactions. Cases of fatal aganulocytosis have been reported, although the absolute incidence is low (1 in 50,000 persons). Besides agranulocytosis, aplastic anemia, thrombocytopenia, increased prothrombin time, and leukopenia are potential effects of this drug. Patients with a history of bone marrow depression should not receive this drug.

More common yet less severe reactions to carbamazepine than those previously mentioned include drowsiness, dizziness, unsteadiness, nausea, and diplopia. Other adverse reactions include activation of latent psychosis, confusion in elderly patients, hepatic and renal damage, and dermatologic problems. Meador et al. (1991) found that cognitive changes associated with carbamazepine were not significant.

Implications

Therapeutic versus toxic levels. Therapeutic serum levels are 4 to 12 μg/ml. Levels above 12 μg/ml are potentially toxic. A lethal dose of carbamazepine ranges from 5 g in small children to 30 g in adults. The first signs of overdose appear within 3 hours of administration and tend to be neuromuscular. Muscle restlessness, twitching, exaggerated reflexes, and, finally, reflex depression are among the initial indications of overdose. Large overdoses lead to respiratory difficulties, cardiovascular symptoms such as arrhythmias, tachycardia, and hypotension or hypertension, and seizures.

Although there is no specific antidote for carbamazepine, supportive care and elimination of the drug from the body can save the life of the patient. Supportive care might include elevating the patient's legs when hypotension develops, monitoring blood pressure, continued surveillance of vital signs until full recovery, and intubation for respiratory difficulty.

Gastric lavage, even after several hours have passed, can help the patient recover from overdose. If alcohol is involved, gastric lavage is even more significant. Vomiting should be induced immediately after discovering an overdose unless otherwise indicated. Activated charcoal via a nasal gastric tube is warranted as well. Hemodialysis for the treatment of severe overdose, replacement therapy in small children, and the administration of an osmotic-based diuretic to hasten renal excretion are other interventions for carbamazepine poisoning. Parenteral diazepam or phenobarbital is indicated to control acute seizures brought on by carbamazepine overdose but may cause additional respiratory depression.

Use in pregnancy. Carbamazepine is not recommended for use during pregnancy. Breast-feeding is usually discouraged because breast milk can contain a level of the drug as high as 60% of the mother's drug serum level (Vestermark and Vestermark, 1991).

Side effects. Complete blood cell counts, hepatic and renal function tests, and eye examinations should be performed before carbamazepine therapy begins and routinely thereafter. If a significant abnormality in any of the preceding areas should develop, the patient's condition should be carefully monitored or the drug discontinued and a new antiepileptic ordered, to prevent exacerbation of seizure activity. Since fatal aganulocytosis has been reported, when carbamazepine is discontinued based on hematologic grounds, blood levels should be determined regularly, perhaps as often as daily. In the elderly patient confusion and CNS symptoms necessitate special attention.

Interactions. Carbamazepine interacts with many drugs but can effectively be given concurrently with other antiepileptic agents. When given with drugs such as phenytoin, phenobarbital, or primidone, an increase in the respective doses of these drugs may be necessary because carbamazepine speeds their metabolism.

Drugs that increase serum levels of carbamazepine. Cimetidine, erythromycin, fluoxetine, propoxyphen, verapamil, and valproic acid increase the effect of carbamazepine. Increased serum carbamazepine levels do not force the clinician to abandon these combinations; however, careful monitoring of the patient is indicated should any of these drugs be ordered concurrently with carbamazepine.

Drugs that decrease serum levels of carbamazepine. Cortiosteroids, coumadin, oral contraceptives, antipsychotics, phenobarbital, phenytoin, and primidone decrease the effect of carbamazepine.

Drug serum level increased by carbamazepine. Carbamazepine possibly increases the effect of phenytoin.

Drug serum levels decreased by carbamazepine. Carbamazepine decreases the effect of warfarin, oral contraceptives, TCAs, theophylline, valproic acid, alprazolam, clonazepam, and doxycycline.

Additionally, since the interactions of carbamazepine and lithium and carbamazepine and haloperidol can cause a neurotoxic condition, such combinations should be used with caution.

Patient education. As with other antiepileptics, the potential to cause GI tract upset is present, so the patient is advised to take the drug with food to avoid nausea, vomiting, and the like. Since drowsiness, dizziness, and blurred vision can complicate driving, cautions in this area should also be taken. Because of the seriousness of hematologic reactions, the patient should notify the physician or nurse when any of the signs and symptoms of blood dyscrasia are present, that is sore throat, bruising, bleeding, fever, chills, and so forth.

RARELY USED ANTIEPILEPTICS

Phenacemide

Phenacemide (Phenurone), although effective in the treatment of severe forms of mixed complex-partial seizures (psychomotor) refractory to other drugs, is a seldom-used antiepileptic because of the intensity of its side effects. Phenacemide can cause direct toxicity in organs, for example, liver damage.

Phenacemide is well absorbed from the intestine and is metabolized in the liver. Therapeutic serum levels are not established. The average maintenance dose of phenacemide is 2 to 3 grams per day in three equal doses; To reduce side effects, initial doses are much lower. Common side effects include anorexia, weight loss, nausea, drowsiness, dizziness, weakness, and ataxia. More serious effects include nephritis and reported fatal blood dyscrasias. A major concern are the psychologic side effects associated with use of this drug. Aggression, suicidal tendencies, and acute psychosis may necessitate discontinuance of the drug.

Acetazolamide

Acetazolamide (Diamox) is a diuretic that inhibits the enzyme carbonic anyhdrase. This mechanism alkalinizes the urine, causing mild systemic acidosis. This reduction in blood pH reduces seizures in some individuals. Acetazolamide is used adjunctively in the treatment of absence, tonic-clonic, and myoclonic seizures.

Lidocaine

Lidocaine (Xylocaine) is a local anesthetic and an antiarrhythmic drug. Its one significant antiepileptic use is as one of the last treatments to be used when attempting to interrupt status epilepticus. The recommended dose is 50 to 100 mg injected IV. High doses of lidocaine can precipitate status epilepticus in otherwise seizure-free patients.

Magnesium sulfate

Patients with lowered levels of magnesium, that is, eclampsia and alcohol withdrawal syndrome, are subject to seizures. Magnesium sulfate given IM (preferred) or IV can prevent these seizures. Since low serum magnesium levels are ongoing in these conditions, it may be necessary to administer magnesium sulfate frequently.

Paraldehyde

Historically paraldehyde has been used to control seizures associated with alcohol withdrawal. New drugs are now being used for this purpose; however, paraldehyde remains a viable agent for the treatment of status epilepticus when other drugs have failed. It is administered IM or IV.

REFERENCES

Barry K, Teixeira S: The role of the nurse in the diagnostic classification and management of epileptic seizures *J Neurosurg Nurs* 15:243, 1985.

Boudewyns PA et al: Comorbidity and treatment outcome of inpatients with chronic combat-related PTSD, *Hosp Community Psychiatry* 42(8):847, 1991.

Dalessio JD: Seizure disorders and pregnancy, *New Engl J Med* 312:559, 1985.

Delgado-Escueta AV, Treiman DM, Walsh GO: The treatable epilepsies, *New Engl J Med* 308:1508, 1576, 1983.

Delgado-Escueta AV et al: Management of status epilepticus, *New Engl J Med* 306:1337, 1982.

Keltner NL: Anticonvulsant drugs. In Shlafer M, Marieb EN, editors: *The nurse, pharmacology, and drug therapy,* Redwood City, Calif, 1989, Addison-Wesley.

Keltner NL, Folks, DG: Alternatives to lithium in the treatment of bipolar disorder, *Perspect Psychiatric Care* 27(2):36, 1991.

Keltner NL, Schwecke LH, Bostrom CE: *Psychiatric nursing: a psychotherapeutic management approach,* St Louis, 1991, Mosby.

McKenna PJ, Kane JM, Parrish K: Psychotic syndromes in epilepsy, *Am J Psychiatry* 142:895, 1985.

Meador KJ et al: Comparative cognitive effects of carbamazepine and phenytoin in healthy adults, *Neurology* 41(10):1537, 1991.

Norman SE, Browne TR: Seizure disorders, *Am J Nurs* 81:984, 1981.

Olin BR, editor: *Drug facts and comparisons,* St Louis, 1990, JB Lippincott.

Penry JK, Newmark ME: The use of antiepileptic drugs, *Ann Intern Med* 90:207, 1979.

Trimble MR: *The psychoses of epilespsy,* New York, 1991, Raven.

Vestermark V, Vestermark S: Teratogenic effect of carbamazepine, *Arch Dis Child* 66(5):641, 1991.

CHAPTER 8

Sleep Disorders

HISTORICAL CONSIDERATIONS

Among the major groups of sleep disorders the dysomnias (insomnia and hypersomnia), the parasomnias, sleep disturbances resulting from narcolepsy, sleep apnea, or periodic leg movements, and psychophysiologic disturbances are most amenable to drug treatment. This chapter primarily focuses on the pharmacologic aspects of disturbed sleep.

A brief historical review of the evolution of sleep disorders medicine is pertinent. Several factors have led to remarkable developments in the basic aspects of this specialty. Not until the late 1940s and early 1950s did the pioneering work take place of Nathanial Kleitman and his graduate students, Eugene Aserinsky and William Dement, at the University of Chicago (Aserinsky and Kleitman, 1953). Their work led to technologic advances in the production of reliable electrographic recordings obtained from the human brain and a variety of other organs, which allowed investigation of the neurophysiologic changes that occur on the wakefulness-to-sleep continuum.

The milestone discovery was the realization that sleep, as it progressed through the nocturnal period, was not a unitary phenomenon but indeed was characterized by a sequence of sleep stages. It was noted that physiologic changes occurred as one stage gave way to another. Furthermore, these stages were found to alternate rhythmically throughout the night. Rapid eye movement (REM) sleep was found to be a state distinct from non-REM sleep. The first two decades of sleep research reflected interest in the phenomena of REM and non-REM sleep. This research consisted of a number of studies of REM sleep that resulted in a large body of information about the physiologic, biochemical, and pharmacologic aspects of sleep. A recognition of distinct sleep disorders resulted. The basic tool of sleep research was the simultaneous electrographic recording of multiple physiologic variables, now referred to as polysomnography (Holland, Dement, and Raynal, 1974). Valuable to subsequent pharmacologic approaches to insomnia and other sleep disorders were research studies of the effects of hypnotic drugs (Kales et al., 1969).

The study of sleep disturbances has become an interdisciplinary field, perhaps best illustrated in the area of sleep-induced breathing disorders, particularly, obstructive sleep apnea. One half to two thirds of all patients referred to sleep disorder centers in this country have disorders that reduce sleep. These disorders are a major cause of social and work disability, as well as a contributor to systemic hypertension, cardiac arrhythmia, and other cardiovascular consequences (Coleman et al., 1982; Guilleminault and Dement, 1978). Hence pulmonologists, neurologists, psychiatrists, psychiatric nurses, and others (depending on the nature of the patient's problem) work together to assess and diagnose the disorders in patients with disturbed sleep. The ability to help these patients continues to improve. Additionally, the use of questionnaires, sleep diaries, medical history, and physical and laboratory examinations have further improved the basic clinical understanding of sleep disturbances. Together with the polysomnogram, these assessment tools, as well as pharmacologic interventions, help guide the management of sleep disorder.

The polysomnogram, a measure of multiple physiologic functions during sleep, involves the patient sleeping one or sometimes two nights at a sleep center. The patient is placed in a sound-controlled private bedroom at a comfortable, controlled temperature. Electroencephalogram (EEG), eye movements, heart rate, and muscle activity from several sources are recorded to determine physiologic state and the sleep stage. Other values specific to the patient's problems may also be measured, including electrocardiogram (ECG), air flow from the nose and mouth, and blood oxygen saturation. Nighttime recordings are often followed by daytime tests such as multiple sleep latency tests, which are quantitative measures of sleep tendency. A complete review of the physiology of sleep (sleep architecture) and electrophysiology (polysomnography) is beyond the scope of this book; however, for further reading see Mendelson (1987) or Hartmann (1974).

Although the sleep laboratory may not achieve the precise quality and architecture of sleep experienced in the patient's home, surveys indicate that fewer than 1 in 1000 patients sleep so poorly as to invalidate the procedure. Perhaps the most encouraging aspects of the growth of this field have been the high degree of patient satisfaction resulting from the use of current diagnostic and treatment modalities and the many treatment interventions that have been developed to significantly improve the patient's quality of life.

DIAGNOSTIC CONSIDERATIONS

Epidemiologic surveys suggest that 20% to 30% of adults report having sleep difficulties at least occasionally (Kales and Kales, 1984). Approximately 7% of the population use sleeping agents to increase sleep; about 1% use a prescription hypnotic 30 days or more per year (Balter and Bauer, 1975). The incidence of excessive sleepiness has varied from 0.02% to 1% in the general population. Surveys of medical patients suggest that the rate of insomnia is 17% and the rate of hypersomnia is 3% (Bixler, Kales, and Soldatos, 1979). Age and disease tend to increase the prevalence of disturbed sleep.

Quality sleep normally requires good health, comfortable circumstance, and a lengthy daily period that is free of stressful obligations. Also, freedom from the influence of stimulants and other drugs that negatively affect the structure of sleep is required for quality sleep. In short, sleep is easily disrupted. The frenetic demands of an industrial culture may induce a briefer-than-normal average sleeping time. "Adlib" sleepers tend to sleep better than those whose obligations compel abbreviated sleep hours; short sleepers (those who require less sleep than normal) tolerate demanding work schedules better than those requiring 8 hours or more of sleep (Caraskadon and Dement, 1982).

Insomnia is defined as complaint of sleep insufficient to support good daytime functioning. Epidemiologic surveys suggest that about 15% of adults complain of insomnia, whereas only 2% actually take hypnotic medication (Kales and Kales, 1984). The majority of individuals taking hypnotic drugs use them less than 30 times per year. Thus transient insomnia is relatively common, but persistent insomnia is not. Interestingly, most individuals who come to sleep disorders clinics do so because of hypersomnia rather than insomnia (Coleman et al., 1982).

Common, nonspecific disruptions of sleep may precipitate or aggravate insomnia. Thus many individuals can improve the quality of their sleep by instituting sleep hygiene, as shown in the box on p. 172. Institution of a sleep hygiene program requires that the patient's interests and motivations are carefully considered. Some aspects of

Measures Used to Improve Sleep Hygiene

1. Arise at the same time each day.
2. Limit daily in-bed time to "normal" amount.
3. Discontinue use of drugs that act on the central nervous system, e.g., caffeine, nicotine, alcohol, and stimulants.
4. Avoid daytime napping except when sleep diary indicates a better night's sleep as a result.
5. Establish physical fitness with a routine of exercise early in the day, followed by other activity.
6. Avoid evening stimulation; substitute either listening to the radio or leisure reading for watching television.
7. Try a warm 20-minute body bath or soak near bedtime.
8. Eat on a regular schedule; avoid large meals near bedtime.
9. Practice an evening relaxation routine.
10. Maintain comfortable sleeping conditions.
11. Spend no longer then 20 minutes awake in the bed.
12. Adjust sleep hours and routine to optimize daily schedule and living situation.

good sleep hygiene, such as quitting smoking, are difficult to achieve. Other recommendations shown in the box above may be arduous or simply may not be possible.

Persistent insomnia without coexisting medical causes is called *primary insomnia* in the *Diagnostic and Statistical Manual of Mental Disorders, Third Edition-Revised (DSM-III-R)* (American Psychiatric Association, 1987). Although in some persons psychopathologic factors may contribute to the development of primary insomnia, others may not show any comorbid psychiatric condition (Kales and Kales, 1984). Of course, in individuals who are psychologically aroused fears or anxiety may develop or the persons may simply ruminate into the night. All these psychologic factors further disrupt sleep. Hypervigilance, anxiety, neuroticism, introversion, and insomnia all theoretically derive from common central nervous system (CNS) profiles of increased internal arousal (Grey, 1982).

Patients and clinicians alike are quick to attribute insomnia to psychologic problems. Specific psychiatric conditions do predispose persons to insomnia, in particular, mood disorders, anxiety, and the dementias. However, insomnia should not be attributed to these conditions unless reasonably good sleep hygiene measures are in place. Many patients have spent fruitless years seeking dependable sleep by means of anxiety reduction and psychotherapy while concomitantly working late, drinking coffee, and sleeping late on weekends.

Patients may complain loudly of insomnia simply because it is debilitating and because it is socially acceptable or quite easy to focus on the symptom. Whether depressed or anxious, patients who complain primarily about insomnia may do so because of a complex mixture of biopsychosocial factors. For example, many patients ascribe their depression to insomnia rather than vice versa. Patients whose moods are dysphoric in concert with insomnia may be promptly helped by sedative hypnotic drugs; however, long-lasting relief of insomnia is sustained only in a minority of patients with depression. In short, the treatment of insomnia caused by a primary psychiatric disturbance necessitates a full understanding of the patient's psychosocial and mental status, and the clinical approach must appreciate any underlying disorder per se. Moreover, drugs, caffeine, nicotine, and alcohol, so ubiquitously disruptive of sleep, must be discontinued or withdrawn in patients with insomnia, if at all possible (Tan et al., 1984).

Additionally, over-the-counter agents with CNS-stimulating actions may be disruptive of sleep, as may catecholamine blockers such as stimulating antidepressants (fluoxetine and protriptyline), antiarrhythmic drugs, corticosteroids, thyroid preparations, and methysergide. Diuretics may cause cramps or restless leg syndrome, or both. Sleeping pills may paradoxically worsen sleep. Short-acting agents such as triazolam may cause agitation, amnestic episodes, early-morning awakening, or even next-day anxiety. These may merge together with next-night *rebound insomnia* to compound sleeping difficulties (Kales and Kales, 1984). Thus the chronic administration of hypnotics may actually serve to diminish sleep quality.

A variety of sleep difficulties, including insomnia, may result from suboptimal sleep schedules or from medical problems. In individuals who literally have their days and nights mixed up a tendency may develop toward later arising times, which results in delayed sleep-phase syndrome. This syndrome is most likely to occur in those without regular morning obligations. Disruption of the circadian rhythms may follow. Treatment includes progressively shifting the sleep hours incrementally toward a desirable, fixed schedule.

Many shift workers sleep poorly. Some of those individuals who need little sleep may prefer night work and function well on the few hours of sleep that they are able to obtain. However, other shift workers sleep poorly and feel chronically fatigued. Among those in the country's work force, workers on rotating shifts have perhaps the most difficulty. These rotating-shift workers and their employers should consider the problems associated with disruption of circadian rhythms. A potential partial solution is less frequent changing of shifts, for example, changing shifts monthly rather than weekly. Such a common-sense approach may result in a less significant disturbance of sleep. Individuals who are intolerant of shifting work schedules may have chronic fatigue or may ultimately become disabled or debilitated, in some cases necessitating a career change or a significant change in focus of occupation. Professions that are particularly stressful in this regard include nursing, meteorology, and military service.

Although an individual's work hours may normally vary in relation to sleep hours, those with a tendency toward insomnia may make matters worse by sleeping late on weekends. In fact, rising at a predictable hour, going to bed at a regular time, and the previously discussed normal sequencing of sleep may all be compromised by these disruptions in regular sleep hours. Often an examination of a monthly sleep chart results in the astonishment of the patient, who is unaware of his or her irregular sleep schedule. In short, what these individuals need is a regular bedtime.

Symptoms of disease, such as itching or pain, may raise the threshold for sleep. Other symptoms, including dyspnea, nocturia, diarrhea, angina, migraine, or other medical problems, may disrupt sleep significantly. Settings where persons with medical problems are found, such as inpatient hospitals or long-term care settings, may be buzzing with constant activity, enforced sleeping positions, noises, and periodic crises, which hardly encourages adequate sleep. These clinical settings may sometimes actually exceed the Environmental Protection Agency guidelines for healthy noise levels.

The specifics of an individual patient's illness and treatment may further worsen the quality of sleep. For example, the patient in the intensive care unit is interrupted an average of five times per hour, even during the calmest of nights (Dlin et al., 1971). Any nonpsychiatric medical condition that potentially disrupts sleep may increase the risk of insomnia. Fear and worry, together with significant symptoms, may indicate the need for an appropriate therapeutic intervention. Direct effects of disease on sleep-regulating mechanisms can cause sleep disruption. Examples of such disease states include alteration of neurotransmitter systems, unpredictable metabolism associated with liver disease, or cortical dysfunction with primary dementia. Primary sleep problems most often identified with sleep disturbance include obstructive sleep apnea (discussed later); individuals with cardiovascular disorders, especially angina, and those predisposed to breathing impairment; and those with increased metabolic rate in concert with an endocrinopathy such as mild hyperthyroidism or diabetes. Patients with Cushing's disease and individuals with neurologic conditions such as a seizure disorder or Parkinson's disease are at risk for disturbed sleep. Esophageal reflux, chronic renal failure with uremia, other end-organ failure, and urinary frequency, fetal movements, and general discomfort in women in the third trimester of pregnancy all may cause a diminished quantity and quality of sleep.

DRUGS USED TO TREAT INSOMNIA

Currently sleep disorders are categorized as insomnia, hypersomnia, and a variety of sleep disorders related to a psychiatric disturbance, a secondary sleep disorder, or a substance-induced sleep disorder. Insomnia and hypersomnia are conceptualized as being either primary or secondary. Insomnia and hypersomnia, narcolepsy, the parasomnias, periodic leg movements (nocturnal myoclonus), and sleep apnea are among the disorders most frequently responsive to or affected by pharmacologic intervention (see the box on p. 175).

Many drugs, including those used in the treatment of insomnia, alter sleep and daytime function. They may mask wakefulness during sleep or diminish alertness during wakefulness. Changes in sleep may remain unnoticed by the individual, and even with daytime sedation, patients may be unaware of their impaired performance. Thus the effects that many drugs may have on the sleep-wakefulness continuum are of clinical relevance. Moreover, many drugs modify REM activity. For example, with the tricyclic antidepressants this effect may even correlate with a response to therapy.

The following discussion of psychotropic drugs used in the treatment of sleep disorders addresses the mechanisms of neurotransmission and neuromodulation and outlines implications for the use of sedatives or other psychotropics in specified patients with particular diagnostic sleep-wake problems. This chapter is devoted primarily to the clinical pharmacology of hypnotics and their role in therapeutics, but drugs that, although not used primarily for the treatment of insomnia, may be used in the treatment of other disturbances of sleep or daytime alertness are also identified.

The use of hypnotics to relieve insomnia should be temporary. More prescriptions are written for hypnotic and anxiolytic drugs than for any other class of drugs in the United States (Mendelson, 1980). Although the benzodiazepines have almost completely replaced the barbiturates, all known hypnotics promote sleep and inhibit wakefulness. The effects on sleep and wakefulness should not be separated. *All* hypnotic drugs shorten the time that elapses before a person falls asleep (sleep latency), reduce nocturnal wakefulness, increase total sleep time, and decrease body movements during sleep; all also cause difficulty in arousal from sleep. Thus hypnotics are generally viewed as CNS depressants and are specifically viewed as sleep-promoting compounds. This view is supported inasmuch as large doses of long-acting com-

Current Nomenclature of Sleep Disorders

American Psychiatric Association

Dyssomnias

Insomnia related to another mental disorder *or* to known organic factor
Primary insomnia
Hypersomnia related to another mental disorder *or* to known organic factor
Primary hypersomnia
Sleep-wake schedule disorder

Parasomnias

Dream anxiety disorder
Sleep terror disorder
Sleepwalking disorder

American Sleep Disorders Association

Dyssomnias

Intrinsic sleep disorders
Psychophysiological
Narcolepsy
Hypersomnias
Obstructive sleep
Apnea
Central nervous system sleep apnea
Periodic limb movement disorder
Restless leg syndrome
Extrinsic sleep disorders
Inadequate sleep hygiene
Environmental sleep disorder
Hypnotic-dependent sleep disorder
Stimulant-dependent sleep disorder
Alcohol-dependent sleep disorder
Circadian rhythm sleep disorders
Jet lag
Work, shift-related
Delayed sleep-phase
Advanced sleep-phase

Parasomnias

Arousal disorders
Confusional-arousal disorder
Sleepwalking
Sleep terrors
Sleep-wake transition disorders
Sleep-starts disorder
Sleep-talking disorder
REM sleep–related disorders
Nightmares
Sleep paralysis
REM sleep–related behavior disorder
Hypnotic-dependent sleep disorder

Medical and psychiatric sleep disorders

Psychiatric
Psychoses
Mood disorders
Anxiety disorders
Panic disorder
Alcoholism
Neurologic
Dementia
Parkinsonism
Epilepsy
Other medical disorders

Proposed sleep disorders

Fragmentary myoclonus
Menstrual-associated sleep disorders
Others

From American Psychiatric Association *Diagnostic and statistical manual of mental disorders, third edition-revised*, Washington, DC, 1987, The Association.

pounds depress and possibly interfere with the wakening function. Thus there are both short-term and long-term benefits and risks associated with the use of hypnotics. The benefit-to-risk ratio should be weighed carefully with the knowledge that the aim of a good night's sleep should be to improve the vigor of the following day. Rarely has this result been demonstrated as a consequence of the use of hypnotic drugs.

Drug treatment for insomnia is all too often casual, and diagnostic features may be incorrect. Long-term use of sedatives usually relieves only sedative-withdrawal insomnia (that is, the insomnia caused by the sedative itself), not the original insomnia. Of the 3% of adults who use prescribed hypnotics, about 20% use drugs more than 120 days per year (Mellinger, Balter, and Uhlenhuth, 1985). Such drugs are disproportionately prescribed for older adults in whom the drugs can aggravate cortical dysfunction and psychologic regression.

As previously noted, the most appropriate and important management approaches insomnia are removal or treatment of the cause and an alteration of poor sleep habits. Hypnotics, when prescribed, should be administered in short courses and in low doses; alternate or every-other-night therapy is recommended. Treatment should be monitored, and the emergence of nocturnal confusion, agitation, and restlessness, especially in older patients and children, should be carefully considered. As for the patients discussed in Chapters 15, 16, and 17, combining an initial course of pharmacotherapy with a nonpharmacologic approach such as behavioral techniques and then

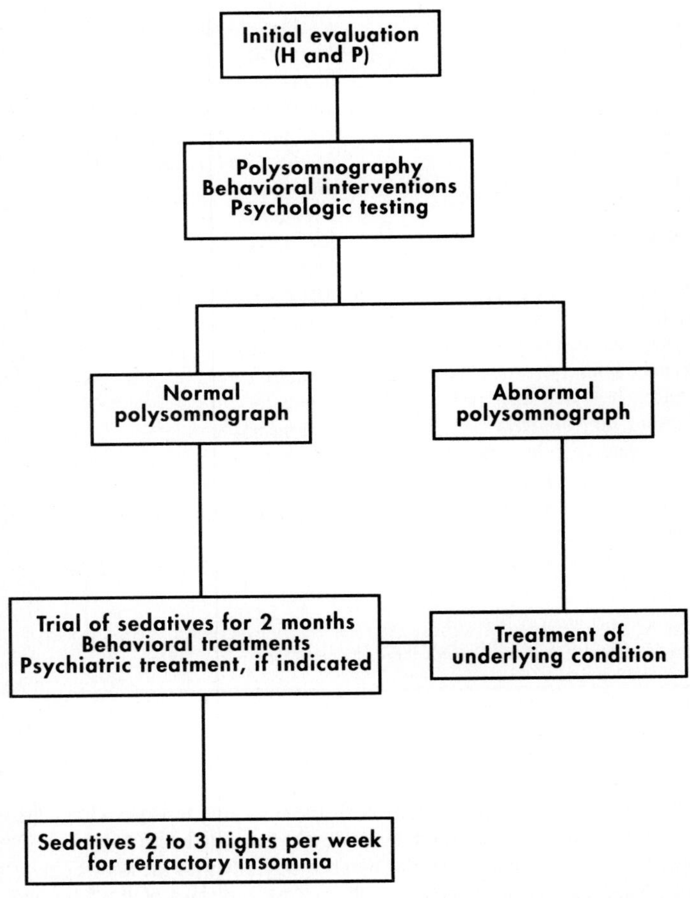

Figure 8-1 Flow chart for the evaluation and treatment of severe insomnia. (From Wooten V: *Psychiatr Ann* 20[8]:466, 1990.)

optimizing the medical and physiologic status of the patient provide an ideal approach.

A useful initial approach to a patient with insomnia is to consider the duration of the complaint. Long-term insomnia (months or years), short-term insomnia (a week or so), and transient difficulties (periodic bouts of insomnia for 2 to 3 days) should be approached quite differently. The duration of the insomnia not only provides an indication of the origin of insomnia but also may help guide the use of psychotropic agents, specifically, hypnotics. Although hypnotics may be appropriately prescribed for patients with long-term insomnia, in these individuals a diligent evaluation is necessary before hypnotics are prescribed. As shown in Figure 8-1, the drugs are most appropriately prescribed when there is clear evidence of disturbed sleep without an apparent and direct intervention. In contrast to long-term insomnia, most other cases involve healthy individuals who wish to carry out their day-to-day activities free from the residual effects of insomnia. For these individuals benzodiazepines and, to a lesser extent, antidepressant medications are most frequently prescribed. Other drug classes that may be considered useful include phenothiazines, which may improve sleep in psychotic patients; phenytoin for the treatment of paroxysmal nightmares associated with psychomotor attacks; beta-adrenergic antagonists for the treatment of disturbed sleep in association with hyperthyroidism; and cimetidine or other H_2-receptor blockers for patients with peptic ulcer disease, nonulcer dyspepsia, or reflux. Many patients have "pseudoinsomnia"; they complain of poor sleep, but polysomnograph studies are normal. These patients benefit best from no drug intervention.

Neurochemical Effects of Hypnotics

As with other psychiatric disturbances, changes in sleep and wakefulness are believed to arise from the activity of chemical agents that influence communication between neurons (see Chapters 2 and 3). In particular, monoamines are synthesized as neurotransmitters and are now known to play a particular role in the control of alert states. Other, less well-known neurotransmitter systems (outlined in Chapter 3) may also ultimately prove important. These neurochemical processes, of course, can be modulated by drugs. Psychotropics that may have some role in the treatment of sleep disturbances are currently divided into the following categories:

1. Neurotransmitter metabolism modifiers, including precursors such as L-tryptophan or levodopa
2. Enzyme inhibitors that effect the synthesis or catabolism of the neurotransmitter
3. Drugs that alter the distribution or utilization of the transmitter, for example, reserpine, alphamethyldopa, or monoamine oxidase inhibitors (MAOIs). (These actions are discussed in detail in Chapter 3.)

Psychotropic drug treatment of sleep disturbance is carried out with the recognition that many drugs have distinct or opposite actions on the CNS at different concentrations; that is, complex dose-response relationships exist. For example, some drugs have a stimulatory effect followed by a sedative effect. Feedback mechanisms that operate within the CNS may also be responsible for complex or paradoxic responses to psychotropics.

Considerable attention recently has been devoted to the pharmacology of the benzodiazepines. As discussed in Chapter 6, these agents modulate gamma-aminobutyric acid (GABA) transmission and interact with specific receptor sites in the brain (Mohler and Okada, 1977). As discussed in Chapter 3, GABA is the most abundant inhibitor neurotransmitter in the CNS and about a third of all synapses are GABAnergic. Most neurons that release this neurotransmitter, however, are interneurons that modulate activity by presynaptic and postsynaptic inhibition. Many intrinsic neurons found within the raphe nuclei and their terminals form inhibitory synapses with serotonergic receptor sites or cells. Terminals are also identified within the locus ceruleus, but the cell bodies of origin are unknown. Although GABA inhibits the activity of the locus ceruleus, the exact mode of action is unclear. A minority of neurons, such as Purkinje's cells in the cerebellum or the GABA-nergic neurons of the striatonigral pathway, project distantly in the brain, probably having complex effects (as noted in Chapters 2 and 3). Moreover, the classic benzodiazepines such as diazepam appear to bind without substantial regional differences. Benzodiazepine-1 receptors located primarily on postsynaptic membranes are distinguished from benzodiazepine-2 receptors, which are presynaptic. The anxiolytic and antiepileptic effects are thought to be related to the agonistic effect on benzodiazepine-1 receptors, whereas sedation may result from activation of the benzodiazepine-2 receptors (Hirsch, Garrett, and Beer, 1985).

BENZODIAZEPINES

Benzodiazepines were first synthesized by Leo Sternback in 1933. In 1956 his colleague Lowell Randell found that chlordiazepoxide (Librium) had tranquilizing effects in animals (Haefely, 1983). Chlordiazepoxide was introduced for clinical use from 1960 to 1961, spawning a series of vastly successful drugs used in the treatment of insomnia. It also is used in the treatment of anxiety, tension, epilepsy, muscle spasm, and neuropsychiatric disturbances. Interestingly, most hypnotic drugs also relieve anxiety (and most CNS stimulant drugs also produce anxiety). As mentioned in Chapter 6, the effects of benzodiazepines on anxiety and alertness are sometimes difficult to distinguish. Most if not all benzodiazepines produce both anxiolytic and hypnotic effects. The selectivity or behavioral effect of benzodiazepines is a product of pharmacokinetic factors. Thus many compounds may have an anxiolytic profile at low doses and a hypnotic profile at high doses. The pattern of metabolism in which many benzodiazepines may be converted to the same metabolite may also account for a specific drug's utility in treatment.

The anxiolytic or hypnotic use of benzodiazepines may have been determined by the pattern of research development or clinical testing. For example, it was found early on that *oxazepam* (Serax) was not an effective sleep inducer but that anxiety was reduced when oxazepam was given in doses that did not cause somnolence (Parkes, 1989). However, two short-acting drugs, *triazolam* (Halcion) 0.5 to 1 mg and *temazepam* (Restoril) 30 mg, were found to cause the least residual impairment (hangover) when used for hypnotic effect (Bond and Lader, 1981). Some studies suggested that the incidence of drowsiness is lower with intermediate half-life benzodiazepines such as *prazepam* (Centrax) and, perhaps, with *lorazepam* (Ativan) and *alprazolam* (Xanax) than with other benzodiazepines of equivalent anxiolytic dose (Cohn, 1981; Dement, Siedel, and Caraskadon, 1982).

The classic benzodiazepines used as hypnotics in the treatment of sleep disturbances are outlined in Table 8-1. These include triazolam, estazolam (ProSom), temazepam, flurazepam (Dalmane), and quazepam (Doral) (Dominguez et al., 1986; Kales, 1990; Greenblatt et al., 1982; Greenblatt et al., 1989). Many conventional antidepressants are also prescribed for the enhancement of sleep because of their sedating properties. The sedative effect and half-life of antidepressants are profiled in Table 8-2. Antidepressants commonly prescribed for the enhancement of sleep include trazodone (Desyrel), amitriptyline (Elavil), doxepin (Sinequan), maprotiline (Ludiomil), imipramine (Tofranil), and nortriptyline (Pamelor). Although these antidepressant compounds are not specifically indicated for use in the treatment of insom-

Table 8-1 Clinical Profile of Commonly Prescribed Benzodiazepine Sedatives

Benzodiazepine sedative	Dosage (mg)	Onset of effect (hr)	Active metabolites	Elimination half-life
Triazolam (Halcion)	0.125-0.25	1-2	None	Rapid
Estazolam (ProSom)	0.5-1	1-2	None	Intermediate
Temazepam (Restoril)	15-30	2-3	Oxazepam	Intermediate
Flurazepam (Dalmane)	15-30	½-1	Hydroxyethylflurazepam, flurazepam aldehyde, desalkylflurazepam	Slow
Quazepam (Doral)	7.5-15	2	2-oxoquazepam N-desalkyl-2-oxoquazepam	Slow

Table 8-2 Antidepressant Sedative Effect and Elimination Half-Life

Agent	Sedative effect*	Half-life (hr)
Trazodone (Desyrel)	+++	4-9
Amitriptyline (Elavil)	+++	31-46
Doxepin (Adapin, Sinequan)	+++	8-24 (51)†
Maprotiline (Ludiomil)	++	21-25
Imipramine (Tofranil)	++	11-25
Nortriptyline (Aventyl, Pamelor)	++	18-44
Amoxapine (Asendin)	+	8-30
Protriptyline (Vivactil)	+	67-89
Desipramine (Norpramin)	+	12-24
Sertraline (Zoloft)	None to +	26-98‡
Fluoxetine (Prozac)	None	48-216
Bupropion (Wellbutrin)	None	8-24

Adapted from Fabre LF: *Trazodone dosing regimen: experience with single daily administration.* Presented at the Eighth World Congress of Psychiatry, Athens, Greece, October 1989.
*+++ = marked; ++ = moderate; + = mild.
†Active metabolite, desmethyldoxepin, has a longer half-life than parent compound (51 hours ± 17 hours).
‡From Roerig: *Psychiatrist's Zoloft sampling program* (manufacturer's pamphlet), New York, 1992, Roerig.

nia, they are often prescribed for that purpose, especially for patients with coexisting depression.

Pharmacologic Effects

The classic benzodiazepines generally shorten sleep latency, reduce the number of awakenings and the duration of wakefulness during the night, and increase total sleep time. The latency to REM sleep is prolonged by the benzodiazepines, but this effect may be due to the suppression of the first episode of REM sleep rather than to a delay in its appearance (Belyavin and Nicholson, 1987). Non-REM sleep is changed considerably by the classic benzodiazepines. The duration of stage 1 is reduced, and that of stage 2 is increased. Moreover, EEGs show slowing of electrophysiologic activity, in particular, the emergence of delta waves, k-wave potentials, and theta activities that are less abundant. (For a complete discussion of the electroencephalographic changes and physiologic correlates see Weitzmann and Pollak, 1982.) Perhaps the most significant effects of benzodiazepines are their effects on stage 4 (deep) sleep. Benzodiazepines may diminish release of growth hormone that is normally released during this stage. This disruption of stage 4 sleep may also decrease REM sleep. Paradoxically some insomniacs may have an increase in REM sleep, since some report having nightmares when taking benzodiazepines. After the withdrawal of benzodiazepines, sleep stages 2 and 4 remain altered much longer than do other sleep stages.

The nonclassic benzodiazepine clonazepam may modify sleep less markedly because it has only a few agonistic effects. Clonazepam is particularly useful as a sleep agent, since it inhibits REM sleep, but stage 4 sleep is actually increased during the night of administration and then decreased during the following night. Clonazepam may be particularly helpful in patients who have a sleep disturbance superimposed on another condition, for example, neurodegenerative disorders such as Alzheimer's or

Parkinson's disease or nocturnal myoclonus with periodic leg movement or restless leg syndrome (discussed later in this chapter).

In general all benzodiazepines alter sleep by binding to the benzodiazepine receptor and the GABA receptor–chloride channel molecular complex (see Chapter 3). Although barbiturates may affect the chloride channels differently from the benzodiazepines, the activity of both classes of drugs has similar neuropharmacologic effects. For example, pentobarbital and phenobarbital exert a hypnotic effect in patients by shortening sleep latency and reducing intermittent awakenings during the night. In contrast to benzodiazepines, barbiturates, when given for an extended period, may induce a rebound REM sleep when discontinued. This REM sleep is often accompanied by nightmares. Thus benzodiazepines have distinct advantages over their predecessors. Further developments in the pharmacologic study of benzodiazepines may provide compounds that are freer of adverse effects than currently used compounds and may improve our knowledge of the mechanisms involved in the regulation of sleep and wakefulness (Gaillard and Phelippeau, 1976).

Pharmacokinetics

The absorption, metabolism, and elimination of benzodiazepines are nearly identical, but distribution is not. Individual differences are characterized in the latter part of this section. The most important factors governing the choice of benzodiazepines in the treatment of insomnia are the dose, the individual rate of absorption, the distribution (most relevant for single-dose effects), and the elimination half-life (most important in the treatment of chronic insomnia). Sleep induction by means of benzodiazepines depends entirely on the rate of absorption from the gut. Most benzodiazepines are rapidly absorbed, but absorption may be slowed by food and antacids. The absorption rate after intramuscular (IM) injection of many benzodiazepines, with the possible exception of lorazepam, is much slower than with oral administration.

The duration of clinical action of benzodiazepines in single doses depends on distribution, whereas accumulation becomes important with multiple doses. This means that absorption rates and distribution to the CNS at the therapeutic level are mostly responsible for a single-dose effect. Long half-life does not necessarily imply long duration of sedation, nor does short half-life imply short duration of action for a hypnotic. Accumulation, of course, is determined by metabolic clearance and elimination half-life. Benzodiazepine metabolism occurs primarily in two ways, conjugation (combining with glucuronic acid and becoming inert) and oxidation (via the hepatic microsomal enzyme system). Some short-acting benzodiazepine derivatives for example, oxazepam and lorazepam, are almost completely inactivated by one-step conjugation in the liver and therefore have few residual morning-after effects. Indeed, benzodiazepines eliminated as rapidly as these may even result in early-morning insomnia, whereas other benzodiazepines may produce persistent long-acting metabolites that cause a lingering impairment in alertness, motor performance, and cognitive functioning (e.g., flurazepam). Benzodiazepine metabolism is largely age dependent; the elimination half-life of diazepam, for instance, may increase three- to four-fold in persons from 20 to 80 years of age, thus increasing the bioavailability of the drug (Tables 8-1 and 8-3).

The action of a benzodiazepine hypnotic depends on its absorption, distribution, and elimination. The rate of absorption determines onset of action because benzodiazepines penetrate the blood-brain bearer easily. The more rapidly absorbed drugs have a faster onset of action, whereas those that are slowly absorbed may not have a desired effect at all. Of the currently marketed hypnotics, *flurazepam* is the most rapidly absorbed, followed by triazolam, which has an intermediate absorption rate, and

Table 8-3 Pharmacokinetic Properties of Some Currently Available Hypnotic Drugs

Significant pharmacokinetic characteristics	Drug (chemical group)	Recommended dose range (mg)	Tmax (h)	T1/2/elim(h)	Comments and indications	References
Slow absorption	Oxazepam (benzodiazepine)	15-30 (in elderly patients, 10-20)	2.2 ± 1.9	6.7 ± 1.7	Free of residual effects, but rather slowly absorbed; used mainly as an anxiolytic but sustains sleep	Greenblatt DJ et al: *J Pharmacol Exp Ther* 215:86, 1980
Slow elimination of parent compound or metabolite	Flurazepam hydrochloride (benzodiazepine): Active metabolites, 1-hydroxyethylflurazepam, desalkylflurazepam	15-30* (in elderly patients, 15)	1.4 ± 0.7 8.0 ± 8.0	0.9 ± 1.1 40 ± 103	Hypnotic effect related to the activity of metabolites; residual effects likely, and accumulation on continued nightly ingestion inevitable; useful for frequent nocturnal awakenings when some daytime sedation is acceptable; 7.5-mg dose may be useful for the elderly patients	Eckert M et al: *Drugs Exp Clin Res* 9:77, 1983

Relatively slow elimination, but marked distribution may lead to a short duration of action	Diazepam (benzodiazepine)	5-10 (in elderly patients, 5)	1.1 ± 0.3	32 ± 11	Free of residual effects when given occasionally, because of marked distribution phase; slow elimination of parent compound and active metabolite leads to accumulation and daytime anxiolytic effect with repeated ingestion	Kaplan SA et al: *J Pharm Sci* 62:1789, 1973
Relatively rapid elimination and marked distribution phase in appropriate formulations	Temazepam (benzodiazepine) soft gelatin capsule	10-60† (in elderly patients, 10-20)	0.8 ± 0.3	8.4 ± 0.6	Soft gel cap formulation in the dose range 10-20 mg is free of residual effects and of significant accumulation on daily ingestion; useful for sleep onset	Divoll M et al: *J Pharm Sci* 70:1104, 1981; Fuccella LM: *Br J Clin Pharmacol* 8:315, 1979
Ultrarapid elimination	Triazolam (triazolobenzodiazepine)	0.250‡ (in elderly patients, 0.125)	1.2 ± 0.5	2.6 ± 0.7	Dose range in some countries is 0.25-0.5 mg, but the higher dose leads to residual effects and rebound insomnia; useful for sleep onset	Jochemsen R et al: *Br J Clin Pharmacol* 16:291S, 1983

*Doses exceeding 15 mg may not be appropriate.
†Doses exceeding 20 mg may not be appropriate.
‡A dose of 0.125 mg may also be useful for adults other than the elderly.

temazepam, with a slow absorption rate. Thus the time at which the medication is given to the patient before the patient retires is of great importance (Greenblatt et al., 1982). Obviously a drug with a slow absorption rate (oxazepam) may be most appropriate for the treatment of anxiety for which a sustained effect with minimal initial drowsiness is sought. Once absorbed, a hypnotic is distributed to the blood and to the highly vascular tissues, that is, the brain, heart, liver, and lungs, and then distributed peripherally to less vascular tissues. This rapid distribution results in an initial drop in the plasma concentration, but the subsequent fall is mainly a result of elimination by metabolism and excretion.

Since a particular pharmacodynamic effect is related to a specific plasma concentration, knowledge of distribution versus elimination half-life can be of great clinical utility. The duration of activity is short when the plasma level is within the phase that predominantly represents distribution but longer when the plasma level is within the elimination phase. In other words, plasma concentration decay occurs more rapidly during the distribution phase than during the elimination phase. Thus both distribution and elimination influence duration of activity, that is half-life. In practical terms this means that a relatively short duration of action may be expected when giving a single dose of a hypnotic that is not rapidly eliminated but is rapidly distributed. Thus, although half-life is a familiar concept and often touted as the most important feature of benzodiazepines, it does have limitations in defining the duration of activity of a single dose.

Most benzodiazepines are metabolized in the liver, some produce numerous active metabolites. The pattern of metabolism of various drugs is similar. Benzodiazepines are mainly transformed in the liver by conjugation of attachment of the molecule to glucuronic acid, then excreted in the urine as pharmacologically inactive metabolites. However, some benzodiazepines form active metabolites, which complicates their pharmacologic properties. In addition, if the hepatic-detoxification system is compromised, as in viral hepatitis, benzodiazepine activity is prolonged and potential exists for physical complications.

The influence of distribution on plasma concentration decay is important. Although using the elimination half-life alone to predict duration of action is taught in most pharmacology courses, this guideline is misleading (Nicholson, 1989). However, it is important to note that with repeated ingestion, the elimination half-life again becomes useful as a concept for predicting the rate and extent of metabolic accumulation. Further, the clinician should recognize that slow elimination of a parent compound or an active metabolite is disadvantageous when drugs are being used on a nightly basis, particularly since freedom from next-day effects is usually sought.

To show how this information can be translated into clinical usefulness, the individual compound temazepam is used as an example. Temazepam has a distribution phase similar to that of its parent compound, diazepam, but an elimination half-life of only 8 hours and insignificant amounts of other metabolite. Thus residual sequelae with temazepam are unlikely unless inappropriately high doses are prescribed.

An important clinical consideration (discussed in Chapter 17) is the comparison of distribution of hypnotics and other agents in the elderly and the young adult. Unless there is severe impairment of renal function, elimination usually is not significantly affected in an adult. However, metabolism may be different (see Chapter 17) and may be slowed in the individual over 65 years of age. Thus the half-lives of compounds may be prolonged in elderly persons and may have a much more profound effect than in the young adult.

Clinical decision-making based on pharmacokinetics. Clearly the benzodiazepines are the sedatives of choice in view of safety and potential for overdose. The more lipid-soluble benzodiazepines readily enter the CNS. For instance, diazepam and flurazepam enter within 10 minutes, whereas oxazepam and clorazepate enter within 18 to 35 minutes, respectively. As shown in Table 8-4, slowly excreted drugs, for example, diazepam and flurazepam, with relatively long half-lives may promote the ease of sleep onset the following day and reduce prolonged anxiety throughout the day. Furthermore, long-acting agents are relatively less likely to provoke untoward reactions on abrupt withdrawal. On the other hand, these long-acting benzodiazepines induce next-day levels of subjective sleepiness and may result in hangover. In short, the difference between the slowly and the rapidly excreted benzodiazepines provides a precarious guide for the individual patient, given large differences in tolerance and sensitivity.

Table 8-4 Older Sedatives (Forerunners of Benzodiazepine Sedatives)

Generic name	Trade name	Comments
Alcohols, aldehydes, and propanediols		
Ethanol	Generic	Not recommended*
Ethchlorvynol	Placidyl	Not recommended*
Chloral hydrate	Generic	1-2 gm to induce sleep
Paraldehyde	Generic	Not recommended*
Meprobamate	Equanil, Miltown, generic	Not recommended*
Tybamate	Tybatran, Solacen, generic	Not recommended*
Barbiturates		
Amobarbital	Amytal, generic	Administer 100-800 mg/h, intravenously in diagnosis or parenterally for emergency sedation
Methohexital	Brevital	Administer 10 mg/5 sec intravenously for electroconvulsive therapy only
Pentobarbital	Nembutal, generic	Can be used for treatment of withdrawal from most sedative addictions†‡
Phenobarbital	Luminal, generic	30-90 mg/day†‡
Secobarbital	Seconal, generic	Not recommended†
Structural relatives of barbiturates (nonbarbiturates)		
Glutethimide	Doriden	Not recommended*
Methyprylon	Noludar	Not recommended*
Methaqualone	Quaalude, generic	Not recommended*
Antihistamines		
Diphenhydramine	Benadryl	25-50 mg parenterally for dystonia§
Hydroxyzine	Atarax, Vistaril	Not recommended*
Promethazine	Phenergan, generic	Not recommended*

*These agents are not recommended for routine use as sedatives.

†Short-acting barbiturates, although not generally recommended, are sometimes used to induce sleep because of their low cost; phenobarbital is an inexpensive sedative and not often abused.

‡Pentobarbital and phenobarbital are often used in the treatment of addiction to sedative-hypnotic drugs.

§Diphenhydramine and other antihistamines are sometimes used as sedatives in pediatric practice. These are not recommended for use in elderly individuals.

The next-day performance and any subjective symptoms of a patient with insomnia are more often influenced by the dose of the drug than by its elimination half-life (Johnson and Cherniak, 1982). Perhaps a choice drug for sleep-onset insomnia is triazolam, and for sleep-maintenance insomnia, temazepam. Early-morning awakening may be best treated by the use of flurazepam, which induces sleep of long duration. That persons with insomnia represent a rather heterogeneous group is implicit in this discussion. Thus the selection of a drug, the prediction of its effects, and the long-range treatment of most types of insomnia must allow for drug variability among patients. Most patients do not need long-term treatment, and in any case benzodiazepines are best given in short courses. The hazards of well-monitored treatment with hypnotic drugs are small, although true physiologic addiction nonetheless may occur (Clift, 1972; Greenblatt and Shader, 1978). Persons who should not take hypnotic agents include pregnant women, alcoholics, those who must arise and function in the middle of the night, and those with symptomatic sleep apnea (Roth et al., 1982).

Side Effects

Benzodiazepines used as hypnotics are unlikely to have severe adverse effects. As noted in Chapter 6, unnecessarily high doses and unnecessarily long treatment periods are the main problems associated with benzodiazepine usage. These problems often result in adverse effects, undoubtedly because of misuse. Impaired performance, anterograde amnesia, and other adverse effects of hypnotics may be particularly troublesome (Nicholson and Ward, 1984).

A number of the adverse effects encountered when these compounds are prescribed for a long period are given in Chapter 6. Also the insomnia on cessation of treatment may arise with the misuse of hypnotics when rebound phenomena emerge, in particular, when short-acting drugs are withdrawn suddenly. Rebound insomnia occurs most often when a relatively high dose of a rapidly eliminated drug is prescribed and used nightly. Rebound insomnia is not observed when benzodiazepine sedatives are used in appropriate doses for a limited time (Roehrs et al., 1986). Drug dependence is also a possibility with the use of hypnotics, as with anxiolytics. The potential for dependence can be minimized by the intermittent use of low doses, together with limited duration of ingestion and gradual withdrawal in the event that continuous treatment has been given for longer than a month (Ladewig, 1983).

Implications

Therapeutic versus toxic levels. Therapeutic levels of benzodiazepines have a comfortable margin of safety in comparison with other sedatives. However, overdoses equivalent to approximately two times a monthly supply or less, when taken with alcohol, have led to death. Moreover, the use of long-acting benzodiazepines, as well as the use of intravenous (IV) diazepam to control seizures or cardiac arrhythmias, is occasionally complicated by respiratory depression, apnea, ventricular arrhythmias, or cardiac arrest. Most deliberate overdoses seem to involve more than one agent; typically alcohol is involved. Thus it is difficult to assess or determine what supply of benzodiazepines would be considered safely dispensed. The continued use of benzodiazepines for more than several weeks should be applied in the context of the critical appraisal of risks and benefits in individual cases.

Use in pregnancy. The safety of benzodiazepines in pregnancy has not been established, and there is no evidence from studies in animals that these drugs are free of hazard. Prolonged administration of benzodiazepines in either low or high dose in the last trimester of pregnancy has been reported to produce irregularities in heart beat, hypertonia, poor sucking, and hypothermia in neonates. Benzodiazepines do cross the placenta and enter milk. Thus ingestion during pregnancy and lactation should be avoided.

Side effects. The most common side effects of benzodiazepines are related to mental alertness. The patient should be cautioned about driving or operating hazardous machinery. Tolerance to most side effects quickly develops. Blood pressure of inpatients should be monitored routinely, and a drop in pressure of 20mm Hg (systolic) on standing warrants withholding the drug and notifying the prescriber.

Interactions. Several of the discussions of drug interactions with benzodiazepines in Chapter 6 are relevant to those prescribed primarily as hypnotics. The sedative effect of benzodiazepines is, of course, increased by combination with centrally acting neuroleptics, tranquilizers, sedating antidepressants, other hypnotics, analgesics, anesthetics, and alcohol. In healthy young adults small doses of temazepam and moderate doses of alcohol may produce no significant additive effect and may not necessarily prolong the effects of benzodiazepines, as they clearly do in elderly patients or in those who, indeed, have alcoholism. The elimination half-life of the benzodiazepines is clearly increased by cimetidine; for other interactions see Chapter 6.

Patient education. Benzodiazepines have a great potential for abuse. Consequently it is important to teach the patient and his or family about these drugs. The nurse or physician should instruct the patient and the family as follows:

Benzodiazepines prescribed for insomnia should be taken as directed.
Over-the-counter drugs may potentiate the actions of benzodiazepines.
Driving should be avoided until tolerance develops.
Alcohol and other CNS depressants potentiate the effects of benzodiazepines.
Hypersensitivity to one benzodiazepine may indicate hypersensitivity to another.
Benzodiazepine treatment should not be stopped abruptly.

Specific Benzodiazepines

Hypnotics, like anxiolytics, are often characterized on the basis of elimination half-life. Triazolam is the most rapidly excreted hypnotic, with an elimination half-life of 1.5 to 5.5 hours. Oxazepam has an elimination half-life of 5 to 20 hours, and the half-lives of lorazepam, temazepam, alprazolam, and chlordiazepoxide are between 10 and 30 hours and generally longer in elderly individuals. Triazolam may be useful when next-day sedation has occurred, but in some patients its rapid washout may provoke rebound insomnia, next-day anxiety, and anterograde amnesia (Kales and Kales, 1984). Another compound, lorazepam, also has a particular propensity for anterograde amnestic effects. The lack of active metabolites may make oxazepam the preferred drug in patients with liver disease and other conditions in which liver function may be compromised. As mentioned in Chapter 6, antacids and anticholinergic drugs may decrease the absorption of benzodiazepines, but cimetidine slows their metabolism to a minor degree. Nevertheless, the near-total replacement of the 50 or more previously available barbiturates by the benzodiazepines has resulted in lower incidence of toxicity and similar but not superior hypnotic effect. These agents cause less respiratory and cardiac depression than do the barbiturates, although overdosage clearly results in respiratory failure. Tolerance of benzodiazepines, in contrast to the barbiturates, is less marked and is never complete.

The choice of an individual hypnotic may depend on the drug's potential to shorten sleep onset when there is difficulty falling asleep, to reduce nocturnal wakefulness or, when insomnia is accompanied by a marked element of anxiety, to provide an anxiolytic effect during the next day. The clinical utility of selected compounds are characterized in Table 8-1 (Nicholson, 1980). Three of specific compounds, designated short-acting (triazolam), intermediate-acting (temazepam), and long-acting (flurazepam), are discussed in detail in the following sections.

Short-acting benzodiazepines: Prototype drug, triazolam. Triazolam is metabolized principally by hepatic microsomal oxidation. Hepatic clearance occurs at a high rate, depending on blood flow in the liver and activity of hepatic microsomal enzymes. This compound is rapidly or very rapidly eliminated after the administration of single doses and does not accumulate. Advantages and disadvantages may occur as a consequence of these properties. The rapid elimination results in no hangover effect, but with the very short-acting compounds early-morning rebound insomnia and anxiety may occur. Furthermore, the complete disappearance of the drug and its metabolites from the blood within a day of discontinuing long-term treatment may result in severe rebound symptoms of drug withdrawal (Kales et al., 1979). Abrupt withdrawal may cause confusion, toxic psychosis, convulsions, or a condition resembling delirium tremor, such as sweating and diarrhea. Long-term treatment should therefore be stopped slowly.

Intermediate-acting benzodiazepines: Prototype drug, temazepam. Among the hypnotics available in alternative formulations with differential rates of absorption is temazepam. Temazepam is available as a soft gelatin capsule with a mean peak plasma concentration time of approximately 1 hour, in contrast to the typical hard gelatin capsule, which is relatively slowly absorbed and has a delay of approximately 2 hours. With temazepam the major metabolite is an inert conjugate. Thus this compound has virtually no active metabolites to prolong its effect.

Because temazepam is metabolized by conjugation rather than by oxidation, its metabolic pathway is less likely to be influenced by factors such as age. Although this knowledge might imply a clinical advantage for temazepam over flurazepam or triazolam among older adults, such an advantage has not been clearly established. The effects of temazepam are thought to be restricted to the night of ingestion as a result of its relatively short half-life. However, with a mean half-life of 13 to 14 hours in some individuals, perhaps longer in others, this drug should be characterized as an intermediate-acting benzodiazepine. Large doses may cause hangover effects.

Long-acting benzodiazepines: Prototype drug, flurazepam. Flurazepam produces a complex mixture of short-acting and long-acting metabolites on repeated dosing. Steady-state levels are reached at 2 to 3 weeks after ingestion. An accumulation may cause impairment of waking performance. Single doses generally cause a full night's sleep with little residual impairment, and the 30-mg dose may result in an anxiolytic effect throughout the day.

Treatment Considerations

Hypnotics have sometimes been introduced in unnecessarily high doses because of dose-ranging studies of persons with chronic insomnia. Such studies may provide information relevant to the use of hypnotics in the treatment of chronic insomnia but are not relevant for the treatment of "normal" insomnia. A further trend toward higher dosing is encouraged when an immediate first-night effect is sought and when high doses of ultrarapidly eliminated drugs are prescribed for the treatment of difficulties in sustaining sleep. Such philosophy and approaches have resulted in significant problems, most recently with triazolam, resulting in both the initial higher dosing recommendations and the 0.5-mg tablet being withdrawn from the market.

Dosage strategies. In prescribing any of the hypnotics shown in Figure 8-1, the clinician should strive to use relatively low doses by choosing the compound with the most suitable pharmacologic profile. The dose should preserve normal sleep architecture to the extent possible during ingestion and after withdrawal, and the pharmacokinetic profile should meet the clinical requirement to shorten sleep onset, to reduce nocturnal wakefulness, or to provide the anxiolytic effect required during the next day. To be as free as possible from the untoward effects on daytime functioning is a goal in every case. The appropriate use of any hypnotic must depend more on whether the profile solves the clinical problems just mentioned and depend less on the particular individual characteristics of the hypnotic.

Effects on electroencephalograms. A significant concern, particularly in patients being evaluated for a primary sleep disorder, may be the effects of benzodiazepines on the EEG. As mentioned earlier, these compounds may cause striking electroencephalographic changes during sleep. There is an overall decrease in the number of sleep-stage shifts throughout the night. Additionally, changes in normal sleep pattern may change and may be manifested differently in different individuals. Clearly benzodiazepines decrease non-REM sleep stages 1, 3, and 4 and increase sleep stage 2, increasing the latency to REM sleep and diminishing REM sleep for the most part. These effects are similar to but less marked than those of the barbiturates.

REM episodes or bursts in REM latency may have considerable inherent variability in response to benzodiazepines or may be erratic with either a decrease or an increase in latency during chronic treatment. REM rebound during drug withdrawal tends to be dose related and most obvious after discontinuance of large doses of benzodiazepines.

Benzodiazepine withdrawal. A full discussion of withdrawal from regimens of benzodiazepines and other similar sedative hypnotic agents may be found in Chapter 6. Indeed, withdrawal of hypnotics after long-term use almost always leads to resurfacing of the original symptoms, difficulties in sleeping, and anxiety. Although there is no doubt that rebound insomnia can occur with the benzodiazepines, the frequency and severity vary (Nicholson, 1980). Withdrawal symptoms may be minimized by tapering rather than stopping treatment, and tapering particularly should be considered with drugs that are short acting; also beta-adrenergic blocking drugs and other agents, for example, clonidine, may be useful in difficult cases (see Chapter 14). Benzodiazepine withdrawal phenomena such as early-morning insomnia and daytime anxiety may occur while the drug is being administered, and on withdrawal such symptoms as rebound insomnia and anxiety may occur. (Kales et al., 1983). Moreover, other undesirable side effects such as impaired memory, anxiety, confusion, depersonalization, and hallucinations may be more related to the direct effect of the drug than to withdrawal itself (van der Kroef, 1979).

Tolerance to effects. Benzodiazepine hypnotics remain the most effective agents for sleep disorders, with clinical effects lasting approximately 6 months with continued use (Oswald et al., 1982). Benzodiazepines do eventually produce adaption intolerance (Greenblatt and Shader, 1978). Some benzodiazepines lose both their anxiolytic and their hypnotic effects over time.

Dependence. Dependence on benzodiazepine hypnotics has not proven to be a major clinical problem, although frequent review is prudent. Dependence and addictions are more likely to occur in patients with a coexisting psychiatric disturbance or a history of an addictive disorder or in patients with personality or somatoform disorders (Folks and Houck, in press).

Benzodiazepine use in elderly individuals. The metabolism and elimination of CNS depressant drugs (discussed in detail in Chapter 17) is decreased in many older adults with low renal glomerular filtration rates, possibly in those with reduced hepatic blood flow, and decreased activity of hepatic drug-metabolizing enzymes. In general, benzodiazepine dosages should initially be *cut in half* and daytime alertness should be monitored for the possibility of serious impairment. The elimination half-life of diazepam, for example, is increased 60% in elderly persons, and the apparent volume of distribution of the drug is also increased (Parkes, 1989). In contrast, the elimination half-life of oxazepam does not alter greatly with aging.

Older adults are also known to rely on or to use sleeping pills much more often than do younger adults (Dunnell and Cartwright, 1972). Ideally a short-acting benzodiazepine given in low dosage should be prescribed for elderly patients. However, some patients may respond poorly to short-acting drugs and prefer longer-acting agents because of their potential to reduce generalized daytime anxiety. As forementioned, the overall choice for young and old alike depends on the individual clinical characteristics in each case.

OTHER DRUGS USED IN THE TREATMENT OF INSOMNIA

Chloral hydrate, the first hypnotic, was developed in 1868 and is still useful today (Table 8-4). Although it is a potent gastric irritant, chloral hydrate in doses of 0.5 to 1 g is widely used and has a rapid onset of action. Chloral hydrate is cross-tolerant with alcohol, is inexpensive, and is available in syrup form for those who have difficulty swallowing pills. Ethchlorvynol (Placidyl) is another hypnotic; in comparison with chloral hydrate, ethchlorvynol stimulates dicumarol metabolism, peaks later, and is more slowly excreted. Glutethimide (Doriden) has a rapid onset of action, rapid metabolism, high mortality when taken as an overdose, and great potential for abuse. Among the over-the-counter agents diphenhydramine (Benadryl), a histamine blocker, also possesses a mild sedative effect and is commonly used and prescribed. L-tryptophan, recently withdrawn from the market, has also been shown to exert mild sedative properties in high doses and is an amino acid precursor to the CNS serotonin production. L-tryptophan has no side effects and results in maximum benefit at doses of approximately 2 to 3 g.

Discussion

The pharmacotherapy of insomnia often occurs in the context of specific pathophysiologic disturbances of sleep or of psychiatric illness. Thus specific treatments of these conditions may also be indicated. Hypnotics may be quite useful when used in the absence of these conditions, or, particularly, when used as an adjunct treatment while patients are receiving behavioral therapy. Daytime residual effects, special problems of elderly patients, interaction with alcohol, dependence, and effects on respiration are just a few of the treatment issues, and a full discussion of these is beyond the scope of this chapter.

Most prescriptions for hypnotics are written for 1 month or less. The vast majority of individuals with insomnia do not take prescribed hypnotic medication; on the other hand, a significant portion of individuals with chronic insomnia self-medicate. Obviously, various disparities exist in the pattern of hypnotic medication prescription, including the disproportionately high rate of prescription among elderly persons. Older sedative hypnotic agents are discussed in Chapter 6, including barbiturates, chloral hydrate, methylquolone, and meprobamate. Other agents, such as antihistamines and heterocyclic antidepressants commonly prescribed because of their hypnotic effect, are also compared with the benzodiazepines in Chapter 6. In general there is rarely a good reason to use the older group of sedative hypnotic agents, with the exception of chloral hydrate. Ironically the triplicate form of prescription now required in New York has discouraged the prescription of benzodiazepines and has led to an increase in the prescription of these older sedative-hypnotic agents, such as meprobamate and barbiturates, for both hypnotic and anxiolytic use in outpatients.

Many so-called *natural* sleep aides and over-the-counter agents are ultimately quite harmful for patients, whereas the benzodiazepines are remarkably nontoxic and safe when used alone. However, most drug-related suicide attempts involve the combination of several agents, including the combination of benzodiazepines with alcohol and other agents that are potentially lethal, for example, the tricyclic antidepressants. Despite the overall safety and efficacy of the benzodiazepines, they may produce unwanted effects, particularly in elderly individuals (see Chapter 17). Long-acting agents may result in daytime impairment, and ultrashort-acting agents may be associated with rebound insomnia and innocent dose escalating. Recently triazolam has received much attention in the popular press because of its alleged profile of severe side-effects. However, data are conflicting and no data regarding its ability to produce daytime anxiety or possible disinhibition resulting in rage, psychosis, or amnesia. For example, a 20% incidence of anterograde amnesia is associated with triazolam but approximately 45% of untreated patients with insomnia also have memory problems, so it is difficult to access the clinical significance of triazolam's effect on memory (Mendelson, 1992).

Newer agents such as quazepam (Doral) may have unique properties; quazepam's parent compound is selective for the benzodiazepine receptor subtype BZ1, located primarily in brain regions associated with sleep. However, one of the metabolites of quazepam is identical to that of flurazepam, suggesting that the selectivity of quazepam may actually be limited or questionable.

Behavioral approaches to insomnia. The use of behavioral techniques, including progressive relaxation, biofeedback, cognitive approaches, stimulus control instructions, sleep restriction therapy, and other attempts to normalize the sleep-wake cycle are of great importance and ideally should be combined with any pharmacologic approach to insomnia. Stimulus control instruction may be especially useful in patients who come to medical attention with a shift in the sleep-wake cycle (see the box on p. 192).

The judicious use of agents to enhance sleep, particularly the benzodiazepines, should continue. The treatment of persistent insomnia should necessitate an integrated approach using both pharmacologic and nonpharmacologic strategies. Accurate diagnosis, review of current medications, behavioral changes, cognitive restructuring, or entrainment of the circadian rhythms, together with the potential use of nonbenzodiazepines such as antidepressants, psychotherapy, exercise, biofeedback, progressive muscle relaxation, dietary changes, and the use of phototherapy and other nonpharmacologic approaches, may be appropriate and effective strategies for sleep enhancement.

Stimulus control therapy instructions, which encourage the individual to lie down with the intention of going to sleep only when he or she is sleepy, may be

Stimulus Control Therapy*

Retire only when sleepy.
Use bed and bedroom only for sleep (and sexual activity).
Go to another room if unable to sleep, and return to bed only when sleepy.
Set alarm at same hour each day, irrespective of amount of sleep attained.
Avoid daytime napping.
Adhere to sleep hygiene guidelines.

Modified from Mendelson WB: *Human sleep,* New York, 1987, Plenum; Wooten V: *Psychiatr Ann* 20(8):466, 1990.
*Method may be repeated as often as needed, and therapy may be continued indefinitely.

more effective than hypnotics. Additionally, individuals should be encouraged not to use the bed for activities other than sleep (except sexual activity). Going to another room and later returning to bed to sleep, if unable to fall asleep, may be a potent intervention. To set the alarm for the same time each morning, regardless of how much sleep is achieved the night before, and to avoid daytime napping are the crucial factors, among others listed, that have led to this nonpharmacologic approach.

Sleep efficiency and sleep hygiene are indeed the key factors in achieving a successful sleep regimen. The sleep laboratory can play a useful role in refractory cases; unsuspected findings of an organic nature such as paroxysmal nocturnal dystonias or sleep apnea may be revealed in as many as 40% of cases. The initial approach outlined in the opening sections of this chapter combined with accurate history, sleep hygiene instruction, and judicious prescription of appropriate hypnotic agents, generally leads to successful patient outcome.

OTHER SLEEP DISORDERS

Hypersomnia

Hypersomnia is a persistent need for excessive sleep. Any disease or drug state affecting the sleep-wake cycle may be responsible. The sleepiness of neurologic, endocrinologic, or psychiatric problems may be accompanied by other stigmata of disease. Sleepiness is typically provoked by prolonged monotony, for example, watching television or attending meetings. Driving for long distances, particularly on interstate highways, may be a culprit. In this section primarily idiopathic hypersomnia is discussed; the primary goal may simply be to ensure that persistent hypersomnia is assessed and hopefully addressed in the context of a careful evaluation in a sleep physiology laboratory.

Idiopathic hypersomnia involves prolonged nocturnal sleep that is normal on polygraphic study, and continuous daytime drowsiness. It commonly develops in young adults who poorly tolerate late-night activities. It may be difficult to identify the onset of hypersomnia, since a change of work requirement or social obligation may precipitate a complaint in an individual who had previously coped with an abnormally increased need for sleep. These individuals often manifest "sleep drunkenness," a period of incapacitating drowsiness on first awakening, sometimes lasting for more than an hour. These individuals often take naps, and the naps are usually prolonged, unlike the shorter naps of narcolepsy. Large sleep requirements often impede fulfilling daytime obligations. Family history of hypersomnia can often be solicited, and hypersomnia may commonly be complicated by depression or impaired daytime concentration in addition to the abnormally prolonged normal night sleep.

The pharmacologic approach to idiopathic hypersomnia involves combining a systematic scheduling of sleep, a prescription of stimulants (discussed in Chapter 13), and the use of a sleep diary with a rigid sleep practice that includes sleep hygiene. Napping is scheduled according to social demands. Stimulants are used primarily as adjuncts in a systematic fashion and are generally prescribed to maintain rather than to restore wakefulness. Pemoline, a long-acting stimulant in 18.75-mg tablets, two to six tablets, are prescribed, to be taken in divided doses in the morning. Amphetamines, including dextroamphetamine and methylphenidate, have short duration of actions and are taken in periodic divided doses on arising and in the presence of sleep drunkenness, before arising (see Chapter 13 for further discussion of these agents). Occasionally, heterocyclic antidepressants, particularly, protriptyline; activating selective serotonin reuptake inhibitors, for example, fluoxetine; or MAOIs are used, with modest clinical response. The outcome of use of these agents often is simply a therapeutic trial in the individual with hypersomnia.

Narcolepsy

Narcolepsy is a sleep disorder with a clear genetic component and occurs in as many as one or two individuals per thousand. Narcolepsy involves features related to REM sleep that suddenly and abnormally intrude on wakefulness during the day. The individual has an irresistible urge to nap for short periods. The paralysis of REM sleep may appear during the daytime with attacks of cataplexy characterized by brief bilateral paresis, which may be brought on by laughter, anger, or surprise. During these periods of cataplexy patients are unable to move, talk, or ambulate. However, consciousness and memory for the event is preserved, distinguishing this event from a seizure episode. Sleep paralysis and hypnagogic hallucinations may also occur with narcolepsy. These dreamlike visual experiences may also be accompanied by apprehension that someone else is present in the room.

The clinical features of narcolepsy may present in a classic case. Paradoxically, wakeful periods may occur during the night. This feature is typically not found in idiopathic hypersomnia. Troublesome dreams and depression are other features seen in association with narcolepsy. Social, familial, and occupational functioning are often impaired. Pharmacologic and clinical approaches to narcolepsy are similar to those for idiopathic hypersomnia. Protriptyline and other conventional antidepressants that suppress REM sleep and therefore narcolepsy symptoms may be especially beneficial. Stimulants, that is, methylphenidate and pemoline, may also be warranted (see Chapter 13). Other cases of narcolepsy may be managed by scheduled naps and small, measured doses of caffeine.

Sleep Apnea

Sleep apnea is a generic term for breathing disorders that occur during sleep. Commonly the clinical picture is of an obese middle-aged or older man who smokes, uses large amounts of caffeine, or drinks alcohol frequently, or has a combination of these behaviors. Mild hypertension or cardiac arrhythmias may be present. The cardinal symptom is snoring. This may, however, be absent when CNS sleep apnea or dysregulation of breathing is present, rather than upper airway obstructive mechanisms. Daytime sleepiness may be mild or may be quite noticeable to others or to the patient. It is common for individuals with sleep apnea to be asymptomatic or to have a tendency to deny that their sleep-related problems exist.

Table 8-5 Sleep Disorders

Disorder	Sleep-laboratory findings	Psychologic evaluation	Management and Treatment
Somnambulism	Incidents occur out of stage-4 sleep; critical skills reactivity are impaired during incident	Psychiatric disturbances infrequent in children and frequent in adults	Prophylactic measures; children frequently outgrow disorders, so parents should be reassured; psychiatry evaluation for adults
Enuresis	Occurs during all sleep stages; dreaming is a frequent causal factor	Psychiatric disturbances infrequent with primary enuresis; psychologic evaluation often indicated for secondary enuresis	Parental counseling and reassurance critical so that parental mishandling does not create psychiatric problems; pharmacologic treatment (imipramine) may be indicated in older children
Night terrors	Occur out of stage-4 sleep; characterized by extreme vocalizations, motility, and autonomic response; recall minimal or absent	Psychiatric disturbances infrequent in children and frequent in adults	Parents should be reassured that children frequently outgrow disorder; for adults psychologic evaluation is often indicated; use of stage-4 suppressants is under investigation

Nightmares	Occur out of REM sleep; characterized by less motility and autonomic response than with night terrors; recall is frequent and elaborate	Frequent nightmares in children or adults may indicate psychopathologic rule out drug withdrawal as a possible cause of nightmares	Parents should be reassured that nightmares in children are often transient: if episodes are frequent in children or adults, psychologic evaluation is indicated
Narcolepsy	Sleep attacks of narcolepsy may be accompanied by three auxiliary symptoms: cataplexy, sleep paralysis, and hypnagogic hallucinations (cataplexy is accompanied by sleep-onset REM periods)	Sleep attacks may be misinterpreted as laziness, irresponsibility, or emotional instability	Establishing diagnosis is critical; stimulants are effective for treatment of sleep attacks; imipramine is effective for treatment of auxiliary symptoms; danger exists in using imipramine and amphetamines simultaneously
Hypersomnia	Sleep-stage patterns normal, but sleep is extended; associated with postdormital confusion and difficulty in awakening; autonomic response variables are increased	Often a symptom of psychologic disorder (e.g., depression)	Stimulant drugs are effective; neurologic and psychologic evaluations are important in establishing diagnosis
Insomnia	Complaints of patients have been verified in sleep laboratory; sleep is more aroused (i.e., heart rate and respiration are increased); most hypnotic drugs lose effectiveness within 2 weeks	Most often a symptom of psychologic disturbance and not a primary disorder; depression a common feature	When insomnia is secondary to medical conditions, pharmacologic treatment may be useful; if psychologic factors are primary, pharmacologic therapy should be combined with psychotherapy

Table 8-5 distinguishes some of the other pertinent clinical characteristics of narcolepsy, idiopathic hypersomnia, insomnia, and other disorders that may be characterized by excessive daytime sleepiness. Although the use of antidepressant medications may be useful and indicated in cases of sleep apnea, perhaps the greatest clinical implication is to *withhold the use of benzodiazepines and other sedative hypnotic agents* that may further depress respiratory drive and contribute to the symptoms. Sleep hygiene and surgical intervention to improve the airway are generally the best approaches to the treatment of sleep apnea.

Parasomnias

Parasomnias are unwanted automatisms or automatic behaviors that occur during deep sleep. These often occur when cortical suppression of fixed-action patterns is lessened compared to other sleep stages. Perhaps the most common type of adult parasomnia is adult enuresis, which may be associated with cystitis, diabetes, or other nonpsychiatric medical conditions. Sleepwalking is another relatively rare parasomnia that occurs during adulthood, although a childhood or family history of sleepwalking is frequently found. Sleepwalking movements are usually slow, poorly coordinated, without integrated purpose, and not recalled by the patient, who rarely hurts himself or herself.

Other sleep automatisms that may be considerations for pharmacologic intervention include bruxism and repetitive movements of the head or extremities. Stereotypic behavior such as sitting, standing, stroking the wall, saluting, or punching can also occur. In addition, night terrors, which rarely occur in adults, are distressing. Night terrors arise during the deep sleep and, like other parasomnias, the details of the event are not remembered. Unlike nocturnal panic attacks, night terrors are not associated with other symptoms of panic or prolapsed mitral valve syndrome. Night terrors are different from nightmares, which may involve upsetting content, occur during REM sleep, and may not cause the individual to awaken (Table 8-5) (Kales and Kales, 1974).

Periodic Leg Movements (Restless Leg Syndrome)

An organic factor that may require further evaluation and clinical management is the presence of periodic leg movements, which may also disrupt sleep and cause an individual to complain of light, broken, or restless sleep. Nocturnal myoclonus entails repetitive, stereotypic leg-muscle jerks. Its incidence increases markedly in individuals over 45 years of age. Although the disorder may be ameliorated by means of benzodiazepines, specifically, clonazepam, it *may worsen with the use of tricyclic antidepressants;* this distinction is crucial, since these agents may be helpful in treating other types of insomnia. Restless leg syndrome is probably a familial disorder. The uncomfortable leg sensations that occur while the patient is at rest are usually relieved by movement. Thus active patients are asymptomatic during the day but are unable to fall asleep at night; they may also have the sleep-related leg movements that further disrupt sleep. The causes of restless leg syndrome are diverse and include underlying conditions such as amyloidosis and iron-deficiency anemia. Benzodiazepines, as forementioned, may be useful only to relieve symptoms.

Comorbid Conditions

The use of psychotropic drugs to treat disorders of sleep has been addressed by largely focusing on insomnia and, to a lesser extent, other disorders. Insomnia and other disturbances often are a harbinger of serious psychiatric illness or are associated with nonpsychiatric medical conditions. Resolution of insomnia may avert subsequent psychiatric morbidity; however, it may be necessary to place the treatment of insomnia in the context of treating associated conditions and comorbid disturbances.

Covert organic factors are the basis for nearly 40% of the cases of insomnia, and if these factors not identified, the patient's condition may actually worsen, even with effective conventional treatment (see the box below). For example, obstructive sleep apnea, as previously characterized, may be associated with cerebral hypoxia and may lead to physical and psychiatric complications. Conventional hypnotic agents may only worsen the condition. Administering tricyclic antidepressants or improving the airway, for example, by use of continuous positive airway pressure, may be extremely helpful.

Several disorders that affect biologic rhythms may result in problems with initiating or maintaining sleep. As described in the discussion of insomnia, sleep-phase syndromes may occur in which the individual is unable to fall asleep at the desired time and then sleeps substantially longer than desired. These syndromes are particularly common among adolescents, college students, and shift workers. Attempting to compensate by sleeping late on weekends is not particularly effective. Elderly individuals may have an advanced sleep-phase syndrome, retiring quite early and awakening af-

Nonpsychiatric Causes of Insomnia

Induced by medical conditions
Cardiovascular disorders
Chronic obstructive pulmonary disease
Conditions associated with pruritus
Endocrine and metabolic disorders
Febrile illnesses and infections
Illnesses associated with pain
Inflammatory bowel disease
Neoplastic disorders
Urinary frequency

Induced by drugs
Antihypertensives
Ace inhibitors
β-adrenergic blockers
Diuretics
Methyldopa
Reserpine
Autonomic agents
Anticholinergics
Cholinergic agonists
Cimetidine
Central nervous system stimulants
Amphetamines
Caffeine
Methylphenidate
Nicotine
Sympathomimetics
Central nervous system depressants
Alcohol
Anxiolytics
Hypnotics
Narcotics
Opiates
Hormones
Corticotropin
Cortisone
Oral contraceptives
Progesterone
Thyroid hormone preparations
Others
Anticancer medications
Antidepressants
Digoxin
Monoamine oxidase Inhibitors
Theophylline

Modified from Erman MK: *Psychiatr Clin North Am* 10:525, 1987.

ter a normal 7 or 8 hours of sleep, for example, at 3 AM. This sleep pattern creates problems in the home or living situation and leads to the inappropriate prescription of medication.

Other cases of insomnia may simply be associated with the use of over-the-counter agents, alcohol, or drugs prescribed for other medical conditions, for example, antibiotics, thyroid preparations, cancer chemotherapeutic agents, and many other medications that can and do affect the sleep-wake cycle (see the box on p. 197).

REFERENCES

American Psychiatric Association: *Diagnostic and statistical manual of mental disorders, third edition-revised,* Washington, DC, 1987, The Association.

Aserinsky E, Kleitman N: Regularly occurring periods of eye motility and concomitant phenomena during sleep, *Science* 118:273, 1953.

Balter MB, Bauer ML: Patterns of prescribing and use of hypnotic drugs in the United States. In Clift AD, editor: *Sleep disturbances and hypnotic drug dependence,* Amsterdam, 1975, Excerpta Medica.

Belyavin A, Nicholson AN: Rapid eye movement sleep in man: modulation by benzodiazepines, *Neuropharmacology* 26:485, 1987.

Bixler EO, Kales A, Soldatos CR: Sleep disorders encountered in medical practice: a national survey of physicians, *Behav Med* 6:13, 1979.

Bond A, Lader M: After-effects of sleeping drugs. In Weatley D, editor: *Psychopharmacology of sleep,* New York, 1981, Raven.

Caraskadon MA, Dement WC: Nocturnal determinants of daytime sleepiness, *Sleep* 5(suppl 2):73, 1982.

Clift AD: Factors leading to dependence on hypnotic drugs, *Br Med J* 3:4, 1972.

Cohn JB: Multicenter double-blind efficacy and safety study comparing aprazolam, diazepam and placebo in clinically anxious patients, *J Clin Psychiatry* 42:347, 1981.

Coleman RM et al: Sleep-wake disorders based on a polysomnographic diagnosis, *JAMA* 247:997, 1982.

Dement W, Siedel W, Caraskadon M: Daytime alertness, insomnia and benzodiazepines, *Sleep* 5(suppl):S28, 1982.

Dlin BM et al: The problems of sleep and rest in the intensive care unit, *Psychosomatics* 12:155, 1971.

Dominguez RA et al: Comparative efficacy of estazolam, flurazepam, and placebo in outpatients with insomnia, *J Clin Psychiatry* 47:362, 1986.

Dunnell K, Cartwright A: *Medicine takers, prescribers and hoarders,* London, 1972, Routledge & Kegan Paul.

Erman MK: An overview of sleep and insomnia, *Hosp Practice* 23(2):6, 1988.

Folks DG, Houck CA: Somatoform disorders, factitious disorders and malingering. In Stoudemire A, Fogel BS, editors: *Principles of medical psychiatry,* ed 2, Oxford (in press).

Gaillard JM, Phelippeau M: Benzodiazepine-induced modifications of dream content: the effect of flunitrazepam, *Neuropsychobiology* 2:37, 1976.

Greenblatt DJ, Shader RI: Dependence, tolerance and addiction to benzodiazepines: clinical and pharmacokinetic considerations, *Drug Metab Rev* 8:13, 1978.

Greenblatt DJ et al: Benzodiazepine hypnotics: kinetics and therapeutic options, *Sleep* 5(suppl):S18, 1982.

Greenblatt DJ et al: Pharmacokinetic determinants of dynamic differences among three benzodiazepine hypnotics: flurazepam, temazepam, and triazolam, *Arch Gen Psychiatry* 46:326, 1989.

Grey JA: *The neuropsychology of anxiety,* New York, 1982, Oxford University.

Guilleminault C, Dement WC: *Kroc Foundation series. V. Sleep apnea syndromes,* New York, 1978, Alan R Liss.

Haefely W: Alleviation anxiety: the benzodiazepine saga. In Parnaham MJ, Bruinvals J, editors: *Discoveries in pharmacology, vol 1. Psycho- and neuro-pharmacology,* Amsterdam, 1983, Elsevier.

Hartmann EL: *The functions of sleep,* New Haven, Conn, 1974, Yale University.

Hirsch JD, Garrett KM, Beer B: Heterogeneity of benzodiazepine binding sites: a review of recent research, *Pharmacol Biochem Behav* 23(4):681, 1985.

Holland G, Dement WC, Raynal DM: *Polysomnography: a response to a need for improved communication.*

Fourteenth annual meeting of the Association for the Psychophysiological Study of Sleep, Jackson Hole, Wyoming, June 1974.

Johnson LL, Cherniak DA: Sedative hypnotics and human performance, *Psychopharmacology (Berlin)* 76:101, 1982.

Kales A: Quazepam: hypnotic efficacy and side effects, *Pharmacotherapy* 10:1, 1990.

Kales A, Kales JD: Sleep disorders: recent findings in the diagnosis and treatment of disturbed sleep, *New Engl J Med* 290:487, 1974.

Kales A, Kales JD: *Evaluation and treatment of insomnia,* New York, 1984, Oxford University.

Kales A et al: Effects of hypnotics on sleep patterns, dreaming and mood state: laboratory and home studies, *Biol Psychiatry* 1:235, 1969.

Kales A et al: Rebound insomnia: a potential hazard following withdrawal of certain benzodiazepines, *J Am Med Assoc* 241:1692, 1979.

Kales A et al: Early morning insomnia with rapidly eliminated benzodiazepines, *Science* 220:95, 1983.

Ladewig D: Abuse of benzodiazepines in Western European society: incidence and prevalence of motives in drug acquisition, *Pharmacopsychiatry* 16:103, 1983.

Mellinger GD, Balter MB, Uhlenhuth EH: Insomnia and its treatment, *Arch Gen Psychiatry* 42:225, 1985.

Mendelson WB: *The use and misuse of sleeping pills,* New York, 1980, Plenum Press.

Mendelson WB: *Human sleep,* New York, 1987, Plenum.

Mendelson WB: Pharmacologic treatment of insomnia. In Pies R, editor: *Advances in psychiatric medicine (Psychiatric Times [suppl]),* Santa Ana, Ca, 1992, CME.

Mohler H, Okada T: Benzodiazepine receptor: demonstration in the central nervous system, *Science* 198:849, 1977.

Nicholson AN: Hypnotics: rebound insomnia and residual sequelae, *Br J Clin Pharmacol* 9:223, 1980.

Nicholson AN: Hypnotics: clinical pharmacology and therapeutics. In Kryger MH, Roth T, Dement W, editors: *Principles and practice of sleep medicine,* 1989,Philadelphia, WB Saunders.

Nicholson AN, Ward J, editors: Psychomotor drugs and performance, *Br J Clin Pharmacol* 18(suppl 1), 1984.

Oswald I et al: Benzodiazepine hypnotics remain effective for 24 weeks, *Br Med J* 284:860, 1982.

Parkes JD: Sleep and its disorders. In Kryger MH, Roth T, Dement WC, editors: *Principles and Practice of Sleep Medicine,* Philadelphia, 1989, WB Saunders.

Prevalence and diagnosis of insomnia. In Pies R, editor: *Advances in psychiatric medicine (Psychiatric Times [suppl]),* Santa Ana, Ca, 1992, CME.

Roehrs TA et al: Dose determinants of rebound insomnia, *Br J Clin Pharmacol* 22:143, 1986.

Roth T et al: Effects of benzodiazepines on sleep and wakefulness, *Br J Clin Pharmacol* 11:315, 1981.

Roth T et al: Pharmacological and medical considerations in hypnotic use, *Sleep* 5(suppl):S46, 1982.

Tan TL et al: Biopsychobehavioral correlates of insomnia. IV. Diagnosis based on DSM-III, *Am J Psychiatry* 141:357, 1984.

van der Kroef C: Reactions to triazolam, *Lancet* 2:526, 1979.

Weitzmann ED, Pollak CP: Effects of flurazepam on sleep and growth hormone release during sleep in healthy subjects, *Sleep* 5(4):343, 1982.

CHAPTER 9

Acute Psychoses and the Violent Patient

SCOPE OF THE PROBLEM

Violence is endemic in the mental health treatment setting and constitutes a bona fide occupational hazard. Physical assaults on mental health professionals have been reported in all clinical settings, including inpatient wards, outpatient clinics, emergency departments, and institutional facilities (Lion, 1983). These patients can usually be successfully treated, if the clinical approach is objective, systematic, and appreciative of the underlying dynamics or psychopathologic factors (Dubin, 1981).

Estimates of the incidence of assault on mental health professionals have been drawn from retrospective questionnaires or reviews of incident reports. The reported incidence varies with the profession sampled, the setting, and survey methods. Using a survey questionnaire, Madden, Lion, and Penna (1976) found that 42% of psychiatrists had been assaulted at some point in their careers, generally while working in their younger years with seriously mentally ill patients. Bernstein (1981) surveyed psychiatrists, psychologists, social workers, and counselors working in both inpatient and outpatient settings. These clinicians reported a 14.2% rate of assault. Although the inpatient setting was more often characterized as having great risk for violent behavior and assault (33%), the largest percentage of the assaults occurred in an outpatient or a private practice setting (47%). Depp (1976) reported that 12% of 379 documented assaults over an 8-month period in an institutional setting involved the staff. Lion, Snyder, and Merrill (1981) reported 203 incidences of assault against nursing staff over a 1-year period in a Maryland state hospital; as many as five times that number of assaults were thought to be unreported to the administration.

THE CLINICAL APPROACH

Patients tend to become violent when they feel helpless or passive. Successful interventions often alleviate these feelings and diminish the chances of loss of behavioral control. Usually a prodromal pattern of behavior precedes overt violence. Sudden, unexpected violence is rare, and most violence is a predictable culmination of a 30- to 60-minute period of escalation (Dubin, 1990).

The patient's posture, speech, and motor activity are key indicators that a violent episode is forthcoming. Most violence is preceded by a period of increasing restlessness and pacing. Hyperactivity may be a sign that immediate intervention is necessary. Patients who are potentially violent are often verbally abusive and using profanity. This verbal abuse should not elicit a response from the staff that is personalized or defensive; such a response serves only to increase the risk of violence. Essentially verbal abuse is most assuredly attempted by the patient to assert autonomy and diminish feelings of helplessness (Dubin, 1990).

POLICIES ON VIOLENCE

Because violent behavior and assault are occupational hazards in all mental health settings, each facility should carefully and thoughtfully develop defined policies and procedures that are appropriate in meeting the problems of its own patient population (Kyser, Diner, and Raulston, 1989). Policies for the care of violent patients who are severely agitated or acutely psychotic should be reviewed, approved, and supported at the highest level of clinical administration. Procedures for the clinical management of a violent patient should be rehearsed by the staff on a regular basis to facilitate safe patient care. Nursing staff and other health care professionals must take the time to learn and practice the steps necessary for the emergency management of a violent patient. This chapter focuses on the emergency pharmacologic management of the violent patient, including diagnostic assessment, diagnostic categories, short-term and long-term treatment, and the implications important for the successful management of the patient.

DIAGNOSTIC CONSIDERATIONS

Assessment and Clinical Approach

The initial clinical approach to the care of the violent patient clearly differs from the customary process of clinical diagnosis and treatment as outlined in previous chapters. Rapid assessment and swift symptomatic relief through immediate intervention are often necessary. Treatment is directed against the target symptoms of the agitated or violent behavior, often with little time for diagnostic sophistication. The primary goal is to ensure the safety of the patient, the staff, and others who may be innocent bystanders (Hanke, 1984). Once the violence is contained, controlled, or concluded, the staff may begin to work on delineating the origin and pathogenesis of violence (Soreff, 1984).

A clinical approach to the care of the violent patient initially makes use of verbal intervention, which may be quite effective. Patients who may be on the verge of losing control frequently respond to a well-timed verbal intervention. Because potentially violent patients are terrified of losing control, they welcome therapeutic efforts and may actually respond to an empathic response that takes charge of the situation. Of course, the nature of the setting, the staff, and the security resources largely determines whether the patient can be safely managed and dictates the level of immediate response.

Therapeutic practices obviously differ among emergency, outpatient, inpatient, and institutional settings and the locked forensic facility. The sophistication and experience of the staff and the philosophy of care ultimately determine the choice of verbal, pharmacologic, or physical control for the patient. The more secure the setting and the more experienced the staff, the less aggressive and restrictive is the preferred intervention likely to be (Soloff, 1987).

During an interview with a violent or potentially violent patient the clinician should focus on the patient's underlying feelings. Rationalization and intellectualization are not generally therapeutic and may serve only to increase the patient's sense of frustration. Ventilating anger reduces agitation. By acknowledging the patient's emotional state, the clinician may accomplish some degree of emotional catharsis in the patient, thereby diminishing the need or desire for further aggression (Lion, Levenberg, and Strange, 1972).

During the assessment and interview of a violent patient, the interviewer should stay at arm's length. The violent patient should never be left alone. Police, security personnel, or family should be asked to remain nearby to help control the patient, if necessary. During the verbal intervention it may be helpful to offer the patient food or drink; hot liquids are avoided, for obvious reasons. Food symbolizes nurturance and caring and may alleviate an angry patient's disruptive behavior. Also the patient's agitated behavior may distinguish the degree of loss of control. For example, the patient who cooperates with the initial verbal intervention and postures himself or herself in a restrained or secure fashion is more likely to comply with treatment.

The experience and skill of the interviewer is clearly important in defusing the violent threat with directable and responsive patients. Staff may contribute to violent episodes, particularly during inpatient services. Countertransference feelings, racial tensions, treatment structures characterized by authoritarianism, underinvolvement by the staff, or a lack of program clarity may contribute to violent outbursts (Soloff, 1987). Conflicts over issues of power, dependency, or self-esteem constitute the psychodynamic themes that respond to verbal and psychotherapeutic crisis intervention. Thus the agitated paranoid, the borderline, or the mildly psychotic patient, through clarifying his or her grievances and ventilating frustrations, may, in fact, be able to "talk it out."

The ultimate threat is posed by a patient with a weapon. Ideally the mental health professional inquires about or explores the fear that led the patient to arm himself or herself. A weapon may symbolize a defense against feelings of helplessness and pas-

Management Approach to Violent Patients

Do	Do Not
Anticipate violence	Ignore gut feelings
Respond to personal fears and feelings	Respond hastily to angry, threatening individuals
Call security at the first sign of violence	Compromise ability to maintain safety and security
Be aware of possible weapons	Antagonize or challenge a patient with a weapon
Offer food, drink, or medication	Touch or Startle the Individual
Restrain with an organized format	Restrain without a plan or without sufficient personnel
Offer injectable medicines if oral medicines are refused	Neglect "organic" causes of violence
Observe restrained or sedated patient	Bargain about restraint, medication, or need for admission
Hospitalize patients who are violent or uncooperative or patients who are psychotic or cognitively impaired	Forget medical and legal concerns and appropriate documentation
Warn potential victims of threatened violence	Overlook the usefulness of family and friends
Evaluate thoroughly	"Carry the coffin" by yourself: *Do* get help

Adapted from Dubin NR. In Stoudemire A, editor: *Clinical psychiatry for medical students*, Philadelphia, 1990, JB Lippincott; Rabins PL, Folks DG, Hollender MH: *Southern Med J* 75:1369, 1982; Weissberg MP: *Am J Psychiatry* 136:787, 1979.

sivity. An immediate request to give up the weapon may heighten these feelings and further exacerbate the threat. Nonthreatening expressions of a desire to help, coupled with an expression of fear, is the response most likely to avert physical harm (Dubin, Wilson, and Mercer, 1988). A similar concern is a threat that may be posed by the staff's potential use of weapons, especially guns carried by police officers and security personnel who may be involved in an intervention. Generally and preferably these employees disarm themselves while in an emergency setting.

Ultimately the violent patient requires symptomatic relief followed by a thorough evaluation as to the origin and pathogenesis of the violent or aggressive behavior. A number of algorithms and techniques have appeared in the literature regarding the initial clinical approach to these patients. A standard set of techniques outlining the exchange with an agitated or aggressive patient in the emergency department is generally applicable to other settings, as summarized in the box on p. 202. Additionally, many guidelines for the initial assessment of violent patients with respect to the clinical setting and the appropriate goals of intervention are outlined in the box below. Many of these suggested techniques and guidelines are appropriately combined with the administration of medication or followed by seclusion or restraint of the patient.

The use of drugs to treat violent behavior in a patient may occur without clear identification of symptomatic, syndromal, or diagnostic features. The diagnostic features of these patients are summarized in the box on p. 204. The specific drug prescribed varies with the clinical problem but always involves some consideration of short-term versus long-term treatment, restraint, and seclusion. Drug treatment is directed toward acute affective or cognitive symptoms responsible for the imminent loss of behavioral control. Thus agitation, hostility, belligerence, suspiciousness, and conceptual disorganization are initially treated, regardless of the underlying process.

Interview Techniques Used with Potentially Violent Patients

1. Secure a private but safe interview environment.
2. Approach the patient respectfully, professionally, and politely.
3. Maintain a nonthreatening, passive clinical approach.
4. Clarify, reassure, and gather data without interpretation or confrontation.
5. Listen uncritically and empathically in an unhurried fashion.
6. Offer food and drink as a symbol of help, assurance, and nurturance.
7. Involve family or friends in the clinical dialogue.
8. Communicate positive expectations for the patient, but prepare for the worst.
9. Provide the patient with options and the opportunity for making choices for treatment.
10. Assist the patient in focusing anger and grievances; for example, the staff is not usually a legitimate target.
11. Offer medication to maintain control, as appropriate.
12. Ask security officers to stand by or sit in, as appropriate (show of force).

Adapted from Dubin WR. In Stoudemire A, editor: *Psychiatry for medical students,* Philadelphia, 1990, JB Lippincott; Soloff PH. In Hales RE, Frances AJ, editors: *American Psychiatric Association annual review,* vol 6, Washington, DC, 1987, American Psychiatric.

Diagnostic Features Frequently Associated with Violence

Symptoms of agitation, confusion, or anxiety
Syndromes of mixed anxiety-depression or psychosis
Disorders of mood, thought, cognition, or perception
Disorders of drug and alcohol use
Disorders of personality or interpersonal functioning
Cases involving malingering and noncompliance

In some cases drug treatment addresses symptoms of primitive or disruptive forms of personality disorders such as borderline, narcissistic, histrionic, antisocial, schizotypal, or paranoid disorders. In other cases drug treatment relieves symptoms that reflect an acute exacerbation of schizophrenia, bipolar disorder, delusional disorder, or psychotic or agitated depression. Occasionally medication may simply represent the "chemical restraint" for short-term treatment of violence in progress (Monroe, 1970). Thus incidents of violence resulting from psychotic ideation, cognitive impairment or manic excitement, extreme anxiety, or irritability or explosive behavior may all represent cases in which drugs are required to manage the violent behavior.

DRUG TREATMENT

Short-Term Treatment

The acute drug treatment of the violent patient generally involves one of the following classes of agents: (1) the anxiolytic or sedative-hypnotic class, usually a benzodiazepine administered orally, (2) the neuroleptic or antipsychotic class, appropriately reserved for patients who are wildly agitated or psychotic, and (3) intravenous sedative-hypnotics (barbiturates), benzodiazepines (diazepam), or antipsychotics (haloperidol), reserved for cases of extreme violence in progress in which other medications are not effective. The pharmacologic characteristics of these drugs are described in Chapters 4 and 6.

The benzodiazepines are clearly efficacious in the treatment of acute anxiety, but their use in the violent patient is somewhat controversial. In fact, anxiolytics may result in disinhibition or further loss of control over feelings and may contribute further to rage, hostility, or aggression. Patients who have a history of outbursts, belligerence, or assaultive or impulsive behavior should probably not be given benzodiazepines except with extreme caution (Salzman, Kochausky, and Shader, 1974). For example, patients with borderline personality disorder have shown marked disinhibition of self-directed and other-directed violence, including suicide attempts and mutilation, when given benzodiazepines (Gardner and Cowdry, 1985). However, widespread acceptance of and familiarity with anxiolytics, as well as the usefulness of a pill "to take the edge off," may well prevent the escalation of anxiety in a patient who is violent or potentially violent and may facilitate interpersonal interaction (Lion, 1979). Some clinicians recommend the use of low-potency agents, for example, oxazepam or diazepam, in doses of 15 to 30 mg and 5 to 10 mg, respectively.

Neuroleptic or antipsychotic medication is often given electively to a potentially violent or agitated patient in the spirit of facilitating an evaluation. However, prompt intervention for the patient who is progressively more agitated is the most common circumstance in which a neuroleptic is prescribed. The patient's treatment at this point may no longer be entirely voluntary. Thus the medication may be presented to the patient in a firm but kind manner that indicates to the patient that his or her behavior is slipping out of control and that the medication is now needed to prevent further loss of control. However, the patient may be given a choice of oral elixir or parenteral medication to preserve self-esteem. Therapeutic work or evaluation can then continue after administration of the medication. On the other hand a lack of response on the patient's part may suggest the need for a "show of force," physical restraint, or seclusion. A lack of response may also suggest the need for rapid neuroleptization.

Although verbal intervention is the mainstay, the preferred method of evaluation and treatment for an acutely agitated or aggressive patient, neuroleptics continue to represent the most effective drug treatment of the acutely violent patient. Rapid neuroleptization is defined as the "careful titrated administration of parenteral high-potency antipsychotic drugs" (Anderson and Kuehnle, 1976). This therapeutic technique, used during the last 25 years, has been effectively carried out in acutely psychotic, agitated, or violent patients. Rapid neuroleptization has demonstrated both safety and efficacy as an emergency treatment of violent behavior. Rapid tranquilization essentially requires varying doses of medication given at 30- to 60-minute intervals; patients most often begin to respond within 30 to 90 minutes (Dubin, Weiss, and Dorn, 1986).

The technique of rapid neuroleptization is outlined in the box below. Medication and dosages are depicted in Table 9-1. Target symptoms of tension, anxiety, restlessness, hyperactivity, and motor excitement, as well as core psychotic symptoms such as hallucinations, delusions, and disorganized thought, are ultimately addressed. However, rapid tranquilization does not fully relieve psychotic symptoms until 7 to 10 days of appropriate antipsychotic drug treatment has been given. Thus the goal of rapid neuroleptization is to calm patients so that they may cooperate in the evaluation, treatment, and disposition of their cases. Similarly sedation may not necessarily be an end point, especially since drowsiness may delay evaluation and disposition. Although rapid neuroleptization may indeed obscure the patient's mental status or result in sedation, withholding this effective intervention may serve only to prolong the risk of violence.

Clinical response to rapid neuroleptization is usually amazingly rapid. Improvement in symptoms of hostility and belligerence may be noted within 20 minutes of an

Technique of Rapid Neuroleptization

Use a high-potency neuroleptic.*
Medicate at 4-hour intervals for a low-dose strategy.
Medicate at 30- to 60-minute intervals for a high-dose strategy.
Note response 20 minutes after a dose.
Observe for nontherapeutic effects after each dose.
Document levels of consciousness and vital signs before each dose.
Maintain close observation for patients in seclusion or restraint, as appropriate.

From Dubin WR, Weiss KJ, Dorn JM: *J Clin Psychopharmacol* 6:210, 1986.
*Low-potency neuroleptics and sedative-hypnotics are sometimes employed but are not recommended (see Table 9-1).

Table 9-1 Rapid Tranquilization: Medications and Doses*

Medication	Parenteral (mg)	Oral (mg)	Range of usual daily dose (mg)	Maximum daily dose (mg)
High-potency neuroleptics				
Haloperidol (Haldol)	5	10	15-100	100
Thiothixene (Navane)	10	20	30-100	100
Trifluoperazine (Stelazine)	10	20	30-100	100
Loxapine (Loxitane)	10	25	30-200	200
Low-potency neuroleptics				
Chlorpromazine (Thorazine)	25	50	100-400	400
Mesoridazine (Serentil)	25	50	50-200	200
Benzodiazepines†				
Diazepam (Valium)	5-10 (IV or IM)	5-10	5-40	40
Chlordiazepoxide (Librium)	25-50	25-50	100-400	400
Lorazepam (Ativan)	0.5-2	1-2	1.5-8	8
Sedative-hypnotic‡				
Sodium amytal (Brevital)	1 ml/min (IV)	—	150-500	—

Adapted from Soloff PH. In Hales RE, Frances AJ, editors: *American Psychiatric Association annual review*, vol 6, Washington, DC, 1987, American Psychiatric.
*Doses are arbitrary and not recommended for routine use but have been found effective by the authors. Doses for elderly individuals should be half the recommended doses for adults. Adverse effects may occur and should be monitored.
†Benzodiazepines are absorbed erratically or incompletely when given intramuscularly, with the possible exception of lorazepam.
‡Use of sodium amytal is reserved for extreme cases of violence-in-progress.

initial injection of haloperidol 10 mg, with some improvement of core symptoms of psychosis within 6 hours (Donlon et al., 1980). Response rates of 50% to 95% have been reported in acutely psychotic patients within 48 hours of treatment with modest doses of neuroleptic (Anderson and Kuehnle, 1974; Slotnick, 1971). The most important variables in this technique are the choice of agent, the loading dose, the frequency of injection, and the time frame for titration (see the box on p. 205 and Table 9-1). Although low-potency agents such as chlorpromazine or mesoridazine may be used, they are not preferred because of the potential for nontherapeutic effects (see Chapter 4). The exception may be when the intent is true chemical restraint such that excessive sedation and parkinsonian slowing, which are usually undesirable in routine treatment, are useful elements of physical control. However, if the goal is continuation of assessment or psychiatric intervention, the preference must be given to high-potency, nonsedating neuroleptics. Thus haloperidol or an equivalent dose of a high-potency antipsychotic in single doses of 2.5 mg to 10 mg every 30 to 60 minutes in total maximum daily doses of 100 mg is standard, as outlined in the box on p. 205 and Table 9-1. Studies of low-dose versus high-dose medication indicate that optimal efficacy occurs in the middle range of 15 to 60 mg (Anderson, Kuehnle, and Catanzano, 1976; Donlon et al., 1980).

Baldessarini, Katz, and Cotton (1984) have recently described the tendency toward the use of massive doses of high-potency neuroleptics. This phenomenon generally occurs after rapid neuroleptization, when oral doses far in excess of the actual clinical need are given for maintenance. Salzman et al. (1986) have recommended the simultaneous use of parenteral lorazepam to reduce the total neuroleptic dosage required in managing violent behavior. A ratio of 5 mg of haloperidol to 1 or 2 mg of lorazepam has been found effective for the acute control of disruptive and violent patients. Thus the patient is spared the long-term use of high doses of neuroleptic medication.

Rapid neuroleptization is an effective approach to the care of the violent patient across all diagnostic categories. Whether the violent or disruptive presentation is secondary to a major psychiatric syndrome such as schizophrenia or mania, a disorder of cognitive impairment, or alcohol or substance abuse, this approach is quite effective (Dubin, Weiss, and Dorn, 1986). In patients with substance abuse or alcohol abuse disorders rapid neuroleptization serves only to treat loss of behavioral control; cross-tolerant agents such as the benzodiazepines are preferred for the actual treatment of the withdrawal syndrome.

Patients receiving intensive care or critical care sometimes require a different or alternative treatment approach. Patients with burns, debilitated patients, and post-surgical patients may benefit from intravenous administration of medication. Other patients may simply benefit from the rapid intravenous effect (Clinton et al., 1987). Patients receiving intravenous haloperidol may actually possess a lower incidence of extrapyramidal symptoms than patients receiving oral medication (Menza et al., 1987). Goldstein (1987) provides an excellent review of rapid neuroleptization in the intensive care unit and gives guidelines for intravenous use, as summarized in Table

Table 9-2 Guidelines for the Use of Intravenous Haloperidol in Critical Care Settings*

Degree of agitation	Dose (mg)
Mild	0.5-2.0
Moderate	2-10
Severe	Boluses up to 40

Titration and maintenance

Start with a low dose and titrate in increments of 25% to 100%.

Allow 30 minutes before repeating a dose.

If agitation is unchanged, double the inital dose every 30 minutes until patient becomes calms.

If patient calms down, repeat the effective dose at regular dosing intervals, for example, every 2 to 8 hours.

Adjust dose and interval to patient's clinical course. Gradually increase the interval between doses until the interval is every 8 hours.

Once the patient's condition is stable for 24 hours, administer doses on regular schedule with supplemental doses as needed.

Once the patient's condition is stable for 36 to 48 hours, attempt to gradually taper dosage.

If agitation is severe, high boluses (up to 40 mg) may be required.

Adapted from Dubin WR. In Stoudemire A, editor: *Clinical psychiatry for medical students*, Philadelphia, 1990, JB Lippincott; Tesar GE, Murray GB, Cassem NH: *J Clin Psychopharmacol* 5:344, 1985.

*Haloperidol is not specifically approved by the Food and Drug Administration for the intravenous route; careful documentation of the necessity and rationale must be achieved.

9-2. However, the use of intravenous haloperidol has not been specifically approved by the Food and Drug Administration. Thus documentation of the rationale for this technique must be provided.

Side effects resulting from rapid neuroleptization are generally uncommon and reversible. Muscle rigidity, drooling, dystonia, akathisia, bradykinesia, and the like may occur in the first 24 hours after treatment. Extrapyramidal side effects that are not dose related may occur early, as may dystonic reactions. The most serious form of dystonia is laryngospasm, which compromises the airway by contraction of the muscles of the larynx and leads to severe respiratory distress.

The sedative or anticholinergic effects of neuroleptics may mask or aggravate certain delirious or toxic metabolic confusional states. In general these effects are more common with low-potency neuroleptics, whereas the extrapyramidal symptoms are more typical of high-potency agents. Akathisia is a sometimes subtle or unrecognized side effect that is too frequently misdiagnosed in a patient who is agitated or is having psychotic decompensation. The inability to sit still, restlessness, or an inner feeling of anxiety induced by akathisia is relieved only by pacing. The patient is literally wound up like a spring; he or she is irritable and feels like "jumping out of his or her skin" (Van Putten and Marder, 1987). This drug-induced phenomenon can literally worsen the patient's clinical outcome and has been reported to lead to acts of suicide, violence, or homicide. Thus the patient who has received rapid tranquilization and appears to be worsening, the patient who responds initially but becomes agitated subsequently, or the patient who complies with drug treatment but has an apparent relapse should be considered a likely prospect for akathisia. (See Chapter 14 for a discussion of treatment of this side effect.)

Less common problems that may emerge with rapid neuroleptization are discussed in Chapter 4. Neuroleptic malignant syndrome, the potential for tardive dyskinesia (not well defined in these patients), the possibility of sudden death, or other potentially serious side effects generally develop with long-term neuroleptic use. A final concern with rapid neuroleptization arises when low-potency drugs are used, for example, chlorpromazine, requiring large volumes of injectable medication. As much as 25 mg/ml, when resulting in local tissue irritation, requires adequate nursing techniques and prohibits the administration of individual volumes any larger than 3 ml per site. Of course, a high-concentration, high-potency neuroleptic is preferred for this practical reason alone.

Sedative-hypnotic agents may be useful in situations involving violence in progress. Acutely violent patients under temporary physical control or restraint may benefit greatly from sedatives, if the goal is immediate sedation. Sodium amytal in doses of 200 to 500 mg may be given by slow intravenous push as a 2.5% or 5% solution at the rate of 1 ml per minute until sleep is induced. The advantage of this technique is rapid and total control of behavior through sedation. Complications include potentiation of excitement when insufficient doses are given, laryngeal spasm, or respiratory depression. Barbiturates may potentiate the effects of other central nervous system depressants, including alcohol or other sedative hypnotic agents, as discussed in Chapter 6. Another alternative is the use of intravenous diazepam in 5- to 10-mg doses (Tupin 1975).

Other sedative-hypnotic agents that may be used in the treatment of alcohol or sedative-hypnotic withdrawal in less profoundly ill patients or when neuroleptics are ineffective include diazepam, chlordiazepoxide, and lorazepam (Table 9-1). The intramuscular use of lorazepam in 1- to 2-mg doses is discussed in Chapter 6 and is given in Table 9-1. Side effects may include ataxia, nausea, vomiting, amnesia, and confusion. Aggression is usually well controlled by means of a regimen of 10 mg or less of lorazepam in a 24-hour period, but sedative-hypnotics are not particularly effective in psychotic patients. Lorazepam or an equivalent dose of clonazepam may be especially useful in the management of acute mania (Lenox et al., 1992), as discussed in Chapter 5.

A discussion of the use of restraints and seclusion is beyond the scope of this text. However, some general guidelines for the use of restraints with or without seclusion are provided in Table 9-3. When verbal intervention and voluntary medication are refused or fail to benefit the violent patient, seclusion and restraint are measures that may be necessary to ensure safety and facilitate treatment. The task force on seclusion and restraint (American Psychiatric Association, 1985) has noted that seclusion or restraint may be necessary in the following instances: (1) to prevent imminent harm to the patient or other persons when other means of control are ineffective or inappropriate, (2) to prevent serious disruption of the treatment program or significant damage to the physical environment, (3) for treatment as part of an ongoing plan of behavior therapy, (4) to decrease the stimulation that a patient is receiving, and (5) at the request of the patient. Thus "the containment of the violent impulse, the isolation from frightening or confusing external stimuli, and the definition of disrupted ego boundaries may result in a therapeutic response" (Soloff, 1987). An emergency setting may include patients brought by the police in handcuffs; in such cases restraint is necessary so that a further measure of security and control is provided while assessment is carried out or treatment begins.

Physical control such as seclusion and restraint are used when the patient's behav-

Table 9-3 Intensive Care of the Violent Patient: Guidelines for Restraint With or Without Seclusion

Guideline	Comment
Personnel and approach	A team of four or five personnel approach the patient confidently and calmly with a firm but kind "show of force"; an explanation is provided for the seclusion and restraint; reassurance and clarification are provided throughout the process.
Technique	Restraint is achieved by use of leather straps, with patient's legs "spread eagle," one arm to one side, and one arm above the head with the head slightly raised.
Monitoring	Restraints are checked every 5 to 15 minutes as appropriate; toileting occurs at least every 4 hours, and requests for food and beverage are promptly met; the attending physician is notified of the restraint within 1 to 3 hours and attends the patient, in keeping with established policies.
Treatment	Verbal or drug intervention ensues immediately, and rapid tranquilization is carried out, if appropriate, per protocol; restraint and then seclusion are discontinued only after the patient is calm, communicative, and cooperative.
Removal	Restraints are removed one at a time, except for the last two, which are removed simultaneously; the patient is debriefed, that is, given a clear explanation for the use of seclusion and restraint.

Adapted from Binder RL, McCoy SM: *Hosp Community Psychiatry* 34:1052, 1983; Dubin WR. In Stoudemire A, editor: *Clinical psychiatry for medical students,* Philadelphia, 1990, JB Lippincott; Dubin WR, Weiss KJ. In Michels R et al: *Psychiatry,* vol 2, Philadelphia, 1985, JB Lippincott.

ior exceeds the tolerance of the setting, a tolerance which may be defined by staffing patterns, patient population, or philosophy of care (Gerlock and Solomons, 1983). With rare exception mechanical restraint or seclusion is, indeed, an involuntary treatment requiring the use of force and suspension of the patient's right to refuse (Outlaw and Lowery, 1992; Keltner and Folks, in press). The choice of either seclusion or restraint as a means of control is all too often made on the basis of legal rather than clinical wisdom (Phillips and Nast, 1983). The mental health professional should be familiar with the legal aspects of seclusion and restraint, as well as the clinical advantages and disadvantages of both. Further discussion of this topic may be reviewed in Soloff, Gutheil, and Wexler (1985).

Long-Term Treatment

Long-term treatment of the violent patient is generally carried out in treatment settings such as a state hospital or another institution. Management of violence in patients may also be carried out in an outpatient setting, especially within the community or in a public setting. The mentally retarded, psychotic, or cognitively impaired patient may represent the majority of these cases.

The long-term drug treatment of violent behavior often and ideally combines medication with psychosocial interventions. Psychotherapy for patients with personality disorders, as well as medication and social intervention for those who may be cognitively impaired, has proven quite beneficial. Compliance with medical regimen may also be a significant problem in such cases. The motivation of the patient, the patient's ability to achieve self-control, issues regarding transference and countertransference, the development of affective awareness and insight, and the appreciation of the consequences of violence all represent psychotherapeutic tasks that are imperative in these cases.

Generally there is no one drug treatment for long-term management in the case of the violent patient, who may be potentially disruptive or aggressive. A variety of drugs have been suggested, depending on the underlying cause. Neuroleptics, lithium, carbamazepine, propranolol, and, potentially, other beta blockers, as well as the anxiolytics, have been used effectively, as depicted in Table 9-4. Most recently buspirone has emerged as a potentially beneficial long-term medication. Also, the novel antidepressant trazodone has been suggested as possibly useful in a variety of patients, including those with mixed mood disorders, cognitive impairment, and bipolar disorder (Folks, 1990; Folks and Fuller, in press).

As outlined in Table 9-4, neuroleptics are mostly useful for the treatment of schizophrenia, mania, and other organic syndromes in which delusional thinking, significant agitation, or psychotic symptoms are present. Haloperidol is particularly popular because it can be administered rapidly in high doses and is safe for use in epileptic patients (Donlon, Hopkin, and Tupin, 1979). Also, haloperidol and fluphenazine may be reasonable choices for the patient in whom depot administration is desirable in aftercare, for example, the patient with paranoid schizophrenia. With long-term treatment patients are subject to the long-term side effects of tardive dyskinesia, as outlined in Chapter 4.

Lithium is particularly effective for the treatment of aggression or hypersexuality, or both, in manic patients and for the prophylaxis of manic depressive disorder. Lithium is useful in decreasing agitation, aggression, and the potential for violence in these and other patients. However, no study has shown that lithium has been effective in the treatment of aggression associated with epilepsy (Lion and Tardiff, 1987). Lithium has been successfully applied to the treatment of children and adolescents with chronic aggressive behavior and conduct disorders (Campbell et al., 1982). Al-

Table 9-4 Long-Term Psychopharmacologic Treatment of Aggression

Agent	Indications	Approximate dose* (mg)	Special clinical considerations†
Neuroleptic	Aggression directly related to psychotic symptoms; management of violence or aggression by use of single dose or rapid neuroleptization	Standard antipsychotic doses	Oversedation; multiple side effects, including risk of tardive dyskinesia when used long-term
Carbamazepine	Aggression related to seizures; aggression possibly related to other organic disorders	300-800 mg/day in divided doses (to maintain serum levels at 6-12 μg/ml	Monitor for evidence of bone marrow suppression, hematologic abnormalities, or liver toxicity; watch for microsomal induction and drop in serum level
Lithium	Aggression and irritability related to manic excitement or cyclic mood	300 mg bid (to maintain serum levels at 0.6-1.2 mEq/L)	Effective for treatment of aggression in institutional settings; may augment effects of antidepressants, antipsychotics, or carbamazepine
Antianxiety Agents			
Benzodiazepines	Acute management of agitation by use of sedative-hypnotic properties	Standard anxiolytic doses	Possible induction of paradoxic rage; problems with oversedation
Buspirone	Long-term management by use of antianxiety and serotonergic properties	15-60 mg in divided doses	Onset of action up to 30 days at sufficient dose; may be used secondarily as an adjunct to another agent
Beta-blockers	Chronic or recurrent aggression in patients with cognitive impairment or brain injuries; chronic or recurrent aggression or irritability when aggression is not directly related to psychosis	50-400 mg/day propranolol in divided doses	Latency period before onset of action may be 4-6 weeks; metaprolol, atenolol, and nadolol are alternative agents

Modified from Maletta GJ: *Psychiatr Ann* 20:454, 1990.
*Doses for geriatric patients should be started at lower levels and individually titrated over time.
†Trazodone in 25- to 50-mg doses may also be useful alone or as an adjunct to another agent.

though no significant difference is evident between lithium and haloperidol, the advantages of lithium with respect to short-term and long-term side effects are obvious in these patients. Generally lithium produces the best results in children or adolescents with a strong affective component related to the aggressive or violent behavior. Also, lithium is not currently approved for uses other than the treatment of manic depressive illness and is not generally recommended for use in children under the age of 12 years, as noted in Chapters 15 and 16.

Carbamazepine has recently been reported to be useful in the treatment of aggression in psychiatric patients without epilepsy. This drug is discussed in detail in relation to bipolar disorder (Chapter 5) and epilepsy (Chapter 7). Psychotic patients, predominantly patients with schizophrenia associated with aggression and excitability, benefit greatly from the use of carbamazepine with or without haloperidol as an adjunct (Luchins 1983; Klein et al., 1980). Carbamazepine may be particularly useful in patients with temporal lobe abnormalities on electroencephalogram (Folks et al., 1982; Luchins, 1984). Carbamazepine may also be useful in decreasing agitation, aggressiveness, and emotional lability in patients with episodic dyscontrol syndrome (Monroe, 1970; Stone et al., 1986).

Propranolol may be useful in the treatment of chronic or recurrent aggression, especially in patients with organic brain syndrome. Chronic or recurrent aggression or irritability in patients whose aggression is not directly related to psychotic ideation may also benefit particularly from this class of drug. Silver and Yudofsky (1985) have reviewed the use of the beta blockers, noting their successful use for the treatment of aggression in patients with head trauma, seizures, Wilson's disease, mental retardation, minimal brain dysfunction, Korsakoff's psychosis, and other neuropsychiatric disorders. Doses lower than 640 mg per day and a response time of 2 days to 6 weeks are typical. Side effects include lowered blood pressure, decreased pulse rate, and rarely respiratory difficulties, nightmares, ataxia, and lethargy. Most patients receive concomitant treatment with haloperidol or other neuroleptic medication. Some adverse effects, including central nervous system intoxication, severe sedation, and cardiovascular reactions, have been reported (Alexander, McCarty, and Giffen, 1984). Thus a careful medical examination should be performed to identify any patients with cardiopulmonary distress, asthma, insulin-dependent diabetes mellitus, cardiac disease, severe renal disease, or hyperthyroidism.

The initial dosages of propranolol are 20 mg three times a day; dosages may be increased by 60 mg every 3 to 4 days, usually to a dose of no more than 640 mg per day. Dizziness, wheezing, and ataxia are all indications for decreasing the dosage. The highest tolerated dose should be given for at least 1 month before concluding that the patient is nonresponsive. Plasma levels of neuroleptics and antiepileptics should also be monitored in concert with beta-blocker treatment. Prospective studies and further use of propranolol and other, similar agents are needed. Recently Ratey et al. (1992) showed a significant decline in the frequency of nadolol-treated aggression when compared to controls. Thus nadolol and other beta blockers may prove to be of significant benefit in the treatment of aggression in psychiatric patients with chronic conditions.

IMPLICATIONS AND TREATMENT ISSUES

There are many special concerns about the treatment of violence in patients with psychiatric disorders, particularly in an outpatient setting. Lion and Tardiff (1987) have noted that countertransference issues, inappropriate response, safety concerns for staff and bystanders, the duty to protect potential victims, and other ongoing issues must be addressed. As patients become less violent, a risk of despondency ensues.

Aggressive patients presumably value being aggressive. To relinquish such behaviors is to be confronted with passivity, dependence, and the helplessness inherent in being weak. Thus the therapeutic task in the treatment of violence both short-term and long-term, includes consideration of these aspects of management of patient care. These considerations, together with the drug treatment, supportive interventions, and use of seclusion, restraint, and maintenance medication, are intended to culminate in improved therapeutic outcome and to reduce the potential for harm.

REFERENCES

Alexander HE, McCarty K, Giffen MD: Hypotension and cardiopulmonary arrest associated with concurrent haloperidol and propanalol therapy, *JAMA* 252:87, 1984.

American Psychiatric Association: *Report of the Task Force on Psychiatric Uses of Seclusion and Restraint of the Council on Governmental Policy and the Law of the American Psychiatric Association*, Task Force Report No 22, Washington DC, 1985, The Association.

Anderson WH, Kuehnle JC: Strategies for the treatment of acute psychosis, *JAMA* 229:1884, 1974.

Anderson WH, Kuehnle JC, Catanzano DM: Rapid treatment of acute psychosis, *Am J Psychiatry* 133:1086, 1976.

Baldessarini RJ, Katz B, Cotton P: Dissimilar dosing with high-potency and low-potency neuroleptics, *Am J Psychiatry* 141:748, 1984.

Bernstein HA: Survey of threats and assaults directed toward psychotherapists, *Am J Psychother* 35:542, 1981.

Campbell M et al: Lithium and haloperidol in hospitalized aggressive children, *Psychopharmacol Bull* 18:126, 1982.

Clinton JE et al: Haloperidol for sedation of disruptive emergency patients, *Ann Emerg Med* 16:319, 1987.

Depp FC: Violent behavior patterns on psychiatric wards, *Aggressive Behavior* 2:295, 1976.

Donlon PT, Hopkin J, Tupin JP: Overview: efficacy and safety of the rapid neuroleptization method with injectable haloperidol, *Am J Psychiatry* 136:273,1979.

Donlon PT et al: Haloperidol for acute schizophrenic patients: an evaluation of three oral regimes, *Arch Gen Psychiatry* 37:691, 1980.

Dubin WR: The evaluation and management of the violent patient, *Ann Emerg Med* 10:481, 1981.

Dubin WR: Psychiatric emergencies: recognition and management. In Stoudemire A, editor: *Clinical psychiatry for medical students*, Philadelphia, 1990, JB Lippincott.

Dubin WR, Weiss KJ, Dorn JM: Pharmacotherapy of psychiatric emergencies, *J Clin Psychopharmacol* 6:210, 1986.

Dubin WR, Wilson S, Mercer C: Assaults against psychiatrists in outpatient settings, *J Clin Psychiatry* 49:338, 1988.

Folks DG: Clinical approaches to anxiety in the medically ill elderly, *Drug Ther Suppl*, August 1990, p 72-80.

Folks DG, Fuller WC: Uses of anxiolytics and sedatives in geriatric practice: clinical selection and treatment considerations. In Smith DA, editor: *Psychotropic therapy in the elderly patient*, New York, Marcel Dekker (in press).

Folks DG et al: Carbamazepine treatment of selected affectively disordered inpatients, *Am J Psychiatry* 139:115, 1982.

Gardner DL, Cowdry RW: Alprazolam-induced dyscontrol in borderline personality disorder, *Am J Psychiatry* 142:98, 1985.

Gerlock A, Solomons HC: Factors associated with the seclusion of psychaitric patients, *Perspect Psychiatr Care* 21:47, 1983.

Goldstein MG: Intensive care unit syndromes. In Stoudemire A, Fogel BS, editors: *Principles of medical psychiatry*, Orlando, Fla, 1987, Grune & Stratton.

Hanke N: *Handbook of emergency psychiatry*, Lexington, Mass, 1984, DC Health.

Keltner NL, Folks DG: Legal considerations in the administration of psychotropic drugs, *Perspect Psychiatr Care* (in press).

Klein DF et al: *Diagnosis and drug Treatment of Psychiatric disorders: adults and children*, ed 2, Baltimore, 1980, Williams & Wilkins.

Kyser JG, Diner BC, Raulston GW: A practical approach to the assessment and management of psychiatric emergencies, *Jefferson Psychiatry* 7:81, 1989.

Lenox RH et al: Adjunctive treatment of manic agitation with lorazepam versus haloperidol: a double-blind study, *J Clin Psychiatry* 53:47, 1992.

Lion JR: Benzodiazepines in the treatment of aggressive patients, *J Clin Psychiatry* 40:70, 1979.

Lion JR: Special aspects of psychopharmacology. In Lion JR, Reid WC, editors: *Assaults within psychiatric facilities,* New York, 1983, Grune & Stratton.

Lion JR, Levenberg LB, Strange RE: Restraining the violent patient, *J Psychosoc Nurs and Ment Health Serv* 10:9, 1972.

Lion JR, Snyder W, Merrill GL: Underreporting of assaults on staff in state hospitals, *Hosp Community Psychiatry* 32:497, 1981.

Lion JR, Tardiff K: The long-term treatment of the violent patient. In Hales RE, Frances AJ, editors: *Psychiatry update: American Psychiatric Association annual review,* Vol 6, Washington, DC, 1987, American Psychiatric.

Luchins DJ: Carbamazepine for the violent psychiatric patient, *Lancet* 1:766, 1983.

Luchins DJ: Carbamazepine in psychiatric syndromes: clinical and neuropharmacological properties, *Psychopharmacol Bull* 20:569, 1984.

Madden DJ, Lion JR, Penna MW: Assaults on psychiatrists by patients, *Am J Psychiatry* 133:422, 1976.

Menza MA et al: Decreased extrapyramidal symptoms with intravenous haloperidol, *J Clin Psychiatry* 48:278, 1987.

Monroe RR: *Episodic behavioral disorders,* Cambridge, Mass, 1970, Harvard University.

Outlaw FH, Lowery BJ: Seclusion: the nursing challenge, *J Psychosoc Nurs and Ment Health Serv* 30:13, 1992.

Phillips MA, Nast SJ: Seclusion and restraint and prediction of violence, *Am J Psychiatry* 140:229, 1983.

Ratey JJ et al: Nadolol to treat aggression and psychiatric symptomology in chronic psychiatric inpatients: a double-blind, placebo-controlled study, *J Clin Psychiatry* 53:41, 1992.

Salzman C, Kochansky GE, Shader RI: Chlordiazepoxide-induced hostility in a small group setting, *Arch Gen Psychiatry* 31:401, 1974.

Salzman C et al: Benzodiazepines combined with neuroleptics for management of severe disruptive behavior, *Psychosomatics* 27(suppl):17, 1986.

Silver JM, Yudofsky S: Propranolol for aggression: literature review and clinical guidelines, *Int Drug Ther Newsletter* 20:9, 1985.

Slotnick VB: *Management of the acutely agitated psychotic patient with parenteral neuroleptics: a comparative symptoms effectiveness profile of haloperidol and chlorpromazine.* Paper presented at the Fifth World Congress of Psychiatry, Mexico City, Nov 1971.

Soloff PH: Emergency management of violent patients. In Hales RE, Frances AJ, editors: *American Psychiatric Association annual review* vol 6, Washington, DC, 1987, American Psychiatric.

Soloff PH, Gutheil TG, Wexler DB: Seclusion and restraint in 1985: a review and update, *Hosp Community Psychiatry* 36:318, 1985.

Soreff SM: Violence in the emergency room. In BS Comstock et al, editors: *Phenomenology and treatment of psychiatric emergencies,* New York, 1984, Spectrum.

Stone JL et al: Episodic dyscontrol disorder and paroxysmal EEG abnormalities: successful treatment with carbamazepine, *Biol Psychiatry* 21:208, 1986.

Tupin JP: Management of the violent patients. In Shader RI, editor: *Manual of psychiatric therapeutics,* Boston, 1975, Little, Brown.

Tupin JP: The violent patient: a strategy for management and diagnosis, *Hosp Community Psychiatry* 34:37, 1983.

Van Putten T, Marder SR: Behavioral toxicity of antipsychotic drugs, *J Clin Psychiatry* 48(suppl 9):13, 1987.

CHAPTER 10

Alcoholism and Other Substance Abuse Disorders

SCOPE OF THE PROBLEM

Abuse of drugs and alcohol in American society is widespread, despite concerted efforts to educate the public and curb their use. Dependence on alcohol and drugs has moved to the forefront of issues in psychiatric medicine and nursing. Many new developments have taken place in the field. Studies of genetic and environmental influences, neurobiologic contributors, and the clinical approach have provided important insights about treatment. Moreover, a greater understanding of individuals with dual diagnoses and sequelae resulting from alcohol or drug use has further improved the ability to develop effective treatment strategies. This chapter focuses on pharmacologic agents used to ameliorate withdrawal syndromes, modify drug-seeking behavior, and treat psychiatric disorders in drug-dependent individuals. Chapter 12 examines drugs of abuse without reference to treatment considerations. Although there is some overlap in the content of these two chapters, there is little redundancy.

EPIDEMIOLOGY

Accurate assessment of the extent and character of substance abuse and dependence patterns is difficult because of several significant measurement problems. Since the use of most drugs is illicit or unacceptable, most surveys are likely to provide conservative estimates of prevalence as a result of underreporting by respondents. Because drug-taking patterns change rapidly, national survey data may also be outdated by the time they are reported. Also, marked variation exists in patterns among persons from various cultural groups and different geographic regions. Further, data from emergency departments and other treatment facilities, as well as data from arrest records or reports of overdose deaths, measure only those individuals who are largely unsuccessful in their drug use patterns. Despite these limitations, it is possible to outline some of the trends in substance abuse that are pertinent to pharmacologic interventions.

Historical Perspective

Before the 1960s the abuse of all psychoactive drugs except alcohol was relatively rare and confined primarily to certain underprivileged inner-city populations, individuals within the entertainment world, or criminals. The use of marijuana began to increase in the 1960s, particularly among urban men. This use increased with the emergence of a counterculture that rejected traditional values and sought to find meaning, truth, or escape in pharmacologically induced altered states of consciousness. Subsequently the civil rights movement, the Vietnam war, birth control pills, and the development of a range of legitimate psychotropic medicines were contributing factors in a sharp rise in nonmedical psychoactive drug taking. For example, during the 1960s and 1970s the use of marijuana spread to rural areas, increasing the incidence of use at least once in a lifetime (lifetime experience incidence) in 1979 to 31% in 12- to 17-year-olds and 68% in young adults (Fishburne, Abelson, and Cisin, 1980). During the 1980s a decrease in the use of marijuana and other hallucinogens was observed. Also, the nonmedical use of sedative-hypnotic agents, in particular, barbiturates, appeared to level off. Cocaine became a more frequently used drug of abuse, its use rising in 1982 to a lifetime experience rate of 28.3% among young adults. Since the mid-1980s the use of cocaine has appeared to remain stable or to decrease slightly. Heroin use has remained stable, although moving from predominantly inner- city, impoverished groups to more affluent populations (Johnston, Bachman, and O'Malley, 1984; Miller, et al., 1983). Also during the 1980s a major shift in the gender pattern of substance abuse took place. Traditionally men were more likely to smoke, drink alcoholic beverages, or use drugs, but in recent years more women are noted to be drug users than in the past (Clayton, 1984).

National Surveys

The National Institute on Drug Abuse sponsors two key national surveys, The National Survey of High School Seniors and the National Household Survey on Drug Abuse. The National Survey of High School Seniors has noted a steadily declining annual prevalence of substance abuse since 1987, to an annual incidence of 5.3% in 1990 (Johnston, Bachman, and O'Malley, 1991). The use of crack cocaine, an inexpensive freebase form of the drug, has steadily decreased from a lifetime experience incidence of 5.4% in 1987 to 4.7% in 1989 and 3.5% in 1990. Despite the general overall decreases and the decline in the use of crack cocaine, 48% of high school seniors in 1990 had tried one illicit drug and almost a third had tried an illicit drug other than marijuana (Johnston, Bachman, and O'Malley, 1991). One problem with such surveys is that they do not include high school dropouts, among whom there is a higher incidence of drug abuse.

Data from the National Household Survey on Drug Abuse (1991) indicated that in general, substantial declines in the prevalence of drug use had occurred, beginning in 1985. Marijuana appears to be the most widely abused illegal drug in the United States; an estimated 67.7 million Americans having used marijuana at least once in their lifetimes (National Household Survey on Drug Abuse, 1991). Some critics challenge the validity of the National Household Survey on Drug Abuse because homeless individuals, prison inmates, and others living in institutions or treatment centers are not counted. The segment of the population that is not counted by the survey is, perhaps, the one most affected by drug addiction. Many scientists, educators, and politicians have expressed the fear that the numbers reported by the National Institute on Drug Abuse will be used to underestimate the amount of resources needed to combat the drug problem (Kaufman and McNaul, 1992).

Pregnancy Considerations

Drug abuse, particularly, the use of cocaine, in pregnant women and its impact on the fetus and infant is also an epidemiologic concern. The consequences of cocaine use during pregnancy include complications both prenatally and during delivery, as well as other toxic effects that can result in congenital malformations and drug withdrawal symptoms in infants, which may last for several weeks beyond birth (Dixon, 1989; Neerhof et al., 1989; Little et al., 1988; Giacoia, 1990).

Psychologic Considerations

Psychologic alterations induced by drug abuse may have significant influences on the personalities of those exposed persistently to drugs. Drug-related nonfatal emergencies, deaths, and emergency room visits for the treatment of alcohol abuse are well-known phenomena. Thus there is the need to continue studying determinants of drug and alcohol abuse and to further develop pharmacologic agents that may be useful in treatment.

GENETIC, ENVIRONMENTAL, AND OTHER INFLUENCES

Genetic Influences

The study of genetic contributors to alcohol and substance abuse is just beginning. The lack of knowledge about the genetic aspects of drug addiction is marked, in contrast to the wealth of knowledge about the genetic aspects of alcoholism, for which a hereditary relationship has been well established for years. Adoption studies and twin studies focusing on drug abuse have begun to improve our understanding of genetic and environmental factors that contribute to drug abuse (Cadoret et al., 1986; Grove et al., 1990; Pickens and Svikis, 1989). Generally drug abuse is highly correlated with antisocial personality disorder, and antisocial personality disorder in turn is often predicted by the presence of antisocial personality behavior in a first-degree relative. Alcohol problems among biologic relatives often predict increased drug or alcohol abuse, or both, in those without antisocial personality disorder who are adopted but not in adoptees with the disorder (Cadoret et al., 1986). Offspring of tobacco smokers are more likely to become tobacco smokers and to become tobacco dependent than is the general population (Krasnagor, 1979). A higher rate of opiate dependence is found among the siblings and relatives of opiate addicts than among the general population (Kaufman, 1981). Interestingly a recent pilot study measured euphoric response to a single 1-mg oral dose of alprazolam in a sample of 12 nonalcoholic sons of alcoholics (Ciraulo et al., 1989). Nine of the men with a family history of alcoholism experienced euphoria, whereas only two of the 12 control subjects without a family history of alcoholism had a euphoric response.

Other studies of risk or possible genetic contributors to substance abuse include the longitudinal study of Kandel, Simcha-Fagan, and Davis (1986), who found that delinquency was highly predictive of drug abuse in adolescents and young adults. Wallace (1990) has found that 61% of a sample of individuals referred for crack cocaine detoxification were adult children of alcoholics and that another 36% had dysfunctional family characteristics other than alcoholism. Another recent study identified the influence of older brothers, peers, and parents on younger brothers' drug use (Brook et al., 1990). The results showed that older brothers who did not use drugs could offset the effects of parental drug use on younger brothers. Also, younger brothers were least likely to use drugs if both older brothers and peers served as models for abstinence.

Environmental Influences

Drug-taking patterns are apparently influenced by factors relating to the family constellation and psychosocial environment. Possibly the lack of realistic, rewarding alternatives and the paucity of legitimate role models may render drug-taking behaviors more attractive (Millman and Khuri, 1981). Peer influence plays a central role in the initiation, development, and maintenance of drug abuse patterns (Sadava, 1973). The media may also have a profound impact on substance abuse patterns. Alcohol, marijuana, and tobacco have been romanticized such that engaging in these behaviors sometimes may confer on the user a variety of attributes perceived to be positive. Although the dangers of cocaine, alcohol, and tobacco use are receiving a great deal of attention in newspapers and magazines and on television, these drugs also are portrayed as an exciting province of the rich, the famous, and the popular. Moreover, young individuals growing up in families with parents or older siblings who are substance abusers tend to become substance abusers themselves. Parental attitudes or perceived parental attitudes influence the adolescent's decision to start drinking alcoholic beverages or taking drugs. Other familial factors possibly related to drug abuse include family instability, parental rejection, and divorce (Maloff et al., 1982; Millman, 1986).

Psychiatric Influences

Whether drug abuse or dependence results from specific personality factors or psychodynamics and whether particular drug-use patterns are associated with certain personality types remain controversial (Millman, 1986). Youthful drug abusers have been characterized as having external locus of control (Williams, 1973), and lowered self-esteem and increased anxiety and depression have been noted among abusers (Braucht et al., 1973; Weider and Kaplan, 1969). Psychodynamic conceptualizations have suggested that abuse of alcohol and drugs is an attempt to self-medicate a variety of dysphoric states. In addition, the muting and antiaggression properties of the opiates and other compounds may diminish painful psychic states, at least temporarily, and allow the narcotic-dependent individual to cope (Khantzian, 1974; Wurmser, 1974).

Sometimes it is difficult to tell whether the psychopathologic features associated with alcohol or substance abuse are secondary or primary to the pharmacologic effect of the chronic use of the particular drug. Also, the adaptation to the experience of becoming and being a drug-dependent person in a society that stigmatizes and punishes such behavior must be appreciated (Zinberg, 1975). Most likely, substance abusers vary markedly in premorbid personality patterns and in psychopathologic features. Systematic studies of narcotic addicts in methadone treatment have demonstrated the heterogeneity of psychiatric diagnoses in these populations (Rounsaville, Gawin, and Kleber, 1985; McLellan, Woody, and O'Brien, 1979). Perhaps the choice of drug may reflect personality patterns or psychopathology, thus whether stimulants, narcotics, opiates, alcohol, or other sedative-hypnotic depressants are used may depend on the specific individual's makeup and may account for great heterogeneity among substance-abuse populations. As noted in Chapters 6 and 8, alcohol or other depressants may be used to suppress or treat symptoms of anxiety or, by contrast, to allow expression of long-suppressed anger (Millman, 1986). Some individuals may avoid the use of marijuana, hallucinogens, or stimulants that weaken the connection to reality and amplify paranoid, psychotic, or anxiety states. Generally a careful drug-use history with particular emphasis on which drugs are perceived as pleasant and beneficial and which have led to adverse reactions may facilitate the clinical approach.

Drug-Related Influences

All too often the sense of control that derives from drug abuse is related to the effect of a rapid rate of change of consciousness or perception in almost any direction (Millman, 1985). For example, cocaine is perceived to be more desirable than an oral amphetamine; a rapidly acting benzodiazepine may be more subject to abuse than are drugs that are slower in onset. Moreover, the conditioned learning important in maintaining drug abuse patterns and in initiating relapse may also be an important environmental influence. For example, the dysphoric symptoms that the drug-taking behavior allayed or controlled or certain situations that have come to be associated with drug-taking behaviors become in time the conditioned stimulus for the experience of drug craving and drug-seeking behavior. Learning may be an important determinant of the subjective perception of the drug experience; for example, marijuana is used in some cultures as a work enhancer and an appetite suppressant, in contrast to its publicized effects in America as a drug that decreases motivation and stimulates the appetite for sweet food.

Regarding the neurobiologic contributors, most recent neurochemical research has focused on opioids and cocaine. Cocaine and other abusable stimulants have varied actions on multiple neurotransmitter systems. Essentially these compounds exert their primary effect on dopaminergic systems, but they also affect noradrenergic, serotonergic, and cholinergic systems (Gawin, 1988). Cocaine increases dopamine concentration in the synaptic cleft, resulting in increased neurotransmission in brain reward systems. Chronic use of cocaine or other stimulants causes catecholamine receptor supersensitivity. Autoreceptor feedback systems may ultimately decrease dopaminergic transmission. This action may explain the anhedonia seen in chronic cocaine users. Cocaine may also impair the ability of neurons to use dopa (Baxter et al., 1988; Volkow et al., 1990). Also, the benzodiazepine receptor may be affected by cocaine through complex interactions. Studies of these receptors and their interactions with the gamma-aminobutyric acid (GABA) neurotransmitter systems may further explain some of the phenomena seen in both cocaine and benzodiazepine withdrawal (Kolata, 1982). In addition to the opiates, a receptor specific for tetrahydracannabinol (THC), the active ingredient in marijuana, has recently been identified in human brain (Culhane, 1990). This discovery may lead to a better understanding of the effects of marijuana, both positive, for example, appetite stimulation and nausea prevention, and negative, such as perceptual and memory disturbance. The toxic effects of marijuana may be due to its effect on the cells of the hippocampus, which are known to be important in learning and memory (Schuster, 1990).

Endogenous Opiate Receptors

Endogenous opiate receptors were discovered in the mid-1970s. Three distinct opiate receptors, mu, kappa, and delta, have been well characterized, and subtypes of these receptors are likely to be found. These endogenous opiate receptor systems are undoubtedly complex, affecting a wide range of important physiologic functions. Pain perception, behavioral manifestations, and a role in schizophrenia, headache, depression, and other mood disturbances may be partially explained through a better understanding of these systems (Terenius, 1982). Ultimately a better understanding of the opioid, benzodiazepine, GABA, and the other neurotransmitter systems (reviewed in detail in Chapter 3) may lead to improved pharmacologic strategies for the treatment of withdrawal symptoms, drug-seeking behavior, or psychiatric disorders common among drug-dependent individuals.

DIAGNOSTIC CONSIDERATIONS

The appropriate treatment of an individual with substance abuse or dependence depends not only on the characterization of the specific drug and pattern of use but also on an understanding of the psychologic set and social situations attendant to the behavioral patterns. The nature and degree of drug-induced psychoactive effects, as well as the presence of abstinence phenomena, should be evaluated, which requires careful history and physical assessment, including a complete history of drug use.

The recognition and treatment of alcoholism and other types of substance abuse and dependence require knowledge of the pharmacokinetics and pharmacodynamics of specific psychoactive substances. The presence of substance abuse or dependence must be considered with respect to known therapies for the acute management of intoxication and withdrawal and options for long-term rehabilitation. Several aspects of substances that are often abused have been reviewed in a previous chapter. However, some consideration of the diagnostic approach is necessary in examining those pharmacologic agents that are used in the treatment of alcohol and drug abuse and dependence.

Frequently no clear delineation distinguishes the appropriate use of a psychoactive substance from misuse, abuse, or dependence. Although the scope of this problem has been considered with respect to epidemiologic, genetic, environmental, and neurobiologic contributors, most of the factors determining an individual's susceptibility to substance abuse are not well understood. Studies of populations at risk for developing substance abuse have identified factors that foster the development and continuance of substance abuse. However, the relative contribution of these factors varies among individuals and no single factor appears to account entirely for the risk. Diagnosis and classification of substance abuse disorders reflect prevailing cultural attitudes and theoretic biases. In recent years it has become recognized that these disorders may exist independent of other psychiatric conditions. Thus the current nomenclature permits the independent diagnosis of substance use and dependence apart from other psychiatric disorders (American Psychiatric Association, 1987).

American Psychiatric Association Considerations

The *Diagnostic and Statistical Manual of Mental Disorders, Third Edition-Revised (DSM-III-R)* has brought sweeping changes in the diagnosis of drug dependence, reflecting a redefinition of the concept of dependence that has evolved over the past decade. The movement toward a multifocal approach and away from reliance solely on physiologic dependence has gained much support. Thus the diagnostic description now considers the nature and severity of dependence, the degree and type of disability, and the personal and environmental factors that influence substance abuse. Also the concept of a generic drug-dependency syndrome applies to all psychoactive substances and allows comparison of symptomatology in a variety of drugs of abuse. (Barbor et al., 1990). Thus an individual might be diagnosed as having substance dependence without having the classic symptoms of withdrawal, tolerance, or physical effects. *DSM-IV* is likely to continue along similar lines with increased emphasis on biologic markers and potential roles of social and behavioral factors (Kaufman and McNaul, 1992).

Defining Key Factors

The American Psychiatric Association has considered the problem of psychiatric substances to be a medical disorder when the use of psychoactive substances constitutes or meets a certain set of criteria. From a pharmacologic perspective dependence is a state in which a syndrome of specific withdrawal signs and symptoms follows reduction or cessation of the drug use. This definition is in keeping with the generic diagnosis outlined in *DSM- III-R* (American Psychiatric Association, 1987) and shown in the box on p. 221. *Tolerance* refers to a state in which the physiologic or behavioral effects of repeated doses of a psychoactive substance decrease over time or a greater

Criteria for Substance Dependence

At least *three* of the following persist for at least 1 month or have occurred repeatedly over a significant period of time.

- Substance taken in larger amounts or over a longer period than originally intended
- Substance use to relieve or avoid stress (may not apply to cannabis, hallucinogens, or PCP)
- One or more unsuccessful attempts to cut down or to control substance use or a persistent desire to do so
- Considerable time spent in activities necessary to obtain the substance, using the substance, or recovering from its effects
- Symptoms of intoxication or withdrawal occur when expected to fulfill major obligations at work, school, or home
- Important activities or obligations are reduced or unmet due to the substance use
- Continued substance use despite knowledge that a persistent or recurrent social, psychological, or physical problem is related to use of the substance
- Marked tolerance with increased amount of the substance (at least 50%) to achieve intoxication or a desired effect: markedly diminished effect with use of the same amount of substance
- Characteristic withdrawal symptoms

From American Psychiatric Association: *Diagnostic and statistical manual of mental disorders, third edition- revised,* Washington, DC, 1987, American Psychiatric Association.

dose of drug is necessary to achieve the same effect. *Withdrawal* is a physiologic state that follows cessation or reduction in the amount of the drug used. *Abuse* is a residual category for patterns of drug use that do not meet the criteria for dependence. Psychoactive substance abuse is therefore defined as a pattern of substance use of at least 1 month's duration that causes impairment in social or occupational functioning and the presence of psychologic or physical problems or situations in which use of the substance is physically hazardous, for example, driving while intoxicated. "Addiction" is often used as a synonym of "dependence" but carries a more negative and pejorative connotation.

The acute and chronic effects of psychoactive substances are classified by *DSM-III-R* under two major categories. The first category, psychoactive substance–induced organic mental disorders, describes the direct effects of the drug on the central nervous system, such as intoxication, withdrawal, delirium, delusion, or mood changes. The second category is psychoactive substance use (dependence and abuse) that results from maladaptive behaviors caused by the acute or chronic effects of the drug. *DSM-III-R* designates 11 distinct classes or categories of psychoactive substances, described in the box on p. 222. All of these classes except nicotine are associated with abuse and dependence; dependence is defined only for nicotine. Individuals who use three categories or more of substances are said to be polysubstance abusers or polysubstance dependent (Swift, 1990).

Psychoactive Substances

Alcohol*
Amphetamines (sympathomimetics)
Caffeine
Cannabis
Cocaine*
Hallucinogens
Inhalants
Nicotine*
Opioids*
Phencyclidine (arylcyclohexylamines)
Sedative-hypnotics* (anxiolytics)

From American Psychiatric Association: *Diagnostic and statistical manual of mental disorders, third edition-revised*, Washington, DC, 1987, American Psychiatric Association.
*Represents a significant class with respect to drug interventions.

Comorbidity

Much of the current treatment approach to alcoholism and other substance use disorders has focused on the association with other psychopathologic features (Meyer, 1986; Butcher, 1988; Kosten and Kleber, 1988). Dually diagnosed patients constitute 30% to 50% of psychiatric patients and up to 80% of substance abusers. The comorbid pathologic characteristics found consist of both axis I and axis II disorders within the *DSM-III-R* nomenclature. Although a complete discussion of the comorbid pathologies found among substance abusers and substance-dependent individuals is beyond the scope of this book, the most prevalent disorders include mood disorders, disorders within the affective spectrum, psychotic disorders, attention deficit and conduct disorders, and personality disorders, particularly those that fall within the cluster characterized as antisocial, histrionic, borderline, and narcissistic (Kaufman and McNaul, 1992). Several personality characteristics measured by the Minnesota Multiphasic Personality Inventory (MMPI) have been shown to be associated with substance abuse. Interestingly substance use disorders are the only psychiatric illness in which a known environmental agent (the abused drug) is necessary to the development of the disorder. Khantzian's self-medication hypothesis of addiction (1985) postulates that individuals seek out specific classes of drugs to defend against and cope with painful affective states; thus affected individuals may experiment with multiple substances but tend to settle on a single drug of choice.

DRUG TREATMENT

The pharmacologic approach to the treatment of alcohol and drug use or dependence ideally includes a combination of psychotherapy, behavioral techniques, and adjunctive interventions that may also serve to improve compliance with the medical regimen. To provide appropriate treatment, it is necessary to consider the psychosocial characteristics of the patient, as well as the pharmacology and pattern of abuse of the particular psychoactive substance. Treatment should be conceptualized as including initial and long-term phases.

Short-Term Treatment Objectives

During the initial phase, termination of drug use and establishment of a stable, drug-free state must be the primary therapeutic goal. Identifying the substance use problem and helping the patient accept the proposed intervention may require some degree of confrontation in a family, work, social, or school setting (Blume, 1984). During the initial treatment phase, provisions must be made for long-term interventions. Whereas the therapeutic relationship and trust are essential to the treatment process, patients often resume their abuse without informing the therapist. Thus intermittent or routine screens may be performed and objective data on drug abuse status may actually facilitate an open and trusting therapeutic alliance. In the context of this relationship the following objectives of short-term treatment have been outlined by Swift (1990):

1. Relieving subjective symptoms of distress and discomforts resulting from intoxication or withdrawal
2. Preventing and treating serious complications of intoxication, withdrawal, or dependence
3. Establishing a drug- or alcohol-free state
4. Preparing for and referral to longer-term treatment or rehabilitation
5. Engaging the family in the treatment process

Long-Term Treatment Objectives

The objective of long-term treatment or rehabilitation is to maintain the alcohol- or drug-free state through ongoing psychologic, family, and vocational interventions. Long-term treatment involves behavioral and psychologic interventions to maintain abstinence. Changes in life-style, work, or friendships may be necessary. Halfway houses, therapeutic communities, and other residential treatment situations may also be useful. Treatment of underlying psychiatric or medical illnesses may reduce the impetus for self-medication. Self-help groups such as Alcoholics Anonymous (AA) and Narcotics Anonymous (NA) provide education, emotional support, and hope to substance abusers and their families. Many patients who come to medical attention for treatment do so in the context of a family structure that is dysfunctional. For these individuals, involving the family, particularly spouses and children, may provide great benefit.

Drugs Used in the Treatment of Alcoholism

An estimated 5% to 7% of Americans have alcoholism in a given year; 13% have alcoholism at some time during their lives. Simply defined, alcoholism is a repetitive but inconsistent and sometimes unpredictable loss of control of drinking that produces symptoms of serious dysfunction or disability (Clark, 1981). There are marked sex differences in alcohol dependence and abuse; the prevalence is about 5% to 6% for men and 1% to 2% for women. The prevalence is highest among men from 18 to 64 years of age and women from 18 to 24 years of age, with a gradual drop afterward (Regier et al., 1988). Alcoholism is believed to account for 20% to 50% of all hospital admissions but is diagnosed in less than 5% (Lewis and Gordan, 1983; Holden, 1985). Alcohol use is also highly correlated with suicide, homicide, and accidents (Goodwin, 1967).

Drug treatment of alcohol intoxication or withdrawal (short-term). Patients who come to medical attention for treatment of alcohol intoxication or withdrawal may show various types of impairment. Many alcoholics have profound social and financial problems that our health care system is ill equipped to handle. Particularly frustrating is the alcoholic with profound social needs who does not require medical treatment or who refuses medical treatment. The acute alcohol withdrawal syndrome varies greatly in severity. Although severity of withdrawal is generally proportional to the level and duration of alcohol intake, many other factors such as previous episodes of dependence and concurrent medical illness influence the syndrome's severity. Most episodes are mild and require neither hospitalization nor pharmacologic intervention (Whitfield, 1980).

Although prescribing sedative-hypnotic agents to manage withdrawal on an ambulatory basis may seem taboo, these drugs are quite useful among hospitalized alcoholics (Jaffe and Ciraulo, 1985). Generally, comprehensive nursing care, the routine use of nutritional supplements, and prompt attention to complicating illnesses are responsible for the present low rates of delirium tremens and mortality resulting from alcohol withdrawal. Although the benzodiazepines, paraldehyde, chloral hydrate, barbiturates, and other sedative hypnotic agents are effective in suppressing the alcohol withdrawal syndrome, the benzodiazepines are superior when given in adequate dosage for sufficient periods of time (Sellers and Kalant, 1982). Available benzodiazepines vary greatly in complexity, as outlined in Chapters 6 and 8.

Use of benzodiazepines. In the use of the benzodiazepines to treat alcohol withdrawal, the basic principle is rapid substitution of a sufficient amount to suppress withdrawal, followed by a gradual tapering of drug level over several days. Drugs with long-acting properties, such as chlordiazepoxide (Librium) and diazepam (Valium), are useful in that they self-taper. Parenteral administration must be considered for patients who cannot take drugs by mouth. Lorazepam (Ativan), which is promptly and reliably absorbed from intramuscular sites, may be preferred. If suppression of withdrawal is delayed and hallucinosis develops, dopaminergic blockers such as haloperidol may be required in addition to the benzodiazepines (Sellers and Kalant, 1982).

Other agents. Barbiturates may be preferred for the treatment of alcohol withdrawal. Chloral hydrate and paraldehyde, however, should be considered obsolete because of toxic effects. Phenytoin is sometimes used as a part of the treatment of alcohol withdrawal, but there is no evidence that it should be used routinely except in patients who have a history of seizures unrelated to alcohol withdrawal. Unlike phenytoin, valproic acid does suppress alcohol withdrawal seizures in animals and may be useful in treating alcohol withdrawal in humans. Carbamazepine and buspirone may be of future interest in the management of acute alcohol withdrawal syndrome (Jaffe, 1987).

Thiamine should be administered to all alcohol users as soon as possible (and before the administration of glucose) to prevent the development of Wernicke's encephalopathy, which is characterized by ataxia, nystagmus, ophthalmoplegia, and changes in mental status. The encephalopathic symptoms tend to improve with thiamine repletion. Levels of magnesium and other electrolytes should be determined and deficits replaced. Other details of detoxification management are beyond the scope of this chapter.

Long-term treatment of alcoholism (abstinence). The goal of long-term treatment of alcoholism is to maintain abstinence through a comprehensive treatment program that includes psychologic, family, and social interventions. Pharmacologic agents can deter alcohol consumption by making the ingesting of alcohol aversive (sensitizing agents) or by producing unpleasant effects that deliberately lengthen the metabolism of alcohol to create an aversion to alcohol (conditioning agents). Although many drugs alter the response to alcohol and make its ingestion unpleasant, only *disulfiram (Antabuse)* has been widely used in the treatment of alcoholism. This agent inhibits the enzyme aldehyde oxyseductase dehydrogenase, which metabolizes acetaldehyde to acetic acid. When acetic acid is inhibited, ingestion of alcohol causes a rise in the acetaldehyde level and brings on an unpleasant syndrome characterized by facial flushing, tachycardia, pounding in the chest, decreased blood pressure, nausea, vomiting, shortness of breath, sweating, dizziness, and confusion (Sellers, Naranjo, and Peachey, 1981). Recently the toxic effects of disulfiram have resulted in the question of whether it is justified in the therapeutic use under any circumstances. Patients taking disulfiram must be informed about the danger of the combination with even small amounts of alcohol. Alcohol present in foods, shaving lotion, mouthwashes, or over-the-counter medications may produce a reaction. The usual dose of disulfiram is 250 to 500 mg daily. Disulfiram may interact with other medications, notably, anticoagulants and phenytoin. Its use is contraindicated in patients with liver disease. Contraindications may include myocardial disease, severe pulmonary insufficiency, renal failure, disorders of cognitive impairment, neuropathy, psychosis, or difficulty with impulse control or suicidal ideation. Certain medications such as vasodilators, beta-adrenergic agonists, monoamine oxidase inhibitors (MAOIs), or antipsychotic agents may also represent relative contraindications.

Emetic-induced nausea coupled with the ingestion of alcohol has been used for more than 40 years to induce aversion to alcohol. Controlled studies in the 1980s have demonstrated that conditioned aversion to alcohol can, in fact, be established and that such conditioning contributes to a positive clinical outcome (Jaffe, 1987). The use of lithium as an emetic can also produce aversion. Efforts to demonstrate useful alcohol aversions associated with electric shocks have not been successful (McClellan and Childress, 1985). Apomorphine, which can produce emesis, has also been used as a conditioning agent, but it has been used primarily for other pharmacologic treatments, which are discussed later.

A number of drugs other than lithium that have been useful in the treatment of postwithdrawal anxiety and depression associated with reduction of alcohol consumption include tricyclic antidepressants (TCAs), MAOIs, benzodiazepines, propranolol, dopaminergic antagonists such as haloperidol, and other dopaminergic blockers. The TCAs are frequently prescribed, but there is little firm evidence for their efficacy, even in alcoholics with primary depression. However, it is now clear that alcoholics metabolize imipramine much more rapidly than do controls, and in all probability in most previously made studies insufficient dosages were used. Thus the use of TCAs in the postwithdrawal syndrome may be useful (Jaffe and Ciraulo, 1985). Recent studies with selective serotonin reuptake inhibitors, for example, fluoxetine and sertraline, have shown efficacy in reducing alcohol use in nondepressed heavy drinkers (Swift, 1990; Schuckit, 1986).

Drugs Used to Treat Narcotic (Opioid) Dependence and Abuse

Estimates of the incidence and prevalence of narcotic or opioid use and dependence have been relatively stable over the last several years. Generally the use of the term *addict* has been used to mean someone with severe dependence on opiate drugs. The term *opioid* generally refers to a large number of chemically diverse substances that have in common the capacity to bind specifically and to produce actions at several distinct types of opioid receptors. The term *narcotic analgesic* has also been used to describe this class of drugs.

The physiologic effects of opiates are due to stimulation of receptors that modulate endogenous hormones, enkephalins, endorphines, and dynorphines. Mu, kappa, sigma, delta, and epsilon opioid receptors, as forementioned, have been identified

(Jaffe and Martin, 1985). Morphine, heroin, and methadone act primarily through mu receptors and produce analgesia, euphoria, and respiratory depression. Drugs that appear to be mediated through the kappa receptors include the so-called mixed agonist-antagonists, butorphanol and pentazocine, which produce analgesia but less respiratory depression. The sigma receptor appears to imitate the receptor for the hallucinogen phencyclidine (PCP). The delta receptor binds endogenous opioid peptides. At high doses opioid drugs lose their receptor specificity and have agonist or antagonist properties at multiple receptor subtypes.

No single accepted standard of treatment exists for opioid dependence. Treatment may involve inpatient, residential, day care, or outpatient settings; the qualifications of therapists may range from advanced degrees to a personal history of recovery from dependence. Patients are often treated for withdrawal from opioids on either an inpatient or an outpatient basis. The use of opioid drugs to treat withdrawal or to stabilize patients is regulated by federal and state governments. New regulations permit the use of decreasing doses of opioids, and methadone is the only drug approved for use in a certified program and may be given for 6 months or more.

Methadone. Methadone (Dolophine) maintenance continues to be a major modality for treating opioid dependence. The maintenance approach achieves the effect of alleviating drug hunger with high doses of methadone, blocking the dependency by means of cross-tolerance. Decreases in criminal activity and increases in legitimate productive work have been shown to be outcomes of this type of treatment. Methadone is typically administered by the oral route, and because of its reliable absorption and delay in peak plasma levels of 2 to 6 hours after ingestion, the patients are protected against sharp peaks in serum levels and continuation of tolerance. Administration of methadone can ultimately result in a once-daily administration, and opioid maintenance programs using methadone can be administered with confidence. Patient progress is monitored by means of interviews and urine testing.

The objective in managing withdrawal is to suppress severe withdrawal symptoms. However, some discomfort is almost always experienced; the discomfort and associated craving can sometimes be reduced by gradual reduction in opioid dosage. Hospitalized patients are generally more able than outpatients to tolerate rapid dosage reductions, often starting with 15 to 20 mg of methadone repeated after 2 to 4 hours when withdrawal symptoms are not suppressed or if they reappear. The dosage is generally not more than 40 mg per day, and dosage reductions of approximately 10% to 20% per day can be started and the entire process completed within 1 to 2 weeks (Fultz and Senay, 1975). Some low-level withdrawal symptoms, including sleep and mood disturbance, may persist for weeks after the last dose. Constipation and sweating are side effects of methadone and may persist.

Patients who have been on a maintenance regimen of high doses of methadone or professionals with access to pure opioids may have more severe degrees of physical dependence. They may require higher stabilization doses and may be unable to tolerate a rapid withdrawal protocol. Successful detoxification is more difficult to achieve on an outpatient basis. Some clinicians recommend a slow dose reduction of 10% dosage reduction per week, then 3% per week after the dosage is less than 20 mg per week (Senay et al., 1977; Jaffe, 1986).

Clonidine. The alpha-2 agonist clonidine (Catapres) has been used to facilitate opioid withdrawal in both inpatient and outpatient settings (Charney et al., 1981). This drug acts by means of interaction with presynaptic noradrenergic nerve endings in the locus ceruleus and blocks adrenergic discharge produced by opiate withdrawal. Clonidine in divided doses totaling up to 2 mg per day may reduce many of the autonomic effects of the opioid withdrawal syndrome, although craving, lethargy, insomnia, restlessness, and muscle aches are not well suppressed (Gold et al., 1979). Clonidine detoxification has also been used to facilitate the initiation of naltrexone (Trexan) treatment (Charney et al., 1982).

Narcotic antagonists. The use of opioid antagonists in treating opioid dependence was originally based on the high relapse rate after detoxification. Naltrexone is a long-acting, orally effective agent that, when given either daily as 50 mg per day or 3 times weekly in doses of 100 mg, produces substantial blockade of the effects of large doses of injected opioid drugs (Resnick, Schuyten-Resnick, and Washton, 1980). Naltrexone is contraindicated in patients with acute hepatitis or liver failure. Patients must be free of opioid dependence for 1 week before naltrexone can be used.

Opioid overdose, a life-threatening emergency, should be suspected in any patient who comes to medical attention with coma and respiratory suppression. Treatment of suspected overdose includes emergency support of respiration and cardiovascular functions. Parenteral administration of the opioid antagonist, naloxone (Narcan), 0.4 to 0.8 mg, rapidly reverses the coma and respiratory suppression but does not result in the depression caused by other sedatives such as alcohol or barbiturates. Naloxone can precipitate opioid withdrawal, causing the patient whose life has just been saved to be extremely ungrateful.

Drugs Used to Treat Effects of Central Nervous System Stimulants

Drugs used to treat cocaine abuse and dependence. The use of cocaine and crack cocaine has undergone an epidemic increase. Cocaine has emerged as a major drug of abuse after a relatively long quiescent period during which its use was limited to a small subgroup of the population. The pure drug has been available for only approximately 100 years, but chewing coca leaves has been a practice for 2000 years. Cocaine is an alkaloid extracted from the leaves of the native South American plant. Cocaine is a local anesthetic that blocks the initiation and propagation of nerve impulses and is a potent sympathomimetic agent that potentiates the actions of catecholamines in the autonomic nervous system, causing tachycardia, hypertension, and vasoconstriction. Cocaine is also a central nervous system (CNS) stimulant, increasing arousal and producing mood elevation and psychomotor activation.

There has been a major shift from snorting cocaine to intravenous injection and smoking freebase cocaine. Freebase cocaine, known as crack, is inexpensive and widely available. Thus the dramatic increases in hospital admissions for treatment, emergency care, and deaths reflect not only the increased number of users but also new ways of ingesting this drug.

Cocaine intoxication is characterized by elation, euphoria, excitement, pressured speech, restlessness, stereotypic movements, and bruxism. Sympathetic nervous system stimulation occurs, including tachycardia, mydriasis, and sweating. Paranoia, suspiciousness, and psychosis may occur with prolonged use. Overdosage produces hyperpyrexia, hyperreflexia, seizures, coma, and respiratory arrest (Swift, 1990).

Cocaine has a short plasma half-life of 1 to 2 hours, which correlates with its behavioral effects (Van Dyke et al., 1978). Along with the decline in plasma levels, most users experience a period of dysphoria, which often leads to additional cocaine use within a short period. The dysphoria of the "crash" is intensified and prolonged after repeated usage. Abusers uniformly report control over early stimulant usage. As use continues, however, the individual binges until immediate supplies are exhausted

(Gawin and Kleber, 1985). This compulsive use pattern and impairment of self-control are the best indicators of stimulant abuse and of the severity of abuse.

Clinical presentations involving cocaine abuse and dependence include a mixture of acute and chronic symptoms with different intensities. Cocaine intoxication, delirium, delusions, postuse dysphoria, and withdrawal may be present. Cocaine may cause severe drug intoxication or death through an extension of its sympathomimetic properties. Chronic medical complications may include malnutrition, anorexia, nutritional deficiencies, dehydration, endocrine abnormalities, and complications linked to the route of administration (Cohen, 1981).

The major new developments in the area of pharmacologic treatment of substance abuse are in the treatment of cocaine abuse and dependence. Before the 1980s the scientific evaluation of the treatment of cocaine abuse was sparse and no consensus existed regarding optimal treatment strategies. Clearly, accurate psychiatric characterization of the cocaine abuser is important because symptoms appearing during abstinence might provide guides to when and what pharmacologic adjuncts are indicated. Treatment generally focuses on one of three areas, acute sequelae, craving, and withdrawal. Psychologic supports and behavioral therapy are generally applied in the treatment of these patients. Hospitalization may be required for individuals who are chronic freebase or intravenous cocaine users or concurrent alcohol users, or for individuals who have significant psychiatric or medical comorbidity, psychosocial impairment, or lack of motivation or who were not successfully treated as outpatients (Kleber and Gawin, 1986; Rounsaville, Gawin, and Kleber, 1985).

Although no panacea exists for the treatment of cocaine dependence, a wide range of psychotropic medications have been used, including stimulants, antidepressants, precursors to neurotransmitters, neuroleptics, and other agents that have multiple effects on brain neurotransmission. Pharmacologic agents that aid the recovering addict may be divided into those that are useful as anticraving agents and those that may be more useful in the phases of maintaining abstinence and preventing relapse. Agents that have a relatively rapid onset of action, including amantadine, bromocriptine, levodopa (L-dopa), carbidopa, methylphenidate, and carbamazepine, may be useful; in addition, the TCAs may be useful for the treatment of craving. Although no long-term, placebo-controlled, double-blind studies have been made of any of these agents, their efficacy has been touted in case reports and in some single-dose placebo cross-over trials (Gawin and Ellinwood, 1988; Giannini and Baumgartel, 1987; Tennant and Segherian, 1987).

Dopaminergic drugs. Amantadine (Symmetrel) may exert its therapeutic effect by releasing neuronal stores and delaying uptake of dopamine and norepinephrine, thereby increasing availability to the postsynaptic receptor sites. This drug theoretically could be given with L-dopa, carbidopa, or tyrosine to enhance the clinical effect. Although amantadine initially is effective without significant side effects, its usefulness appears to be limited to the acute withdrawal phase (Gawin et al., 1989b).

Bromocriptine, a dopamine antagonist, also appears to reduce the density of the inhibitory receptors or autoreceptors on dopamine neurons that exert a rapid anticraving effect (Giannini et al., 1989). Doses of 0.5 to 1.5 mg per day may be useful. Abstinent cocaine users report an antagonist effect of bromocriptine when using cocaine. Thus bromocriptine might be useful in abstinent cocaine abusers as an antagonist, similar to the way disulfiram or naltrexone is used with alcoholics or opiate addicts, respectively.

Carbamazepine. Carbamazepine (Tegretol) has been used in treatment-resistant addicts. Theoretically carbamazepine, through its ability to reverse cocaine-induced kindling, reverses cocaine receptor supersensitivity that results from chronic cocaine use (Halikas et al., 1989). Patients receiving treatment in an open trial have shown significant reductions in cocaine craving with use of this drug.

Tricyclic antidepressants. Tricyclic antidepressants have had success in the treatment of cocaine users, but because of the delayed onset of action of TCAs, their use may be better suited for the later phases of maintaining abstinence and preventing relapse (Kosten, 1989; Gawin et al., 1989b). The rationale for their effectiveness is that they reduce dopaminergic receptor sensitivity and thereby reduce cocaine-induced supersensitivity. Most of the better-controlled studies of drug treatment of cocaine dependence have used the TCAs. Several trials have used desipramine, resulting in significant decreases in cocaine use and craving. However, desipramine was found useful only when given in adequate doses for sufficient duration. Daily doses of 2.5 mg per kg body weight for up to 6 weeks may result in the full therapeutic effect. The effect of lower doses such as 75 to 100 mg daily may not be much better than that of a placebo (Kaufman and McNaul, 1992).

The anhedonia, anergia, and consequences of chronic cocaine abuse can result in a syndrome known as *intracranial self-stimulation.* Desipramine, imipramine, and amitriptyline treatment have been employed, and use in an animal model seems to reverse the changes that occur at catecholamine receptors as a result of repeated stimulant use. In essence the TCAs restore hedonic capacity and decrease cocaine craving. Whether desipramine and, possibly, other tricyclic or heterocyclic antidepressants, for example, trazodone, have some ability to block the physiologic effects of cocaine has been the subject of speculation (Rowbotham et al., 1984). However, to determine conclusively whether antidepressants block cocaine's effects or have anticraving effects, or both, remains a subject of further study.

Other agents. The central role of depression in cocaine abuse is demonstrated not only by the striking resemblance of the cocaine withdrawal syndrome to depression but also by findings that depressive disorders predict increased cocaine use in follow-up. Because depression predicts subsequent cocaine abuse, pharmacologic treatment of depression may, indeed, be an important preventive strategy. Methylphenidate (Ritalin) may be a useful agent in treatment for the abstinent cocaine abuser but is not recommended because of its ability to stimulate cocaine craving (Khantzian, 1983). Lithium may also diminish craving, particularly in persons who meet *DSM-III-R* criteria for cyclothymia or who have family history of bipolar disorder. However, lithium is not generally considered a blocking agent for cocaine euphoria and has not been established as a particularly useful agent for these patient.

Cocaine has no specific antagonist for the treatment of acute sequelae. Management of overdose is largely symptomatic and is aimed at reversing epileptogenic, cardiorespiratory, and metabolic effects (Gay, 1982). Diazepam for transient agitation, together with propranolol, may be useful for persistent symptoms. Suicidal ideation and depressive symptoms that often occur during the post-cocaine "crash" are transient and require no acute treatment other than close observation. Neuroleptics may be used briefly for severe psychotic symptoms; chlorpromazine, because of its sedative effects and potential to antagonize the lethal effects of cocaine, may be particularly useful (Kleber and Gawin, 1986). Haloperidol may also be used effectively for the treatment of cocaine-induced psychosis (Smith, 1984). However, psychotic symptoms seem to be short-lived and usually remit after sleep normalization. Symptoms of depression or psychosis that do not remit within approximately 3 days may necessitate conventional treatment.

In summary, several pharmacologic agents have shown promise as adjuncts in the treatment of cocaine abuse, both for craving and for withdrawal. Imipramine, desipramine, trazodone, and lithium may reduce craving or usage, or both. Dopamine antagonists, bromocriptine and amantadine, may block craving as well. Many treatment facilities provide short-term intensive psychologic treatment and drug education in a drug-free environment. Ideally this approach, followed by a long-term residential drug-free program for those with more severe difficulties, may be most efficacious. Self-help groups such as Narcotics Anonymous may also be useful as a primary treatment modality or as an adjunct to another treatment. Certain psychiatric disorders such as depression, cyclothymia, and attention deficit disorder may be common in cocaine users and should be treated. In addition, many cocaine users also use alcohol or other drugs, particularly sedatives and heroin, and may require treatment for abuse of these substances as well.

Drugs used to treat amphetamine dependence. Although the subjective effects of amphetamines are quite similar to those of cocaine, there are important differences in their mechanisms of action. It is not clear why cocaine epidemics have stimulated so many more attempts at pharmacologic intervention than did the amphetamine epidemic that occurred in the 1960s. Nevertheless, remarkably little is known about the pharmacologic treatment of amphetamine dependence or its complications (Jaffe, 1987).

Amphetamines as a group are structurally related to the catecholamine neurotransmitters norepinephrine, epinephrine, and dopamine. These drugs release endogenous catecholamines from nerve endings and are catecholamine agonists at receptors in the peripheral, autonomic, and central nervous systems. Thus intoxication with stimulants such as amphetamines, methylphenidate, or other sympathomimetics produces a clinical picture similar to that of cocaine intoxication or amphetamine psychosis. Agitation, paranoia, delusions, and hallucinosis may follow the chronic use of these drugs (Ellinwood, 1969; Swift, 1990). Chronic users engage in a pattern similar to that of chronic cocaine abusers, escalating doses for several days, then abstaining. Paranoid psychosis similar on diagnosis to schizophrenia may result. Underlying psychiatric illnesses such as affective disorder may also be present, as in cocaine dependence.

Over-the-counter sympathomimetic amines may be abused. Use of these medications, sold as appetite suppressants, decongestants, or bronchodilators, may become evident with signs of intoxication similar to those present with amphetamine intoxication. However, a greater tendency for autonomic effects is present with use of these over-the-counter sympathomimetic amines and may result in a hypertensive crisis.

Dopaminergic blockers such as haloperidol are generally preferred for treating amphetamine-induced paranoid and psychotic states that do not subside spontaneously within a few days. Lithium may be useful to blunt or block the euphoric effects of amphetamines. However, this agent tends to be useful in patients with affective symptoms or alcoholism. The use of TCAs has been recommended to reduce postamphetamine depression and drug craving. However, there are no definitive reports of success with the use of TCAs, not even in cases in which depression was a significant motivating factor for the use of the amphetamines (Jaffe, 1987).

Drugs used to treat caffeine dependence. The use of caffeine and related compounds such as theophylline is ubiquitous in the United States. Caffeine is present in chocolate and a variety of prescription and over-the-counter agents that are used as stimulants, appetite suppressants, analgesics, and cold and sinus preparations (Dews, 1982). The physiologic effects of these agents include cardiac stimulation, diuresis, bronchodilation, and CNS stimulation. These compounds may augment the actions of neurotransmitters such as norepinephrine and may have a direct stimulatory effect on nerve endings. Central nervous system effects of caffeine include psychomotor stimulation, increased attention and concentration, and suppression of the need for sleep. Caffeine may exacerbate the symptoms of anxiety disorders and increase requirements for neuroleptic or sedative medications (Charney, Henninger, and Jatlow, 1985). In moderate to heavy users a withdrawal syndrome characterized by lethargy, hypersomnia, irritability, and severe headache may ensue. Treatment of caffeine dependence consists of limiting consumption and substituting decaffeinated forms of beverages such as coffee or cola. No other definitive treatments are available.

Drugs Used to Treat Tobacco Dependence

Heavy or persistent smokers who abruptly stop smoking typically experience tobacco withdrawal syndrome, consisting of craving, irritability, impatience, hostility, restlessness, anxiety, depression, difficulty in concentrating, confusion, disturbed sleep patterns, increased appetite, decreased heart rate, and increased slow waves on the electroencephalogram (EEG). As with individuals dependent on alcohol and opioids, pharmacologic treatments for tobacco dependence are divided into the following groups: (1) agents that produce some of the effects produced by nicotine, (2) agents that deliver nicotine but with reduced toxicity, and (3) agents intended to block the reinforcing effects of smoking or to make smoking aversive.

Nicotine is an alkaloid drug present in the leaves of the tobacco plant. Nicotine addiction and tobacco use are legally sanctioned forms of substance abuse. Tobacco is clearly the most lethal substance in our society. The percentage of Americans who smoke has declined (Swift, 1990); however, the number of young women who smoke tobacco products has increased, since tobacco companies continue their unscrupulous practice of marketing tobacco as a chic product.

Nicotine has several effects on the peripheral, autonomic, and central nervous systems. It agonizes the nicotinic cholinergic receptor sites and stimulates autonomic ganglia in the parasympathetic and sympathetic nervous systems, producing salivation, increased gastric motility and acid secretion, and increased catecholamine release. Thus tobacco is a mild psychostimulant, producing increased alertness, increased attention and concentration, and appetite suppression. Tobacco can be used to prevent weight gain, which makes the use of this drug attractive, particularly to some individuals concerned about weight control. Repeated use of nicotine produces tolerance and dependence. The degree of dependence is considerable: 70% of those who quit using tobacco relapse within 1 year.

The treatment of nicotine-dependent patients follows the general principles common to treatment of dependence on all psychoactive substances. Short-term goals consist of reducing or stopping the tobacco use, followed by treatment designed to support and encourage abstinence. Few patients can reduce tobacco use on their own; most require a smoking cessation program (Greene, Goldberg, and Ockene, 1988). The most successful treatment combines pharmacologic and behavioral therapies.

Generally attempts to produce stimulation, appetite suppression, or other amphetamine-like effects in smokers do not reduce the use of tobacco. The use of sedatives, tranquilizers, or propranolol have not been of substantial aid in smoking cessation. Lobeline, an alkaloid that is structurally similar to nicotine, has been proposed as a treatment for tobacco dependence and withdrawal. Although this compound has some cross-tolerance with nicotine and is marketed as an over-the-counter preparation, it is not significantly superior to placebo in helping smokers stop smoking (Jaffe, 1987).

There is evidence that nicotine in the form of chewing gum can suppress important components of tobacco withdrawal and be practically useful in achieving long-term success. Symptoms that are relieved include irritability and impatience, with some reduction in restlessness, anxiety, hunger, insomnia, and changes in heart rate. The gum is a sweet-flavored resin containing 2 mg of nicotine, which is released slowly when the gum is chewed. Proper use of the gum can somewhat reduce the craving for tobacco and decrease the discomfort during the withdrawal period (Jarvik and Schneider, 1984; Schneider, Jarvik, and Forsythe, 1984). It is not clear whether the failure to relieve all symptoms of tobacco withdrawal is related to the dose or to the route of administration. However, nicotine gum does *not* substantially alleviate craving and generally must be combined with careful instruction on its use and a smoking cessation program.

In addition to nicotine gum, other means of delivery of nicotine itself have been developed, such as nicotine nasal sprays or skin patches (Jaffe, 1987). Currently three types of nicotine patches are available for use, as depicted in Table 10-1. Use of these patches significantly increases abstinence rates when combined with a behavioral or a smoking cessation program. Their use significantly reduces craving for cigarettes or other tobacco products. They maintain a steady blood level of nicotine by means of a simple, convenient, once-daily therapy. Nicotine patches are generally prescribed beginning with the highest dosing system, except for individuals weighing less than 100 pounds. Regardless of the product choice, Prostep, Habitrol, or Nicoderm, each is prescribed for a period of 4 to 6 weeks, with subsequent weaning to the next lower dose for a period of 2 to 4 weeks. Generally the weaning process takes from a minimum of 6 weeks to a maximum of 12 weeks. Again, these treatments are best combined with a behavioral or a smoking cessation program, since psychologic factors such as stress and negative emotions can trigger the urge for tobacco, as do social and behavioral factors of dependence (Bonowitz, 1988; Stitzer and Gross, 1988). The box on p. 233 presents guidelines for nicotine patch use.

The use of nicotine patches requires absolute motivation and abstinence during the treatment phase. Adjustments in the dosages of concomitant medications may be necessary, for example, decreases in benzodiazepines, TCAs, beta blockers, theophylline, insulin, or beta-adrenergic antagonists. By contrast, an increase in dose of adrenergic agonists such as phenylephrine may be necessary at the cessation of smoking.

Nontherapeutic effects such as allergic reactions and topical effects may occur as a

Table 10-1 Nicotine Transdermal Systems

Agents (trade name)	Dosages (delivery rate in vivo)	Comments (apply to all three systems)
Nicoderm	21 mg/day	
	14 mg/day	
	7 mg/day	
Habitrol	21 mg/day	Rotate skin sites; consider nontherapeutic effects, i.e., nicotine excess versus withdrawal symptoms; topical reactions are most common side effect; other side effects, in descending order of frequency, are diarrhea, dyspepsia, muscle ache, abnormal dreams, and insomnia.
Prostep	14 mg/day	
	7 mg/day	
	22 mg/day	
	11 mg/day	

Guidelines for Use of the Nicotine Patch (Nicotine Transdermal Systems)

The goal of the program is complete abstinence.
Patients must read instructions and have questions answered for appropriate use.
Quality, frequency, and intensity of support and a formal smoking cessation program are recommended.
Patients who fail to quit using nicotine should be given a "therapy holiday" before another attempt.
Symptoms of withdrawal and excess overlap and should be considered assiduously.*
Nicotine transdermal systems should not be used for longer than 3 months.
Patches should be applied to a nonhairy, clean, dry site.
Skin sites should be alternated and should not be reused for 1 week.

*Excess nicotine causes abnormal dreams, insomnia, and gastrointestinal symptoms. Withdrawal form nicotine causes anxiety, somnolence, and depression, including somatic symptoms.

result of the patch itself. The regimen for patients with cardiovascular and peripheral vascular diseases should be started carefully, and the benefits of nicotine replacement should be considered in the context of the cardiovascular disease. Patients with ischemic heart disease, severe cardiac arrhythmia, and vasospastic diseases should be carefully screened and evaluated before nicotine replacement is prescribed. Nicotine patches should be used with caution in patients with hyperthyroidism, pheochromocytoma, or insulin-dependent diabetes, since nicotine causes the release of catecholamines by the adrenal medulla. Nicotine may delay the healing of peptic ulcers and accelerate hypertension. Data regarding the teratogenic effects of nicotine in humans are inconclusive. Nicotine has been shown to produce skeletal abnormalities in the offspring of mice and therefore is not recommended for use during pregnancy. Because dependence on nicotine chewing gum has been reported, the use of a patch system beyond 3 months should be discouraged. To minimize the risk of dependence, the patient should also be encouraged to gradually withdraw from the treatment after 4 to 6 weeks of usage, progressively decreasing the dosage every 2 to 4 weeks, as previously noted. Recently the alpha-2 receptor agonist clonidine has been reported as partially efficacious in reducing nicotine withdrawal symptoms (Glassman et al., 1988). Nonetheless, the most successful treatment of nicotine dependence combines pharmacologic and behavioral approaches.

Many former smokers have adopted the use of oral tobacco in the form of snuff or chewing tobacco. This practice may reduce the hazards associated with smoke inhalation but does not qualify as a pharmacologic treatment of tobacco dependence.

Drugs Used to Treat Cannabis (Marijuana) Dependence

Some individuals use cannabis on a daily or an almost-daily basis. In many of these persons the capacity to function normally is seriously impaired. A withdrawal syndrome that is not life threatening but resembles mild sedative withdrawal has been reported. The relationship of this syndrome to marijuana-seeking behavior remains unclear (Jaffe, 1987). There are no specific therapeutic agents for cannabis withdrawal or dependence.

Drugs Used to Treat Abuse of Phencyclidine and Similar Agents

Phencylidine (PCP) is used as an anesthetic in veterinary medicine and pediatrics. The mechanism of action is not well understood, although recently this drug has been shown to bind the so-called sigma opioid receptor in the brain.

Phencyclidine intoxication has several definitive features based on empirical data. Phencyclidine and other similar agents produce amnestic, euphoric hallucinatory states, and their effects may be unpredictable, resulting in a prolonged agitated psychosis with impulsive violence directed at self and others (Peterson and Stillman, 1979; Walker, Yesavage, and Tinklenberg, 1981). The general approach to detoxification also includes isolation in a quiet environment, supportive measures to prevent patients from harming themselves, maintenance of cardiorespiratory functions, and drug treatment that ameliorates psychotic symptoms. The removal of PCP, which is sequestered in acidic gastric fluids, can be aided by judicious use of gastric drainage. Acidification of urine accelerates excretion but is no longer routinely used. Dopamine blockers such as haloperidol appear to be of value in the treatment of PCP-induced acute psychotic states. Opioids such as meperidine and morphine may be valuable in certain cases but are not conventionally prescribed. In addition to haloperidol, benzodiazepines have been described as useful in decreasing agitation and psychosis. Psychiatric hospitalization may be necessary in those individuals with prolonged psychosis.

Drugs Used to Treat Sedative-Hypnotic and Anxiolytic Abuse and Dependence

Sedatives, unlike heroin, cocaine, amphetamines, marijuana, and other abusable substances, are produced almost entirely by pharmaceutical companies. Thus the diversion of these substances originates primarily from pharmaceutical and medical sources. Many adverse effects of sedative abuse may result, including acute drug effects and bodily damage resulting from accidents or overdoses. Discussion of the chronic effects of sedative-hypnotics is beyond the scope of this chapter. The treatment of sedative abuse or dependence usually occurs in two stages, detoxification and long-term treatment. The primary goal of treatment is abstinence.

The type of detoxification recommended is determined by evaluation of the patient's medical condition and social and personal circumstances. Patients may be treated in an outpatient setting, if no physical dependence exists. However, hospitalization is usually necessary for successful detoxification. Abrupt withdrawal from sedatives can lead to seizures or to toxic psychosis; deaths have been reported as a consequence (O'Brien and Woody, 1986). Several detoxification techniques are used; each involves substituting a prescribed sedative for that which has been abused. Once the patient's condition has been stabilized on a substitute drug regimen, the drug is reduced by approximately 10% per day, a generally acceptable rate of detoxification. The pentobarbital challenge test, as presented in Table 10-2, involves the oral administration of 200 mg of pentobarbital followed by close observation to assess the degree of tolerance. Based on the patient's condition after the test dose, an estimated 24-hour pentobarbital requirement is determined; similarly a phenobarbital substitution technique may be carried out with the oral substitution of 30 mg phenobarbital for each 100 mg of the estimated pentobarbital requirement. Medication is administered

Table 10-2 Pentobarbital Challenge Test: Initial Response to 200 mg of Pentobarbital

Patient's condition	Degree of tolerance	24-hour pentobarbital requirement* (mg)
Asleep and sedate	None	None
Drowsy; marked intoxication	Mild	400-600
Comfortable; minimal intoxication	Marked	600-1000
No effect	Extreme	1000

*Phenobarbital may be preferred and substituted at a dose of phenobarbital 30 mg for pentobarbital 100 mg.

every 6 hours for approximately 24 hours. If a stabilization dose is reached, the substituted agent may then be reduced as previously described. Phenobarbital is generally preferred because it is longer acting and has better anticonvulsant activity than does pentobarbital.

The condition of patients who are addicted to both sedatives and narcotics must be stabilized on a regimen of both types of drugs before detoxification can occur. It is important to remember that patients are restless and anxious and often have insomnia during and after detoxification. Given the significant heterogeneity of sedative abusers, it is essential to attempt to categorize the social and psychologic correlates of drug use in each patient so that a long-term treatment plan can be formulated (Wesson and Smith, 1975; Wikler, 1968).

Long-term treatment of sedative abuse is customized and may include residential drug-free programs or self-help groups such as AA and NA, or a combination of these. Some patients may be found to have an underlying psychiatric disorder. If pharmacologic treatment is deemed necessary, the use of antidepressant medication or a nondependence-producing anxiolytic such as buspirone should be considered.

REFERENCES

American Psychiatric Association: *Diagnostic and Statistical Manual of Mental Disorders, Third Edition-Revised,* Washington, DC, 1987, The Association.

Barbor TF et al: From basic concepts to clinical reality: unresolved issues in the diagnosis of dependence, *Recent Dev Alcohol* 8:85, 1990.

Baxter LR et al: Localization of neurochemical effects of cocaine and other stimulants in the human brain *J Clin Psychiatry* 49(suppl):23, 1988.

Blume SB: Psychotherapy in the treatment of alcoholism: psychiatry update. In Grinspoon L, editor: *The American Psychiatric Association annual review,* vol 3, Washington, DC, 1984, American Psychiatric.

Bonowitz NI: Pharmacologic aspects of cigarette smoking and nicotine addiction, *New Engl J Med* 319:1318, 1988.

Braucht G et al: Deviant drug use in adolescence: a review of psychosocial correlates, *Psychol Bull* 79:92, 1973.

Brook JS et al: The role of older brothers in younger brothers' drug use viewed in context of parent and peer influences, *J Genet Psychol* 151:59, 1990.

Butcher JN: *Personality factors in drug addiction,* NIDA Research Monograph Series, No 89, Rockville, Md, 1988, National Institute on Drug Abuse.

Cadoret RJ et al: An adoption study of genetic and environmental factors in drug abuse, *Arch Gen Psychiatry* 43:1131, 1986.

Charney DS, Henninger GR, Jatlow PI: Increased anxiogenic effects of caffeine in panic disorders, *Arch Gen Psychiatry* 42:233, 1985.

Charney DS et al: The clinical use of clonidine in abrupt withdrawal from methadone, *Arch Gen Psychiatry* 38:1273, 1981.

Charney DS et al: Clonidine and naltrxone: a safe, effective, and rapid treatment of abrupt withdrawal from methadone therapy, *Arch Gen Psychiatry* 39:1327, 1982.

Ciraulo DA et al: Parental alcoholism as a risk factor in benzodiazepine abuse: a pilot study, *Am J Psychiatry* 146:1333, 1989.

Clark WD: Alcoholism: blocks to diagnosis and treatment, *Am J Med* 71:275, 1981.

Clayton R: Extent and consequences of drug abuse. In *Drug abuse and drug abuse research*, Rockville, Md, 1984, National Institute on Drug Abuse.

Cloninger CR: Neurogenetic adaptive mechanisms in alcoholism, *Science* 236:410, 1987.

Cohen S: *Cocaine today*, New York, 1981, American Council on Drug Education.

Culhane C: Marijuana's brain receptor found, *US Journal*, Dec. 11, 1990, p 11.

Dews PB: Caffeine, *Annu Rev Nutr* 2:323, 1982.

Dixon SD: Effects of transplacental exposure to cocaine and methamphetamine on the neonate, *Western J Med* 150:436, 1989.

Ellinwood EH: Amphetamine psychosis: a multidimensional process, *Semin Psychol* 1:208, 1969.

Fishburne PM, Abelson HI, Cisin I: *National survey on drug abuse. Main finding: 1979*, Department of Health and Human Services Pub No ADM-80-976, Washington DC, 1980, US Government Printing Office.

Fultz JM Jr, Senay EC: Guidelines for the management of hospitalized narcotic addicts, *Ann Intern Med* 82:815, 1975.

Gawin FH: Chronic neuropharmacology of cocaine: progress in pharmacotherapy, *J Clin Psychiatry* 49(suppl):11, 1988.

Gawin FH, Ellinwood EH: Cocaine and other stimulants: actions, abuse, and treatment, *New Engl J Med* 318:1173, 1988.

Gawin FH, Kleber HD: Cocaine abuse in a treatment population: patterns and diagnostic distinctions. In Kozell NJ, Adams EH, editors: *Cocaine use in America: epidemiologic and clinical perspectives*, NIDA Research Monograph Series, No 61, Rockville, Md, 1985, National Institute on Drug Abuse.

Gawin FH et al: Desipramine facilitation of initial cocaine abstinence, *Arch Gen Psychiatry* 46:117, 1989a.

Gawin FH et al: Double-blind evaluation of the effect of acute amantadine on cocaine craving, *Psychopharmacology* 97:402, 1989b.

Gay GR: Clinical management of acute and chronic cocaine poisoning, *Ann Emerg Med* 11:562, 1982.

Giacoia GP: Cocaine in the cradle: a hidden epidemic, *Southern Med J* 83:947, 1990.

Giannini AJ, Baumgartel PD: Bromocriptine therapy in cocaine withdrawal, *J Clin Pharmacology* 27:267, 1987.

Giannini AJ et al: Bromocriptine and amantadine in cocaine detoxification, *Psychiatr Res* 29:11, 1989.

Glassman AH et al: Heavy smokers, smoking cessation and clonodine: results of a double-blind, randomized trial, *JAMA* 259:2863, 1988.

Gold MS, Redmond DE Jr, Kleber HD: Noradrenergic hyperactivity in opiate withdrawal suppressed by clonidine, *Am J Psychiatry* 136:100, 1979.

Gold MS et al: Opiate withdrawal using clonidine: a safe, effective and rapid non-opiate treatment, *JAMA* 234:343, 1979.

Goodwin DW: Alcohol in homicide and suicide, *Q J Stud Alcohol* 28:517, 1967.

Goodwin DW: Alcoholics and genetics: the sins of the fathers, *Arch Gen Psychiatry* 42:517, 1985.

Greene HL, Goldberg R, Ockene JK: Cigarette smoking: the physician's role in cessation and maintenance, *J Gen Intern Med* 3:75, 1988.

Grove WM et al: Heritability of substance abuse and antisocial behavior: a study of monozygotic twins reared apart, *Biol Psychiatry* 27:1293, 1990.

Halikas J et al: Carbamazepine for cocaine addiction? (letter), *Lancet* 1:623, 1989.

Hansen HJ, Caudhill SP, Boone DJ: Crisis in drug testing: results of the CDC blind study, *JAMA* 253:2382, 1985.

Holden C: The neglected disease in medical education, *Science* 229:741, 1985.

Jaffe JH. Opiods. In Frances AJ, Hales RE, editors: *American Psychiatric Association Annual Review*, vol 5, Washington, DC, 1986, American Psychiatric.

Jaffe JH: Pharmacological agents in treatment of drug dependence. In Meltzer HY, editor: *The third generation of progress*, New York, 1987, Raven.

Jaffe JH, Ciraulo D Drugs used in the treatment of alcoholism. In Mendelson JH, Mello NK: *The diagnosis and treatment of alcoholism*, New York, 1985, McGraw-Hill.

Jaffe JH, Martin WR: Opioid analgesics and antagonists. In Gilman AG et al: *The pharmacological basis of therapeutics* ed 7, New York, 1985, Macmillan.

Jarvik ME, Schneider NG: Degree of addiction and the effectiveness of nicotine gum therapy for smoking, *Am J Psychiatry* 141:790, 1984.

Johnston LD, Bachman JG, O'Malley PM: *Drug use, drinking, and smoking: national survey results from high school, college, and young adult populations, 1975-1990*, Rockville, Md, 1991, National Institute of Mental Health.

Johnston LD, Bachman JG, O'Malley PM: *1983 highlights: drugs and the nation's high school students*, Washington DC, 1984, US Government Printing Office.

Kandel D, Simcha-Fagan O, Davis M: Risk factors for delinquency and illicit drug use from adolescence to young adulthood, *J Drug Issues* 16:67, 1986.

Kaufman E: Family structures of narcotic addicts, *Int J Addictions* 16:273, 1981.

Kaufman E, McNaul JP: Recent developments in understanding and treating drug abuse and dependence, *Hosp Community Psychiatry* 43:223, 1992.

Khantzian EJ: A critique of therapy and some implications for treatment, *Am J Psychother* 28:59, 1974.

Khantzian EJ: Extreme case of cocaine dependence and marked improvement with Ritalin, *Am J Psychiatry* 140:784, 1983.

Khantzian EJ: The self-medication hypothesis of addictive disorders: focus on heroin and cocaine dependence, *Am J Psychiatry* 142:1259, 1985.

Kleber HD, Gawin FH: Cocaine. In Frances AJ, Hales RE, editors: *American Psychiatric Association annual review*, vol 5, Washington, DC, 1986, American Psychiatric.

Kolata G: New Valiums and anti-Valiums on the horizon, *Science* 216:604, 1982.

Kosten TR: Pharmacotherapeutic interventions for cocaine abuse: matching patient to treatments, *J Nerv Ment Dis* 177:379, 1989.

Kosten T, Gawin F, Shumann B: *Treating cocaine-abusing methadone patients with desipramine*, NIDA Research Monograph Series, No 81, Rockville, Md, 1988, National Institute on Drug Abuse.

Kosten TR, Kleber HD: Differential diagnosis of psychiatric comorbidity in substance abusers, *J Subst Abuse Treat* 5:201, 1988.

Krasnagor NA, editor: *The behavioral aspects of smoking*, NIDA Research Monograph Series, No 26, Rockville, Md, 1979, National Institute on Drug Abuse.

Lewis D, Gordon A: Alcoholism and the general hospital: the Roger Williams intervention program, *Bull N Y Acad Med* 59:181, 1983.

Little BB et al: Cocaine use in 46 pregnant women in a large public hospital, *Am J Perinatol* 5:206, 1988.

Maloff D et al: Informal social controls and their influence on substance use. In Zinberg N, Hardin WM, editors: *Control over intoxicant use*, New York, 1982, Human Sciences.

McLellan AT, Childress AR: Aversive therapies for substance abuse: do they work? *J Subst Abuse Treat* 2:187, 1985.

McLellan AT, Woody GE, O'Brien CP: Development of psychiatric illness in drug abusers, *New Engl J Med* 201:1310, 1979.

Meyer RE: *Psychopathology and addictive disorders: how to understand the relationship between psychopathology and addictive disorders*, New York, 1986, Guilford.

Miller JD et al: *National survey of drug abuse. Main findings: 1982*, Department of Health and Human Services Pub No ADM-83-1263, Washington DC, 1983, US Government Printing Office.

Millman R: Drug abuse and dependence. In Wyngaarde JB, Smith LH, editors: *Textbook of medicine*, ed 17, Philadelphia, 1985, WB Saunders.

Millman RB: General principles of diagnosis and treatment. In Frances AJ, Hales RE, editors: *American Psychiatric Association annual review*, vol 5, Washington, DC, 1986, American Psychiatric.

Millman RB, Khuri ET: Adolescence and substance abuse. In Lowinson JH, Ruiz P, editors: *Substance abuse: clinical problems and perspectives,* Baltimore, 1981, Williams & Wilkins.

National Household Survey on Drug Abuse, Rockville, Md, 1991, National Institute of Mental Health.

Neerhof MG et al: Cocaine abuse during pregnancy: peripartum prevalence and perinatal outcome, *Am J Obstet Gynecol* 161:633, 1989.

O'Brien CP, Woody GE: Sedative-hypnotics and antianxiety agents. In Frances AJ, Hales RE, editors: *American Psychiatric Association annual review,* vol 5, Washington, DC, 1986, American Psychiatric.

Peterson RC, Stillman RC, editors: *PCP (phencyclidine) abuse: an appraisal,* NIDA Research Monograph Series, No 21, Department of Health, Education, and Welfare, Washington DC, 1979, US Government Printing Office.

Pickens RW, Svikis DS: *The twin method in study of vulnerability to drug abuse,* NIDA Research Monograph Series No 89, Rockville, Md, 1989, National Institute on Drug Abuse.

Regier DA et al: One-month prevalence of mental disorders in the United States, *Arch Gen Psychiatry* 45:977, 1988.

Resnick RB, Schuyten-Resnick E, Washton AM: Assessment of narcotic antagonists in the treatment of opioid dependence, *Annu Rev Pharmacol Toxicol* 20:463, 1980.

Rounsaville BJ, Gawin FH, Kleber HD: Interpersonal psychotherapy adapted for ambulatory cocaine users, *Am J Drug Alcohol Abuse* 11:171, 1985.

Rowbotham MC et al: Trazodone–oral cocaine interactions, *Arch Gen Psychiatry* 41:895, 1984.

Sachs DPL: Advances in smoking cessation treatment, *Curr Pulmonol* (in press).

Sadava SW: Initiation to cannabis use: a longitudinal social psychological study of college freshmen, *Can J Behav Sci* 5:371, 1973.

Schneider NG, Jarvik ME, Forsythe AB: Nicotine vs placebo gum in the alleviation of withdrawal during smoking cessation, *Addict Behav* 9:149, 1984.

Schuckit MA: Genetic and clinical implications of alcoholism and affective disorder, *Am J Psychiatry* 143:140, 1986.

Schuckit MA: Genetics and the risk for alcoholism, *JAMA* 254:2614, 1985.

Schuster CR: The National Institute on Drug Abuse in the decade of the brain, *Neuropsychopharmacol* 3:315, 1990.

Sellers EM, Kalant H. In Kaufman E, Pattison EM, editors: *Encyclopedic handbook of alcoholism,* New York, 1982, Gardner.

Sellers EM, Naranjo CA, Peachey JE: Drug therapy: drugs to decrease alcohol consumption, *New Engl J Med* 305:1255, 1981.

Senay EC et al: Withdrawal from methadone maintenance: rate of withdrawal and expectation, *Arch Gen Psychiatry* 34:361, 1977.

Skinner HA et al: Identification of alcohol abuse using laboratory tests and a history of trauma, *Ann Intern Med* 101:847, 1984.

Smith DE: *Treatment and aftercare for cocaine dependency.* Presented at the Institute of Alcoholism and Drug Abuse Studies Conference on Cocaine: Problems and Solutions, Baltimore, January 1984.

Stitzer ML, Gross J: Smoking relapse: the role of pharmacological and behavioral factors, *Prog Clin Biol Res* 261:163, 1988.

Swift RM: Alcoholism and substance abuse. In Stoudemire A, editor: *Clinical psychiatry for medical students,* Philadelphia, 1990, JB Lippincott.

Tennant FS, Segherian AA: Double-blind comparison of amantadine and bromocriptine for ambulatory withdrawal from cocaine dependence, *Arch Intern Med* 147:109, 1987.

Terenius L: Clinical aspects. In Malick JB, Bell RMS, editors: *Endorphins: chemistry, physiology, pharmacology, and clinical relevance,* New York, 1982, Marcel Decker.

Van Dyke C et al: Oral cocaine: plasma concentration and central effects, *Science* 200:211, 1978.

Volkow ND et al: Effects of chronic cocaine abuse on postsynaptic dopamine receptors, *Am J Psychiatry* 147:719, 1990.

Walker S, Yesavage JA, Tinklenberg JR: Acute phencyclidine (PCP) intoxication: quantitative urine levels and clinical management, *Am J Psychiatry* 138:674, 1981.

Wallace BC: Crack cocaine smokers as adult children of alcoholics: the dysfunctional family link, *J Subst Abuse Treat* 7:89, 1990.

Weider H, Kaplan E: Drug use in adolescents, *Psychoanal Study Child* 24:339, 1969.

Wesson DR, Smith DE: A new method for the treatment of barbiturate dependence, *JAMA* 231:294, 1975.

Whitfield C. In Frann WE et al, editors: *Phenomenology and treatment of alcoholism*, New York, 1980, Spectrum.

Wikler A: Diagnosis and treatment of drug dependence of the barbiturate type, *Am J Psychiatry* 125:758, 1968.

Williams AF: Personality and other characteristics associated with cigarette smoking among young teenagers, *J Health Soc Behav* 14:374, 1973.

Wurmser L: Psychoanalytic considerations of the etiology of compulsive drug use, *J Am Psychoanal Assoc* 22:820, 1974.

Zinberg NE: Addiction and ego function. In Fissler BS et al, editors: *The psychoanalytic study of the child*, New Haven, 1975, Yale University.

UNIT III

Drug Issues Related to Psychopharmacology

CHAPTER 11

Drugs Used for Electroconvulsive Therapy

"ECT's effectiveness in rescuing severely ill patients from the despairing depths of depression or perilous heights of uncontrolled mania is well accepted by psychiatrists. However, ECT, like treatments for every other illness, is not 100% effective, it is not a cure and it does have some adverse effects."
Herbert Pardes, President, American Psychiatric Association*

Treatments that make use of physiologic or physical interventions to effect a behavioral change are called somatic therapies. There are several types of somatic therapy, including psychosurgery (lobotomy), flurothyl (Indoklon) therapy, insulin coma therapy, and electroconvulsive therapy (ECT). Electroconvulsive therapy is the most frequently used somatic therapy. Drugs that are used to facilitate effective ECT are the focus of this chapter. However, before those drugs are discussed, an overview of ECT is presented.

HISTORICAL CONSIDERATIONS

Electroconvulsive therapy has now been used for more than half a century (Hay, 1991) and has proven to be a remarkably safe treatment (American Psychiatric Association, 1990). During those 50 years a number of critics emerged and affected public and professional perceptions of this treatment form. Because of its efficacy, however, and for no other reason, ECT has weathered these misperceptions and continues to be used effectively today.

Electroconvulsive therapy, also referred to as electroshock therapy (EST) or "shock therapy," emerged as a treatment form in 1938. It was introduced by Ugo Cerletti and Luciano Bini, two Italian psychiatrists. Although ECT has proven to be effective, paradoxically the theoretical premise on which it was built was faulty. Early twentieth-century psychiatrists believed schizophrenia and epilepsy were incompatible. Although we now know that this is not true, the conceptual extension of this false belief led to the development of an effective treatment form.

The early advocates of ECT envisioned a dramatic relief from the curse of mental illness. Over time, inappropriate use and disappointing results, coupled with growing distrust of psychiatric hospitals, created a climate of hostility toward ECT. When psychopharmacologic agents emerged in the 1950s, the use of ECT began to decline (Coffey and Weiner, 1990). Eventually, in the 1960s and early 1970s, the use of ECT came under harsh criticism and legislation was passed to limit its use. By 1980 the use of ECT had come to a virtual standstill (Thompson and Blaine, 1987).

During the 1980s ECT once again emerged as a viable treatment alternative when more conventional treatment approaches failed. With the application of rigid treatment criteria and careful pretreatment evaluation many psychiatric patients, particularly those with depression, have responded to ECT. Currently ECT is again recognized as an effective treatment for a variety of affective disorders.

*Quoted in the Los Angeles Times, December 22, 1989, p. A39.

Historical Perspective on the Negative View

To appreciate the safety and effectiveness of modern ECT, it is important to understand why the "old" ECT procedure caused such great distress. The "old" ECT was literally applied as an electric current that passed through the brain, causing epileptic, or grand mal, seizure. The convulsion was accompanied by various complications, including muscle soreness, fractures, dislocations, sprains, and tongue lacerations. In its heyday ECT was given to almost every patient who did not respond to other treatment forms. In large state hospitals ECT was given on Mondays, Wednesdays, and Fridays to as many as 20 or more patients on a psychiatric ward. One patient after another—some under their own power, others literally overpowered and held—would take his or her place on the bed to be given ECT. Nursing staff would hold the patient in place (to decrease fractures, dislocations, and the like), insert the mouth guard (to prevent tongue bites), put paste on the electrodes and hold the electrodes in place on each side of the head (usually the temple area), and hold the chin and jaw in proper alignment (similar to cardiopulmonary resuscitation (CPR) positioning to prevent dislocation and maintain the airway); the physician in the background would deliver the shock. A full grand mal seizure would occur. After convulsion activity stopped, the patient would be turned on his or her side and tied in place (to prevent aspiration) while a staff member or "helper patient" would stay at the bedside until consciousness returned. The ECT team would then move on to the next patient.

This unforgettable scene, the media (including novels and films), and reports from former patients contributed to the stigma and public fear of ECT. Despite this historically negative view of ECT, the addition of several important drugs and refinements in the delivery of the stimulus have revitalized the technique. Many psychiatric professionals view ECT as the treatment of choice for major depression, finding it safe and economical (Markowitz et al., 1987).

MODERN ELECTROCONVULSIVE THERAPY

During ECT an electrical current (60 to 150 volts) is passed through the brain for 0.5 to 2 seconds. The seizure resulting from ECT should be between 20 and 120 seconds in duration to be of therapeutic value. The events performed before, during, and after the treatment, including primarily nursing, medical, or shared responsibilities, follow in roughly sequential order and are outlined in the box on pp. 244 to 245.

Seizure activity is monitored by an electroencephalograph (EEG). Blood pressure and heart rate are also monitored. Oxygen is administered immediately before and after the treatment because of interruption of breathing caused by the succinylcholine and the electrically induced seizure. Typically patients are given ECT two to three times per week up to a total of six to twelve treatments (or until the patient improves or is obviously not going to improve).

Indications

Electroconvulsive therapy is most useful in the treatment of major depression; these patients respond better (Bowden, 1985) and faster (Coffey and Weiner, 1990) to ECT than to other treatments. Patients with depression that has not responded to other treatments, suicidal tendencies, acute mania, catatonia, and some types of schizophrenia in which catatonia or affective symptoms are prominent are significantly helped by ECT (American Psychiatric Association, 1978; Hay, 1991). Weiner and Coffey (1988) found an 80% response rate with ECT. Electroconvulsive therapy seems to be particularly suited to the elderly patient because there are no drug side

Electroconvulsive Therapy Administration

Preparation

Medical

The patient must have a pretreatment evaluation, including physical examination, electrocardiogram, laboratory work (blood cell count, blood chemistry studies, and urinalysis), and baseline mental status examination that includes a formal assessment of cognition. A computed tomography scan or magnetic resonance imaging of the head may also be indicated and performed.

Nursing

A consent form must be signed. Since ECT is often given as a treatment of last resort, some patients are so profoundly depressed by the time ECT is ordered that obtaining the "informed consent" of the patient is not possible. In such cases, involving family members and requesting assistance from the facility's legal staff may be necessary.

Medical

1. Eliminate the routine use of benzodiazepines or barbiturates for nighttime sedation because of their ability to raise the seizure threshold and cause shorter seizures (less than 25 to 30 seconds in duration).* Chloral hydrate may be used as an alternative drug regimen. A subconvulsive stimulus may be harmful to the patient.† Discontinue antidepressant and lithium regimens to avoid adverse effects or the potential for neurotoxicity.‡
2. Obtain the services of a trained electrotherapist and an anesthesiologist. Whether an anesthesiologist provides care significantly different from that of a psychiatrist is a subject of debate. The new American Psychiatric Association guidelines on ECT§ carefully skirt this issue. Pearlman, Loper, and Tillery† found no deaths attributable to ECT in surveying 9 years of psychiatrist-administered anesthesia (N = 8161).
3. Obtain an ECT treatment device (e.g., MECTA SA-1 (MECTA, Inc., Portland, Oregon) or Medcraft B-25).

Before treatment

Nursing

1. The patient should receive nothing by mouth from the midnight preceding treatment until after the treatment.
2. Give atropine as ordered. Atropine can be given 1 hour before treatment or given by intravenous (IV) administration immediately before treatment. Atropine reduces secretions and subsequent risk of aspiration. Metoclopramide (Reglan) may also be given in concert with atropine or as an alternative agent.
3. Ask the patient to urinate before the treatment. (Seizure-induced incontinence is common.)
4. Remove the patient's hairpins and dentures.

*Fink M: *Am J Psychiatry* 144:1195, 1987.

†Pearlman T, Loper M, Tillery L: *Am J Psychiatry* 147:1553, 1990.

‡Coffey CE, Weiner RD: *Hosp Community Psychiatry* 41:515, 1990.

§American Psychiatric Association: *APA Task Force on Electroconvulsive Therapy,* task force no. 14, Washington, DC, 1990, The Association.

‖Coffey CE et al: *Am J Psychiatry* 147:579, 1990.

Electroconvulsive Therapy Administration—cont'd

5. Take the patient's vital signs.
6. Be positive about the treatment, and attempt to reduce the patient's pre-treatment anxiety.

During treatment

Medical or nursing

1. Insert an intravenous (IV) line.
2. Attach electrodes to the proper place on the head. Electrodes are typically held in place with a rubber strap.

Nursing

Insert bite-block.

Medical

1. Give methohexital (Brevital) 1.5 mg/kg body weight or another short-acting barbiturate (occasionally, thiopental sodium 3.5 mg/kg body weight) by the intravenous route (IV) for anesthesia. The barbiturate causes immediate anesthesia, preempting the anxiety associated with waiting for the "jolt to hit" and the anxiety caused by succinylcholine (Anectine). (Succinylcholine causes paralysis but not sedation, thereby leaving the patient conscious but unable to breathe.)
2. Give succinylcholine IV. Succinylcholine prevents the external manifestations of a grand mal seizure, thus minimizing the risk of fractures, dislocations, and the like while not affecting the "brain seizure."
3. The anesthesiologist mechanically ventilates the patient with 100% oxygen immediately before the treatment.
4. Give the electrical impulse: up to 150 volts for 0.5 to 2 seconds.
5. Observe the length of the seizure. The seizure must be greater than 20 to 30 seconds in duration to be of therapeutic value. If the seizure is less than 30 seconds long, a decision must be made to stimulate another seizure or not. Coffey et al.[‖] augmented ECT with the administration of caffeine (242 mg IV push pretreatment) to maintain or increase seizure duration.

Medical or nursing

1. Monitor the patient's heart rate, heart rhythm, and blood pressure; electroencephalography is also used.
2. Ventilation and monitoring should continue until the patient recovers.

After treatment

Medical

The anesthesiologist mechanically ventilates the patient with 100% oxygen until the patient can breathe on his or her own.

Nursing

1. Monitor for respiratory problems.
2. Since ECT causes confusion and disorientation, it is important to help re-orient the patient (to time, place, and person) as he or she emerges from this groggy state.
3. Observe the patient until he or she is oriented and is steady on his or her feet.

Medical and nursing

Carefully document all aspects of the treatment for the patient record.

effects and it is safe and effective (Alexopoulos, Young, and Abrams, 1989; Fogel, 1988; Hay, 1989; Hay, 1990).

Electroconvulsive therapy is *not* useful in the treatment of mild depressions, behavior disorders, phobias, anxiety, somatoform disorders, or personality disturbances.

The majority of ECT patients (about 75%) are severely depressed. Tancer et al. (1989) found that affective disorders accounted for 85% to 89% of all ECT patients. Traditionally it was thought that depressed individuals who were candidates for ECT should have endogenous symptoms: insomnia, anorexia, immobility, muteness, early morning awakening, anhedonia, and delusional experiences. Prudic et al. (1989) indicated that these symptoms may be unrelated to outcome.

Contraindications

Electroconvulsive therapy is relatively contraindicated for patients with cerebrovascular accidents or space-occupying tumors and absolutely contraindicated for patients with increased intracranial pressure.

Advantages

"Even with the host of psychotropic agents now available, ECT still represents for some patients the safest, most rapid, and most effective form of treatment . . ." (Frances, Weiner, and Coffey, 1989).

Electroconvulsive therapy is a safe procedure. Death as a result of ECT is rare. Mortality rates for ECT (.002% to .004% per treatment) are lower than mortality rates for childbirth (.01%) or anesthesia induction (.003% to .04%) (Coffey and Weiner, 1990). Mortality is most often associated with cardiovascular complications; however, even these complications are less problematic with ECT than with tricyclic antidepressants (TCAs). Runck (1985), after developing a major report for the National Institute of Mental Health, found only 2.9 deaths per 10,000 patients receiving ECT. Electroconvulsive therapy is not only safe but also appears to be more effective than antidepressants. Black, Winokur, and Nasrallah (1987) found that 70% of depressed patients and 85% of patients diagnosed as schizoaffective showed marked improvement with ECT, whereas only 48% of those receiving treatment with TCAs had similar improvement.

Additionally, because ECT works faster than TCAs, it is more economical. Markowitz et al. (1987) found that patients receiving ECT stayed in the hospital an average of 13 fewer days than did depressed patients receiving treatment with antidepressants, at a savings of $6,405 per patient. Electroconvulsive therapy is also safer than TCAs for patients with heart problems, since it does not produce the cardiovascular side effects associated with TCAs.

Disadvantages

The major disadvantage of ECT is that treatment provides only temporary relief: it does not provide a permanent cure. Certainly many patients are able to remain depression free for long periods, and still others may never need treatment again. However, for some patients receiving ECT, another series of treatments may be needed within a few months. Some psychiatrists order maintenance or continuation ECT (once per month for 6 to 12 months); however, the benefits of this approach are not clear.

Memory impairment, both retrograde (memory before treatment) and anterograde (ability to learn new things and memory after treatment), has been frequently cited as a side effect of ECT. Memory of events closest in time to ECT is most frequently affected. Although it is true that memory is impaired for events that occur before and after each treatment and that confusion occurs immediately after each treatment, there seems to be no substantial loss of mental function once the treatment series is completed. Furthermore, since depression, too, can cause memory loss, it is not always clear whether memory impairment is related to ECT or to depression.

Unilateral electrode placement has been shown to reduce anterograde memory loss and disorientation after treatment. Frances, Weiner, and Coffey (1989) reported that memory actually improved after unilateral nondominant-hemisphere stimulation ECT was begun. When the unilateral approach is used, both electrodes are placed on the nondominant hemisphere (usually the right hemisphere) instead of one being placed on each side of the head. This approach is now a recommended method of delivering ECT.

HOW ELECTROCONVULSIVE THERAPY WORKS

It is not clear how ECT works or why it is so effective. The following hypotheses, some more reasonable than others, have been advanced to explain its efficacy:

Patients recover because they view ECT as punishment or atonement for their guilt.

Patients recover because they no longer remember why they are depressed.

Electroconvulsive therapy causes some of the same biochemical changes that antidepressant drugs cause (i.e., the 5-HT_2 serotonin receptor is affected by both ECT and TCAs [Brown and Mann, 1985]).

Although the preceding explanations may or may not be convincing, the fact remains that ECT is an effective treatment modality for major depression, depression resistant to psychophamacology and psychotherapy, mania, catatonia, and some variants of schizophrenia.

DRUGS USED IN ELECTROCONVULSIVE THERAPY

Basically three drugs are used to enhance ECT: atropine, methohexital (Brevital), and succinylcholine (Anectine). Before treatment atropine is given to reduce secretions and to minimize aspiration. Atropine can be given 1 hour before treatment by mouth or may be given intravenously immediately before the treatment. Once the patient is ready for the treatment, methohexital is given intravenously. Methohexital induces anesthesia. Anesthesia reduces pretreatment anxiety. One can easily imagine the fear associated with waiting for the "jolt" to hit that patients in the premodern ECT era experienced. A second and perhaps more important rationale for the use of methohexital is that it induces anesthesia before succinylcholine is given. Succinylcholine is a muscle relaxant that prevents the external manifestations of seizure activity long associated with ECT. Although brain seizures continue to occur and can be measured by EEG, tonic and clonic seizures do not occur, sparing the patient from the physical consequences associated with convulsions.

SUCCINYLCHOLINE

Succinylcholine is an ultrashort-acting, noncompetitive neuromuscular blocker used for several short-duration procedures, including ECT. Succinylcholine is a depolarizing blocker, as opposed to most neuromuscular blockers, which are nondepolarizing. Nondepolarizing agents block the nicotinic receptors on the muscle cell, thus preventing muscle activation by acetylcholine (ACh). Depolarizing agents such as succinylcholine are ACh agonists that mimic ACh but are longer acting. Initially the muscle is highly stimulated, but since succinylcholine is longer acting, the depolarized muscle becomes insensitive to further stimulation by the ACh. The initial stimulation caused by succinylcholine lasts about 30 seconds and produces strong muscle contractions. It has been reported to cause bone fractures in a few weakened individuals.

Pharmacokinetics and Interactions

Succinylcholine is given intravenously and is metabolized rapidly by plasma and liver pseudocholinesterases; however, because succinylcholine is noncompetitive, the paralysis it induces cannot be reversed by pharmacologic treatment. Succinylcholine has the shortest duration of all neuromuscular blockers, about 5 minutes. For ECT an intravenous dose of 0.6 mg/kg succinylcholine is given. Propranolol, quinidine, and other drugs, including phenelzine, promazine, oxytocin, procainamide, lithium carbonate, and furosemide, can prolong paralysis, leading to hypotension; digoxin increases the risk of cardiac arrhythmias; and lidocaine enhances respiratory depression when combined with succinylcholine. An important interaction is the one succinylcholine has with neostigmine, a drug that inhibits the destruction of ACh and is used as an antidote for nondepolarizing neuromuscular blockers. When combined with succinylcholine, neostigmine inhibits succinylcholine metabolism and intensifies the initial depolarization of muscles. Neostigmine should not be used with succinylcholine.

METHOHEXITAL

Methohexital is an ultrashort-acting barbiturate used to induce anesthesia and is the preferred agent for inducing a light coma preceding delivery of ECT. Less often, thiopental sodium (Pentothal) is used for this purpose. Although the primary efforts in modern ECT have been directed at eliminating the overt manifestations of seizure activity, induction of anesthesia is the first step in that process. Succinylcholine provides the sought after muscle relaxation needed to reduce observable convulsions, but it does not induce anesthesia. Consequently, if succinylcholine alone were to be given to the patient, the patient would experience muscle paralysis, including respiratory paralysis, while conscious. The emotional reaction to suffocation would be panic; therefore, anesthesia induction with methohexital is required.

Pharmacokinetics

Methohexital is given intravenously just before the intravenous administration of succinylcholine. Methohexital rapidly crosses the blood-brain barrier and quickly depresses the central nervous system (CNS), causing unconsciousness within 10 to 15 seconds. The duration of effect is relatively short (5 to 7 minutes) as a result of a natural redistribution to adipose tissue and other less vascular sites. Methohexital is metabolized by the liver, excreted in the urine, and has a half-life of 3 to 8 hours.

The dose of methohexital for ECT is typically 50 to 120 mg IV (or 1.5 mg/kg body weight) for adults. Pettinati et al. (1990) recommended a dose of 0.9 mg/kg for their ECT patients.

Side Effects

The major side effects of methohexital are respiratory depression, hypotension, myocardial depression, and decreased cardiac output. Consequently methohexital is used cautiously in persons with asthma, hypotension, and severe cardiovascular disease. Other potentially life-threatening reactions include anaphylactic reactions, cardiac arrhythmias, peripheral vascular disease, apnea, laryngospasm, and bronchospasm. Bothersome and occasionally serious side effects include prolonged unconsciousness, headache, restlessness and anxiety, nausea and vomiting, dyspnea, hiccups, and a variety of skin rashes.

Interactions

Methohexital has several potentially serious drug interactions. Most notably, other CNS depressants increase CNS and respiratory depression. Furosemide (Lasix), a commonly prescribed drug in older patients, interacts with methohexital to cause substantial orthostatic hypotension. In addition, a number of drugs have decreased effectiveness when given concurrently with methohexital.

ATROPINE

Atropine is the prototype anticholingeric agent. Anticholingeric drugs inhibit the effects of ACh on the parasympathetic system. Atropine is derived from a common plant, Atropa belladonna. Atropine and all anticholinergics have a wide effect in the body; however, atropine is given before ECT for several specific responses, including the inhibition of salivation and respiratory tract secretions (decreasing potential for aspiration respiratory problems) and vagal stimulation (decreasing the potential for cardiovascular depression resulting from succinylcholine and methohexital).

Pharmacokinetics

Atropine is well absorbed when given orally (onset 30 minutes) or IM/SC (onset 15 minutes) 1 hour before ECT and can be given IV (onset 1 minute) just before delivery of ECT. Atropine readily crosses the blood-brain barrier, is metabolized in the liver, and is excreted primarily in the urine. It has a duration of action of 4 hours and a half-life of 2 to 3 hours. A typical dose ranges from 0.4 to 0.6 mg.

Side Effects

The most common side effects associated with atropine are dry mouth, blurred vision, constipation, urinary hesitancy, and, possibly, urinary retention. More serious reactions include paralytic ileus, mydriasis, and anaphylactic reactions. Occasional adverse responses include nervousness, flushing, confusion, fever, restlessness, tremor, bradycardia, palpitations, nausea and vomiting, photophobia, and skin rashes.

Atropine is used cautiously when a patient is known to have a history of glaucoma, prostatic hypertrophy, cardiac arrhythmias, current fever, or obstructive uropathy. Interventions for anticholinergic side effects are found in Chapters 4 and 5.

Interactions

When atropine is given concurrently with other anticholinergic drugs, an additive effect occurs. Particularly common drug-drug interactions are found between atropine and the following drugs with anticholinergic properties: antihistamines, antipyschotics, antiparkinson agents, TCAs, amantadine, benzodiazepines, and monoamine oxidase inhibitors. Caution should also be used when atropine is concurrently given with sympathomimetics (an increased sympathomimetic response), cholinesterase inhibitors (decreased cholinesterase effect), digitalis, slow-release digoxin, and neostigmine (an increased potential for side effects).

Patients with hypertension or cardiovascular disease or those who are frail or medically ill can usually be safely treated with ECT. However, additional drugs to reduce the autonomic or cardiac effects may be used to protect the patient. Beta blockers or calcium channel blockers, nitroglycerin, and lidocaine may be useful to maintain cardiac integrity. Other agents routinely employed by anesthesiologists to maintain homeostasis may also be used in complicated cases, which are beyond the scope of this chapter.

REFERENCES

Alexopoulos G, Young R, Abrams RC: ECT in the high-risk geriatric patient, *J Am Geriatr Soc* 32:651, 1989.

American Psychiatric Association: *APA Task Force On Electroconvulsive Therapy*, task force no. 14, Washington, DC, 1978, The Association.

American Psychiatric Association: *The practice of electroconvulsive therapy, recommendations for treatment, training, and privileging: a task force report of the American Psychiatric Association*, Washington, DC, 1990, The Association.

Black DW, Winokur G, Nasrallah A: The treatment of depression: electroconvulsive therapy v. antidepressants: a naturalistic evaluation of 1,495 patients, *Comprehensive Psychiatry*, 28:169, 1987.

Bowden CL: Current treatment of depression, *Hosp Community Psychiatry* 36:1192, 1985.

Brown, RP, Mann JJ: A clinical perspective on the role of neurotransmitters in mental disorders, *Hosp Community Psychiatry* 36:141, 1985.

Coffey CE et al: Caffeine augmentation of ECT, *Am J Psychiatry* 147:579, 1990.

Coffey CE, Weiner RD: Electroconvulsive therapy: an update, *Hosp Community Psychiatry* 41:515, 1990.

Fogel B: Electroconvulsive therapy in the elderly: a clinical research agenda, *Int J Geriatr Psychiatry* 3:181, 1988.

Frances A, Weiner RD, Coffey CE: ECT for an elderly man with psychotic depression and concurrent dementia, *Hosp Community Psychiatry* 40:237, 1989.

Hay DP: Electroconvulsive therapy in the medically ill elderly, *Convulsive Ther* 5(1):8, 1989.

Hay DP: Electroconvulsive therapy. In Sadavoy J, Lazarus LW, Jarvik LF, editors: *Comprehensive review of geriatric psychiatry*, Washington, DC, 1991, American Psychiatric.

Markowitz J et al: Reduced length and cost of hospital stay for major depression in patients treated with ECT, *Am J Psychiatry* 144:1025, 1987.

Pearlman T, Loper M, Tillery L: Should psychiatrists administer anesthesia for ECT? *Am J Psychiatry* 147:1553, 1990.

Pettinati HM et al: Evidence of less improvement in depression in patients taking benzodiazepines during unilateral ECT, *Am J Psychiatry* 147:1029, 1990.

Prudic J et al: Relative response of endogenous and nonendogenous symptoms to electroconvulsive therapy, *J Affect Disorders* 16:59, 1989.

Runck B: NIMH report: concensus panel backs cautious use of ECT for severe disorders, *Hosp Community Psychiatry* 36:943, 1985.

Tancer ME et al: Use of electroconvulsive therapy at a university hospital: 1970 and 1980-1981, *Hosp Community Psychiatry* 40:64, 1989.

Thompson JW, Blaine JD: Use of ECT in the United States in 1975 and 1980, *Am J Psychiatry* 144:557, 1987.

Weiner RD, Coffey CE: Indications for use of electroconvulsive therapy. In Frances AJ, Hales RE, editors: *American Psychiatric Press review of psychiatry*, vol 7, Washington, DC, 1988, American Psychiatric.

CHAPTER 12

Drugs of Abuse

This chapter represents a departure from the intervention model used in this book. The scope of alcohol and substance abuse and diagnostic guidelines relevant to the pharmacologic interventions for drug abuse are discussed in Chapter 10. For nonpharmacologic interventions the reader is referred to other sources.

Drug abuse is perhaps the single most significant issue of our day, and it is underrecognized and undertreated. The cost to the United States in terms of cost of treatment, reduced productivity, mortality, criminal justice expenditure, and other related costs is thought to exceed $161 billion (National Foundation for Brain Research, 1992). For example, in 1991, 27% of the men and 48% of the women with AIDS were intravenous (IV) drug users (Kaufman and McNaul, 1992). Tables 12-1, 12-2, and 12-3 capture the categories of drugs of abuse and provide information on key variables. The box below provides selected facts about drug abuse in the United States.

Smith et al. (1986) defined dependence as a pathologic process involving a compulsion to use a psychoactive drug, loss of control over use of the drug, and continued use of the drug despite adverse consequences. The term *dependency* has replaced *addiction* for describing compulsive drug use because it more precisely defines the condition. The *Diagnostic and Statistical Manual of Mental Disorders, Third Edition-Revised (DSM-III-R)* (American Psychiatric Association [APA], 1987) differentiates

Facts About Drug Abuse in the United States

General illicit drug use within the past month: 6.2% of population in 1991, including the following:
- 15.4% of persons 18-25 yr
- 16.8% of unemployed persons
- 9.4% of blacks
- 8.1% of persons in large western cities

Marijuana use: 67.7 million persons have used marijuana during their lifetime (33.4%)

Cocaine use: 1.8 million persons are current users and 855,000 persons are heavy users*; 2.4 million persons were current users in 1990, according to the U.S. Senate Judicial Committee†

Crack: 1 million users in 1991*

Heroin: 200,000 users*; 1 million users†

Cocaine-related deaths: 2496 in 1989†

*National Institute on Drug Abuse: National Household Survey on Drug Abuse, Rockville, Md, 1991, National Institute of Mental Health.

†Kaufman E, McNaul JP: *Hosp Community Psychiatry* 43(3):223, 1992.

Table 12-1 Drugs of Abuse: Trade or Other Names

Drugs, Controlled Substance Act schedules	Trade or other names
Narcotics	
Opium: II, III, V	Dover's Powder, Paregoric, Parepectolin
Morphine: II, III	Morphine, MS-Contin Roxanol, Roxanol-SR
Codeine: II, III, V	Tylenol with codeine, Empirin with codeine, Robitussan A-C, Fiorinal with codeine
Heroin: I	Diacetylmorphine, Horse, Smack
Hydromorphone: II	Dilaudid
Meperidine: II	Demerol, Mepergan
Methadone: II	Dolophine, Methadone, Methadose
Other narcotics: I, II, III, IV, V	Numorphan, Percodan, Percocet, Tylox, Tussionex, Fentanyl, Darvon, Lomotil, Talwin
Depressants	
Chloral hydrate: IV	Noctec
Barbiturates: II, III, IV	Amytal, Butisol, Fiorinal, Lotusate, Nembutal, Seconal, Tuinal, Phenobarbital
Benzodiazepines: IV	Ativan, Dalmane, Diazepam, Librium, Xanax, Serax, Valium, Tranxene, Verstran, Versed, Halcion, Paxipam, Restoril
Methaqualone: I	Quaalude
Glutethimide: III	Doriden
Other depressants: III, IV	Equanil, Miltown, Noludar, Placidyl, Valmid
Stimulants	
Cocaine: II	Coke, Flake, Snow, Crack
Amphetamines: II	Biphetamine, Delcobase, Desoxyn, Dexedrine, Obetrol
Phenmetrazine: II	Preludin
Methylphenidate: II	Ritalin
Other stimulants: III, IV	Adipex, Cylert, Didrex, Ionamin, Melfiat, Plegine, Sanorex, Tenuate, Tepanil, Prelu-2
Hallucinogens	
LSD: I	Acid, Microdot
Mescaline and peyote: I	Mexc, Buttons, Cactus
Amphetamine variants: I	STP, MDA, MDMA, DOM, DOB
Phencyclidine: II	PCP, Angel Dust, Hog
Phencyclidine analogues: I	PCE, TCP
Other hallucinogens: I	DMT, psilocybin, psilocin
Cannabis	
Marijuana: I	Pot, Acapulco Gold, Grass, Reefer, Sinsemilla, Thai Sticks
Tetrahydrocannabinol: I, II	THC
Hashish: I	Hash
Hashish oil: I	Hash oil

DMT, N, N-dimethyltriptamine; *DOB,* 4-bromo-2, 5-dimethoxyamphetamine; *DOM,* 4-methyl-2, 5-dimethoxyamphetamine; *LSD,* lysergic acid diethylamide; *MDA,* 3, 4-methylenedioxyamphetamine (methylene dioxyamphetamine); *MDMA,* 3, 4-methylene dioxymethamphetamine; *PCE,* N-ethyl-1-phenylcyclohexylamine; *PCP,* phencyclidine; *STP,* 2, 5-dimethoxy-4-methyl; *TCP,* 1-[1-phenylcyclohexyl]-pyrrolidine; *THC,* tetrahydrocannabinol.

Table 12-2 Controlled Susbances: Uses and Adminstration

Drugs, Controlled Substance Act schedules	Medical uses	Dependence		Tolerance	Duration (hr)	Method of administration
		Physical	Psychologic			
Narcotics						
Opium: II, III V	Analgesic, antidiarrheal	High	High	Yes	3-6	Oral, smoke
Morphine: II, III	Analgesic, antitussive	High	High	Yes	3-6	Oral, smoke, inj
Codeine: II, III, V	Analgesic, antitussive	Moderate	Moderate	Yes	3-6	Oral, inj
Heroin: I	None	High	High	Yes	3-6	Inj, sniff, smoke
Hydromorphone: II	Analgesic	High	High	Yes	3-6	Oral, inj
Meperidine: II	Analgesic	High	High	Yes	3-6	Oral, inj
Methadone: II	Analgesic	High	High-low	Yes	12-24	Oral, inj
Other narcotics: I, II, III, IV, V	Analgesic, antidiarrheal, antitussive	High-low	High-low	Yes	Vary	Oral, inj
Depressants						
Chloral hydrate: IV	Hypnotic	Moderate	Moderate	Yes	5-8	Oral
Barbiturates: II, III, IV	Anesthetic, anticonvulsant, sedative, hypnotic	High-moderate	High-moderate	Yes	1-16	Oral
Benzodiazepines: IV	Antianxiety, anticonvulsant sedative, hypnotic	Low	Low	Yes	4-8	Oral
Methaqualone: I	Sedative, hypnotic	High	High	Yes	4-8	Oral

ADHP, Attention deficit hyperactivity disorder; *LSD*, lysergic acid diethylanide; *inj*, injection.

Continued.

Table 12-2 Controlled Susbances: Uses and Adminstration—cont'd

Drugs, Controlled Substance Act schedules	Medical uses	Dependence		Tolerance	Duration (hr)	Method of administration
		Physical	Psychologic			
Glutethimide: III	Sedative, hypnotic	High	Moderate	Yes	4-8	Oral
Other depressants: III, IV	Antianxiety, sedative, hypnotic	Moderate	Moderate	Yes	4-8	Oral
Stimulants						
Cocaine: II	Local anesthetic	Possibly	High	Yes	1-2	Sniff, smoke, inj
Amphetamines: II	ADHD, narcolepsy, obesity	Possibly	High	Yes	2-4	Oral, inj
Phenmetrazine: II	Obesity	Possibly	High	Yes	2-4	Oral, inj
Methylphenidate: II	ADHD, narcolepsy	Possibly	Moderate	Yes	2-4	Oral, inj
Other stimulants: III, IV	Obesity	Possibly	High	Yes	2-4	Oral, inj
Hallucinogens						
LSD: I	None	None	Unknown	Yes	8-12	Oral
Mescaline and peyote: I	None	None	Unknown	Yes	8-12	Oral
Amphetamine variants: I	None	Unknown	Unknown	Yes	Vary	Oral, inj
Phencyclidine: II	None	Unknown	High	Yes	Days	Smoke, oral, inj
Phencyclidine analogues: I	None	Unknown	High	Yes	Days	Smoke, oral, inj
Other hallucinogens: I	None	None	Unknown	Pos	Vary	Smoke, oral, inj
Cannabis						
Marijuana: I	None	Unknown	Moderate	Yes	2-4	Smoke, oral
Tetrahydrocannabinol: I, II	Cancer chemotherapy	Unknown	Moderate	Yes	2-4	Smoke, oral
Hashish: I	None	Unknown	Moderate	Yes	2-4	Smoke, oral
Hashish oil: I	None	Unknown	Moderate	Yes	2-4	Smoke, oral

Table 12-3 Controlled Substances: Effects

Drugs, Controlled Substance Act schedules	Possible effects	Effects of overdose	Withdrawal syndrome
Narcotics Opium: II, III, V Morphine: II, III Codeine: II, III, V Heroin: I Hydromorphone: II Meperidine: II Methadone: II Other narcotics: I, II, III, IV, V	Euphoria, drowsiness, respiratory depression, constricted pupils, nausea	Slow and shallow breath, clammy skin, convulsions, coma, possible death	Watery eyes, runny nose, yawning, loss of appetite, irritability, tremors, panic, cramps, nausea, chills, and sweating
Depressants Chloral hydrate: IV Barbiturates: II, III, IV Benzodiazepines: IV Methaqualone: I Glutethimide: III Other depressants: III, IV	Slurred speech, disorientation, drunken behavior without odor of alcohol	Shallow respiration, clammy skin, dilated pupils, weak and rapid pulse, coma, possible death	Anxiety, insomnia, tremors, delirium, convulsions, possible death
Stimulants Cocaine: II Amphetamines: II Phenmetrazine: II	Increased alertness, excitation, euphoria, increased pulse rate and blood pressure, insomnia, loss of appetite	Agitation, increase in body temperature, hallucinations, convulsions, possible death	Apathy, long periods of sleep, irritability, depression, disorientation

From *Federal Register* 55(159):33590, Washington, DC, August 16, 1990.

Continued.

Table 12-3 Controlled Substances: Effects—cont'd

Drugs, Controlled Substance Act schedules	Possible effects	Effects of overdose	Withdrawal syndrome
Methylphenidate: II Other stimulants: III, IV			
Hallucinogens Lysergic acid diethylamide (LSD): I Mescaline and peyote: I Amphetamine variants: I Phencyclidine: II Phencyclidine analogues: I Other hallucinogens: I	Illusions and hallucinations, poor perception of time and distance	Longer, more intense "trip" episodes; psychosis, possible death	Withdrawal syndrome not reported
Cannabis Marijuana: I Tetrahydrocannabinol: I, II Hashish: I Hashish oil: I	Euphoria, relaxed inhibitions, increased appetite, disoriented behavior	Fatigue, paranoia, possible psychosis	Insomnia, hyperactivity, decreased appetite occasionally reported

between substance dependence and substance abuse. Dependence is more severe and indicates physiologic dependence. Heroin "addiction" and alcoholism are correctly referred to as drug dependencies. In 1987 the American Medical Association declared all drug dependencies to be diseases. Such a view seems to reduce the guilt and blame traditionally associated with chemical dependency, thereby facilitating treatment.

Although not all psychiatrists and psychiatric nurses embrace the disease concept of drug dependencies, there are convincing arguments for accepting the disease hypothesis. Using alcoholism as an example, Ohlms (1988) points out that alcoholism (1) causes the person to function abnormally, (2) has a characteristic chain of symptoms reflecting specific stages of the disease that are both reliable and predictable, and (3) has the inevitable outcome of death, if continued. These characteristics satisfy the definition of a disease model.

Many clinicians avoid the dependency-abuse debate. For those professionals, chemicals are a problem for the person when their use interferes with and disrupts family, work, or social relationships and treatment is warranted.

ALCOHOL

Alcohol abuse is the number one problem in North America and is addressed separately because of the enormity of the problem. The cost to the United States in health problems, lost work hours, family disruption and disintegration, and criminal activity is currently estimated at more than $90 billion for 1991. An estimated 12.1 million Americans have one or more symptoms of alcoholism (Noble, 1985); after cardiovascular disease and cancer, alcoholism ranks third among the causes of death and disability in the United States (Whitfield, Davis, and Barker, 1986). Alcoholics have a death rate two to four times higher than that of nonalcoholics. Approximately 100,000 deaths each year are directly related to alcohol (Institute of Medicine [IOM], 1992). Cirrhosis and other medical problems, motor accidents (50% [IOM, 1992]), homicides and suicides (35% [IOM, 1992]), and nonvehicular accidents are leading causes of death associated with alcohol. Low to moderate drinking produces a pleasant, uninhibited feeling; higher amounts result in significant impairment. The legal blood alcohol level for drunkenness is 0.1% in most states. Several states have lowered the legal blood alcohol level to 0.08% in the hope of reducing highway deaths caused by drunken drivers.

The effects of alcoholism are commonly found among medical and psychiatric patients. It is estimated that among general hospital inpatients, 15% to 42% of the men and 4% to 35% of the women are alcoholics (Lewis and Gordon, 1983). Regans (1985) reported that one third of American adults (56 million persons) have been adversely affected by alcohol.

Etiologic Theories

Psychodynamic theories. A number of psychologic theories have attempted to explain how people become alcoholics. Traditionally alcoholics have been viewed as psychologically weak-willed, irresponsible, selfish, self-destructive, and morally bankrupt individuals who easily succumb to the escape provided by alcohol. Psychoanalytic theory describes alcoholics as having strong oral tendencies related to unresolved issues from the oral stage of development. Drinking alcohol is thought to be an unconscious attempt to satisfy these oral needs. More recent theories have described alcoholics as premorbidly (before they became addicted to alcohol) more phobic, inferior-feeling, dependent, and feminine than nondrinkers. Over time the search for an "alcoholic personality" has given way to a multivariate model that incorporates the biopsychosocial components of the disease (Hough, 1989). Current researchers think that many of the stereotypic characteristics found among alcoholics, such as dependency, low self-esteem, passivity, and introversion, are the result of, not the cause of, alcoholism.

Biologic theories. Heredity as an etiologic factor has been studied for many years and continues to provide insight into understanding the genesis of alcoholism. Genetic predisposition is considered to be the single most significant piece of information in identifying alcoholism (Ohlms, 1988). Children of alcoholic parents, even if raised in an alcohol-free environment, are more likely to become alcoholics than are the children of nonalcoholic parents (Goodwin et al., 1973). Mueller and Ketcham (1987) found that even when the child of the alcoholic does not drink, an inherited susceptibility to alcoholism is passed on to his or her children. Hereditary explanations provide a good basis for understanding the vulnerability to alcohol apparent in alcoholics.

Pharmacokinetics

The chemical name for alcohol is ethanol (CH_3CH_2OH). It is primarily metabolized in the liver. The oxidation process can be described chemically as follows:

$$\underset{\text{(ethanol)}}{CH_3CH_2OH} \rightarrow \underset{\text{(acetaldehyde)}}{CH_3CHO} + H_2 \longrightarrow \underset{\text{(acetic acid)}}{CH_3 - C - OH - O} \longrightarrow \underset{\text{(carbon dioxide [water])}}{CO_2 - H_2O}$$

At each step of the metabolizing process an enzyme breaks down the chemical. Ethanol is broken down by alcohol dehydrogenase to acetaldehyde and hydrogen. The hydrogen molecule causes the liver to bypass normal energy sources (the hydrogen from fat) and to use the hydrogen from ethanol. Fat accumulates and leads to fatty liver, hyperlipemia, hepatitis, and cirrhosis. Acetaldehyde is toxic to the body. It compromises normal cell function in the liver. If the metabolism of acetaldehyde is impaired, it accumulates in the liver, causing cell death and necrosis. Liver cell loss continues to cirrhosis. Acetaldehyde interferes with vitamin activation. Aldehyde dehydrogenase breaks down acetaldehyde to acetic acid, which in an innocuous substance. When enzymatic action on acetaldehyde is blocked by the aldehyde dehydrogenase blocker disulfiram (Antabuse), acetaldehyde accumulates, causing severe sickness and potentially death. Recent research confirms an age-old suspicion that women become intoxicated more easily than men, even when studies are controlled for size differences. Frezza et al. (1990) have discovered that the gastrointestinal tissue of women and of alcoholic men contains little alcohol dehydrogenase. The alcohol dehydrogenase in the gastrointestinal tissue of nonalcoholic men oxidizes a significant amount of the alcohol in the gut before it enters the bloodstream. The inability of women's bodies to make this "first-pass metabolism" accounts for their enhanced vulnerability to alcohol.

Some researchers think that some of the excess acetaldehyde travels to the brain and reacts chemically with neurotransmitters to make tetrahydroisoquinolines (TIQs) and beta-carbolines (Figure 12-1). Tetrahydroisoquinolines are similar to the addictive substance found in heroin and morphine (Mueller and Ketcham, 1987). When TIQs are infused into the brains of monkeys, the monkeys develop an irreversible preference for alcohol over water. Beta-carbolines have been shown to cause severe anxiety, and it is hypothesized that alcoholics use alcohol to attempt to reduce the anxiety caused by previous drinks of alcohol (Wallace, 1985).

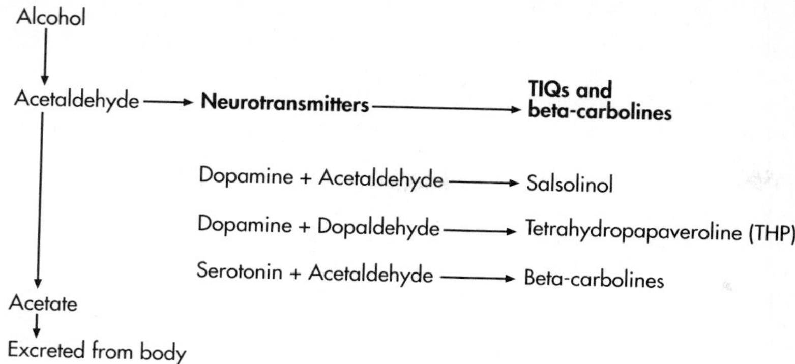

Figure 12-1 How addictive products, tetrahydroisoquinolines (TIQs), and beta-carbolines are formed in the body. Alcohol is metabolized to acetaldehyde. Acetaldehyde and other aldehydes condense with neurotransmitters to produce TIQs and beta-carbolines. These compounds, formed when we drink alcohol, appear to be highly addictive brain substances similar to morphine precursors. Infused into animal brains, they produce what seems to be irreversible addictive drinking. (From Wallace J: *Alcoholism: new light on the disease*, Newport, RI, 1985, Edgehill.)

Alcohol is absorbed partially from the stomach but mostly from the small intestine. Within *20 minutes* it is in the bloodstream, if it is ingested by a person with an *empty stomach*. The rate of absorption is affected by the form of alcohol consumed. Alcohol in beer and wine is absorbed more slowly than alcohol in liquor. This may be partially due to dilution. Beer contains 4% ethanol; wine, 12% ethanol; and whiskey, 40% to 50% ethanol. However, slower absorption cannot be totally accounted for by dilution of the alcohol. Food also slows alcohol absorption.

Ethanol is distributed equally in all body tissue according to water content. Large persons or persons with great amounts of body water can ingest more alcohol than small persons or persons with less body water. Alcohol affects the cerebrum and cerebellum before it affects the spinal cord and the vital centers because the former areas contain more water.

The rate of absorption largely determines how quickly a person will become intoxicated, but the metabolic rate largely determines how long alcohol will affect the body. The metabolic rate is constant. The body can metabolize 10 ml of alcohol (1 ounce of whiskey or 1 glass of beer) every 90 minutes. In persons who drink alcohol frequently over a number of years, hepatic drug-metabolizing levels are increased to hasten alcohol metabolism. Hot coffee, "sweating it out," and other home remedies do not increase alcohol metabolism, nor do they speed the "sobering-up" process. Attempts by scientist to develop a drug to prevent or decrease intoxication have been unsuccessful. In late-stage alcoholism tolerance decreases as the abused liver finally can no longer adequately metabolize the alcohol.

Tolerance to alcohol occurs and is probably related to elevated hepatic enzyme levels and to cellular adaptations. The normal drinker might be noticeably drunk after 10 to 12 drinks, whereas the long-term drinker with a tolerance might walk around almost unaffected by drinking the same amount. This is an example of tolerance. "Drinking someone under the table" is a function of "practice" rather than "manhood" (Scavnicky-Mylant and Keltner, 1991).

Physiologic Effects

Initially individuals drink because alcohol causes a reaction that they desire. Disinhibition, impaired judgment, and fuzzy thinking are initial responses to alcohol ingestion. These signs represent cerebrum intoxication. In many situations this mental relaxation is pleasant. Alcohol also depresses psychomotor activity. Alcohol has been described as a social lubricant because it relaxes self-imposed barriers that tether sociability. Anxiety and tension are relieved, usually for a couple of hours after a drink is taken. Eventually, at least for the alcoholic, drinking becomes defensive; that is, the alcoholic often drinks to avoid the effects of many years of drinking. For instance, once the anxiety-reducing effect wears off, more tension and anxiety are caused, so the drinker must consume more alcohol to regain the "anxiety-free" state again. Many alcoholics, even after drinking all they "can hold," are not able to quell the psychomotor rebound upheaval caused by years of alcohol-related central nervous system (CNS) irritation.

The adverse effects of alcohol can be categorized as central (CNS) or peripheral nervous system (PNS). Central nervous system effects are related to sedation and toxicity. As the vital centers become affected, a slower, stuporous-to-unconscious mental state develops. Large amounts of alcohol can cause sleep, coma, deep anesthesia, and death. Other common symptoms of intoxication include slurred speech, a short retention span, loud talk, and memory deficits. Blackout is a period in which an alcoholic functioned socially and for which he or she has no memory.

Historically the brain damage associated with alcoholism was thought to be caused by alcohol-related nutritional deficiencies. Alcoholics do eat poorly, and no doubt such behavior leads to pathologic change. It is now known, however, that brain damage occurs when drinking, even when a nutritious diet is maintained. In fact, all alcoholics have some brain cell loss.

Increased psychomotor activity as a consequence of alcohol is called the alcohol-withdrawal syndrome. Sedation is the predominant effect of alcohol, but as sedation wears off, psychomotor activity increases. This is referred to as a rebound phenomenon. As the CNS becomes more irritated, the normal drinker feels sick and irritable (a hangover) but lives through it, perhaps vowing, "never again." The heavy drinker and the alcoholic have to drink again to "resedate" the psychomotor system. Eventually alcoholics have to drink large amounts of alcohol, just to feel somewhat "normal." Some reach the point at which they cannot drink enough and CNS irritability is not "sedatable." Alcoholic tremors, sweating, palpitations, and agitation then occur. Most often these symptoms occur when alcohol ingestion has stopped, but in some cases they occur while the alcoholic is drinking.

Alcoholic hallucinosis, a state of auditory hallucinations, is a phenomenon that alcoholics sometimes experience. The brain begins to "invent" sensory input. Alcoholic hallucinations usually begin 48 hours or so after drinking has stopped. Usually within the context of a clear sensorium, frightening voices or sounds are heard.

The ultimate level of CNS irritability is delirium tremens (DTs). In DTs the body not only invents sensory input but also has extreme motor agitation. Hallucinations become visual (e.g., the proverbial pink elephants), and the sufferer is tremulous and terrified. Tonic-clonic seizures (grand mal) can occur.

Wernicke-Korsakoff syndrome is an organic mental disorder characterized by amnesia, clouding of consciousness, confabulation (falsification of memory) and memory loss, and peripheral neuropathy. This disorder results from the poor nutrition of alcoholics (specifically, inadequate amounts of thiamine and niacin in the diet) and from the neurotoxic nature of the alcohol.

Peripheral nervous system involvement is varied and causes great suffering. For a complete discussion of these various processes the reader is directed to a pathophysiology textbook.

Cirrhosis and peripheral neuritis are the physical health problems most commonly associated with alcohol. Cirrhosis is the fifth leading cause of death in the United States. As the alcoholic's liver function becomes impaired, he or she is less able to "tolerate" alcohol. The man who once boasted of his drinking exploits is drunk after only a few beers. Physical consequences of cirrhosis include obstructed blood flow (which leads to portal hypertension, ascites, and, finally, to esophageal varices) and decreased liver cell function, low protein levels, high ammonia and bilirubin serum levels, and clotting problems. Peripheral neuritis causes numbness and the subsequent injury in the legs, as well as changes in gait.

Alcohol is also an irritant. It burns the mouth and throat and prompts the stomach to secrete more hydrochloric acid. Gastric ulcers are caused and then worsened by alcohol. Alcoholics experience ulcers, gastritis, bleeding, and hemorrhage in the stomach. Ulcers can eventually perforate, creating a life-threatening situation.

The pancreas is affected by alcohol in many direct and indirect ways. Pancreatitis and diabetes are not uncommon consequences of alcoholism. A malabsorption syndrome is caused by irritation of the intestinal lining. This seems to affect B vitamins generally and to lead to a deficiency of vitamin B1 (thiamine) in particular. Thiamine deficiency contributes to peripheral neuritis. Alcohol also has a direct effect on muscle tissue, a condition known as alcohol myopathy. Other organs affected by alcohol include the eyes (loss of peripheral and night vision), the heart (hypertension, enlarged left ventricle), and reproductive organs (as a depressant, alcohol can cause impotence).

Related Issues

Overdose. People die of overdoses of alcohol because it depresses the CNS. Vital centers become anesthetized, compromising breathing and heart rate, leading to a comatose state or death. Gastrointestinal bleeding or hemorrhage can occur. Alcohol also causes heat loss, and many people have succumbed to hypothermia in cold climates. People consistently underestimate the potency of alcohol, and deaths have occurred simply because individuals have drunk too much. At least yearly, newspapers report the death of a college student coerced into drinking too much alcohol. Although alcohol used alone can kill, most alcohol-related deaths are the result of combining alcohol with CNS depressants.

Disulfiram. Disulfiram (Antabuse) inhibits the breakdown of acetaldehyde by the enzyme aldehyde dehydrogenase (see Chapter 10). Because acetaldehyde is toxic to the body, the person who drinks alcohol while taking disulfiram becomes ill (sweating, flushing of the neck and face, a throbbing headache, nausea and vomiting, palpitations, dyspnea, tremor, and weakness). This combination can also cause arrhythmias, myocardial infarction, cardiac failure, seizures, coma, and death. The unpleasant response to alcohol reinforces the alcoholic's efforts to stop drinking.

Interactions. Alcohol taken with other CNS depressants causes profound CNS depression, often leading to death. For instance, diazepam, which is seldom lethal when taken alone (even in large doses), can lead to death when it is combined with alcohol. Alcohol should be avoided when a person is taking barbiturates, antipsychotic drugs, antidepressants, benzodiazepines, and other CNS depressants. Chloral hydrate and lorazepam (Ativan) have been associated with intentional sedating of un-

Table 12-4 Withdrawal Courses for Addictive Drugs

Drug	Intoxication signs and symptoms	Withdrawal signs and symptoms	Length of acute detoxification	Recurring withdrawal symptoms	Common detoxification agents
Narcotics	Pinpoint pupils, euphoria, nodding, sleepiness, anxiety, depressed blood pressure and respiration, elevated pulse rate	Yawning, dilated pupils, gooseflesh, vomiting, diarrhea, runny nose and eyes, sleeplessness, anxiety, irritability, elevated blood pressure and pulse rate, craving for narcotics			Methadone or other tapering opiate or nonopiate withdrawal regimens
Heroin			3-5 days	Common	
Morphine			3-5 days	Common	
Demerol			3-5 days	Common	
Methadone			2 wk or longer	Common	
Depressants	Slurred speech, poor coordination, confusion, drowsiness, clumsiness, depressed respirations and blood pressure	Anxiety, sweats, tremors, flushed face, irritability, sleeplessness, confusion, seizures, delirium			
Alcohol			3-5 days	Not usual	Chlordiazepoxide, oxazepam, hydroxyzine, diazepam, alcohol*
Valium			Slow drug taper up to 2 wk	Common	Chlordiazepoxide, diazepam

Phenobarbital			Slow drug taper for 2-4 wk	Common	Chlordiazepoxide, phenobarbital
Stimulants	Rapid pulse, elevated blood pressure, dilated pupils, sweats, tremors, hyperactivity, loss of appetite, irritability, sleeplessness, delirium, seizures	General fatigue, apathy, depression, drowsiness, irritability, paranoia			
Amphetamines			3-5 days	Common	Drug intervention usually not required
Cocaine			3-5 days	Common	
Marijuana	Rapid pulse rate, elevated blood pressure, dilated pupils, flushed face, red conjunctivae, anxiety, hallucinations, time-space disorientation, rambling speech	Few signs of withdrawal, craving for marijuana, general anxiety, restlessness	2-3 days	Possible prolonged craving	Usually none

From Mueller LA, Ketcham K: *Recovering: how to get and stay sober*, New York, 1987, Bantam.

*Low-dose alcohol withdrawal: Traditionally, alcohol was used by laymen to taper a drunk off a binge. With the advent of sedative medication, this practice was discouraged. The use of general sedatives was thought to be more "clinical" and to achieve better control with less toxicity. In recent years, however, the alcohol withdrawal model has been revived. Leading the way in this detoxification method is Dr. Walter Gower, M.D., of North Central Alcoholism Research Foundation, Inc., Fort Dodge, Iowa.

Treatment regimen: 0.5 oz vodka (80-100 proof) with 0.5 oz water every 1-6 hr for detoxification control; indications for use are the same as for sedatives intervention; can be used alone or in combination with sedatives such as chlordiazepoxide; patients with seizure histories are better protected during withdrawal with the combined regimen

Other opiate-withdrawal protocol: propoxyphene-N 100: 1-2 every 4-6 hr to control detoxification signs and symptoms, taper to discontinue in 3-4 days; clonidine: 0.1 mg initially; repeat in 1 hr, if needed, then 0.1-0.2 mg every 6-8 hr as long as blood pressure is no lower than 90/60 mm Hg; can be used for 7-14 days to control opiate withdrawal symptoms suspecting persons in bars. A chloral hydrate and alcohol combination (the legendary "knock-out drops") was used years ago to "recruit" men for ship duty or for robbery. The combination of lorazepam and alcohol has been used in recent days by prostitutes to debilitate their clients so they can rob them.

Use in elderly persons. Individuals with impaired liver function do not metabolize alcohol efficiently and therefore can tolerate little of the drug. Decreased liver function is a product of aging; consequently many older persons cannot drink much alcohol without becoming inebriated, confused, and sedated. The nurse or physician should be particularly watchful for combinations of alcohol with other CNS depressants in members of this age group.

Fetal alcohol syndrome. Pregnant women who drink alcohol run the risk of seriously harming their unborn children. Fetal alcohol syndrome (FAS) is the result of alcohol's inhibition of fetal development during the first trimester. Fetal alcohol syndrome is the third most commonly recognized cause of mental retardation and has been particularly devastating among some American Indian tribes. Characteristic signs of FAS include microcephaly, cleft palate, altered palmar creases, cardiac defects, anomalous genitalia, severe mental retardation, and a depressed sucking reflex. The risk of FAS is directly related to the amount of alcohol the mother drinks.

Withdrawal and detoxification. Withdrawal from alcohol can be painful, scary, and even lethal. As the person abstains from alcohol, he or she begins to reap the consequences of the CNS irritation caused by alcohol: tremulousness, nervousness, anxiety, anorexia, nausea and vomiting, insomnia and other sleep disturbances, rapid pulse rate, high blood pressure, profuse perspiration, diarrhea, fever, unsteady gait, difficulty concentrating, exaggerated startle reflex, and a craving for alcohol and other drugs. As the withdrawal symptoms become more pronounced, hallucinations can occur. The body is experiencing alcohol intoxication and needs detoxification. Table 12-4 provides an overview of the withdrawal courses for addictive drugs (Mueller and Ketcham, 1987). Treatment for alcoholism is further discussed in Chapter 10.

OTHER CENTRAL NERVOUS SYSTEM DEPRESSANTS

Central nervous system depressants are relatively new pharmacologic agents. Barbiturates were first used medicinally as sedatives in the last half of the nineteenth century. It was not until 1950 that researchers were able to confirm the ability of CNS depressants to produce physical dependence. CNS depressants decrease the awareness of and response to sensory stimuli. Two classes of CNS depressants discussed in this chapter are barbiturates and inhalants. Antipsychotic drugs and antianxiety agents, which also depress the CNS, are discussed in previous chapters.

BARBITURATES

Barbiturates are used to relieve anxiety or to produce sleep (see Chapter 8). They have a narrow therapeutic index, the lethal dose being only slightly higher than the therapeutic dose. These drugs produce both physical and psychologic dependence.

Barbiturates are classified according to the duration of action as follows: ultrashort (30 minutes to 3 hours), short (3 to 4 hours), intermediate (6 to 8 hours), and long (10 to 12 hours). Uses range from anesthesia (ultrashort-acting barbiturates such as thiopental) to long-term use in epilepsy (long-acting barbiturates such as phenobarbital).

Pharmacokinetics

Barbiturates are usually taken orally. They are metabolized by the liver and excreted by the kidneys. When barbiturates are combined with alcohol, dangerous levels of CNS depression can occur.

Physiologic Effects

Barbiturates cause CNS depression, thus decreasing awareness of external stimuli, shortening the attention span, and decreasing intellectual ability. Regular sleep patterns are changed, with a loss of rapid eye movement sleep. Barbiturates are used to treat insomnia, to soften withdrawal from heroin, and as anticonvulsants. Drug abusers take barbiturates to maintain a state of relatively anxiety-free living. These drugs are also taken to counteract the effects of amphetamines, "to come down," or to replace heroin when it is not available. The acutely intoxicated person has an unsteady gait, slurred speech, and sustained nystagmus. Chronic users have mental symptoms that include confusion, irritability, and insomnia. A tolerance to barbiturates develops in persons who regularly use them.

Related Issues

Overdose. The toxic dose of barbiturates varies; in general, an oral dose of 1 g results in serious poisoning and doses of 2 to 10 g can be fatal. Acute overdose is manifested by CNS and respiratory depression. Coma and death are possible. Treatment is supportive.

Interactions. Barbiturates interact with many drugs, but the most significant are those that increase CNS depression. Central nervous system depressants such as alcohol, sedatives, tranquilizers, and antihistamines can cause serious CNS depression.

Use in elderly persons. Barbiturates frequently cause excitement in elderly individuals. Elderly persons are also prone to confusion caused by barbiturates.

Use during pregnancy. Barbiturates can cause fetal abnormalities. These drugs cross the placental barrier, and fetal serum levels approach maternal blood levels. Infants born to mothers who take barbiturates during the last trimester of pregnancy have withdrawal symptoms.

Withdrawal and detoxification. Symptoms of withdrawal from barbiturates are severe and can cause death. Symptoms usually begin 8 to 12 hours after the last dose. Minor withdrawal symptoms include anxiety, muscle twitching, tremor, progressive weakness, dizziness, distorted visual perception, nausea and vomiting, insomnia, and orthostatic hypotension. More serious withdrawal symptoms include convulsions and delirium beginning approximately 16 hours after the last dose and lasting up to 5 days. Untreated, withdrawal symptoms may not decline in intensity for some time. Detoxification requires a cautious and gradual reduction of these drugs. One approach is to reduce the patient's regular dose by 10% each day. Barbiturates can be detected in the urine for up to 3 weeks (Table 12-5).

INHALANTS

Three basic forms of inhalants are hydrocarbon solvents (gasoline), aerosol propellants (the propellants in spray cans), and anesthetics (chloroform and nitrous oxide). Inhalants usually depress the CNS and increase hilarity. They are particularly dangerous because the amount inhaled cannot be controlled. Deaths resulting from asphyxiation have been reported. Inhalants cross the blood-brain barrier quickly. Common side effects include mouth ulcers, gastrointestinal problems, anorexia, confusion, headache, and ataxia.

NARCOTICS (OPIOIDS)

Narcotics or opioids are widely abused and include heroin, morphine, codeine, meperidine (Demerol), methadone, and fentanyl. Until the relatively recent "cocaine crisis" the general public viewed heroin as the most significant drug of abuse. Although heroin abuse has been relegated to "back-page" status for some time, it is again becoming the focus of attention, since drug users find it less expense than cocaine. Illicit drugs can be swallowed, smoked, snorted, injected into soft tissue (skin popping), and mainlined (injected intravenously). Parenteral use of heroin, for example, involves (1) "cooking" the substance in a spoon or bottlecap, (2) filtering it with a cotton ball, (3) "sterilizing" a needle with a match, and (4) injecting the drug into a vein. Initially veins in the antecubital space are used, but as vein membranes break down and sclerosis ("tracks") develops, other veins are "used up." The needle is frequently passed from one user to another. Infections, including acquired immunodeficiency syndrome (AIDS) and hepatitis, are known to be associated with intravenous drug abuse.

Pharmacokinetics

Opioids are metabolized in the liver and excreted by the kidneys. They are not absorbed well in the gut but are readily metabolized there and in the liver. Opioids can be given orally but are usually given parenterally. Drugs that compete for liver metabolism increase the effect of opioids.

Physiologic Effects

Opioids relieve pain by increasing the pain threshold and by reducing anxiety and fear. They do this by stimulating specific neurotransmitter receptor sites in the brain. These naturally occurring neurotransmitters, the endorphins, among other responses, mediate pain and regulate mood. The opioids are endorphin agonists. It is their effect on mood (a feeling of euphoria) that attracts drug abusers. Drug abusers frequently refer to the euphoric mood created by heroin as "better than sex." In addition to the euphoria, an overall CNS depression occurs. Drowsiness or "nodding" and sleep are common effects.

Heroin has a higher abuse potential than morphine because it more readily passes the blood-brain barrier. Once heroin enters the brain, its chemical structure is changed to that of morphine, so it becomes "trapped" in the brain. This property of heroin causes a more sustained high than that of morphine.

Central nervous system effects of opioids include respiratory depression related to decreased sensitivity to carbon dioxide stimulation by the medullary center for respiration. Respiratory depression is the primary cause of death among opioid abusers. Peripheral nervous system effects include constipation; decreased gastric, biliary, and pancreatic secretions; urinary retention; hypotension; and reduced pupil size. Pinpoint pupils are a sign of opioid overdose. Morphine also causes vomiting.

Related Issues

Overdose. At therapeutic doses prescribed and administered by professionals, morphine is a helpful and safe analgesic. Drug abusers, however, are never sure of the amount of the drug they are taking. Street purchases are not standardized, and occasionally users obtain "more pure" drug than they anticipated. Inadvertent overdose occurs. The primary effect of overdose is respiratory depression. A respiratory rate below 12 breaths per minute is cause for concern. The following recognizable symptom pattern for overdose is documented:

The person becomes stuporous and then sleeps.
The skin is wet and warm.
Coma develops, accompanied by respiratory depression and hypoxia.
The skin becomes cold and clammy.
The pupils dilate.
Death quickly ensues.

Provision of adequate airway and assisted ventilation, if needed, are treatment priorities. A narcotic antagonist (see Chapter 10) is administered to reverse the effects of opioids.

Narcotic antagonists. The opioids are the only class of commonly abused drugs that has a specific antidote. Naloxone (Narcan), a narcotic antagonist, is the drug of choice when opioid overdose is suspected. Naloxone blocks the neuroreceptors affected by opioids, so the patient responds in a few minutes to an intravenous injection of naloxone. Respirations improve, and the patient consciously responds. However, since most opioids have a longer-lasting effect than naloxone has, it is often necessary to repeat the antagonist to maintain adequate respirations. The nurse administering naloxone must carefully observe the patient to determine whether additional antagonist will be needed. Nalorphine (Nalline) is also a narcotic antagonist. Narcotic antagonists do not interrupt the effects of nonnarcotics. The treatment strategy with these agents is further discussed in Chapter 10.

Interactions. The effects of opioids are increased when they are combined with other CNS depressants. Since the use of multiple drugs is common among drug abusers, the potential for deadly combinations is real. If it is known that heroin has been taken and naloxone does not reverse CNS depression, it can be safely assumed that other depressants were also taken. In such cases supportive care is indicated.

Use in elderly persons. Elderly persons are particularly at risk for decreased pulmonary ventilation associated with opioids.

Use during pregnancy. Pregnant women who abuse opioids give birth to babies who have withdrawal symptoms. These drugs can cross the placental barrier and produce respiratory depression in neonates.

Withdrawal and detoxification. The unassisted withdrawal from alcohol or barbiturates can be fatal, but the unassisted withdrawal from opioids is rarely fatal. Withdrawal symptoms are related to the degree of dependence and the abruptness of the discontinuance. Maximum intensity is reached within 36 to 72 hours and subsides in

Table 12-5 Period of Time After Ingestion That Drugs Can Be Detected in Urine

Drug	Detection period
Narcotics	
Heroin	2-4 days
Morphine	2-4 days
Meperidine (Demerol)	2-4 days
Methadone	2-4 days
Fentanyl	Can be <1 h
Depressants	
Barbiturates	12 h-3 wk
Benzodiazepines	Up to 1 wk
Stimulants	
Amphetamines	2-4 days
Cocaine	2-4 days
Hallucinogens	
Marijuana	3 days to >1 mo
Phencyclidine (PCP)	1 day-1 mo

Adapted from Sullivan E, Bissell L, Williams E: *Chemical dependency in nursing*, Redwood City, Calif, 1988, Addison-Wesley, 1988.

5 to 10 days. Withdrawal symptoms can be categorized as early, intermediate, and late appearing. Early symptoms of withdrawal include yawning, tearing, rhinorrhea, and sweating. Intermediate symptoms include flushing, piloerection, tachycardia, tremor, restlessness, and irritability. Symptoms that are late appearing include muscle spasm, fever, nausea, diarrhea, vomiting, repetitive sneezing, abdominal cramps, and backache. Treatment is primarily symptomatic and supportive.

Specific Drugs

Drugs related to morphine include hydromorphone (Dilaudid), a derivative of morphine and more potent; levorphanol (Levo-Dromoran), a drug whose action is identical to that of morphine but that is used for less severe pain; meperidine, a synthetic narcotic analgesic, pentazocine (Talwin), which has weaker analgesic effects than other narcotic drugs, is less addicting, and does not cause euphoria; and several related drugs such as oxymorphone (Numorphan), alphaprodine (Nisentil), anileridine (Leritine), butorphanol (Stadol), and nalbuphine (Nubain). Fentanyl (Sublimaze), an anesthetic, is similar to but 100 times stronger than morphine and 20 to 40 times stronger than heroin. It is said to produce an "unbelievable" high.

Morphine. Morphine is the prototype opioid; as stated previously, it is useful in the alleviation of pain. Oral administration has a variable onset, but intravenous morphine provides a fast effect. It is metabolized in the liver, excreted in the urine, and has a half-life of 2.5 to 3 hours.

Methadone. Methadone (Dolophine), although an opioid similar to morphine, is used to prevent withdrawal symptoms. Methadone is given orally and is poorly metabolized in the liver. Accordingly, it has a much longer half-life (15 to 30 hours) than morphine has (2.5 to 3 hours). Because of the long half-life, once-a-day dosage is effective and conducive to outpatient care.

Heroin. Heroin is derived from morphine and is referred to as a semisynthetic drug. It was originally thought to be a cure for morphine addiction but proved to be far more addictive than morphine.

Codeine. Codeine is used primarily as a cough suppressant. Its abuse preceded the general drug abuse of the mid-to-late 1960s because codeine was easily available in over-the-counter cough syrups. Ease of access was eliminated at about the same time that drug abuse became recognized as an emerging national problem. It is not a drug choice for many substance abusers today.

STIMULANTS

Use of stimulants by Americans is widespread, for instance, in caffeine-containing drinks. Many people, if they cannot start their day with a cup of coffee, feel absolutely sluggish. Should they remain caffeine free all day, they have the withdrawal symptoms associated with stimulant withdrawal, that is, headache, nausea, and vomiting. Tobacco is also a stimulant.

COCAINE

Coca leaves have been used as stimulants for thousands of years. Coca plants grow high in the Andes, and the Inca Indians chewed coca leaves long before the Spanish explorers arrived. Cocaine is extracted from the coca plant and is a fine, white, odorless substance with a bitter taste. It was introduced to Western medicine as an anesthetic in 1858. Freud was known to use cocaine and believed it to be a remedy for morphine addiction. It was once used in Coca-Cola, and advertisements extolled Coke's ability to "refresh." After the Pure Food and Drug Law was passed in 1906, cocaine was eliminated from Coca-Cola. Cocaine and its offspring, *crack,* cause perhaps the biggest drug problem today. The list is long of famous and not-so-famous persons struck down in their youth by these stimulants. The problems associated with these drugs extend to every level of society. The United States Senate Judiciary Committee has said that the rising murder rate in America can be blamed on rising stockpiles of assault weapons and shrinking supplies of cocaine. In a 1-year study of suicides in New York City, fully 20% of suicide victims under the age of 61 years had taken cocaine within days of their deaths (Marzuk et al., 1992).

Pharmacokinetics

Cocaine passes the blood-brain barrier quickly, causing an instantaneous high. When administered intravenously, cocaine is rapidly metabolized by the liver, so the "rush," although exhilarating, does not last long. Cocaine exerts both CNS and PNS effects because of its ability to block norepinephrine and dopamine reuptake into neurons. It depletes these neurotransmitters. Cocaine can also be swallowed (but is poorly absorbed this way) and snorted. Snorting, in which cocaine is absorbed through the nasal mucus, is the preferred route for drug abusers. Freebasing is another way of using cocaine. Freebasing is a process used to rid "street cocaine" of its adulterants and reduce it to a pure cocaine base. The cocaine base is volatile, and explosions have occurred (e.g., Richard Pryor was burned severely as a result of freebasing cocaine). Freebase cocaine is smoked and produces incredibly powerful feelings of euphoria instantaneously. Euphoria is quickly followed by discomfort, so more smoking is required to relieve the discomfort. A vicious cycle ensues.

Crack, or "rock," a form of cocaine, may be the most addictive drug on the streets today. It is produced in a relatively uncomplicated procedure (mixed with baking soda and water, heated, and hardened) and then smoked. It produces an instantaneous high and a "crash" almost as instantaneous. An intense desire to smoke again is produced. Crack is cheap (as low as $5 to $10 a purchase) and easy to find.

Tolerance to CNS and PNS effects develops quickly because neuronal norepinephrine stores are depleted (and, of course, decreased norepinephrine levels is one explanation for depression), causing a need to increase drug amounts to create the desired effect. Tolerance develops to otherwise lethal amounts.

Physiologic Effects

Cocaine and its derivatives are addictive stimulants. Although physical dependence is less severe than with opiate abuse, psychologic dependence is intense. Abusers become tongue-tied when attempting to describe the sensations of cocaine. Euphoria, increased mental alertness, increased strength, anorexia, and increased sexual stimulation are major desired effects of cocaine and its derivatives. The number of persons who have tried cocaine at least once increased from 5.4 million in 1974 to 30 million in 1989 (DiGregorio, 1990). The primary effect is a dopaminergic stimulation of mesolimbic and mesocortical reward pathways (Kaufman and McNaul, 1992). Chronic cocaine use leads to cathecholamine receptor supersensitivity and probably the eventual destruction of dopaminergic neurons. This result may account for the anhedonia found in some chronic cocaine users (Kaufman and McNaul, 1992).

Increased motor activity, tachycardia, and high blood pressure are PNS effects. Sensory and motor nerve endings are numbed, causing blood vessels to contract. Decreased stimulation occurs. CNS effects include stimulation of the medulla, resulting in deeper respirations, euphoria, increased mental alertness, dilated pupils, anorexia, and increased strength. The cocaine user also talks a lot and is stimulated sexually. This latter characteristic, no doubt, adds to the drug's overall appeal. Less common reactions are specific hallucinations and delusions. Cocaine users report "bugs" crawling beneath the skin (formication) and foul smells. Nasal septum perforation is associated with snorting cocaine and is due to extreme vasoconstriction, which impedes blood supply to this area and thus causes nasal necrosis.

AMPHETAMINES

Amphetamines were developed in 1887. They have medicinal uses, such as short-term treatment of obesity, attention deficit hyperactivity disorder in childhood (Chapters 15 and 16), and narcolespy (Chapter 8). Although not technically addictive by *DSM-III-R* criteria, they are highly abused. The *San Francisco Chronicle* on May 30, 1989,* ran a front-page story entitled "Speed Makes a Comeback on Bay Area Drug Scene." "Speed," sometimes known as crank, is called the poor man's cocaine. Some notable quotations from the article follow:

> Everybody's predicting that it's going to be the next big drug problem . . . Only cocaine and marijuana are used more often. Speed is gaining on cocaine because it produces a longer high . . . It is also cheaper . . . A lot of people arrested for doing crank say they would never do coke. For some reason they think crank isn't as addicting . . . The greatest percentage of new patients seeking help for speed addiction are teenagers who cannot afford more expensive drugs . . .

*Pages A-1 and A-11.

Pharmacokinetics

Amphetamines (speed) are indirect-acting sympathomimetics that cause the release of norepinephrine from nerve endings. Amphetamines also block norepinephrine reuptake in presynaptic nerve endings. Amphetamines are well absorbed from the gastrointestinal tract. They are given orally. Therapeutic parenteral administration is illegal in the United States, but many "speed freaks" self-administer amphetamines intravenously.

Physiologic Effects

As with cocaine, individuals take amphetamines because amphetamines make them feel good. Central nervous system effects include wakefulness, alertness, heightened concentration, energy, improved mood to euphoria, insomnia (sometimes desired, sometimes not), and amnesia.

The most common side effects of amphetamine use are restlessness, dizziness, agitation, and insomnia. Peripheral nervous system effects are palpitations, tachycardia, and hypertension. Respirations are also increased because, like cocaine, the amphetamines stimulate the medulla. A psychiatric side effect of amphetamine use is amphetamine-induced psychosis. In the emergency room this psychotic presentation can be almost indistinguishable from paranoid schizophrenia.

Related Issues

Overdose. Cocaine overdose has resulted in a number of deaths, primarily due to arrhythmias and respiratory collapse. Freebasing adds to the problem because large amounts reach the system quickly. Toxic levels of amphetamines causes severe hypertension, cerebral hemorrhage seizures, and coma. Treatment includes induction of vomiting, acidification of the urine, and forced diuresis. In patients with amphetamine psychosis related to toxic levels of these drugs, chlorpromazine or haloperidol given intramuscularly antagonizes the amphetamine effect.

Interactions. The effects of cocaine and amphetamines are augmented when they are combined with other CNS stimulants. Many over-the-counter products such as hay fever medications and decongestants contain stimulants. Urinary alkalinizing agents such as sodium bicarbonate decrease the elimination of stimulants, whereas urinary acidifying agents increase the elimination of stimulants.

Use during pregnancy. Amphetamines should be used during pregnancy only when clearly needed because harm to the fetus has been demonstrated. Cocaine-addicted mothers give birth to addicted babies with multiple problems. The use of cocaine and crack among pregnant women in New York City is responsible for a dramatic decrease in the birth weight of infants in that city (Joyce, 1990). Consequences of cocaine use include abruptio placentae, preterm delivery, premature rupture of membranes, microcephaly, and increased neonatal morbidity (Kaufman and McNaul, 1992).

Withdrawal and detoxification. Although cocaine and amphetamines are highly addictive, physical withdrawal is relatively mild. Psychologic withdrawal is severe, however, because the drugs are so pleasurable. For persons withdrawing from amphetamines under medical supervision the withdrawal process is gradual and safe. "Cold turkey" withdrawal without medical supervision causes agitation, irritability, and severe depression. As a rule of thumb, the "low" of withdrawal will be inversely proportional to the "high" experienced. Withdrawal from cocaine causes intense craving for the drug. A number of approaches are used, all aiming to restore depleted neurotransmitters. Amino acid precursors such as tyrosine and phenylalanine, TCAs, and the dopamine agonist bromocriptine are three approaches used to increase the availability of neurotransmitters.

HALLUCINOGENS

Hallucinogens, also referred to as psychotomimetics or psychedelics, alter perception. There are two basic groups of hallucinogens: natural and manufactured, or synthetic. Natural hallucinogenic substances include mescaline (peyote [from cactus]), psilocybin (psilocin [from mushrooms]), and marijuana *(Cannabis sativa)*. Synthetic or semisynthetic substances include lysergic acid diethylamine-25 (LSD), 2,5-dimethoxy-4-methyl amphetamine (STP), phencyclidine (PCP), N,N-dimethyltryptamine (DMT), and methylene dioxyamphetamine (MDA).

In general hallucinogens can heighten awareness of reality or can cause a terrifying psychosis-like reaction. Users report distortions in body image and a sense of depersonalization. Particularly frightful is a loss of the sense of reality. Hallucinations depicting grotesque creatures such as a "dog with a snake for a tongue" can be extremely frightening. Emotional consequences of such effects are panic, anxiety, confusion, and paranoid reactions. Some person have had frank psychotic reactions after minimal use. In the jargon of the hallucinogens, such an experience is a "bad trip."

MESCALINE AND RELATED SYNTHETIC SUBSTANCES

Mescaline (peyote) is derived from cactus plants found in America. Native Americans harvested peyote "buttons" from cacti and used them in their religious ceremonies. This religious practice is still protected by law and is part of their worship. Manufactured forms of mescaline are STP, DMT, and MDA.

Pharmacokinetics

Mescaline, whether naturally occurring or synthetically produced, is taken orally and is quickly absorbed. Its site of action is probably the norepinephrine synapses. Mescaline passes the blood-brain barrier within 2 hours and usually takes effect within 30 to 40 minutes. Its effects last up to 12 hours. It is excreted in the urine.

Physiologic Effects

With mescaline use, colors are vivid, music is more beautiful, and sounds are more intense. When the user closes his or her eyes, colors and images can be seen. A distorted sense of space and time occurs. A young man who drove his car after taking peyote stated that it seemed to take an eternity to reach a stop sign no more than 50 feet away. The experience is directly related to preingestion expectations. "Good" experiences include hilarity and joy. The user may feel especially insightful. The answers to such questions as those involving the "meaning of life" may seem quite clear. Such insights can easily add to a sense of religious experience.

"Bad trips" are the side effects of concern. Although less potent than LSD, peyote, nonetheless, can cause panic, paranoid thinking, and anxiety when the "trip" is too intense. Dependence does not occur in the strict sense, yet users enjoy the experience and seek to repeat it. Pupil dilation and tremors sometimes occur.

PSILOCYBIN, PSILOCIN

Psilocybin is derived from mushrooms (*Psilocybe mexicana*).

Pharmacokinetics

Psilocybin is taken orally. Once in the stomach, it is converted to psilocin by enzymatic action. Psilocybin decreases the reuptake of serotonin in the brain. Onset of action is experienced in 25 to 40 minutes. Effects last up to 8 hours.

Physiologic Effects

Hallucinations and time, space, and perceptual alterations are experienced and are the sensations that caused American Indians to continue to use psilocybin. Psilocybin dilates the pupils and increases heart rate, blood pressure, and body temperature. Tingling of the skin and involuntary movements can occur. As with other hallucinogens, a sense of unreality can occur. An inability to concentrate may add to feelings of anxiety and lead to panic and paranoia. Hallucinations and illusions may occur. Although no deaths resulting from psilocybin intoxication have been reported, deaths related to perceptual distortions have occurred.

MARIJUANA

Marijuana is probably the drug most widely used illegally in the United States; typically it is used by teenagers and young adults. Marijuana (*Cannabis sativa*) and other related drugs (hashish and tetrahydrocannabinol [THC]) come from a hemp plant. Marijuana is difficult to categorize. Placement with the hallucinogens seems appropriate, but other categorizations are defensible.

Pharmacokinetics

The active ingredient in marijuana is Δ−6−3,4−THC. Tetrahydrocannabinol is changed to metabolites in the body and is stored in fatty tissues. It remains in the body for up to 6 weeks after it is smoked and can be detected in blood and urine for 2 weeks. The effects of smoked marijuana last between 2 and 4 hours. If marijuana is ingested, effects may last up to 12 hours.

Physiologic Effects

Marijuana produces a sense of well-being, is relaxing, and alters perceptions. Euphoria results and is the cause of drug-seeking behaviors. Increased hunger ("munchies") is an effect that makes it useful for anorexic persons (e.g., cancer patients). Marijuana's antiemetic properties make it useful for treating nausea and vomiting associated with chemotherapy.

Balance and stability are impaired for up to 8 hours after marijuana use. Short-term memory, decision making, and concentration are also impaired. Recent research has found that marijuana is toxic to hippocampal cells, cells that are important to these cognitive functions (Schuster, 1990).

Dry mouth, sore throat, increased heart rate, dilated pupils, conjunctival irritation, and keener sight and hearing are physical responses to marijuana. It has been thought to be amotivational, but not all research supports this thinking.

Other effects associated with the use of marijuana include harmful pulmonary effects (bronchitis), weakening of heart contractions, immunosuppression, and reduction of serum testosterone and sperm count. Anxiety, impaired judgement, paranoia, and panic are not uncommon reactions to marijuana. These terrifying experiences may culminate in some health-compromising behavior.

Flashbacks, more commonly associated with LSD, have also been reported with marijuana use. A flashback is a spontaneous reliving of feelings experienced during a "high."

LYSERGIC ACID DIETHYLAMIDE

Pharmacokinetics

Lysergic acid diethylamide stimulates the sympathetic nervous system by inhibiting the reuptake of serotonin. It is taken orally, and onset of action occurs within 30 to 40 minutes. Effects are experienced for up to 12 hours. Extremely small amounts of LSD, usually only 50 to 300 μg, produce these effects.

Physiologic Effects

Lysergic acid diethylamide causes a phenomenon known as synesthesia. Synesthesia is the blending of senses (for example, smelling a color or tasting a sound). Expectations and environment govern the "quality" of the LSD "trip."

Lysergic acid diethylamide causes an increase in blood pressure, tachycardia, trembling, and dilated pupils. Central nervous system effects include a sense of unreality, perceptual alterations and distortion, and impaired judgement. Another problem associated with LSD is flashbacks. Flashbacks are scary and can heighten a sense of "going crazy." Bad trips from LSD use cause anxiety, paranoia, and acute panic. Some persons have had psychotic "breaks" as a result of LSD use and have never fully recovered. A number of persons have killed themselves while under the influence of LSD.

PHENCYCLIDINE

Phencyclidine (PCP), a synthetic drug, traditionally has been used as an animal tranquilizer. Many emergency room nurses are familiar with this drug because PCP-intoxicated persons are often brought to the emergency room: their unpredictable outbursts of violent behavior are legendary. They literally change from coma to violent behavior and back. Caution must be exercised when one is providing care to these patients because of their unpredictable behavior.

Pharmacokinetics

Phencyclidine acts on the brain. It is taken orally and intravenously and is smoked and snorted. Oral PCP takes effect in 5 minutes. Injected or snorted PCP takes effect immediately; effects from smoking PCP take longer. Phencyclidine is well absorbed by all routes. Effects last for 6 to 8 hours. Phencyclidine can be found in the blood and urine for up to 10 days after intake.

Physiologic Effects

The user experiences a "high." Euphoria and a peaceful, easy feeling can occur and are sought. Perceptual distortions are common.

Undesired effects of PCP are many and serious. Blood pressure and heart rate are elevated. Other PNS effects include ataxia, salivation, and vomiting. Psychologic symptoms include hostile, bizarre behavior, a blank stare, and agitation. A catatonic type of muscular rigidity alternating with violent outbursts is particularly frightening to bystanders.

Related Issues

Overdose. High doses of mescaline are not generally toxic, but high doses of STP and MDA can cause hyperexcitability. Deaths have occurred because of these drugs. Psilocybin overdose has not been associated with any deaths, and usually a calm environment is all that is needed to assist withdrawal. LSD- and PCP-related deaths are not uncommon. Deaths can be caused by overdose but are more likely to be associated with perceptual disorientation and unresponsiveness to environmental stimuli. Confusion and acute panic can result from an overdose of marijuana. Diazepam (Valium) can be administered for psilocybin, LSD, and mescaline overdoses. Phencyclidine presents greater problems. Diazepam may be given for seizures and agitation, and haloperidol (Haldol) for psychotic behavior. Acidifying the urine to a pH of 5.5 accelerates excretion of PCP. Urine screening is the best means of identifying abused substances.

Interactions. Mescaline, psilocybin, and LSD can potentiate sympathomimetics. Marijuana should not be used with alcohol, because marijuana masks the nausea and vomiting associated with excessive alcohol consumption. Respiratory depression, coma, and death can occur.

Use during pregnancy. A number of birth defects have been associated with these drugs.

Withdrawal and detoxification. Hallucinogens do not produce physical dependence, so there are no withdrawal symptoms. Symptoms of withdrawal from marijuana are insomnia, restlessness, and hyperactivity. One of the biggest concerns for the clinician is development of an approach for dealing with the intoxicated person. Basically, one should provide a calm, reassuring environment.

REMARKS

The goal of treatment for the chemically dependent person is abstinence from alcohol and drugs. The person who is dependent on one substance can easily become cross-dependent on another. Since patients are rarely "cured," most clinicians view treatment as a lifelong process in which the person is continually "recovering." The term *recovering* indicates an ongoing and dynamic process but also indicates the ever-present possibility of "slipping."

In the psychiatric hospital every patient should be assessed for chemical dependency. It is estimated that one third to one half of all psychiatric patients abuse alcohol or drugs (Carey, 1989, Ananth et al., 1989). Always ask whether the patient drinks or uses other drugs, whether he or she has had problems associated with alcohol and drugs, and whether any relative has had alcohol-related or drug-related problems.

Estes and Heinemann (1986) recommended avoiding the terms *alcoholic* or *addict* early in the assessment process and instead suggested the use of phrases such as "problem with drinking" or "difficulties with drug use." It may also be helpful initially to focus on legal drugs or more culturally accepted drugs such as caffeine and nicotine.

If the patient's responses indicate that he or she is at risk, a more definitive screening tool should be used.

The best known intervention programs are Alcoholics Anonymous (AA) and Narcotics Anonymous (NA). These programs use self-help, a support group model made up of fellow users in various stages of "recovery." Philosophically AA and NA view psychosocial problems as stemming from substance abuse and reject the idea that an underlying psychopathologic disease or disorder is responsible for drinking or drug abuse. Alcoholics Anonymous has established the twelve-step system, which starts with a man or woman admitting his or her powerlessness over alcohol and ends with the person's making himself available, night or day, to another alcoholic in need. The popular bumper sticker slogan "Easy does it" reflects a philosophy of taking life one day at a time and avoiding a frenetic life-style. Alcoholics Anonymous and NA subscribe to the belief that only total abstinence can free the chemically dependent person from the bondage of alcohol and drugs.

Screening Tests

Several screening questionnaires have been developed to assist the health care professional in diagnosing chemical dependency. The Michigan Alcoholism Screening Test (MAST) is a reliable screening test that can be given without extensive training (Powers and Spickard, 1984). It can be modified to identify other drug problems.

The acronym *CAGE*, a questionnaire, is another valid instrument and is easier to use but less discriminating than the MAST. The following questions make up the *CAGE* questionnaire:

1. Have you ever felt you should *Cut* down on your drinking?
2. Have people *Annoyed* you by criticizing your drinking?
3. Have you ever felt bad or *Guilty* about your drinking?
4. Have you ever had a drink first thing in the morning *(Eye-opener)* to steady your nerves or get rid of a hangover?

Two positive responses are suggestive of alcoholism, and three or four positive responses are diagnostic (Whitfield, Davis, and Barker, 1986). Schofield (1988) pointed out that questions 1 and 3 assess introspection and reflection on personal drinking, and question 2 provides reinforcement of this introspection by external cues. Question 4 reflects a change in behavior.

Another tool that distinguishes severity of alcoholism is the Drinking and You self-report instrument (Harrell and Wirtz, 1988). It was specifically developed for use with adolescents and taps four areas: loss of control and social, psychological, and physical symptoms.

The problem with most screening tests has been their susceptibility to faking and denial on the part of the patient (Creager, 1989). The MacAndrew Scale (MacAndrew, 1965), made up of appropriate items from the Minnesota Multiphasic Personality Inventory (MMPI) scale (Allen, Eckardt, and Wallen, 1988), and the Substance Abuse Scale have been developed to overcome denial and lying. The Substance Abuse Scale requires only 10 minutes to complete and claims 90% accuracy of diagnosis (Creager, 1989).

REFERENCES

Allen JP, Eckardt MJ, Wallen J: Screening for alcoholism: techniques and issues, *Public Health Rep* 103:6, 1988.

American Psychiatric Association: *The diagnostic and statistical manual of mental disorders, third edition-revised*, Washington, DC, 1987, The Association.

Ananth J et al: Missed diagnosis of substance abuse in psychiatric patients, *Hosp Community Psychiatry* 40:297, 1989.

Carey KB: Emerging treatment guidelines for mentally ill chemical abusers, *Hosp Community Psychiatry* 40:341, 1989.

Creager C: SASSI test breaks through denial, *Professional Counselor*, July-August, 1989, p 65.

DiGregorio GJ: Cocaine update: abuse and therapy, *Am Fam Physician* 41:247, 1990.

Estes N, Heinemann ME: Issues in identification of alcoholism. In *Alcoholism: development, consequences, and interventions*, ed 3, St Louis, 1986, Mosby.

Frezza M et al: High blood alcohol levels in women: the role of decreased gastric alcohol dehydrogenase activity and first-pass metabolism, *New Engl J Med* 322(2):95, 1990.

Goodwin DW et al:Screening adolescents in adoptees raised apart from alcoholic biological parents, *Arch Gen Psychiatry* 28:238, 1973.

Harrell AV, Wirtz PW: *Screening adolescents for drinking problems*. Paper presented at 1988 National Alcoholism Forum, Arlington, Va, April 1988.

Hough ESE: Alcoholism: prevention and treatment, *J Psychosoc Nurs* 27(1):15, 1989.

Institute of Medicine: Prevention and treatment of alcohol-related problems: research opportunities, *J Stud Alcohol* 53(1):5, 1992.

Joyce T: The dramatic increase in the rate of low birthweight in New York City: an aggregate time-series analysis, *Am J Public Health* 80:682, 1990.

Kaufman E, McNaul JP: Recent developments in understanding and treating drug abuse and dependence, *Hosp Community Psychiatry* 43(3):223, 1992.

Lewis DC, Gordon AJ: Alcoholism and the general hospital: the Roger Williams Intervention Program, *Bull N Y Acad Med* 59:181, 1983.

MacAndrew C: The differentiation of male alcoholic outpatients from non-alcoholic psychiatric outpatients by means of the MMPI, *Q J Stud Alcoholism* 26:238, 1965.

Marzuk PM et al: Prevalence of cocaine use among residents of New York City who committed suicide during a one-year period, *Am J Psychiatry*, 149(3):371, 1992.

Mueller LA, Ketcham K: *Recovering: how to get and stay sober*, New York, 1987, Bantam.

National Foundation for Brain Research: *The cost of disorders of the brain*, Washington, DC, 1992, National Foundation for Brain Research.

Noble J: *Working paper: projections of alcohol abusers, 1980, 1985, 1990*, Washington DC, 1985, NIAAA, Department of Biometry and Epidemiology, National Association of Private Psychiatric Hospitals.

Ohlms D: *The disease of alcoholism* [videotape], Millstadt, Ill, 1988, Gary Whitaker.

Powers JS, Spickard A: Michigan alcoholism screening test to diagnose early alcoholism in a general practice, *Southern Med J* 77:852, 1984.

Regans P: *ABC News and Washington Post poll*, survey no. 0190, Washington, DC, 1985, Washington Post.

Scavnicky-Mylant M, Keltner NL: Chemical dependency. In Keltner NL, Schwecke LH, Bostrom C, editors: *Psychiatric nursing: a psychotherapeutic management approach*, St Louis, 1991, Mosby.

Schofield A: The CAGE questionnaire and psychological health, *Br J Addict* 83:761, 1988.

Schuster, CR: The National Institute on Drug Abuse in the decade of the brain, *Neuropharmacology* 3:315, 1990.

Smith AR et al: Trends in psychotropic prescribing in general practice and general medical patients, *Postgrad Med J* 62:637, 1986.

Wallace J: *Alcoholism: new light on the disease*, Newport, R.I., 1985, Edgehill.

Whitfield C, Davis J, Barker L: Alcoholism. In Barker LR, Burton JR, Zieve PD, editors: *Principles of ambulatory medicine*, Baltimore, 1986, Williams & Wilkins.

CHAPTER 13

Drugs Used to Stimulate the Central Nervous System

Two basic categories of drugs that stimulate the central nervous system (CNS) are cerebral stimulants that mainly affect the cerebral cortex, and analeptics that primarily stimulate the brain stem. Analeptics are used to increase respirations in patients who are having difficulty with breathing. Analeptics do so by stimulating the medullary respiratory control center in the brain stem and by actions on the peripheral carotid chemoreceptors that regulate respiration by sensing blood carbon dioxide levels. A discussion of analeptics is not consistent with the objectives of this book. More information on these drugs can be found in a basic pharmacology text.

The drugs to be considered in this chapter are the cerebral stimulants, commonly referred to as psychostimulants. These agents affect the cerebral cortex and have a number of beneficial psychopharmacologic effects. The potential therapeutic use of cerebral stimulants is compromised by their great potential for abuse. Specific therapeutic uses of cerebral stimulants are also presented in Chapters 8, 15, 16, and 17; specific abuses are discussed in Chapters 10 and 12.

CEREBRAL STIMULANTS

The amphetamines and amphetamine congeners (chemical derivatives of amphetamines) are the major classes of cerebral stimulants, but other drugs are used in a similar manner. Caffeine in beverages; drugs for attention deficit hyperactivity disorder (ADHD), such as methylphenidate (Ritalin) and pemoline (Cylert); and phenylpropanolamine and other related compounds found in many over-the-counter cold, hay fever, stimulant, and anorectic preparations are examples of other cerebral stimulants. Amphetamines are addressed most thoroughly in this chapter, since understanding these drugs enables understanding of other CNS stimulants.

AMPHETAMINES

The amphetamines were first synthesized in 1887, but not until 40 years later were their stimulant effects discovered (Lovgren, 1985). They were first marketed in the United States in 1932 as nasal inhalers, were later used as respiratory stimulants (indicating a broader range of effect than just the cerebral cortex), and in 1937 gained acceptance as a treatment for narcolepsy (Roccaforte and Burke, 1990; Lovgren, 1985).

Amphetamines gained popularity during World War II because they were helpful in overcoming battle fatigue for soldiers. Close to 200 million amphetamine tablets were issued to American soldiers stationed in Britain during the war (Warneke, 1990). Psychostimulants were used in the 1950s in the treatment of depression (Arana and Hyman, 1991). By 1970, 10 billion stimulants were being legally manufactured in the United States (Warneke, 1990).

Today stimulants are the only Food and Drug Administration–approved drugs for the treatment of ADHD (see Chapters 15 and 16), narcolepsy (see Chapter 8), and refractory obesity. Although formerly a preferred treatment approach for obesity, the aforementioned propensity to abuse these drugs coupled with pronounced tolerance and tachyphylaxis (unusually rapid tolerance) have made the prescription of amphetamines for obesity all but unheard of.

Three amphetamines are used for clinical purposes: dextroamphetamine (Dexedrine), racemic amphetamine or amphetamine sulfate, and methamphetamine (Desoxyn). The two forms of amphetamine that are molecular "mirror images" are designated as *d* (dextro) form and *l* (levo) form. These forms are more correctly referred to as isomers and have different pharmacologic properties. To explain the "mirror-image" metaphor, visualize pointing your hand directly into a mirror. Your actual thumb is farthest away from the mirror, and the mirror image of your thumb is set most deeply into the mirror image. This identical yet opposite molecular configuration accounts for a difference in effect. Thus the d-isomer amphetamine (i.e., dextroamphetamine and methamphetamine) is three to four times more potent than the l-isomer amphetamine (Roccaforte and Burke, 1990) and is a more potent CNS stimulant. The *l* form is a more effective cardiovascular system stimulator. "Racemic" amphetamine is a mixture of *d* and *l* forms.

Pharmacologic Effect

Amphetamine is a potent catecholamine agonist that causes the release of biogenic amines and blocks their reuptake (Goldberg et al., 1991; Kuczenski, 1983). Amphetamines have both a CNS and a peripheral nervous system (PNS) effect. These effects are caused "indirectly" through the release of norepinephrine, dopamine, and serotonin from the nerve endings. The concept of indirect action is important, simply meaning that amphetamines stimulate the body by causing the release of these neurotransmitters, which in turn trigger neuronal firing. Examples of direct-acting sympathomimetics include norepinephrine bitartrate (Levophed), epinephrine (Adrenalin), and phenylephrine hydrochloride (Neo-Synephrine). Amphetamines increase catecholamine bioavailability by blocking the reuptake of norepinephrine and dopamine back into the presynaptic nerve ending.

Central nervous system effects. Amphetamines stimulate the cerebral cortex, the brain stem, and the reticular activating system (RAS). The RAS provides sensory neuronal communication between the medulla and the cerebral cortex. Amphetamine cortical effects that account for its abuse potential include wakefulness, alertness, increased concentration, increased motor activity, improved physical performance, decreased fatigue, improved mood, inhibited sleep, and an anorexigenic effect. As noted in the section on side effects, an exaggeration of these pharmacologic effects is precisely the element of amphetamine usage associated with adverse outcomes.

Amphetamines appear to stimulate the reward center of the brain; this stimulation accounts for the great appeal of these drugs. The nucleus accumbens, a small subdivision of the basal ganglia, appears to be a major component of the reward center (Fischbach, 1992). By stimulating the reward center, amphetamines produce a sense of well-being usually reserved for accomplishment, love, or some other rewarding external source of gratification. Amphetamines and other stimulants essentially enhance or perpetuate this sense of well being. Obviously abuse of stimulants can result, as discussed in Chapters 10 and 12.

Research seems to indicate that the euphoric properties of amphetamines may be more closely related to their effects on dopaminergic systems than on norepinephrine or serotonin systems, as formerly thought, This hypothesis stems from the ability of haloperidol (a dopamine antagonist) to block euphoria, which noradrenergic blockers do not do. Amphetamine's anorectic effect probably results from the stimulation of the hypothalamus.

Because of medullary stimulation, respirations are increased by psychostimulants. Such an effect serves to illustrate the well-known fact that drugs have many intersystem and intrasystem effects and that, although the amphetamines produce primarily a cortical effect, they also stimulate subcortical areas.

Paradoxically, in low doses amphetamines may depress the CNS. Occasionally individuals report a sedative effect after taking a low dose. Nonetheless, CNS activity is really a balancing of opposing actions between excitatory and inhibitory neurons and low doses of amphetamines appear to show a preference for inhibitory neurons, consequently causing a shift in the "norm" toward an overall inhibitory response, i.e., CNS depression. This "paradox" is particularly beneficial in normalizing hyperkinetic motor activity and behavior.

Low doses of amphetamines and related drugs such as methylphenidate apparently stimulate the immature RAS in children with ADHD; thus improved functioning results. Normalization of this system presumably enables the ADHD patient to sit and listen, to tune out extraneous stimuli, and to control bothersome motor activity. The precise mechanism of amphetamines and other stimulants used to treat ADHD is not clear.

As the effects of amphetamines wear off, a reversal of the sought-after effects begins to emerge. A sense of well being gives way to despair, concentration turns to irritation and distractibility, and improved physical performance and alertness become fatigue. Some have viewed this reversal of emotions as a roller-coaster ride with the "downs" roughly paralleling the "ups." For many beginning users such swings in emotion discourage further experimentation, but others find the "highs" irresistible and endure the "lows," as discussed in Chapter 12.

Peripheral nervous system effects. The PNS effects of psychostimulants with greatest potential for harm are the cardiovascular effects. Amphetamines may increase blood pressure and heart rate. Tachycardia and tachyarrhythmias can also have serious implications in individuals with preexisting conditions. Paradoxically amphetamines can decrease heart rate through activation of the baroreceptor reflex as a result of increased blood pressure. This baroreceptor reflex increases parasympathetic input to the heart, thus causing bradycardia. Amphetamines also dilate the pupils and cause a decongestion of mucous membranes. Other effects related to abuse are outlined in Chapter 12, and treatment of abuse is discussed in Chapter 10.

Pharmacokinetics

Amphetamines given orally are well absorbed from the gut, are distributed throughout the body, and are highly lipophilic, crossing the blood-brain barrier readily (Chiarello and Cole, 1987). When given orally (the only legally approved route in the United States), they exert both CNS and PNS effects within 30 to 60 minutes. Amphetamines are available in several oral forms, including timed-release capsules, immediate-acting tablets, and an elixir. Other amphetamines come in a chewable, slow-release form.

Amphetamines are not metabolized per se and continue to produce an effect until excreted. Drug effect is terminated by elimination from the body through renal excretion. Renal excretion of dextroamphetamine and other amphetamines is altered by urine pH; acidic urine expedites excretion (a pH of less than 5.6 equals a half-life of

7 hours), whereas urine alkalinization slows elimination (a half-life of up to 30 hours) (Olin, 1990). The average half-life of an amphetamine is 12 hours (Roccaforte and Burke, 1990). Urinary alkalinization extends half-life because molecules are unchanged and hence diffuse quickly back into the bloodstream. An average 7-hour increase in amphetamine half-life results from every one-unit increase in pH (Olin, 1990). Thus the clinician may seek to avoid the use of dietary and pharmacologic substances that alkalinize the urine.

Side Effects

Amphetamine side effects are to a large extent extensions of effects previously mentioned (see the box below). Through the CNS these drugs cause anorexia and consequent weight loss (sometimes desired), insomnia (sometimes desired), overly anxious behavior and moodiness, euphoric feelings that can lead to inappropriate or overly ambitious decisions, and irritability or dysphoria. Growth retardation is a concern in children who are given these drugs for ADHD (see Chapters 15 and 16). Other CNS effects include restlessness, tremor, talkativeness, aggressive behavior, confusion, panic, and increased libido (Clark, Queener, and Karb, 1982).

A toxic paranoid psychosis or toxic delirium, or both, can develop in some individuals. Traditionally the toxic psychosis caused by amphetamines has been viewed as a schizophrenia-like manifestation, in keeping with amphetamine's dopamine-potentiating properties. Some clinicians think that such an analysis, although tempting in light of the dopamine hypothesis of schizophrenia, is oversimplified and argue that this phenomenon closely parallels a dysphoric manic episode. Because amphetamines increase norepinephrine, psychotic symptoms arising from amphetamine intoxication could be attributable to increased norepinephrine bioavailability as well (Breier et al., 1990).

Peripheral nervous system effects, as mentioned previously, include cardiovascular effects (more pronounced with racemic amphetamine) with elevated blood pressure, chilling, palpitations, and, less frequently, tachycardia and tachyarrhythmias. Some

Side Effects of Central Nervous System Stimulants

Central nervous system
Restlessness, dizziness, insomnia, overstimulation, euphoria, anorexia, weight loss

Eye
Mydriasis, photophobia

Metabolic
Hyperglycemia, worsening of diabetic symptoms

Cardiovascular
Palpitations, tachycardia, hypertension, angina, arrhythmias

Gastrointestinal
GI upset, diarrhea

patients have died of circulatory collapse (Clark, Queener, and Karb, 1982). Headaches, pallor, facial flushing, mucous membrane decongestion, mydriasis and photophobia, diarrhea, cramps, vomiting, dry mouth, and abdominal pain are also potential side effects of amphetamines.

Implications

Therapeutic versus toxic levels. Toxic effects generally reflect autonomic overstimulation and cause an extreme exaggeration of side effects previously mentioned. Therapeutic blood levels of amphetamines range from 5 to 10 μg/dl (Olin, 1990). Some individuals can ingest much more than the recommended levels of amphetamines without serious effects, because of tolerance and tachyphlaxis.

Tolerance, as defined in Chapter 10, is an important dimension of treatment with amphetamines. Tolerance to amphetamines occurs in two ways, one more significant than the other. The more significant mechanism is the depletion of norepinephrine from the nerve endings. As norepinephrine is depleted, more and more amphetamine is required to maintain a consistent response. Tolerance to amphetamine can occur after only one or two doses. The second mechanism of amphetamine tolerance is ketosis, a byproduct of amphetamine-caused anorexia. As the individual stops eating, an alteration in metabolism occurs, resulting in ketosis that in turn leads to an acidic urine. As noted previously, acidic urine hastens the excretion of amphetamine.

Although tolerance to almost all of the CNS and PNS effects can occur, no tolerance is observed for the psychotic effects of amphetamines. What this means is that abusers can take doses of amphetamines hundreds of times greater than therapeutic doses without harmful physical effects but remain vulnerable to amphetamine psychosis. High levels of amphetamine ingestion would kill someone who has not developed amphetamine tolerance (Keltner, 1989).

Overdose results in sympathetic hyperactivity, that is, hypertension, tachycardia, and hyperthermia accompanied by the delirium and toxic psychosis previously mentioned (Arana and Hyman, 1991). Grand mal seizures can occur as a physiologic response to an overdose of amphetamine. Deaths have been reported when tachycardias, tachyarrhythmias, hyperthermia, and seizures have converged to compromise body systems (Arana and Hyman, 1991).

Acute overdose treatment includes emptying of stomach contents, the administration of activated charcoal 1 g/kg, and urine acidification. Strategies to treat overdose of amphetamines should also include the use of adrenergic blockers such as phentalomine, to reduce blood pressure and lower pulse rate. Other measures for overdose are supportive. Airway support is critical for patients who are unconscious, and external cooling approaches, including the use of cooling blankets, are required for hyperthermia. Seizures can be controlled with intravenous (IV) benzodiazepine, for example, lorazepam (Ativan) 1 to 2 mg or diazepam (Valium) 5 to 10 mg (Arana and Hyman, 1991). Fluids should be administered until urine flow reaches 3 to 6 ml/kg/hr (Olin, 1990).

Use in pregnancy. Amphetamines are highly lipophilic and cross the placental barrier. Although the d-amphetamines have a federal pregnancy category C rating (potential risk to the fetus), racemic amphetamine is in category X, which is an absolute prohibition against use during pregnancy.

Side effects. Side effects can be minimized somewhat by the following sensible yet conventional supportive measures:

Mydriasis and photophobia: Wearing of protective eyewear out of doors
Weight loss: Taking medication after meals minimizes anorectic effect
Insomnia: Take the last dose at least 6 hours before bedtime; insomnia and restlessness associated with overdose can be treated with lorazepam 1 to 2 mg or diazepam 5 to 10 mg every 1 to 2 hours as needed (Arana and Hyman, 1991)
Cardiovascular effects: Monitor blood pressure and vital signs frequently; guard against other subtle sympathomimetic substances such as coffee and colas that could add to existing system stimulation; severe hypertension and tachyarrhythmias can be treated with IV propranolol 1 mg every 5 to 10 minutes as needed, up to a total of 8 mg (Arana and Hyman, 1991) or with an IV vasopressor (Olin, 1990)
Gastrointestinal upset: Taking amphetamines with meals reduces gastrointestinal upset
Central nervous system effects: When patients become too restless, euphoric, or agitated, reduce the dosage until therapeutic effects are experienced but these side effects are minimized
Toxic psychosis or delirium: Chlorpromazine (Thorazine) 50 mg four times a day IM or haloperidol (Haldol) 5 mg two times a day IM has proven to be an effective intervention (Arana and Hyman, 1991); since chlorpromazine also has antiadrenergic properties, it has the added benefit of reducing blood pressure and pulse rate

Interactions. The major concern with drug interactions is the additive effect of other CNS stimulants (Table 13-1). Prescription, nonprescription, and common dietary substances can potentiate the stimulating effects of amphetamines. Some of the more common interactions include the following:

Table 13- 1 Major Interactions Between Central Nervous System Stimulants and Other Drugs

Interactant	Result of interaction
Acidifying agents (urinary) (ascorbic acid, fruit juices, etc.)	Decreased CNS and PNS effects of cerebral stimulants
Alkalinizing agents (urinary) (sodium bicarbonate)	Increased CNS and PNS effects of stimulants
Antidepressants	Increased antidepressant blood levels
Antihypertensives	Decreased antihypertensive effect with most CNS stimulants
Antipsychotic drugs	Decreased cerebral stimulant effect, decreased peripheral sympathomimetic effect
Central nervous system depressants, including alcohol	Antagonism of desired stimulant effect
Hypoglycemic drugs (insulin, oral hypoglycemics)	Increased or decreased blood glucose levels; poor diabetes control
Lithium	Decreased effect of one or both interactants, poor control of psychiatric disorder
Monoamine oxidase inhibitors	Risk of severe hypertensive episode, stroke
Sympathomimetics	Increased and potentially serious cardiac effects; CNS stimulation; hypertension

Common dietary substances: Coffee, tea, and colas can potentiate the effects of amphetamines

Over-the-counter sympathomimetics such as cold, cough suppressant, allergy, and appetite suppressant medications: These agents enhance the effects of amphetamines

Monoamine oxidase inhibitors: Monoamine oxidase inhibitors (MAOIs) generally should not be given with amphetamines because this combination floods the peripheral synapses with norepinephrine, causing a potential hypertensive crisis

Tricyclic antidepressants: Tricyclic antidepressants (TCAs) in combination with amphetamines may cause increased anticholingergic effects and increased cardiac stimulation

Guanethidine: Amphetamines decrease the antihypertensive effect of guanethidine

Urinary acidifiers: These agents *decrease* the half-life, hence the effect of amphetamines; higher doses of amphetamine might be needed; ascorbic acid and fruit juices acidify the urine

Urinary alkalinizers: These agents *increase* the half-life, hence the effect of amphetamines; lower doses of amphetamine might be indicated; sodium bicarbonate (used for heartburn, particularly in elderly persons) and acetazolamide are examples of urinary alkalinizers

Antipsychotic drugs: These drugs antagonize the effects of amphetamines

Patient education. The patient and family should be taught the following:

To take these drugs early in the day to avoid insomnia

To decrease caffeine consumption

To avoid over-the-counter preparations, as previously described

To avoid alcohol consumption

To observe for rest deficits, since these agents tend to cause an avoidance of rest behaviors

To avoid chewing sustained-released forms of the drug

To increase dosage only on the advice of the prescriber

That amphetamines can mask extreme fatigue, so care should be observed when undertaking potentially hazardous tasks

That these agents can cause nervousness, restlessness, insomnia, dizziness, anorexia, and GI disturbances but that by notifying the prescriber, measures may be developed that can modify these effects

OTHER PRESCRIPTION CENTRAL NERVOUS SYSTEM STIMULANTS

Two other prescription CNS stimulants are available for clinical use. Methylphenidate (Ritalin) and pemoline (Cylert) are two drugs frequently prescribed for both ADHD (see Chapters 15 and 16) and narcolepsy (see Chapter 8).

METHYLPHENIDATE

Methylphenidate (Ritalin) is the most commonly prescribed drug for ADHD and is structurally related to amphetamine (Figure 13-1). It is a milder cortical stimulant than amphetamine (Chiarello and Cole, 1987), being about half as potent, and appears to have a greater effect on mental activities than on motor activities. Its mechanism of action is not fully understood; however, tolerance to the effects of this drug does occur to some extent.

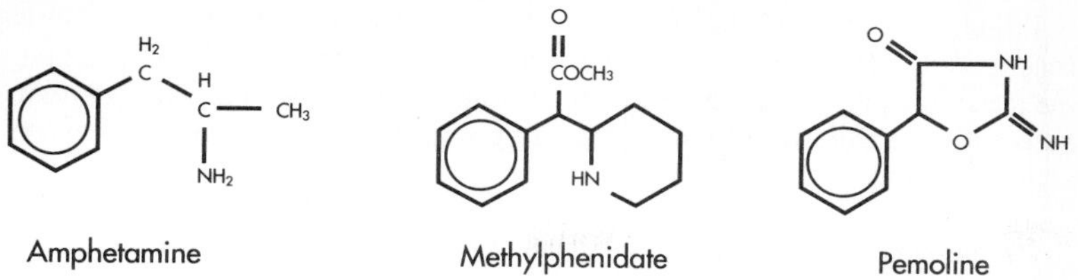

Amphetamine Methylphenidate Pemoline

Figure 13-1 Chemical structures of amphetamine, methylphenidate, and pemoline.

Pharmacokinetics

Methylphenidate is well absorbed from the gastrointestinal tract and reaches peak blood levels within 1 to 3 hours. Its half-life ranges from 1 to 3 hours, but effects last up to 6 hours. Methylphenidate is metabolized in the liver to inactive products (unlike the amphetamines), so urinary acidification or alkalinization does not have an impact on its stimulatory effects. It is excreted in the urine. Methylphenidate is also available in a slow-release form (Ritalin SR).

Side Effects

The side effects of methylphenidate are similar to those of the amphetamines already discussed. Insomnia, restlessness, and nervousness are the most common effects. Anorexia and consequent weight loss are of particular concern to parents of children with ADHD. This concern is addressed in Chapters 15 and 16. In a few individuals anemia and other blood dyscrasias have been linked to methylphenidate treatment. Periodic complete blood cell counts can help the clinician monitor for an untoward effect on the hematologic system.

Implications

Therapeutic versus toxic levels. An overdose of methylphenidate manifests as CNS overstimulation, i.e., agitation, tremors, muscle twitching, euphoria, confusion, hallucinations, delirium, headache, facial flushing, fever, and cardiovascular stimulation such as palpitations, tachycardia, tachyarrhythmias, and hypertension. Treatment is supportive. The patient's environment should be controlled to guard against excessive stimulation that would aggravate physiologic stimulation. If the patient is conscious and if not too much time has elapsed since ingestion, gastric lavage or forced emesis is appropriate. Maintenance of adequate circulation and airway are important. External cooling is appropriate should hyperpyrexia occur.

Use in pregnancy. Although no evidence of fetal malformation has been documented, methylphenidate should not be given to a pregnant woman unless the benefits outweigh the risk to the fetus.

Side effects. The side effects of methylphenidate are similar to those of amphetamines, and interventions discussed for amphetamines are appropriate for methylphenidate. One notable exception is that since methylphenidate is metabolized, acidifying the urine does not hasten its excretion.

Interactions. Most of the interactions associated with amphetamines are also of concern with methylphenidate (Table 13-1). However, methylphenidate also inhibits the metabolism of several antiepileptics, for example, phenobarbital and phenytoin. Essentially the half-lives of these drugs are prolonged, leading to increased effects such as sedation.

Patient education. Patients and families should be taught the following:

To take the last dose of methylphenidate in the afternoon, to avoid methylphenidate-induced insomnia

To take methylphenidate with meals to reduce anorectic effects

To use caution when driving and the like because methylphenidate can mask fatigue

To notify the prescriber when nervousness, insomnia, palpitations, vomiting, and fever occur

To refrain from chewing timed-release capsules

PEMOLINE

Pemoline (Cylert) is an FDA-approved drug for the treatment of ADHD. It is only remotely similar to amphetamine and has minimal sympathomimetic activity (Warneke, 1990). Pemoline is well absorbed from the stomach, and peak serum levels occur within 2 to 4 hours. The half-life is 12 hours, which facilitates once-per-day dosage. About half of each dose is excreted unchanged in the urine; the rest is metabolized before excretion (Keltner, 1989).

Pemoline apparently causes its effect by increasing storage or synthesis of dopamine. A beneficial effect does not occur for 3 to 4 weeks. Pemoline causes less cerebral stimulation than do the amphetamines and methylphenidate; it also has fewer peripheral sympathomimetic effects. Side effects, adverse responses, toxic effects, and appropriate interventions are similar to those for amphetamines (Keltner, 1989). The abuse potential for pemoline is less than that for amphetamines and methylphenidate.

OTHER STIMULANTS: CAFFEINE AND AMPHETAMINE-LIKE ANORECTICS

Many other drugs with stimulant qualities are available. Most of these drugs are sold as anorectics (also referred to as anorexigenics or anorexiants), which are drugs used for weight loss. Other stimulants can be found in foodstuff (caffeine), headache tablets, hay fever and cold remedies, and decongestants. Although some anorectics require a prescription, many other stimulants can be purchased over the counter.

Caffeine

Caffeine is the most widely "abused" drug in the United States. It can be found in coffee, tea, or colas and is an ingredient in more than 1000 over-the-counter medications (Lecos, 1984). Many persons in the United States could not start their day without their eye-opening cup of coffee. In fact, 85% of Americans ingest caffeine daily, with an average consumption of 200 mg/day (Schreiber et al., 1988). Coffee's CNS-stimulating potential with the accompanying "mini-euphoria" makes it popular (Greden, 1974; Greden et al., 1978).

The psychiatric significance of caffeine is related to its ability to produce a sustained anxiety-like syndrome in individuals hypersensitive to its sympathomimetic effects. The *Diagnostic and Statistical Manual of Mental Disorders, Third Edition-Revised (DSM-III-R)* identifies this disorder as *caffeinism*. "The essential features of this disorder include symptoms of restlessness, nervousness, excitement, insomnia, flushed face, diuresis, and gastrointestinal complaints" (American Psychiatric Association [APA] 1987). These symptoms can occur with doses as small as 250 mg per day, but in individuals diagnosed with caffeinism higher doses are usually required. When doses have exceeded 10 grams per day, deaths have been reported (APA, 1987). Table 13-2 lists sources of caffeine.

DSM III-R (APA, 1987) succinctly notes that coffee contains 100 to 150 mg of caffeine per cup, tea about half that amount, and colas about one third. Caffeine containing headache powders contain one third to one half the amount of caffeine in a cup of coffee. Between 20% and 30% of persons in the United States ingest between 500 and 600 mg of caffeine per day (Pilette, 1983) and about 10% consume more than 750 mg per day, the defining point for overuse (Hughes et al., 1992). As many as 10% of persons in the United States could be described as having caffeinism. Hughes et al. (1992) suggested that caffeine withdrawal but not caffeine abuse or dependence be added to the *DSM-IV*.

Excessive caffeine intake is prevalent among psychiatric patients (Hughes et al., 1992). A number of inpatient units across the country have gone "caffeine free" in an attempt to reduce the synergistic impact of too much caffeine on other diagnostic conditions. Anecdotal summaries indicate improvement in patient interactions, a decrease in aggressive outbursts, and facilitation of treatment strategies.

Caffeine stimulates the CNS and heart and relaxes smooth muscle in blood vessels and the bronchi. A faster heart rate coupled with vasodilation leads to increased urine output. Gastric acid and other secretions are also increased, leading to a variety of GI tract ailments. Not all the GI tract disorders associated with coffee are caffeine related. Oils found in coffee, for example, are irritating to the stomach; however, such a discussion lies outside the objectives for this text. The basal metabolism rate of regular coffee drinkers is increased by about 10% (Greden, 1974).

Caffeine's effect apparently is caused by its ability to inhibit the breakdown of cyclic adenosine monophosphate (cAMP), a second messenger in norepinephrine and dopamine neurotransmitter systems. The increase in cAMP bioavailability intensifies other CNS and PNS sympathominetic effects (Keltner, 1989).

Caffeine withdrawal. Caffeine withdrawal is accompanied by headache (and occasionally, vomiting), decreased arousal, and fatigue. Withdrawal effects are reversible with readministration of caffeine.

Phenylpropanolamine

Phenylpropanolamine is a ingredient in over 100 prescription and over-the-counter anorectics, nasal decongestants, psychostimulants, and treatments for premenstrual syndrome (Dilsaver, Votolato, and Alessi, 1989). Table 13-3 lists several well-known compounds that are sold as anorectics. Phenylpropanolamine is often combined with caffeine but can be the only stimulant in the product. The amount of phenylpropanolamine ranges from 25 mg to 75 mg per tablet and should be used only by adults. At somewhat lower doses (i.e., 12.5 mg) it is used in allergy, cough suppressant, and cold medications.

Psychiatrically phenylpropanolamine is important because it intensifies stimulant properties of other sympathomimetics or antagonizes the effects of other psychotropic agents. Phenylpropanolamine is molecularly similar to amphetamine; however, it is a direct-acting sympathomimetic. It acts as a pressor agent because of a strong al-

Table 13-2 Sources of Caffeine

Source	Caffeine content (approximate)
Beverages	
Coffee, brewed (drip)	60-180 mg/5 oz
Coffee, brewed (percolator)	40-170 mg/5 oz
Coffee, instant	30-120 mg/5 oz
Coffee, decaffeinated, brewed	2-5 mg/5 oz
Tea, brewed, major US brands	20-90 mg/5 oz
Tea, instant	25-50 mg/5 oz
Tea, iced	67-76 mg/12 oz
Cocoa	2-20 mg/5 oz
Soft drinks*	
Sugar-free Mr. Pibb	59 mg/12 oz
Mountain Dew	54 mg/12 oz
Tab	47 mg/12 oz
Coca-Cola	46 mg/12 oz
Diet Coke	46 mg/12 oz
Mr. Pibb	41 mg/12 oz
Dr. Pepper	40 mg/12 oz
Big Red	38 mg/12 oz
Pepsi-Cola	38 mg/12 oz
Diet Pepsi	36 mg/12 oz
RC Cola	36 mg/12 oz
Over-the-counter analgesics*	
Anacin, Midol, Vanquish	32 mg/tablet
Excedrin Extra Strength	65 mg/tablet or capsule
Over-the-counter cold preparations*	
Dristan	16 mg/tablet
Triaminicin†	32 mg/tablet
Over-the-counter stimulants*	
No Doz	100 mg/tablet
Vivarin	200 mg/tablet
Prescription medications*	
Darvon compound	32 mg/capsule
Fiorinal	40 mg/tablet or capsule
Cafergot	100 mg/tablet

From Keltner NL. In Schlafer M, Marieb E, editors: *The nurse, pharmacology, and drug therapy,* Redwood City, Calif, 1989, Addison-Wesley.

*A representative sampling of the caffeine-containing preparations in these categories.

†These products also contain phenylpropanolamine.

Data for beverages; over-the-counter analgesics, cold preparations, and stimulants; and prescription medications adapted from Lecos C: *FDA Consumer* 18:14, 1984.

Table 13-3 Representative Over-the-Counter Weight-Loss Products Containing Phenylpropanolamine

Product	Phenylpropanolamine content (mg)
Acutrim	75 (tablet)
Appedrine*	35 (tablet)
Dexatrim capsules*	25, 75 (capsule)
Grapefruit diet plan with Diadax	12.5, 30, 75 (capsule)
Phenoxine	25 (tablet)
Unitrol	75 (capsule)

*Also contains caffeine.

pha-1 effect and a relatively weak beta effect. Subsequent hypertension associated with phenylpropanolamine is often accompanied by a reflex bradycardia (Dilsaver, Votolato, and Alessi, 1989). The box below lists signs and symptoms associated with phenylpropanolamine use in descending order, from most common to least common.

Other anorectics include drugs containing phentermine, phenmetrazine, benzphetamine, phendimetrazine, diethylpropion, mazindol, and fenfluramine (Olin,

Clinical Signs and Symptoms Associated with Phenylpropanolamine Use*

Hypertension
Throbbing bilateral headache
Nausea and emesis
Anxiety
Palpitations
Seizures
Paresthesias
Stroke
Tremor
Hallucinations
Tachycardia
Ventricular ectopy or tachycardia
Myalgias
Reversible renal failure
Increased intracerebral pressure verified by lumbar puncture
Disorientation to person, place, or time
Paranoid psychosis
"Bizarre" behavior (e.g., disrobing in public)
Suicidal behavior

From Dilsaver SC et al: *Am Fam Physician* 39(4):201, 1989.
*Listed in order of decreasing frequency.

1990). These prescription drugs have effects and precautions similar to amphetamine.

TREATMENT CONSIDERATIONS

Amphetamines, methylphenidate, and pemoline are used primarily in the treatment of ADHD and narcolepsy (Table 13-4). Of children with ADHD, 60% to 70% remain symptomatic into their adult years (Garfinkel and Amrami, 1992) and drug dosages given in Chapter 16 may be applicable. Information on the pharmacologic treatment of ADHD is found in Chapters 15 and 16. Information on the treatment of narcolepsy is found in Chapter 8.

Treatment of Depression

Psychostimulants have been prescribed for the treatment of depression (Levin, 1991; Masand, Pickett, and Murray, 1991). Although anecdotal reports are encouraging, research does not tend to support the use of psychostimulants over more conventional antidepressant approaches (Arana and Hyman, 1991). After an extensive review of the literature beginning with the first article by Myerson (1936), Chiarello and Cole (1987) concluded that treating depression with stimulants ". . . is intriguing but clearly insufficient to warrant consideration for FDA approval." In a case study (N = 1) Gupta, Ghaly, and Dewan (1992) reported that a combination of dextroamphetamine and fluoxetine resulted in a "robust response" in only 6 days in a woman previously considered refractory to treatment. A number of other studies support the augmentation role for stimulants in depression (Metz and Shader, 1991; Warneke, 1990).

Treatment of Depressed Medically Ill Patients

Myers and Stewart (1989) reported that methylphenidate has shown promising results with or without TCAs in the treatment of depressed medically ill patients. As an example of a dosing strategy, they reported that 25 mg of desipramine twice a day

Table 13-4 Dosages of Major Central Nervous System Stimulants

Drug	Indications	Usual adult dose (mg/day)
Dextroamphetamine (Dexedrine), schedule II	ADHD	10-30*
	Narcolepsy	5-60 in divided doses
Racemic amphetamine, schedule II	ADHD	10-30*
	Narcolepsy	5-60 in divided doses
Methamphetamine (Desoxyn, Gradument SR), schedule II	ADHD	10-30*
Methylphenidate (Ritalin), schedule II	ADHD	20-40*
	Narcolepsy	20-60 in divided doses
Pemoline (Cylert), schedule IV	ADHD	56.25-75.0*

*Adapted from Arana GW, Hyman SE: *Handbook of psychiatric drug therapy*, Boston, 1991, Little, Brown.

coupled with 10 mg of methylphenidate every morning successfully launched a depressed cancer patient on an appropriate antidepressant regimen. Arana and Hyman (1991) concurred that stimulants have a role in this population and added that stimulants have fewer and less powerful cardiovascular side effects than do traditional antidepressants.

Use as a Challenge Test for Predicting a Response to Antidepressants

Arana and Hyman (1990) suggested that a positive response (a euphoric response) to a dose of amphetamine may be an indication that a particular patient will respond positively to TCAs. However, research on this topic is not conclusive.

Use in Elderly Persons

Roccaforte and Burke (1990) in a review of the literature have found evidence to support the notion that psychostimulants can be particularly helpful in elderly persons who have an amotivational syndrome and depression. Effects on cognition were less remarkable. Kaplitz (1975) and Pickett, Masand, and Murray (1990) found that methylphenidate and dextroamphetamine, respectively, were helpful in treating apathetic and withdrawn elderly patients. This topic is further discussed in Chapter 17.

Caffeine Augmentation of Electroconvulsive Therapy

Coffey et al. (1990) and Ancill and Carlyle (1992) have indicated that giving pretreatment caffeine can facilitate the lengthening of ECT-induced seizure time without necessitating an increase in electrical stimulus (see Chapter 11). Clinical efficacy does not appear to be compromised; furthermore, Coffey et al. (1990) reported a higher response rate in the pretreatment caffeine group (95%) than in the control group (80%).

Treatment of Schizophrenia

Goldberg et al. (1991) sought to improve mood and cognition by the coadministration of dextroamphetamine and haloperidol. Although the theoretic underpinnings of their effort seems reasonable (that amphetamine would selectively stimulate D_1 receptors in the frontal cortex), patients in the study did not improve. Chiarello and Cole (1987) reviewed 10 studies of stimulant-treated schizophrenia (N = 430). Ninety-six patients improved and 162 patients were either unaffected or worse. The authors remained hopeful that a role exists for stimulants in the treatment of schizophrenia. A more recent study (Carpenter, Winsberg, and Camus, 1992) found no benefit when methylphenidate augmentation therapy was used with schizophrenic patients.

Miscellaneous Uses

Central nervous system stimulants have been used in the treatment of mania, neurasthenia, pathologic fatigue, and obsessive-compulsive disorder. Further studies may reveal a more important role for this group of psychotropic drugs than now realized.

REFERENCES

Ancill MB, Carlyle W: Oral caffeine augmentation of ECT, *Am J Psychiatry* 149(1):137, 1992.

American Psychiatric Association: *Diagnostic and statistical manual of mental disorders, third edition-revised,* Washington, DC, 1987, The Association.

Arana GW, Hyman SE: *Handbook of psychiatric drug therapy,* Boston, 1991, Little, Brown.

Breier A et al: Plasma norepinephrine in chronic schizophrenia, *Am J Psychiatry* 147(11):1467, 1990.

Burgess KE Understanding the spectrum of cerebral stimulants *Nursing* 85:50, 1985.

Carpenter MD, Winsberg BG, Camus LA: Methylphenidate augmentation therapy in schizophrenia, *J Clin Psychopharmacol* 12(4):273, 1992.

Chiarello RJ, Cole JO: The use of psyhcostimulants in general psychiatry, *Arch Gen Psychiatry,* 44:286, 1987.

Clark JB, Queener SF, Karb VB: *Pharmacological basis of nursing practice,* St Louis, 1982, Mosby.

Coffey CE et al: Caffeine augmentation of ECT, *Am J Psychiatry* 147(5):579, 1990.

Dilsaver SC, Votolato NA, Alessi NE: Complications of phenylpropanolamine, *Am Fam Physician* 39(4):201, 1989.

Fischbach GD: Mind and brain, *Scientific American* 267(3):48, 1992.

Garfinkel BD, Amrami KK: A perspective on the attention-deficit disorders, *Hosp Community Psychiatry* 43(5):445, 448, 1992.

Goldberg TE et al: Cognitive and behavioral effects of coadministration of dextroamphetamine and haloperidol in schizophrenia, *Am J Psychiatry* 148(1):78, 1991.

Greden JF: Anxiety or caffeinism, *Am J Psychiatry* 131(10):1089, 1974.

Greden JF et al: Anxiety and depression associated with caffeinism among psychiatric inpatients, *Am J Psychiatry* 135(8):963, 1978.

Gupta S, Ghaly N, Dewan M: Augmenting fluoxetine with dextroamphetamine to treat refractory depression, *Hosp Community Psychiatry* 43(3):281, 1992.

Hughes JR et al: Should caffeine abuse, dependence, or withdrawal be added to DSM-IV and ICD-10? *Am J Psychiatry* 149(1):3340, 1992.

Kaplitz SE: Withdrawn apathetic geriatric patients responsive to methylphenidate, *J Am Geriatr Soc* 23:271-276, 1975.

Keltner NL: Central nervous system stimulants. In Shlafer M, Marieb E, editors: *The nurse, pharmacology, and drug therapy,* Redwood City, Ca, 1989, Addison-Wesley.

Kuczenski R: Biochemical actions of amphetamines and other stimulants. In Creese I, editor: *Stimulants: neurochemical, behavioral, and clinical perspectives,* New York, 1983, Raven.

Lecos C: The latest caffeine scorecard, *FDA Consumer* 18:14, 1984.

Levin R: Psychostimulants for depression (letter), *Am Fam Physician* 44(3):758, 763, 1991.

Lovgren K: Amphetamines, *Emergency* 17(6):10, 1985.

Masand P, Pickett P, Murray GB: Psychostimulants for secondary depression in medical illness, *Psychosomatics* 32(2):203, 1991.

Metz A, Shader RI: Combination of fluoxetine with pemoline in the treatment of major depressive disorder, *Int Clin Psychopharmacology* 6(2):93, 1991.

Myers WC, Stewart JT: Use of methylphenidate, *Hosp Community Psychiatry* 40(7):754, 1989.

Myerson A: The effect of benzedrine sulfate on mood and fatigue in normal and neurotic persons, *Arch Neurology Psychiatry* 36:816-822, 1936.

Olin BR: *Facts and comparisons,* Philadelphia, 1990, JB Lippincott.

Pickett P, Masand P, Murray GB: Psychostimulant treatment of geriatric depressive disorders secondary to medical illness, *J Geriatr Psychiatry Neurology* 3(3):146, 1990.

Pilette WL: Caffeine: psychiatric grounds for concern, *J Psychosoc Nurs* 21:19, 1983.

Roccaforte WH, Burke WJ: Use of psychostimulants for the elderly, *Hosp Community Psychiatry* 41(12):1330, 1990.

Schreiber GB et al: Measurement of coffee and caffeine intake: implications for epidemiologic research, *Prevent Med* 17:280, 1988.

Warneke L: Psychostimulants in psychiatry, *Can J Psychiatry* 35:3, 1990.

Weisman RS, Lewin N: The toxic emergency: over-the-counter weight loss, *Emerg Med* 16(11):169, 1984.

CHAPTER 14

Drugs Used to Treat Extrapyramidal Side Effects

The discussion of material in this chapter should, perhaps, precede the chapter on antipsychotic drugs. Generally the understanding of the primary group of drugs presented here, that is, anticholinergic and antiparkinson drugs, can better delineate and characterize the pharmacologic effects of neuroleptic agents. The mention of antipsychotic drugs is deliberate because that class of drug is most often responsible for side effects that are routinely treated with other drugs.

Antipsychotic drugs cause a number of side effects ostensibly created by a reduction in central nervous system (CNS) dopamine. These undesired effects are referred to as extrapyramidal side effects (EPSEs) and include akathisia, dystonia, akinesia, drug-induced parkinsonism, dyskinesia and tardive dyskinesia, and neuroleptic malignant syndrome. A narrative review of these reactions is given in Chapter 4. The box on p. 294 summarizes the information found in Chapter 4 and provides a ready reference in this chapter. The authors think the best approach to understanding EPSEs is, first, to review the biochemical mechanisms associated with parkinsonism and then, based on that discussion, to trace the concept of EPSEs.

REVIEW OF PARKINSONISM

Parkinsonism is a chronic and progressive neurodegenerative disorder. Degeneration is known to occur in pigmented brain-stem nuclei, particularly in an area of the brain referred to as the substantia nigra, a major dopamine-generating portion of the brain. About 1% of these neurons are lost per year (Scherman et al., 1989), and total cell loss can approach 90% in severely impaired patients with Parkinson's disease (Agid, 1991). A certain cell-depletion threshold of about 50% to 60% in the substantia nigra must occur before symptoms become evident (Agid, 1991). Increased activity by remaining healthy cells and hypersensitivity of dopaminergic receptors account for the lack of symptoms in individuals with dopaminergic cell loss below this threshold.

The substantia nigra is part of a larger system, the extrapyramidal system. Reductions in dopamine synthesis capability in the substantia nigra cause a profound effect on posture, walking, balance, and other muscle-dependent activities. For an individual to successfully negotiate everyday movement, a balance is needed between two neurotransmitter systems, dopamine and acetylcholine (ACh). In parkinsonism there is too little dopamine and a relative excessive level of ACh (a relative excess because a "normal" level of ACh biochemically reacts as such when dopamine is below "normal" levels).

The three primary symptoms of parkinsonism, tremor, bradykinesia, and rigidity, are caused by massive destruction of nigrostriatal dopaminergic neurons (Agid, 1991). Many secondary symptoms are also present. Tremors are common, affecting about 75% of all patients with parkinsonism. Tremors can usually be detected in at least one arm or hand when the person is at rest. Tremors are typically more amena-

Extrapyramidal Side Effects (EPSEs)

Akathisia	Restless legs, "jitters," "nervous energy," motor agitation, most common of all EPSEs (50% or more)
Akinesia	Weakness (hypotonia), fatigue, painful muscles, anergy (lack of energy), absence of movement
Dystonias, Dyskinesias	Grimacing, torticollis, intermittent spasms, opisthotonus, oculogyric crisis, head-neck syndromes, myoclonic twitches, laryngeal-pharyngeal dystonia, which can be life-threatening
Drug-induced parkinsonism	Loss of associated movements, tremor, dysphagia, dysarthria, loss of facial expression, sialorrhea, festinating gait, increased muscle tone, rigidity
Tardive dyskinesia	"Late appearing" (in voluntary muscles), not related to dopamine-acetycholine imbalance, affects 15% to 25% of patients receiving neuroleptics, affects muscles of mouth and face, lipsmacking, grinding of teeth, rolling or protrusion of tongue, tics, diaphragmatic movements that may impair breathing, severity fluctuates, disappears during sleep
Neuroleptic malignant syndrome	Hyperthermia (up to 108° F reported), muscular rigidity, impaired ventilations, muteness, altered consciousness, autonomic hyperactivity, occurs in up to 1% of patients receiving neuroleptics, can be fatal

ble to treatment than are other symptoms. Bradykinesia is a generalized motor slowing. Masked facies (the slowing down of face movements); slowed arm swing; and difficulty initiating, maintaining, and stopping movement are several dimensions of bradykinesia. Rigidity, sometimes referred to as lead-pipe or cogwheel rigidity, impairs movement and makes the simple acts of getting out of a chair or gripping a pen so difficult that patients sometimes defer rather than attempt them.

Other important symptoms include postural difficulties, a gait disorder characterized by shuffling steps, and orthostatic hypotension. Falls are a major source of injury. Gait and postural disturbances seem to be the most treatment-resistant symptoms and are probably caused by nondopaminergic lesions "downstream" from the dopaminergic nerve terminals. Depression and dementia (15% to 20%) (Clough, 1991) are not uncommon and in the case of depression can be partially explained by the decreased levels of dopamine, a precursor to norepinephrine. Figure 14-1 depicts the synthesis of norepinephrine from dopamine. Although dopamine deficiency constitutes the bulk of parkinsonian abnormalities, other neuronal systems are also in-

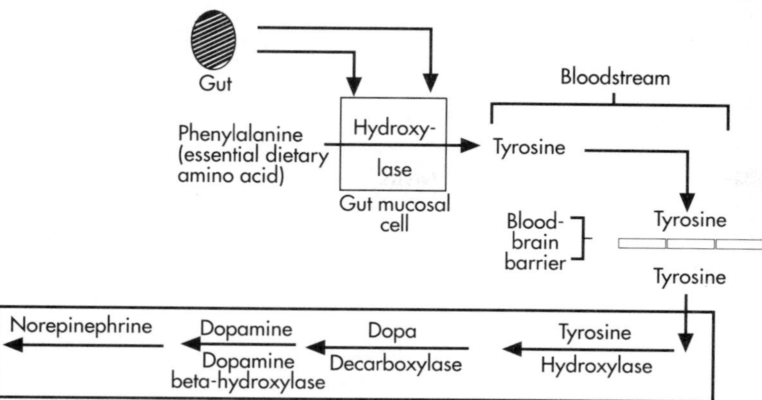

Figure 14-1 The dietary amino acid phenylalanine diffuses through mucosal cells in the GI tract and is metabolized to tyrosine. Tyrosine crosses the blood-brain barrier, enters brain neurons, and is metabolized to dihydroxyphenylalanine (Dopa), which is chemically identical to levodopa, and then to dopamine. Dopamine is converted further to norepinephrine, epinephrine, or both. In Parkinson's disease dopaminergic nerves degenerate, creating an imbalance with opposing effects of acetylcholine that is released from nearby nerves (not shown). In drug-induced parkinsonism, dopaminergic nerves may be intact but postsynaptic dopamine receptors are blocked.

volved (Agid, 1991). Norepinephrine, serotonergic, and cholinergic systems are also disrupted and contribute to symptoms of depression and disturbed cognition.

Secondary symptoms include dysphagia that creates difficulty with eating and can cause excessive accumulation of saliva leading to drool (sialorrhea). Weight loss and choking are two important consequences of dysphagia. The combined effect of bradykinesia and rigidity impair respirations (rigid, immobile respiratory muscles), bladder emptying (rigidity and retarded initiation of stream), and bowel evaluation (a rigid and immobile bowel, leading to constipation or incontinence).

Although the previously mentioned symptoms are common among patients with idiopathic parkinsonism (referred to as Parkinson's disease with cause unknown), the symptoms can also be caused by a parkinson-like condition related to the use of antipsychotic drugs. Antipsychotic drugs block dopamine receptors, frequently causing EPSEs. Many symptoms associated with Parkinson's disease, such as tremor, rigidity, and bradykinesia, are present in drug-induced parkinsonism, along with such related symptoms as akathisia, dystonic reactions, and dyskinesias. These symptoms contribute to the discomfort, anxiety, and frustration of individuals who are already suffering tremendous psychologic anguish. Patients taking antipsychotic drugs can experience EPSEs gradually over time or can have a sudden, dramatic onset of symptoms. The following case history illustrates the latter point:

> A 19-year-old male patient who was taking the antipsychotic drug fluphenazine (Prolixin), was brought to the nurse's station by another patient. The young man was screaming that he could not see. The patient's eyes were rolled upward in such an extreme way that severely limited vision resulted. The patient was experiencing oculogyric crisis. He was in a state of panic and other patients were beginning to feel very anxious and frightened. An "as needed" order for benztropine (Cogentin) 5 mg, was administered intramuscularly. Within 15 minutes the patient responded.

Some clinicians think that a minimal level of EPSEs is related to a therapeutic response (Bitter, Scheurer, and Volavka, 1992).

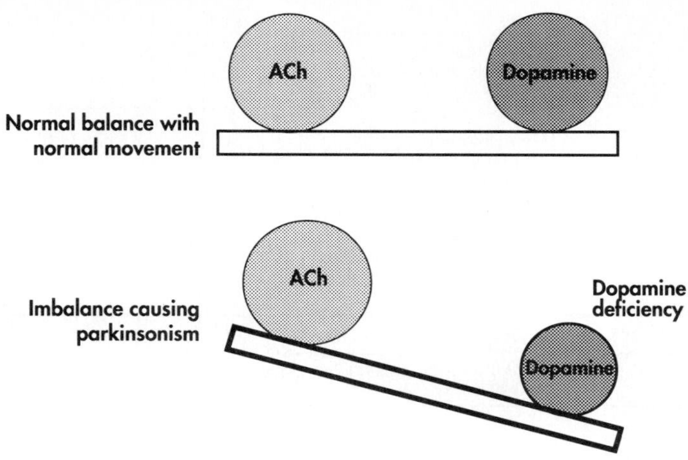

Figure 14-2 Normal and imbalanced states of acetylcholine (ACh) and dopamine.

Drugs Used to Treat Parkinsonism

If the proposed model of parkinsonism is correct (Figure 14-2), it would seem that a reasonable approach could occur in one of two ways. One could attempt to increase dopamine availability or one could attempt to decrease the availability of ACh (Figure 14- 3). The two approaches basically capture the existing approaches to treat parkinsonism. Consequently two classes of antiparkinson drugs exist for the treatment of these patients, dopaminergic antiparkinson agents (those that increase dopamine) and anticholinergic antiparkinson agents (those that block ACh). Parkinsonism caused by neuroleptic drugs is treated most often with the anticholinergic antiparkinson drugs, and much of this chapter is devoted to those agents. However, dopaminergic drugs can be used and are also discussed. Dopaminergic drugs are discussed first.

Dopaminergic antiparkinson drugs. Since parkinsonism is caused by a deficiency in dopamine, it would seem reasonable to give the patient dopamine. However, because dopamine does not pass the blood-brain barrier easily, the large amounts that must be given to achieve therapeutic levels in the brain would produce serious adverse peripheral nervous system (PNS) effects. Therefore, dopaminergic agents, which cross the blood-brain barrier easily and increase dopamine levels in the brain, have been developed to treat parkinsonism. They fall into the following categories:

1. Dopamine precursors, for example, levodopa and carbidopa-levodopa (Sinemet): These drugs *are not* prescribed for drug-induced parkinsonism and interact with most psychotropic medications
2. Dopamine releasers: Amantadine, (Symmetrel) for example, releases the small amounts of dopamine remaining in the dopaminergic neurons in the brain; Amantadine *is used* to treat drug-induced parkinsonism
3. Dopamine agonists: Bromocriptine (Parlodel) and pergolide (Permax), for example, which mimic dopamine at the postsynaptic receptors in the brain; bromocriptine *is used* to treat neuroleptic malignant syndrome

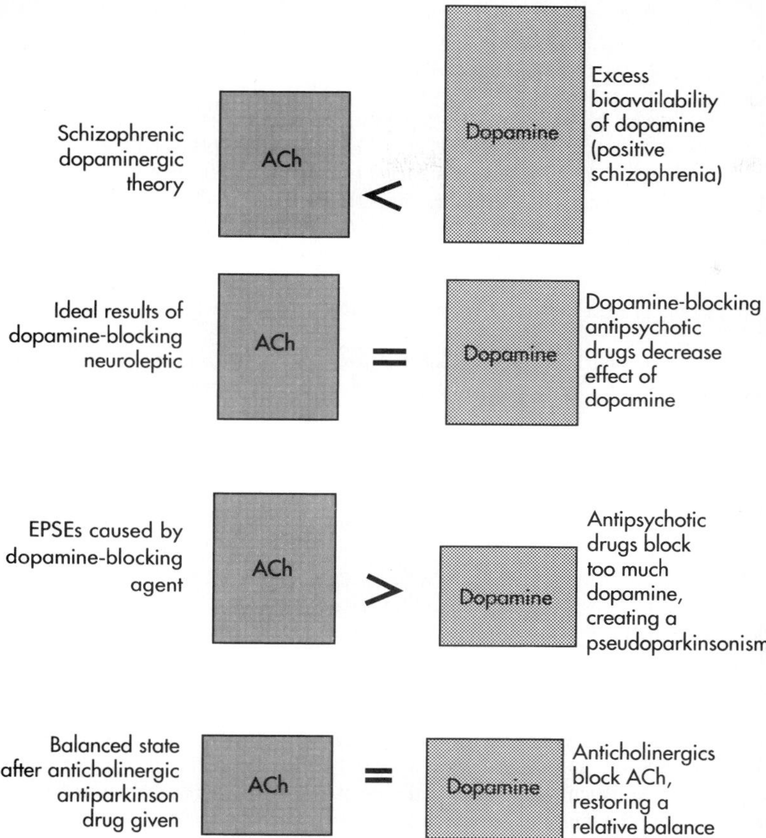

Figure 14-3 Theoretic neurochemical model of schizophrenia.

4. Dopamine metabolism inhibitors: selegiline (Eldepryl), for example, which apparently blocks the metabolism of dopamine by inhibiting monoamine oxidase; Selegiline *is not used* for the treatment of drug-induced parkinsonism

If this were a chapter on the treatment of parkinsonism, it would be important to discuss all the dopaminergic antiparkinson drugs; however, since the focus is primarily on drug-induced parkinsonism, only the dopamine releaser amantadine and the dopamine agonist bromocriptine are discussed.

Dopamine releaser: amantadine. Amantadine (Symmetrel) is a dopamine releaser. It releases the remaining dopamine available in the otherwise dopamine-depleted dopaminergic neurons. It is also thought to inhibit the reuptake of dopamine.

Amantadine was first used as an antiviral drug; however, its application as an antiparkinson drug has been established, even in the treatment of drug-induced parkinsonism (unlike levodopa). Since amantadine has an anticholinergic aspect, it is often used initially in the treatment of parkinsonism and is coming to be used more often in the treatment of drug-induced EPSEs.

Amantadine is absorbed well from the gastrointestinal tract. Peak plasma levels occur about 4 hours after it is administered. The half-life is 18 to 24 hours. Amantadine is excreted unchanged by the kidneys. Impaired renal function slows the excretion of amantadine and can lead to amantadine intoxication. Its excretion is hastened by acidifying the urine.

When used in the treatment of true parkinsonism, amantadine is most effective during earlier stages of the illness because its effectiveness depends on availability of residual dopamine. In more advanced stages amantadine is effective when used adjunctively with levodopa or some other antiparkinson drug. A major drug interaction when administering amantadine is its use with other anticholinergic drugs such as antipsychotic drugs. Theoretically amantadine is less likely to interact with high-potency antipsychotic drugs such as fluphenazine (Prolixin) because they have fewer anticholinergic properties than do the low-potency drugs such as chlorpromazine (Thorazine).

Common side effects of amantadine are drowsiness and confusion. More serious side effects include depression and a psychosis featuring delusions and both visual and auditory hallucinations. The seizure threshold is lowered, and patients with a history of seizures are at risk. Side effects common to anticholinergic drugs, such as blurred vision, orthostatic hypotension, and urinary retention, are also relatively common. A unique side effect of amantadine is the skin reaction referred to as livedo reticularis, a condition in which the skin becomes purple and localized edema develops.

Overdose and toxic effects are treated by stopping drug absorption; that is, induced vomiting, gastric lavage, or administration of activated charcoal. An anticholinergic syndrome is manifested by excitability, delirium, hallucinations, seizures, hypotension, urinary retention, and arrhythmias. Although acidifying the urine theoretically might hasten amantadine excretion, in practice the problem of urinary retention makes this approach risky. There is no specific antidote for amantadine, but physostigmine, a drug traditionally used to treat atropine poisoning, may be beneficial (Olin, 1990).

Adults are usually prescribed an oral dose of 100 mg twice per day up to 400 mg per day for EPSEs. Since the tablet is so large, many geropsychiatric patients are prescribed the syrup form for easy swallowing.

Dopamine agonist: Bromocriptine, for treatment of neuroleptic malignant syndrome. Dopamine agonists are drugs that mimic dopamine by directly stimulating dopaminergic postsynaptic receptors, thus producing a dopamine-like effect. Technically bromocriptine does not add dopamine to the system; it adds a dopamine substitute. Bromocriptine's primary use as a drug to treat the side effects of psychotropic drugs is its usefulness in the treatment of neuroleptic malignant syndrome. Bromocriptine is of obvious benefit in the treatment of Parkinson's disease and is also used to treat endocrine disorders (it inhibits prolactin secretion). Besides bromocriptine, other dopamine agonists include pergolide (Permax) and lisuride; these drugs are not currently used to treat the side effects of psychotropic drugs.

Bromocriptine is not well absorbed from the gastrointestinal tract. The drug is metabolized in the liver and primarily excreted in the feces. Hypotension is a major side effect of bromocriptine. Anxiety, hallucinations, depression, and confusion have been reported. Interaction with antipsychotic drugs may occur because by definition these drugs block dopamine receptors, the site of the agonistic effects of bromocriptine. If bromocriptine is needed, however, antipsychotics have usually been discontinued. When combined with other antihypertensives, bromocriptine can potentiate hypotensive effects. Other bromocriptine interactions pertain more to longer-term use than that associated with the treatment of neuroleptic malignant syndrome. Overdose and toxic effects cause an intensification of the side effects mentioned previously. If overdose is suspected, the drug should be discontinued and supportive, symptomatic care instituted.

Anticholinergic antiparkinson agents. Anticholinergic antiparkinson agents are the agents most often used to treat drug-induced side effects of neuroleptics. Because of their importance, they are discussed here.

ANTICHOLINERGIC ANTIPARKINSON AGENTS

Parkinson's disease, according to the model proposed in Figure 14-3, can be treated by decreasing the availability of ACh. Anticholinergic antiparkinson drugs are presumably effective because they do that very thing. Anticholinergic agents block ACh, thus restoring a relative balance within the dopamine-depleted system. Anticholinergic antiparkinson agents are generally less effective than levodopa but are beneficial in the early stages of parkinsonism and, in fact, are the drugs most often prescribed. Although several of these drugs are used to treat parkinsonism, only three or four are routinely used to treat drug-induced parkinsonism and the related EPSEs.

The anticholinergic antiparkinson drugs used most often in the treatment of drug-induced parkinsonism and other EPSEs are trihexyphenidyl (Artane), benztropine (Cogentin), biperiden (Akineton), and procyclidine (Kemadrin). In addition, antihistamines (e.g., diphenhydramine [Benadryl]), have central anticholinergic effects and are often used substitutively for anticholinergic antiparkinson drugs. The antihistamines have fewer peripheral nervous system (PNS) side effects and may be better tolerated by elderly persons. Trihexyphenidyl is discussed as the prototype anticholinergic antiparkinson drugs.

Pharmacologic Effects

Trihexyphenidyl and the related anticholinergic drugs inhibit the actions of ACh in the brain. Acetylcholine receptors are blocked by these drugs. They may also inhibit the reuptake of dopamine (Olin, 1990). Both effects contribute to restoration of the acetylcholine-dopamine balance. When used to treat Parkinson's disease, trihexyphenidyl is often used adjunctively with dopaminergic drugs. In the treatment of EPSEs trihexyphenidyl is used alone.

Pharmacokinetics

Trihexyphenidyl and the related drugs are usually given orally. Little pharmacokinetic information is available on these drugs; however, it is known that the half-lives of these drugs range from 6 to 10 hours for trihexyphenidyl and from 18 to 24 hours for benztropine. The peak concentration level is achieved in about 1 hour. They are excreted by the renal system. When trihexyphenidyl is used to treat EPSEs caused by antipsychotic drugs, 1 mg is given initially with 1 mg added every few hours until the reaction has been controlled. The usual dosage is 5 to 15 mg per day. In a crisis situation, when an oculogyric crisis or other dystonic reaction occurs, a more aggressive approach with intramuscular injection(s) must be pursued.

Side Effects

The anticholinergic antiparkinson drugs have the side effects associated with atropine. These drugs act both centrally and peripherally. About 19% to 30% of patients taking anticholinergics have CNS effects such as confusion, depression, delusions,

Table 14-1 Side Effects and Interventions for Anticholinergics

Side effects	Appropriate nursing interventions
Dry mouth	Provide sugarless hard candy and chewing gum; frequent rinses
Nasal congestion	Over-the-counter nasal decongestant, if approved by physician
Urinary hesitancy	Running water, privacy, warm water over perineum
Urinary retention	Catheterize for residual urine, encourage fluid intake and frequent voiding
Blurred vision, photophobia	Reassurance; normal vision typically returns in a few weeks; wear sunglasses; caution about driving.
Constipation	Laxatives, as ordered; diet with roughage
Mydraisis	Instruct patient to report eye pain immediately
Orthostatic hypotension	Request patient to get out of bed slowly, to sit on the edge of the bed a short while, then rise slowly
Sedation	Help the patient get up early and get the day started
Decreased sweating	Can lead to fever; take reading of temperature; if fever occurs, reduce body temperature (e.g., sponge baths)

and hallucinations (Olin, 1990). In addition, drowsiness and agitation are common central responses. The cholinergic system is implicated in memory and learning, and anticholinergic drugs can compromise both systems, particularly in elderly persons. Peripheral nervous system effects such as dry mouth, blurred vision, nausea, and nervousness occur in 30% to 50% of these patients. Constipation, a problem for many patients taking antipsychotic drugs, can be worsened by anticholinergics. Urinary hesitancy and retention, decreased sweating, tachycardia, and mydriasis are other PNS effects. Decreased sweating contributes to hyperthermia, a side effect with potentially serious outcome. Table 14-1 summarizes common anticholinergic side effects and appropriate intervention strategies.

Implications

Therapeutic versus toxic drug levels. The therapeutic dosage range for trihexyphenidyl is 5 to 15 mg per day for drug-induced EPSEs. Overdose may result in CNS hyperstimulation, confusion, excitement, hyperpyrexia, agitation, disorientation, delirium, and hallucinations. Convulsions, sometimes fatal, can develop related to hyperthermia associated with atropine poisoning. Overdose can also result in CNS depression, drowsiness, sedation, or coma. The atropine-like effects summarized in Table 14-2 intensify. The mental symptoms of the patient receiving neuroleptics may also intensify. Circulatory collapse, cardiac arrest, and respiratory tract depression or arrest have been reported.

Treatment for anticholinergic antiparkinson drug overdose is similar to that for atropine overdose. The major emphasis is to prevent further absorption. Three mechanisms can be used: gastric lavage, induced vomiting, and ingestion of activated charcoal. The literature seems to support gastric lavage as the preferred approach, particularly when the patient is conscious. If CNS stimulation occurs, a short-acting barbiturate (e.g., thiopental) may be ordered but because stimulation could be preceding CNS depression, caution must be observed. Supportive care (airway maintenance, assisted breathing) and monitoring hyperthermia (rectal temperatures) and vital signs are important. Peripheral nervous system effects can be relieved by giving 5 mg of pilocarpine by mouth and repeating, if necessary (Olin, 1990). More serious or life-threatening situations may require advanced supportive efforts such as treating hyperthermia with a cooling blanket, tepid baths, or ice packs; treatment of seizures with parenteral diazepam; the use of physostigmine (in adults, 1 to 2 mg intramuscularly or intravenously at a rate of no more than 1 mg/min) to reverse cardiac and CNS effects; and fluids and vasopressors for circulatory collapse (Olin, 1990).

Use in pregnancy. Anticholinergics should be used cautiously during pregnancy. Theoretically these drugs decrease milk flow during lactation.

Side effects. Many bothersome side effects are associated with trihexyphenidyl and the other anticholinergics. Table 14-1 lists appropriate interventions. Other considerations include the following:

- Cautious use in patients with tachycardia or other arrhythmias caused by the blocking or "braking" activity of the cholinergic system on the heart
- Cautious use in older men with prostatic hypertrophy caused by the inhibition of the urinary system; anticholinergics relax the detrusor muscle of the bladder and contract trigone muscle and sphincter, thus creating significant mechanical barriers to urination; by definition, men with prostatic hypertrophy already have significant mechanical barriers to urination; thus anticholinergics intensify those problems
- Awareness that anticholinergics may mask the development of EPSEs because of their high anticholinergic properties
- Caution should be followed when administering these drugs during hot weather, particularly in elderly persons; the major culprit is decreased sweating, which prevents the body from cooling down

Interactions. Many over-the-counter drugs have anticholinergic properties and potentiate anticholinergic antiparkinson drugs. Antihistamines, commonly a component of cold medicines, are major interactants. Other major interactants with potential for additive anticholinergic effects are amantadine, antiarrhythmics, antimuscarinics, antipsychotics, monoamine oxidase inhibitors, and TCAs. Elderly persons are most at risk for this additive effects.

Alcohol and other depressants can increase drowsiness and should be avoided, if possible. Antacids and antidiarrheals decrease the absorption of antiparkinson drugs, and 1 to 2 hours should be allowed between doses of these interacting drugs.

Patient Education

Patient education is an important part of the care of patients taking neuroleptics and patients taking antiparkinson agents to decrease drug-induced side effects. Patients should be taught the following:

- To report sudden, marked changes in bowel or bladder function
- To not discontinue the drug suddenly
- To avoid driving or other hazardous activities, if drowsiness is a side effect
- To report eye pain immediately
- To avoid strenuous activities in hot weather
- To avoid the use of over-the-counter and prescription drugs that contain anticholinergic properties (cold and hay fever medications)

Other patient teaching concerns for individual drugs can be reviewed in the Psychotropic Drug Profiles section of this book.

RELATED ANTICHOLINERGIC ANTIPARKINSON DRUGS

Benztropine

Benztropine (Cogentin) is used to treat drug-induced EPSEs and is also prescribed on a prophylactic basis (Table 14-2). It is the most frequently prescribed drug for EPSEs. An intramuscular form is available for noncompliant patients and for emergency intervention during an acute EPSE reaction such as oculogyric crisis. The oral form of the drug should be substituted for parenteral routes as soon as the patient's condition stabilizes. Since benztropine belongs to a different chemical class from trihexyphenidyl, benztropine may be effective when trihexyphenidyl is not. Benztropine causes greater and longer-lasting muscle relaxation and sedation than does trihexyphenidyl. The more intense sedative effect may not be desirable for some patients but may make benztropine more desirable for others. Benztropine is less likely to cause a euphoric effect than is trihexyphenidyl, so benztropine is less likely to be abused. These differences notwithstanding, benztropine should be considered the equivalent of trihexyphenidyl in peripheral anticholinergic effect.

Biperiden

Biperiden (Akineton) is used occasionally to treat drug-induced EPSEs. It is chemically related to trihexyphenidyl. It is usually given orally but can be administered parenterally for acute drug-induced extrapyramidal reactions.

Procyclidine

Procyclidine (Kemadrin) is used infrequently to treat drug-induced EPSEs and is particularly effective in alleviating rigidity. It is not effective in reducing tremor and may actually increase tremors early in treatment. Parenteral forms are not available. It is best given after meals.

Table 14-2 Adult Dosages for Selected Antiparkinson Agents

Agent	Dosage	Intramuscular, intravenous dosage for acute EPSEs
Trihexyphenidyl (Artane)	To start: 1 mg with 1 mg q few hours until symptoms controlled; maintenance or prophylactic, 5-15 mg/day	—
Benztropine (Cogentin)	To start: 1-4 mg qd or bid; prophylactic: 1-2 mg bid or tid	IM/IV 1-2 mg; may repeat; switch to oral dosage as soon as possible
Biperiden (Akineton)	2 mg qd-tid	IM/IV 2 mg qd 30 min prn; do not exceed 8 mg/24 hr
Procyclidine (Kemadrin)	2.5 mg tid; up to 10-20 mg/day	—
Diphenhydramine (Benadryl)	25-50 mg tid-qid	IM/IV 10-50 mg; not to exceed 400 mg/day

Diphenhydramine

Diphenhydramine (Benadryl) is not an anticholinergic antiparkinson agent but is the prototype antihistamine (H_1 antagonist). It has anticholinergic capabilities *and* appears to inhibit dopamine reuptake, providing two means of reestablishing the acetylcholine-dopamine balance. It is better tolerated in older patients who cannot tolerate the more potent anticholinergic antiparkinson agents. It is usually given orally, but can be given parenterally.

ISSUES IN ANTIPARKINSON DRUG ADMINISTRATION

A number of issues exist surrounding the use of antiparkinson agents in the treatment of drug-induced parkinsonism and other EPSEs. These issues are presented in the form of questions and answers.

Is prophylactic antiparkinson treatment necessary and helpful?
Although it is known that these agents are therapeutic for acute EPSEs, it is not known whether they are beneficial as prophylaxis for drug-induced EPSEs. Some practitioners think that proplylactic use prevents the patient from having the annoying and discouraging side effects; other practitioners do not find prophylactic use helpful.

Arguments for prophylactic use include the following:

1. Rectifies poor assessment. Antiparkinson agents are particularly beneficial for akinesias, an extremely annoying EPSE that may contribute the most to noncompliance. Akinesia is often gradual in onset and can provoke listlessness, which in turn can be assessed as an exacerbation of psychosis. Prophylactic use would protect the patient from poor assessment practices.
2. Increases compliance. Extrapyramidal side effects are a major source of noncompliant behavior. If EPSEs can be minimized, the patient will be more likely to comply with the medication regimen.
3. Prevents frightening EPSEs. Antiparkinson agents would prevent the development of frightening dystonic reactions that not only reinforce negative impressions of neuroleptic therapy but also can be health threatening.
4. High prevalence of EPSEs: It is estimated that as many as 75% of all patients taking antipsychotic drugs have some level of EPSEs (Blair, 1990).
5. Depot and high-potency drugs. The extensive use of high-potency and depot drugs during the past decade increases the need for the use of antiparkinson agents as prophylactic agents.

Arguments against prophylactic use include the following:

1. Not needed. Although most patients report EPSEs, only a few have severe symptoms.
2. New problems created. Antiparkinson drugs cause additional side effects, including toxic anticholinergic psychosis.
3. Dangerousness. Antiparkinson drugs mask the development of tardive dyskinesia, which is irreversible.
4. Questionable value. Even maintenance treatment is no guarantee that EPSEs will not occur (Comaty et al., 1990).
5. Decreased effects of neuroleptics. Anticholinergics interfere with the therapeutic effects of neuroleptics by impeding absorption.

Many clinicians think that the disadvantages of prophylactic use of antiparkinson agents for EPSEs outweigh the advantages of their prophylactic use. Hence antiparkinson drugs are often not prescribed until EPSEs occur and then are discontinued as soon as possible (4 to 8 weeks). An exception is use in young men receiving antipsychotic drugs. The rate of EPSEs among this age group is so high that many clinicians who might not consider prophylactic use in an older or female patient do order these drugs for prophylactic use in young men.

What is the potential for abuse or misuse of anticholinergic antiparkinson drugs, and how common is abuse or misuse?

"A review of the literature indicates that the anticholinergic antiparkinson drugs can be abused by some patients to achieve pleasurable effects ranging from a mild euphoria with increased sociability at the lower doses to a toxic anticholinergic psychosis with disorientation and hallucinations at higher doses" (Smith, 1980). Trihexyphenidyl may have the highest abuse potential, but this may be more a function of greater historical availability. Apparently the major effects sought by abusers are (1) a toxic confusional state accompanied by hallucinations, paranoia, and impairment of recent memory and (2) a euphoriant, antidepressant, and socially stimulating state. Abusers use several routes of abuse, such as oral, intravenous, and mixed with tobacco for smoking. Land, Pinsky, and Salzman (1991) reported that 1% to 17% of patients for whom these drugs are prescribed abuse or misuse them. Abuse of anticholinergic drugs increases as the availability of other drugs decreases.

The first case of abuse of these drugs was reported by Bolin (1960). A woman receiving treatment for torticollis (2 mg four times a day) started taking up to 30 mg per day, to achieve a euphoric state: eventually a full-blown toxic psychosis developed. Since that report, many other cases of anticholinergic antiparkinson abuse have been reported.

Misuse is different from abuse and is usually associated with a patient with negative symptoms (i.e., affective blunting) who enjoys the sense of greater sociability.

Anticholinergic abuse can be detered by the following (Land, Pinsky, and Salzman, 1991):

1. Avoid phophylactic use.
2. Do not use with low-potency antipsychotics that have high anticholinergic properties.
3. Treat EPSEs with nonanticholinergic medications (discussed elsewhere in this chapter).
4. When anticholinergic antiparkinson drugs are needed, prescribe the lowest dose possible while still controlling EPSEs.

Does abrupt withdrawal from anticholinergic drugs cause a significant reaction?

Anticholinergic drugs should never be abruptly discontinued, even when abuse is suspected. Abrupt withdrawal causes cholinergic rebound and withdrawal symptoms, including vomiting, malaise, sweating, excessive salivation, vivid dreams, and nightmares (Land, Pinsky, and Salzman, 1991).

What are the characteristics of toxic anticholinergic psychosis, and who is most susceptible?

Mild anticholinergic effects include those mentioned earlier in the chapter, that is, drowsiness, dizziness, constipation, dry mouth, and nervousness. Anticholinergic psychosis or intoxication becomes evident with symptoms of agitation, visual and tactile hallucinations, nightmares, paranoid thinking, confusion, and impairment of recent memory. Toxic PNS symptoms include nausea and vomiting, diarrhea, tachycardia, arrhythmias, hypertension, and bronchospasm. Geriatric and pediatric patients are most sensitive to anticholinergic side effects (Hamdan-Allen and Nixon, 1991).

OTHER AGENTS

Although anticholinergic antiparkinson drugs are the agents most often used to treat drug-induced side effects, several other agents have been successfully administered and continue to enjoy advocates for their use.

Benzodiazepines: Treatment of EPSEs

Benzodiazepines, especially, lorazepam (Ativan) 1.5 to 5 mg, diazepam (Valium) 15 to 40 mg, and clonazepam (Klonopin) 0.5 mg, have been used successfully in the treatment of side effects (Fleischhacker, Roth, and Kane, 1990). These agents may be particularly useful for akinesia and akathisia.

Beta-Adrenergic Antagonists: Treatment of EPSEs

Propranolol (Inderal) 20 to 100 mg and a few other beta-adrenergic antagonists have effectively reduced the side effects of neurologic drugs. These drugs are well tolerated and probably work through the antagonism of central beta-adrenergic receptors; however in current clinical trials these agents are always combined with antiparkinson drugs, so it is difficult to interpret their precise effect on EPSEs.

Clonidine: Treatment of EPSEs

Clonidine (Catapres) is a centrally acting alpha-2 agonist. Clonidine apparently works by decreasing CNS noradrenergic neurotransmission. Dosages from 0.15 to 0.8 mg have been used successfully to treat side effects of antipsychotic drugs, but Fleischhacker, Roth, and Kane (1990) found the alpha-2 agonists more difficult to use without any advantage over other agents.

Nifedipine and Verapamil: Treatment of Tardive Dyskinesia

Nifedipine (Procardia) (30 to 60 mg per day) and verapamil (Calan) (80 mg four times a day) are calcium channel blockers that have been demonstrated to produce statistically significant improvement in patients with tardive dyskinesia (Duncan et al., 1990; Barrow and Childs, 1986). The interaction between the dopamine system in the CNS and calcium antagonist probably explains the improvement noted in patients with tardive dyskinesia.

Tardive dyskinesia, as described in the box on p. 294 and in Chapter 4, is a late-appearing side effect of neuroleptic drugs. It is not satisfactorily amenable to drug therapy; however, as previously mentioned, attempts to find acceptable drug interventions continue. Prevention and careful monitoring of psychotropic medication regimens are crucial to minimizing the effects of tardive dyskinesia.

Dantrolene: Treatment of Neuroleptic Malignant Syndrome

Dantrolene (Dantrium) has been prescribed successfully in patients with neuroleptic malignant syndrome (Shader and Greenblatt, 1992) and lethal catatonia (Pennati, Sacchetti, and Calzeroni, 1991). Dantrolene interferes with intracellular release of calcium necessary to initiate muscle contraction. Dantrolene also exerts a CNS effect (see Psychotropic Drug Profiles for dosage information).

REFERENCES

Agid Y: Parkinson's disease: pathophysiology, *Lancet* 337:1321, 1991.

Barrow N, Childs A: An anti–tardive dyskinesia effect of verapamil, *Am J Psychiatry* 143:1485, 1986.

Bitter I, Scheurer, Volavka J: Are extrapyramidal symptoms necessary? (letter), *J Clin Psychopharmacol* 12(1):65, 1992.

Blair DT: Risk management for extrapyramidal symptoms, *Quality Assurance Rev Bull* 17:116, 1990.

Bolin RR: Psychiatric manifestations of Artane toxicity, *J Nervous Ment Dis* 131:256, 1960.

Clough DG: Parkinson's disease: management, *Lancet* 337:1324, 1991.

Comaty JE et al: Is maintenance antiparkinsonian treatment necessary? *Psychopharmacology Bull* 26(2):267, 1990.

Duncan E et al: Nifedipine in the treatment of tardive dyskinesia, *J Clin Psychopharmacol* 10(6):414, 1990.

Fleischhacker WW, Roth SD, Kane JM: The pharmacologic treatment of neuroleptic-induced akathisia, *J Clin Psychopharmacology* 10(1):12, 1990.

Hamdan-Allen G, Nixon M: Anticholinergic psychosis in children: a case report, *Hosp Community Psychiatry* 42(2):191, 1991.

Land W, Pinsky D, Salzman C: Abuse and misuse of anticholinergic medications, *Hosp Community Psychiatry* 42(6):580, 1991.

Olin BR: *Facts and comparisons,* Philadelphia, 1990, JB Lippincott.

Pennati A, Sacchetti E, Calzeroni A: Dantrolene in lethal catatonia (a letter), *Am J Psychiatry* 148(2):149, 1991.

Scherman D et al: Striatal dopamine deficiency in Parkinson's disease: role of aging, *Ann Neurology* 26:551, 1989.

Shader RI, Greenblatt DJ: A possible new approach to the treatment of neuroleptic malignant syndrome, *J Clin Psychopharmacol* 12(3):155, 1992.

Smith JM: Abuse of the antiparkinson drugs: a review of the literature, *J Clin Psychiatry* 41(10):351, 1980.

UNIT IV

Developmental Issues Related to Psychotropic Drugs

CHAPTER 15

Psychopharmacology for Children

Scope of the Problem

Each year more than 130,000 children (in this chapter, children from birth to 12 years of age) are hospitalized in the United States for psychiatric disturbances (Costello, Dulcun, and Kalas, 1991). Among children with emotional and behavioral problems 5% of the problems develop before the first year of life, 15% before 3 years of age, 25% during the preschool years, another 25% during early elementary school years, and 15% between the ages of 9 and 11 years (News & Notes, 1991). When children have distressing thoughts, feelings, or behaviors, or a combination of these, psychotropic drugs have proven to be beneficial. Concerns about altered pharmacokinetics (absorption, distribution, metabolism, and excretion) and the potential for developmental risk are more pronounced in children because of organ immaturity. As a result, weight-based extrapolations of child dosages from adult dosages are potentially ineffective (Keltner, 1991). As children grow, the reactions and responses to drugs begin to approximate those of adults. Consequently this text provides separate chapters on child and adolescent psychopharmacology.

The history of pediatric psychopharmacology is brief. The box on p. 309 summarizes the benchmarks of this treatment approach.

General Principles

The first principle of pediatric psychopharmacology is to *avoid drug therapy*, except when it is explicitly needed. Need can be determined by correct diagnosis and identification of significant symptoms. Both are based on careful observation and history. When incorrect diagnosis is made, inappropriate medication can be ordered and can have negative consequences. When target symptoms are not identified, evaluation of progress is thwarted.

The second principle of administering psychotropic drugs to children is based on physiologic differences between children and adults. Developmental immaturity can result in a variance in *pharmacokinetics*. Green (1991) noted that children often require larger doses of psychotropic drugs per pound (lb) than do adults, to achieve similar drug serum levels and therapeutic effects. He explained that larger doses are required because liver metabolism is more rapid in children and because glomerular filtration is increased and results in faster elimination. *Pharmacodynamics* may be altered in children also. Teicher and Baldessarini (1987) suggested that less mature neural systems respond differently to drugs than do mature systems. It is thought that the catecholamine systems, for instance, are not mature until late adolesence or early adulthood, thus partially explaining both cause and effective intervention for attention deficit hyperactivity disorder (ADHD).

Green (1991) further pointed out that *cognitive or psychologic factors* can influence drug therapy. For example, consider the depressed child who has not recently experienced "nondepressed" living. It may be difficult for that child to comprehend when

Benchmarks in the History of Pediatric Psychopharmacology

1937	Bradley* uses amphetamines to treat behavioral disorders in children.
1950	Methylphenidate (Ritalin) is prescribed for attention deficit hyperactivity disorder (ADHD).
1952	Soon after Delay and Denikers' report on chlorpromazine (Thorazine), physicians begin ordering this antipsychotic for children.
1953	Heuyer and others describe the value of chlorpromazine in the treatment of psychomotor excitement.
1960	New antipsychotics are prescribed for children, and a new class of drug, the tricyclic antidepressants, are used in the treatment of pediatric depression.
1970s	Antidepressant use expands to include the treatment of separation anxiety, enuresis, and ADHD. Lithium (although not recommended for children under 12) is used in the treatment of bipolar illness, autism, aggression, and conduct disorders.
1980s	Growing concerns about the ethical questions of pediatric psychopharmacology are discussed.
1986	Gadow reports that 15% to 30% of all emotionally disturbed school-aged children receive psychotropic drugs; that 1% to 2% of *all* elementary school children receive drugs for ADHD; and that 5% of moderately retarded children and 13% of mildly retarded children receive psychotropic medication.
1990s	Psychopharmacology remains an important dimension of treatment for children. Research in pediatric psychopharmacology remains a priority among pediatric mental health professionals.

From Campbell M, Palij M: *Psychopharmacol Bull* 21:1063, 1985; Wiener JM, Jaffe SL. In Wiener JM, editor: *Diagnosis and psychopharmacology of childhood and adolescent disorders*, New York, 1985, John Wiley & Sons.

*Bradley C: The behavior of children receiving Benzedrine, *Am J Psychiatry* 94:577, 1937.

he or she is doing "better." Green cautioned mental health professionals who work with children to avoid assuming that both child and clinician understand words and concepts in the same way. He suggested that clinicians should thoughtfully explain meanings to the child.

Parent education is an important principle of pediatric psychopharmacology. Parents are ultimely responsible for compliance with dosage schedules. Parents play an important role in psychopharmacology and need to know general information about their child's medication, side effects, and potential for abuse and overdose. Parent education guidelines for specific psychotropic agents are found in the box on p. 310.

Compliance is important, and parents play a key role in maintaining consistent administration of psychotropic drugs. If the drug regimen is not adhered to, the clinician cannot ascertain agent effectiveness, develop dosing strategies, or make informed decisions. A variety of factors can influence drug-taking behaviors, including the following:

Parent Education for Specific Psychotropic Drugs

Central nervous system stimulants

Parents should be taught the following:

- To be aware of the abuse potential of CNS stimulants, particularly when older siblings are in the home
- To tolerate some hyperactivity in their child
- To avoid increasing the dosage in an attempt to reduce unwanted behavior; even optimal dosages of these stimulants do not always induce immediate acceptable social behavior
- That pemoline's therapeutic effect is not evident for 3 to 4 weeks, hence the lack of immediate improvement does not mean treatment has failed
- To weigh their child weekly because of the potential for appetite suppression and temporary growth retardation; however, long-term growth problems apparently do not occur*
- To provide a "drug holiday" occasionally, to assess whether continued drug treatment is necessary

Antipsychotic agents

Parents should be taught the following:

- To be committed to drug compliance
- Psychotropic drugs are only part of a comprehensive program
- A realistic understanding of the drug's expected effects versus its side effects; this information helps facilitate appropriate parental decision making
- To assess for muscle rigidity, inability to remain still, vague subjective complaints such as a need to move, and any abnormal involuntary movements
- To monitor bowel and bladder function and to encourage appropriate fluid intake
- To seek approval from the clinician before purchasing over-the-counter medications
- That antipsychotic drugs are not addictive
- That the lowest effective dose is used by the clinician because of the relationship between dose and extrapyramidal side effects (EPSEs)

Antidepressants

Parents should be taught the following:

- That a clinical effect takes 3 to 4 weeks to develop
- To provide support to the child during lag time
- To keep the drug away from the child or siblings because of the great risk of overdose and death
- To administer the correct amount of the drug
- To clear the use of all over-the-counter drugs with the clinician before administering them
- To recognize typical side effects

Parent Education for Specific Psychotropic Drugs—cont'd

Lithium

Parents should be taught the following:

- To recognize signs of lithium intoxication and to withhold the drug and report to the physician or nurse should toxic effects appear
- That a lag time of up to 10 days is not unusual before a therapeutic effect is observed
- To give lithium on time
- To refrain from doubling a dose to make up for a missed dose
- To give only the prescribed dose
- To understand the basic information about sodium-lithium excretion, that is, depleted sodium levels lead to increased lithium levels and increased sodium levels lead to decreased lithium levels†

*Vincent J, Carley CK, Leger P: *Am J Psychiatry* 147:501, 1990.
†Olin BR: *Facts and comparisons*, Philadelphia, 1990, JB Lippincott.

- Parental attitude, such as not accepting the child's illness
- Parental surveillance of drug-taking activity (to prevent cheeking and hoarding)
- Parental understanding of drug serum levels
- Parental understanding of how drugs work (for example, that many psychotropic drugs do not act rapidly the way an aspirin does for a headache)

COMMON SYNDROMES

Attention Deficit Hyperactivity Disorder

Attention deficit hyperactivity disorder (ADHD) is the most common pediatric behavioral disorder and, in contrast to most childhood behavioral disorders, is well studied. Attention deficit hyperactivity disorder is characterized by inattention, impulsivity, and hyperactivity. Specific problems include abnormal motor movements, restlessness, emotional problems, social skills deficits, impulsiveness, and learning disabilities. These deficits cause problems for the child in school and may be present in as many as 20% of all school-aged children (LaGreca and Quay, 1984).

Drug treatment. The drugs most commonly used for treatment of ADHD are central nervous system (CNS) stimulants, that is, dextroamphetamine (Dexedrine), methylphenidate (Ritalin), and pemoline (Cylert) (see Chapter 13 for an explanation of these drugs). Although many drugs used in the treatment of childhood behavioral problems simply make children more manageable, CNS stimulants directly affect the problem behavior. Methylphenidate is prescribed most often and, in fact, ranks as the 172nd most prescribed drug in the United States (Kennedy, 1992). When drugs are used in conjunction with counseling, the conditions of approximately 70% to 80% of ADHD patients improve. In an era when outcome measurements are so highly valued, it is important to note that improvement is defined as the ability to control behavior, to pay attention, and to learn. Table 15-1 provides dosage information for dextroamphetamine, methylphenidate, and pemoline.

Indications. Central nervous system stimulants are indicated when a child diagnosed with ADHD exhibits the behavioral, cognitive, and attention problems previously described.

Table 15-1 Pediatric Dosages of Selected Central Nervous System Stimulants for Treatment of ADHD

Drug	Age of child (0-12 yr)	Dosage
Dextroamphetamine (Dexedrine)	<3 yr	Not recommended
	3-5 yr	2.5 mg daily with meals, raise by 2.5 mg/day at weekly intervals;
	>6 yr	5 mg qd or bid with weekly increases of 5 mg/day
Methylphenidate (Ritalin)	<6 yr	Not recommended
	6-12 yr	5 mg before breakfast and lunch; increase by 5- 10-mg increments on weekly basis, if needed; optimal dose 0.3 mg/kg/day; *maximum* dose 60 mg/day
Pemoline (Cylert)	<6 yr	Not recommended
	6-12 yr	37.5 mg in morning; can be increased by 18.75 mg/day at weekly intervals if needed, up to 112.5 mg/day; maintenance dose 56.25-75 mg/day

Mechanism of action. In normal adults CNS stimulants cause stimulation and euphoria. Paradoxically, hyperactive children become less hyperactive. The following theories exist that explain the efficacy of these agents:

1. Some researchers attribute the effect of CNS stimulants to a preferential stimulation of inhibitory efferent neurons in the cerebral cortex at low dosage levels, which causes a decrease in motor activity.
2. Others think that low dosage levels stimulate the afferent neurons of the reticular activating system. Because of increased input constancy, the brain is enabled to concentrate longer on a particular task and is not as easily distracted by other stimuli.

Pharmacokinetics, side effects, and interactions of CNS stimulants are discussed in Chapter 13. Only information specific to pediatric usage is provided here.

Central nervous system stimulants

Dextroamphetamine. Dextroamphetamine (Dexedrine) is not recommended for children under 3 years of age. The dosage for children from 3 to 5 years of age is 2.5 mg daily as a tablet or elixir, taken with or immediately after meals. The dosage may be raised in 2.5-mg per day increments at weekly intervals, as needed. Children 6 years of age and older may be given 5 mg once or twice a day, with an increase of 5 mg per day at weekly intervals, as needed. Spansules (a slow-releasing preparation) may be given once daily in the morning to prevent insomnia. Children should not be given a large supply of dextroamphetamine because of its potential for abuse, especially by those who have access to the child's supply. Amphetamines are Controlled Substance Schedule II drugs, and a new written prescription is required each time these drugs are prescribed.

Methylphenidate. Methylphenidate (Ritalin) is not recommended for children under the age of 6 years. In children over 6 years of age, 5 mg before breakfast and lunch is recommended. If necessary, the daily dose may be increased by 5-10 mg increments at weekly intervals. The optimal daily dose is 0.3 mg/kg. This dose may not correct all behavioral problems, but it will increase learning ability. Children should not receive more than 1 mg/kg/day or a total dose of more than 60 mg per day regardless of weight. A single daily dose of the sustained-release form (Ritalin-SR) can be used instead of divided doses of the regular product. Abuse potential also exists with methylphenidate. It is a Schedule II drug.

Pemoline. Pemoline (Cylert) differs chemically from the amphetamines and methylphenidate. It is used exclusively for ADHD, whereas amphetamines and methylphendate are occasionally prescribed for narcolepsy. Pemoline is well absorbed, has a 12-hour half-life, and 50% is excreted unchanged in the urine.

Pemoline causes less cerebral stimulation than do the other two CNS stimulants. Its side effects are similar to those of the amphetamines and methylphenidate. The dosage for children over 6 years of age is 37.5 mg daily in the morning. Pemoline has a long half-life (12 hours) and can be given once per day. The daily dose may be increased by 18.75 mg at weekly intervals, up to a maximum of 112.5 mg per day. The usual maintenance dose is 56.25 to 75 mg per day. Pemoline has low abuse potential and is a Schedule IV drug.

Other drugs used in treatment of attention deficit hyperactivity disorder. Tricyclic antidepressants (TCAs) have been used for ADHD but have more side effects and shorter-lived results than do the CNS stimulants. The phenothiazine tranquilizers and haloperidol have been tried but are less effective than the stimulants. Lithium, diphendydramine (Benadryl), phenobarbital, and the benzodiazepines have been used with less than satisfactory results. Central nervous system stimulants remain the drugs of choice for ADHD. However, for persons with ADHD who do not respond to stimulants, these drugs are alternatives.

Side effects of central nervous system stimulants. Growth retardation is a major concern when anorexia-causing CNS stimulants are administered. Research indicates that slowed growth is temporary and that children will eventually "catch up" (Klein and Mannuzza, 1988). Anorexia can be reduced by giving these drugs immediately after meals. Insomnia is reduced by giving the last dose at least 6 hours before bedtime. Sometimes ADHD can worsen paradoxically when methylphenidate is used. If this occurs, the drug should be withheld.

Interactions of central nervous system stimulants. A relevant example for the interaction section might be the treatment of a stomachache, a side effect of amphetamines. A parent might unwittingly give a child sodium bicarbonate as a remedy, inadvertently alkalinizing the urine and thereby intensifying the effect of amphetamine. Over-the-counter drugs for colds and hay fever, conditions common in children, often contain sympathomimetic agents that create an additive effect.

Toxic effects. Amphetamine overdose can be fatal. In a typical case of overdose a hyperalert, talkative child comes to medical attention who may have tremors, exaggerated startle reflex, paranoia, hallucinations, confusion, and tachyarrhythmias. If a child seeks medical attention with some of these symptoms, hospitalization is recommended. Overdose procedures enumerated in Chapter 13 should be followed.

Psychotic Disorders

Schizophrenia can occur in children from 5 to 8 years of age. Symptoms may include hallucinations, delusions, thought disorders, anxiety, and inappropriate affect. Speech idiosyncrasies such as mutism, echolalia, and an inability to understand the spoken word may also be present, along with morbid thoughts, a lack of friends, and concrete thinking. Schizophrenia is a rare disorder and more common in boys. There are obvious developmental delays in these children. Some clinicians think that a highly functioning mind is present behind the chaotic exterior; however, evidence seems to indicate the opposite.

Autism is a pervasive developmental disorder differentiated from schizophrenia on diagnosis by its earlier onset (possibly, at birth) and lack of hallucinations, delusions, and schizophrenic thought processes. In contrasting autism and childhood schizophrenia it might be said that the child with schizophrenia experienced a normal or near-normal life at one time, whereas the autistic child never has. The autistic child is unemotional, anxious, unresponsive to normal speech, and has a number of disturbing stereotypic behaviors such as rocking, biting, hand flicking, and head banging. Both diagnostic groups of children exhibit little spontaneous behavior and socially isolate themselves.

Drugs used to treat psychotic disorders. Antipsychotic agents are often the first drugs used to treat childhood psychoses (Wiener, 1985). Antipsychotic drugs are discussed in Chapter 4; only those issues specific to pediatric psychopharmacology are reviewed in this chapter. Table 15-2 provides dosage information for antipsychotic drugs.

Indications. Psychotropic drug intervention for psychotic disorders is embryonic when compared to drug intervention for ADHD. The goal for the schizophrenic child is to decrease thought disorganization so that a normal level of functioning is restored. The goal for the autistic child is to decrease anxiety or stereotypic behaviors. The neuroleptic effect of antipsychotic drugs may be more significant for the autistic child, and the antipsychotic effect is probably more important for the schizophrenic child.

Antipsychotic drugs are also used to manage aggressive, assaultive, or self-destructive behavior. However, psychotropic drugs are never used as the sole treatment measure. Drugs are merely one aspect of a treatment plan that includes therapeutic communication, milieu management, parental involvement, and education.

Antipsychotic drugs

Phenothiazines. Three subclasses of phenothiazines are the aliphatics, the piperidines, and the piperazines (see Chapter 4). *Chlorpromazine* (Thorazine) is an aliphatic phenothiazine and is not recommended for children under 6 months of age. If a child is agitated, overexcited, or overactive, an aliphatic may be preferable because the aliphatics are more sedating than other antipsychotics. Chlorpromazine is usually prescribed at 0.5 mg/kg every 6 to 8 hours and is gradually increased to an oral dose of 50 to 100 mg a day for severely ill and hospitalized children. Rectal suppositories are available. For acutely disturbed children who require immediate treatment, an intramuscular dose of 0.5 mg/kg every 6 to 8 hours is appropriate. A 2- to 5-year-old child should not receive more than 40 mg per day, and a 5- to 12-year-old child should not receive more than 75 mg per day intramuscularly.

Thioridazine (Mellaril), a piperidine phenothiazine, is used by many clinicians. It is not recommended for children under 2 years of age. The dosage for treating psychosis in 2- to 12-year-old children is 0.5 to 3.0 mg/kg/day. This dosage usually translates into 10 mg twice or three times per day for mild symptoms and 25 mg twice or three times per day for severe symptoms. No child should receive more than 3 mg/kg per day.

Trifluoperazine (Stelazine), a piperazine phenothiazine, is not recommended for children under 6 years of age. In 6- to 12-year-old children who are hospitalized or closely supervised, clinicians should start therapy with 1 mg once or twice per day and increase the dosage slowly until the symptoms are resolved or until side effects

Table 15-2 Pediatric Dosages of Selected Antipsychotics

Drug	Disorder	Age of child (0-12 yr)	Dosage
Chlorpromazine (Thorazine)	Psychosis, combativeness, hyperexcitability	0-6 mo	Not recommended
		6 mo-12 yr	*Oral:* 0.5 mg/kg q 4-6 hr up to 200 mg/day; *rectal:* 1 mg/kg q 6-8 hr; *IM:*0.5 mg/kg q 6-8 hr; *maximum IM* dosage for <5 yr or <22 kg is 40 mg/day; *maximum IM* dosage for child 5-12 yr or 22-45 kg is 75 mg/day
Thioridazine (Mellaril)	Psychosis, combativeness, hyperactivity	<2 yr	Not recommended
		2-12 yr	0.5 mg/kg/day up to 3 mg/kg/day; start low and slowly increase; *severely disturbed children:* 25 mg bid or tid
Trifluoperazine (Stelazine)	Psychosis, short-term anxiety	<6 yr	Not recommended
		6-12 yr	Start with 1 mg qd or bid, gradually increase; *maximum* dosage is 15 mg/day
Haloperidol (Haldol)	Psychosis	<3 yr	Not recommended
		3-12 yr	Start with 0.5 mg/day; gradually increase by 0.5 mg q 5-7 days
			Up to 0.15 mg/kg/day
	Tourette's syndrome, severe behavioral disorders	3-12 yr	0.05-0.075 mg/kg/day
Thiothixene (Navane)	Psychosis	12 yr	*Milder symptoms:* start with 2 mg tid, slowly increasing to 5 mg tid; *severe symptoms:* start with 5 mg bid; usual dosage is 20-30 mg/day; *maximum* dosage is 60 mg/day
Chlorprothixene (Taractan)	Psychosis	<6 yr	Not recommended
		6-12 yr	10-25 mg tid or qid
Loxapine (Loxitane)	Psychosis	<16 yr	Not recommended
Fluphenazine (Prolixin, Permitil)	Psychosis	<12 yr	Not recommended
Pimozide (Orap)	Tourette's syndrome	<12 yr	Not recommended
Clozapine (Clozaril)	Psychosis	<16 yr	Not recommended

occur. For rapid control of symptoms, 1 mg (0.5 ml) intramuscularly once or twice a day can be given. Dosage should not exceed 15 mg per day.

Butyrophenenones. *Haloperidol* (Haldol), a high potency antipsychotic, is structurally unrelated to the phenothiazines. It is the most studied treatment for autism. It can be given to children between the ages of 3 and 12 years (weight 15 to 40 kg). Its antipsychotic use in children causes significant EPSEs when compared with chlorpromazine. However, haloperidol is the least sedating antipsychotic. A dose of 0.05 to 0.15 mg/kg/day is recommended for children. Joshi, Capozzoli, and Coyle (1988) found that low maintenance doses of neuroleptics are effective for pervasive developmental disorders. The authors recommended a dosage of 0.04 mg/kg/day. Doses typically should not exceed 6 mg per day.

Thioxanthenes. The two thioxanthenes are structurally related to phenothiazines and are generally less sedating and cause fewer extrapyramidal side effects (EPSEs).

Chlorprothixene. (Taractan) is not recommended for children under 6 years of age, but for children 6 to 12 years of age, 10 to 25 mg three or four times a day is recommended. Thiothixene (Navane) can be given to a 12-year-old (Table 15-2).

Unapproved drugs. Some drugs are used in childhood psychotic disorders that are not approved for pediatric use in the *Physician's Desk Reference (PDR)* (*PDR*, 1990). These drugs should be used with care and with parental approval. A signed informed consent form is advised.

Fluphenazine (Prolixin), a commonly used piperazine in adults, is not recommended for children under 12 years of age. Nonetheless, clinicians prescribe the drug and find it effective for children over 6 years of age. Werry (1978) recommended a starting dose of 0.025 to 0.05 mg/kg up to 0.3 mg/kg per day (3 to 6 mg per day). Joshi, Capozzoli, and Coyle (1988) found low maintenance dosages of 0.04 mg/kg/day to provide significant symptom reduction.

Thiothixene (Navane), although not recommended for use in children under 12 years of age, is sometimes prescribed. Werry (1978) did use the drug in pediatric doses and recommended an average dose of 0.15 to 0.3 mg/kg/day. Molindone (Moban), loxapine (Loxitane), and pimozide (Orap) are not recommended for this age group, and few investigational studies have been completed. Pimozide is used primarily for the treatment of tics.

Side effects of antipsychotic drugs. Only side effects of particular interest for pediatric clinicians are discussed here. For other side effects the reader is referred to Chapter 4.

Extrapyramidal side effects are caused by the imbalance of the acetylcholine-to-dopamine ratio resulting from the dopamine-blocking effects of antipsychotic drugs (see Chapter 14). Dyskinesias, a type of EPSE, are a major concern in children. Facial muscles become motionless, and the eyes stare ahead without blinking or emotion. Although children are clear-headed, they appear dazed (Englehardt and Polizos, 1978). Tardive dyskinesia, an irreversible form, is rare in children. Other side effects and significant drug interactions are discussed in Chapter 4.

Sedation is a particularly prominent side effect in psychotic children taking antipsychotic medications and, although welcomed at times in the agitated child, often interferes with other psychotherapeutic interventions. Changing to a less sedating drug such as trifluoperazine (Stelazine) might be advantageous. Autonomic side effects are not as prominent as in adults, but drowsiness and weight gain are more common (Campbell, 1985). Generally, anticholinergic side effects and antiadrenergic side effects can be resolved by dose modification and by taking antiparkinson-anticholinergic drugs. Downward dosage modification can reduce side effects, but an increase in disturbed behavior is a likely outcome. Such trade-offs are the crux of clinical decision making.

Interactions of antipsychotic drugs. Children taking antipsychotic drugs should not be given medications containing alcohol, including over-the-counter sleeping aids and cough syrups. Clinicians should assess for drowsiness, if such preparations are taken. Over-the-counter anticholinergics such as cold or hay fever medications can compound anticholinergic drug effects. Other interactions previously discussed in Chapter 4 are relevant to pediatric psychopharmacology as well.

Toxic effects. Deaths resulting from antipsychotic drug overdose have been rarely reported in any age group. Overdose usually results in CNS depression, hypotension, and EPSEs. Treatment for overdose is outlined in Chapter 4.

Depression and Mania

Until 10 to 15 years ago many clinicians debated whether depression actually occurred in children. Rutter et al. (1976) carefully studied the 10- to 11-year-old children on the Isle of Wight (2199 children) and found only three who could be described as depressed. Today there is consensus that childhood depression is a mental health problem. However, much less is known about the clinical picture of childhood depression than about the features of adult depression. Childhood depression can be divided into primary and secondary depression. Primary or endogenous depression is defined as a mood disorder in which depression is the presenting problem and the cause cannot be traced to an external event. Secondary or reactive depression is a reaction to a real-life event, situation, or illness and can evolve into a primary depression (Wiener, 1977). The reaction often takes the form of grief or anhedonia, which is a major symptom of the depressed child. Even when surrounded by a series of unpleasant and depressing events, most children display happiness at times.

The existence of mania in children is not as easy to recognize as depression, and its incidence is not clear. Once adolescence is reached, manic symptoms more closely resemble the adult illness. Puig-Antich (1985) identified the following symptoms in children with mania:

Elation
Unrealistic optimism
More activity than usual without fatigue
Grandiosity
Decreased need for sleep
Racing thoughts
Flight of ideas
Distractibility
Motor hyperactivity

Although the psychopharmacologic treatment of depression is known, drug treatment for mania is not as well established. Lithium, an antimania drug and the drug of choice for adult mania, has been used in childhood mania with mixed results. It is not recommended for use in children under 12 years of age.

Drugs used to treat depression. Two major antidepressant drug classes are the tricyclic antidepressants (TCAs) and the monoamine oxidase inhibitors (MAOIs) (see Chapter 5). Monoamine oxidase inhibitors have potentially life-threatening side effects and are not recommended for use in children under 16 years of age. Tricyclic antidepressants were developed in the late 1950s and gained acceptance for treatment of childhood depression in the 1960s. Table 15-3 provides dosage information for TCAs and lithium.

Indications. Antidepressants are indicated for depression, but the *PDR* (*PDR*, 1990) does not recommend any TCA for use in children under 12 years of age for the

Table 15-3 Pediatric Dosages of Selected TCAs and Lithium

Drug	Disorder	Age of child (0-12 yr)	Dosage (unapproved dosage [UAD])
Imipramine (Tofranil)	Depression	<12	Not recommended; see text for UAD
	Enuresis	<6	Not recommended
		6-11	Start with 25 mg one hr before bedtime; if needed, may be increased to 50 mg after 1 week
	Attention deficit hyperactivity disorder		Not recommended
	Separation anxiety		Not recommended; see text for UAD
Nortriptyline (Pamelor)	Depression	<12	Not recommended
Amitriptyline (Elavil, Endep)	Depression	<12	Not recommended
Desipramine (Norpramin, Pertofrane)	Depression	<12	Not recommended
Clomipramine (Anafranil)	Obsessive-compulsive disorder	<10	Not recommended
		10-12	Start with 25 mg/day and gradually increase to *maximum* of 10 mg or 3 mg/kg/day, whichever is less
Fluoxetine (Prozac)		<12	Not recommended
Bupropion (Wellbutrin)		<12	Not recommended
Lithium	Manic depression	<12	Not recommended; see text for UAD

treatment of depression. Imipramine is recommended for children over 6 years of age for the treatment of enuresis. The use of antidepressants not approved for pediatric use in the *PDR* must be carefully discussed with the parent and may require informed consent.

Tricyclic antidepressants. Although the *PDR* does not recommend the use of imipramine for childhood depression, several clinicians use imipramine and their research supports its effectiveness. Puig-Antich, Ryan, and Rabinovich (1985) recommended that dosage be "increased every fourth day from 1.5 to 3, to 4, and to 5 mg/kg per day." Puig-Antich, Ryan, and Rabinovich (1985) and Martin and Agran (1988) indicated that drug serum levels are the crucial variable for clinical effectiveness. Imipramine should have a serum level of 150 to 240 ng/ml, desipramine 115 ng/ml, amitriptyline 100 to 300 ng/ml, and nortriptyline 60 to 100 ng/ml (Newcomb, 1991) for a therapeutic effect. As with adults, a period of 3 to 4 weeks is required before clinical improvement is noted.

Nortriptyline (Pamelor) has been given to children with depression. Geller et al. (1986) found that more than 60% of the patients (ages 6 to 12 yr) in their study responded favorably to nortriptyline. Responders had a daily dosage range of 0.64 to 1.57 mg/kg. Eventually 21 of 22 patients had a favorable response.

Fluoxetine (Prozac), amitriptyline (Elavil), and clomipramine (Anafranil) have been administered to children with depression with some positive results (Green, 1991).

Side effects. Side effects of interest to pediatric clinicians include the multiple expressions of an anticholinergic response. Psychosis resulting from anticholinergic intoxication has been reported in children (Hamden-Allen and Nixon, 1991). Symptoms include agitation, nightmares, and visual hallucinations. Urinary hesistancy, another anticholinergic effect and a blight for older men taking antidepressants, is the effect of interest in the treatment of enuresis. Other anticholinergic effects can be reviewed in Chapter 5.

Cardiovascular side effects are of particular concern in children because they seem to be more sensitive to cardiotoxic metabolites of TCAs. The most significant dimension of cardiac involvement is the conductive slowing of cardiac muscle. Three TCA-related cases of sudden death in children have been reported as recently as 1990 (Medical Letter, 1990). Monitoring vital signs for elevated blood pressure and tachycardia should be routine, a blood pressure greater than 140/90 mm Hg and a heart rate of greater than 130 beats per minute are cause for alarm (Martin and Agran, 1988).

Interactions. Tricyclic antidepressants interact with many other drugs, and these interactions are reviewed in Chapter 5 and the Psychotropic Drug Profiles.

Toxic effects. Children are thought to be more sensitive to overdoses of TCAs than are adults. Although deaths of children for whom TCAs were prescribed have been reported, most TCA poisoning in children is due to their taking a parent's TCA. Imipramine pamoate (Tofranil-PM) is never given to children because the smallest available unit dose is 75 mg. Since TCAs have a narrow therapeutic index, dosage schedules must be followed and these drugs must be made inaccessible to children. Treatment for TCA overdose is found in Chapter 5.

Drugs used to treat bipolar disorder

Indications. Lithium is a naturally occurring element that is indicated in the treatment of bipolar disorder. A full discussion of lithium can be found in Chapter 5.

Lithium. Lithium has been used in children under 12 years of age with a diagnosis of mania, but is not *PDR*-approved for this use. Therefore use of this drug should be carefully discussed with parents. Dosages of 30 mg/kg to 40 mg/kg per day have been reported. The effectiveness of lithium is not clear. Weller, Weller, and Fristad (1986) suggest 900 mg per day in divided doses for children 25 to 40 kg, 1200 mg per day in divided doses for children 40 to 50 kg, and 1500 mg per day in divided doses for children 50 to 60 kg. The effective serum level range is 0.6 to 1.2 mEq/L.

Side effects. Lithium has serious side effects in adults, but children tolerate the drug well. Lithium decreases free thyroxine and triiodothyronine, but increased thyroid-releasing hormone compensates in euthyroid patients. Children should have baseline thyroid hormone levels determined (Puig-Antich, Ryan, and Rabinovich, 1985). After stabilization occurs, monthly drug serum level determinations are adequate. There is a concern among clinicians that long-term use of lithium may cause renal damage, but research does not support this concern (Khandelwal, Vijoy, and Murphy, 1984). Lithium causes sodium diuresis, and the excretion of lithium is tied to sodium excretion. A decrease in sodium intake can lead to lithium intoxication (>1.5 mEq/L).

Campbell, Perry, and Green (1984) reported that the most common side effects of lithium in children are weight gain (44.4%), sedation (27.8%), and decreased activity (25%). Wagner and Teicher (1991) reported loss of hair as a childhood effect to lithium. Other side effects reported in children include weakness, tremor, weight gain, stomachache, and blurred vision. Nausea and vomiting, slurring of speech, and drowsiness may be early indications of intoxication (Puig-Antich, Ryan, and Rabinovich, 1985). Side effects relevant to all patients taking lithium are found in Chapter 5.

Interactions. Interactants with lithium are discussed in Chapter 5.

Toxic effects. Lithium has a low therapeutic index, necessitating frequent serum level analysis. Children may initially require daily determinations of lithium blood levels. If repetitive venipunctures are too traumatic for the child, lithium levels can be determined from saliva specimens, although saliva-to-serum ratios vary among individual children (Green, 1991). Toxic effects of lithium are discussed in Chapter 5.

Other Syndromes

Enuresis. Enuresis is a developmental eliminative disorder in children 5 years of age and older. It is manifested by involuntary urination during sleep. Enuresis is more common in boys. Approximately 20% of these children have psychiatric symptoms. A number of approaches to treatment have been used. Behavioral approaches (for example, buzzer pads) have proven effective for some children, and for others a pharmacologic approach has been beneficial. Imipramine (Tofranil) is approved for the treatment of enuresis in children 6 years of age and older. It is thought that the same anticholinergic effect that causes urinary hesitancy and retention in adults is responsible for imipramine's therapeutic effect in enuretic children. An alternate view is that the enuretic effect is more likely the result of imipramine's effect on stage 4 sleep.

Imipramine (Tofranil). Patients are given 25 mg daily, one hour before bedtime. After 1 week the dosage can be increased to 50 mg in children 6 to 12 years of age. For enuretic children who wet the bed early in the night, it may be more effective to give imipramine earlier and in divided dosages. Children should not be given more than 2.5 mg/kg/day. Imipramine pamoate (Tofranil-PM) is contraindicated in children because the smallest unit dose is 75 mg.

Tourette's syndrome. Tourette's syndrome is characterized by involuntary, repetitive, purposeless muscle movements such as gyrating, hopping, clapping, and kicking, accompanied by multiple verbal tics, including screaming and copralalia (Adkins, 1989). Coprolalia, the utterance of filthy, obscene language, causes numerous social problems for the patient and family and occurs in approximately 40% of patients with Tourette's syndrome. Coprolalia can progress to phrases that are filled with cursing and sexually offensive language. Some patients utter profanities as soon as the thought comes into their minds, without the usual social restraint. Haloperidol is the drug of choice for Tourette's syndrome.

Haloperidol (Haldol). The recommended dosage of haloperidol for Tourette's syndrome is 0.05 mg/kg to 0.075 mg/kg per day. The child should not be given more than 6 mg daily, and EPSEs are significant. Young et al. (1985) recommended an initial dose of 0.5 mg per day, slowly increased to 3 to 4 mg per day. The drug is effective for approximately 80% of patients (Young et al., 1985).

Clonidine (Catapres). Clonidine is an antihypertensive drug that is used by many clinicians, although it is not FDA-approved for use in Tourette's syndrome. Clonidine is an alpha-adrenergic agonist that should be initiated at low doses of 0.05 mg per day and slowly increased for several weeks to 0.15 to 0.30 mg per day. Dosages of over 0.4 to 0.5 mg per day lead to side effects (Gallico, Burns, and Grob, 1988). Clonidine has a slower onset of action than haloperidol, taking up to 3 weeks or more before a therapeutic improvement is noted (Young et al., 1985). Side effects include sedation, dry mouth, and hypotension.

Pimozide (Orap). Pimozide is an antipsychotic drug indicated for managing severe motor or vocal tics in patients with Tourette's syndrome. It is not recommended for use in children under 12 years of age. Clinical experience with children is limited, but favorable results have been reported (Adkins, 1989).

Separation anxiety. Separation anxiety is common, and psychiatric professionals are often consulted when children refuse to attend school (school phobia). The adult equivalent is agoraphobia. When coupled with appropriate psychotherapeutic intervention, imipramine (Tofranil) is recommended for these children. Gittelman-Klein (1975) studied 100 children and stated, "This is one of the few psychiatric treatments that, when successful, induces complete remission." Jaffe and Magnuson (1985) recommended 1.0 to 5.0 mg/kg/day for children with separation anxiety. The dosage should not exceed 200 mg per day (Gittelman-Klein, 1975).

Aggressive behavior. Aggressive behavior is a continual theme in many inpatient psychiatric units. Aggressive behavior among children is not uncommon and can be treated with haloperidol 1 to 6 mg per day (Campbell, Perry, and Green, 1984). Agitation in children 3 to 6 years of age can be managed with a regimen of 0.01 to 0.03 mg/kg/day of oral haloperidol (Olin, 1990). Trazodone (Desyrel) was found to be effective in the treatment of severe behavioral disturbances in children (Zubieta and Allessi, 1992). Sims and Galvin (1990), after retrospectively reviewing the charts of children and adolescents, concluded that a regimen of propranolol (dosages ranging from 30 to 160 mg per day) could be effective in treating aggressive behavior.

Miscellaneous Agents Used in the Treatment of Childhood Emotional Problems

Carbamazepine (Tegretol). An anticonvulsant, carbamazepine is used in a variety of psychiatric diagnoses. It has been effective in the treatment of mania and impulsive behavior. The drug has been used in the treatment of organic mental disease, depression, catatonia, schizophrenia, panic disorder, borderline personality disorder, obsessive-compulsive disorder, hypochondriacal psychosis, explosive disorder, post-traumatic stress disorder, and stuttering.

Benzodiazepines. Benzodiazepines have been used in the treatment of separation anxiety. Benzodiazepines commonly used in children are diazepam (Valium), chlordiazepoxide (Librium), and alprazolam (Xanax). Side effects include sedation and paradoxic agitation or excitement. Reactions occur when these drugs are withdrawn too quickly and may include severe anxiety and seizures.

The recommended dosage of diazepam for children with anxiety is 1 to 2.5 mg three to four times per day. The dosage can be increased as needed and tolerated. Diazepam should not be used in children under 6 months of age.

The recommended dosage of chlordiazepoxide for childhood anxiety is 5 mg two to four times per day. Therapy with chlordiazepoxide should be initiated at the lowest dose and increased as required. Chlordiazepoxide should not be used in children under 6 years of age.

The recommended dosage for alprazolam is 0.25 to 3 mg per day (Gallico, Burns, and Grob, 1988). Withdrawal reactions appear to be especially significant with this drug.

Clomipramine. Clomipramine (Anafranil) has been used in investigations of the treatment of childhood obsessive-compulsive disorder, depression, enuresis, ADHD, and separation anxiety.

REMARKS

Individuals working with children should be careful in the administration of the drugs previously discussed, should understand the side effects of these drugs, should be aware of drug interventions and toxic reactions, and should teach parents about the drugs and the importance of compliance. Although the information about syndromes and psychotropic agents in this chapter is specific to children, much can be gained by referring to other relevant chapters in this book.

REFERENCES

Adkins AS: Helping your patient cope with Tourette syndrome, *Pediatric Nurs* 15:135, 1989.

Campbell M, Perry R, Green WH: The use of lithium in children and adolescents, *Psychosomatics* 25:95, 1984.

Campbell M: Schizophrenic disorders and pervasive developmental disorders/infantile autism. In Wiener JM, editor: *Diagnosis and psychopharmacology of childhood and adolescent disorders*, New York, 1985, John Wiley & Sons.

Costello AJ, Dulcan MK, Kalas R: A checklist of hospitalization criteria for use with children, *Hosp Community Psychiatry* 42(8):823, 1991.

Engelhardt DM, Polizos P: Adverse effects of pharmacotherapy in childhood psychosis. In Lipton MA, DiMascio A, Killam KF, editors: *Psychopharmacology: a generation of progress*, New York, 1978, Raven.

Gallico RP, Burns TJ, Grob CS: *Emotional and behavioral problems in children with learning disabilities*, San Diego, 1988, College-Hill.

Geller B et al: Preliminary data on the relationship between nortriptyline plasma level and response in depressed children, *Am J Psychiatry* 143:1283, 1986.

Gittelman-Klein R: Pharmacotherapy and management of pathological separation anxiety. In Gittelman-Klein R, editor: *Recent advances in child psychopharmacology*, New York, 1975, Human Sciences.

Green WH: *Child and adolescent clinical psychopharmacology*, Baltimore, 1991, Williams & Wilkins.

Hamden-Allen G, Nixon M: Anticholingeric psychosis in children: a case report, *Hosp Community Psychiatry* 42(4):191, 1991.

Jaffe SL, Magnuson JV: Anxiety disorders. In Wiener J, editor: *Diagnosis and psychopharmacology of childhood and adolescent disorders*, New York, 1985, John Wiley & Sons.

Joshi PT, Capozzoli JA, and Coyle JT: Low-dose neuroleptic therapy for children with childhood onset pervasive developmental disorder, *Am J Psychiatry* 145:335, 1988.

Keltner NL: Psychopharmacology. In Clunn P, editor: *Child psychiatric nursing*, St Louis, 1991, Mosby.

Kennedy VP: Relying on Ritalin prescriptions, *Birmingham News*, Nov 11, 1992, p 1A.

Khandelwal SK, Vijoy KV, Murphy RS: Renal function in children receiving long-term lithium prophylaxis, *Am J Psychiatry* 121:278, 1984.

Klein RG, Mannuzza S: Hyperactive boys almost grown up. III. Methylphenidate effects on ultimate height, *Arch Gen Psychiatry* 45(12):1131, 1988.

LaGreca AM, Quay HC: Behavior disorders in children. In Ender NS, Hunt J, editors: *Personality and behavior disorders*, ed 2, New York, 1984, Wiley & Sons.

Martin JE, Agran M: Pharmacotherapy. In Matson JL, editor: *Handbook of treatment approaches in childhood psychopathology*, New York, 1988, Plenum.

Medical Letter: Sudden death in children treated with tricyclic antidepressants, *Medical Letter* 32:53, 1990.

Newcomb P: Tricyclic antidepressants and children, *Nurse Pract* 16(5):26, 1991.

News & Notes: Almost 20 percent of American children have psychological learning problems, survey finds, *Hosp Community Psychiatry* 42(4):438, 1991.

Olin BR: *Facts and comparisons*, Philadelphia, 1990, JB Lippincott.

Physician's desk reference, Oradell, New Jersey 1990, Medical Economics.

Puig-Antich J: Affective disorder. In Kaplan SI, Sadock BJ, editors: *Comprehensive textbook of psychiatry* vol 4, Baltimore, 1985, Williams & Wilkins.

Puig-Antich J, Ryan ND, Rabinovich H: Affective disorders in childhood and adolescence. In Wiener JM, editor: *Diagnosis and psychopharmacology for childhood and adolescent disorders*, New York, 1985, John Wiley & Sons.

Rutter M et al: Research report: Isle of Wight studies, 1964-1974, *Psychol Med* 6:313, 1976.

Sims J, Galvin MR: Pediatric psychopharmacologic uses of propanolol, *J Child Adolesc Psychiatr Ment Health Nurs* 3(1):18, 1990.

Teicher MH, Baldessarrini RJ: Developmental pharmacodynamics. In Popper C, editor: *Psychiatric pharmacosciences of children and adolescents*, Washington, DC, 1987, American Psychiatric Association.

Wagner KD, Teicher MH: Lithium and hair loss in childhood, *Psychosomatics* 32:355, 1991.

Weller EB, Weller RA, Fristad MA: Lithium dosage guide for prepubertal children: a preliminary report, *J Am Acad Child Psychiatry* 25:92, 1986.

Werry J: *Pediatric psychopharmacology*, New York, 1978, Brunner/Mazel.

Wiener JM: *Psychopharmacology in childhood and adolescence*, New York, 1977, Basic Books.

Wiener JM, Jaffe SL: Historic overview of childhood and adolescent psychopharmacology. In Wiener JM, editor: *Diagnosis and psychopharmacology of childhood and adolescent disorders*, New York, 1985, John Wiley & Sons.

Young JG et al: Tourette's syndrome and tic disorders. In Wiener JM, editor: *Diagnosis and psychopharmacology of childhood and adolescent disorders*, New York, 1985, John Wiley & Sons.

Zubietta JK, Alessi NE: Acute and chronic administration of trazodone in the treatment of disruptive behavior disorders in children, *J Clin Psychopharmacol* 12:346, 1992.

CHAPTER 16

Psychopharmacology for Adolescents

The contents of this chapter are closely associated with the topics covered in the previous chapter and with Chapters 4, 5, 13, and 14. To avoid repetition, the authors have decided to refer to those chapters rather than to repeat content. The majority of the content in this chapter, then, is specific to adolescent patients (12 to 17 years of age), and any duplication of previously discussed issues is thoughtfully included for special emphasis. The authors have paid particular attention to dosage variability between the two age groups represented (Chapter 15 [0 to 12 years of age] and Chapter 16 [12 to 17 years of age]).

SCOPE OF THE PROBLEM

Almost 20% of the 25 million adolescents between the ages of 12 and 18 will require mental health care for one or more developmental, learning, or emotional disorders before the end of adolescence (Esman, 1992). A total of seven million persons in this age group have had an emotional or behavioral problem that lasted 3 months or more. About three fourths of the latter group have received treatment or counseling. Twenty-two percent of these problems emerged during adolescence (12-17 years of age). The data were obtained from the 1988 National Health Interview Survey of Child Health, an ongoing effort by the United States government to better understand the scope of the country's pediatric health care needs (News & Notes, 1991).

GENERAL PRINCIPLES OF ADOLESCENT PSYCHOPHARMACOLOGY

Working with adolescent patients is challenging. Psychotropic drug intervention should be viewed as one aspect of a multidimensional treatment approach. Although drug intervention is the best studied treatment form, there are associated risks, including pharmacokinetic variables in the developing body, tendencies among youth to abuse drugs, and emotional fluctuations during adolescence.

Beyond having the ability to work with adolescents and understanding the scientific foundation of drug therapy, the clinician must be aware of the general principles governing adolescent psychopharmacology.

Strategies for Effective Administration

Hogarth (1991) has noted the following strategies for effective administration of psychotropic drugs to adolescents:

1. *Surveillance*, that is, monitoring for response, toxic effects, side effects, interactions, and patient compliance
2. *Teaching* the adolescent and his or her family
3. *Collaboration*, that is, informing other health care providers about the adolescent's response

4. *Advocacy,* that is, establishing appropriate administration and surveillance in other settings

Other Issues of Administration

To Hogarth's list (1991) might be added several other significant principles for working with these young people, including those discussed in the following paragraphs.

Abuse. Abuse of drugs is a major issue when working with adolescent patients. The patient, a friend, or a sibling are potential abusers of these psychoactive drugs. Central nervous system (CNS) stimulants have a particularly high abuse potential.

Assessment. It is important for health care providers and in turn for parents to consistently assess adolescents for extrapyramidal side effects (EPSEs), peripheral anticholinergic effects (constipation, bladder function), and fluid intake. Adolescents are prone to EPSEs, often disregard the body's cues for bowel and bladder evacuation, and by nature do not drink much water. All these factors can develop into serious problems.

Compliance. Psychotropic drugs can be evaluated for effectiveness only if the patient is taking the drug. Parents play an important role in this regard and should be informed about hoarding and "cheeking."

Suicide and overdose. Drug-related emergencies among 6- to 17-year-olds accounted for more than 21,000 emergency room visits in 1988 (Kalogerakis, 1992). Suicide remains the second leading cause of death among adolescents and a significant percentage of adolescent psychiatric patients come to medical attention with some level of suicidal thinking or behavior. Tricyclic antidepressants (TCAs), in particular, are prominent in the accidental and suicidal deaths of children and adolescents. Tricyclic antidepressants have a narrow therapeutic index, and doses only slightly higher than therapeutic doses can result in fatalities. Tricyclic antidepressants account for 25% to 50% of all hospital admissions for overdose (Harsch and Holt, 1988). Many young persons have died of TCA overdose.

Tolerance. Parents should be encouraged to have reasonable expectations for their child's improvement: the hyperactive child may not calm down to the degree the parent would like; the psychotic child may not perform in school at the desired level; and the depressed adolescent taking antidepressants may not respond for 3 to 4 weeks. The clinician should neither discourage the parent nor reinforce unrealistic expectations of drug therapy.

Toxic effects. The clinician and the parent must be aware of signs of toxic effects.

COMMON SYNDROMES

Attention Deficit Hyperactivity Disorder

Until the 1980s it was thought that attention deficit hyperactivity disorder (ADHD) was outgrown at puberty as a result of the developmental changes that take place at that time. Cantwell (1985) found, however, that ADHD symptoms persist into adolescence in 50% to 80% of the cases, indicating a greater incidence of this disorder in adolescents than previously thought. Two thirds of patients with ADHD continue to show signs of this disorder into adulthood (Garfinkel and Amrami, 1992). Boys are three times more likely than girls to have ADHD, and six to nine times more boys than girls seek professional intervention (American Psychiatric Association, 1987). Attention deficit hyperactivity disorder is related to other adolescent problems such as antisocial behavior, substance abuse, and poor school performance. Adolescents with ADHD are about 2 years behind their peers academically (Munoz-Millan and Casteel, 1989).

Drugs used to treat attention deficit hyperactivity disorder. Central nervous system stimulants are the drugs most commonly used to treat ADHD in children but these drugs are used less often in adolescents, particularly in older adolescents. It is a commonly held opinion among many professionals working with ADHD that when the hyperactive individual reaches puberty, stimulants lose their effect. A number of authors have questioned this belief (Cantwell, 1977; Clampit and Pirkle, 1983; Lerer and Lerer, 1977; Safer and Krager, 1988), noting their own and other clinical studies, which indicate that stimulants are as useful for adolescents as they are for younger children. Although ADHD persists into adolescence and adulthood and CNS stimulants continue to be effective, some professionals prefer other psychotropic drugs such as TCAs.

Indications. Attention deficit hyperactivity disorder is characterized by inattention, impulsiveness, and hyperactivity. Fidgeting and restlessness are more prominent in adolescents than is hyperactivity. All these deficits cause a problem for the adolescent in school, who is expected to sit still and listen, and are indications for treatment.

Central nervous system stimulants. Safer and Krager (1988) found that between 1975 and 1987 the percentage of public middle-school students receiving medication for hyperactivity or inattention rose from 0.5% to 3.68% and that between 1983 and 1985 the percentage of public senior high school students receiving medication rose from 0.21% to 0.40%. This research conservatively estimated that 750,000 youths (including 5.96% of all public elementary-school children) received medication for hyperactivity in 1987 and predicted that one million youths will be receiving medication in the early 1990s. Of the school-aged children taking stimulants, 25% are in special education classes (Safer and Krager, 1988).

The most commonly used drugs in the treatment of ADHD are dextroamphetamine (Dexedrine) and methylphenidate (Ritalin). Of the two, methylphenidate is used more often, about 93% of the time (Safer and Krager, 1988). However, these drugs are not as frequently used in adolescents, particularly in older adolescents, partly because of the aforementioned belief that these drugs are not as effective after childhood and partly because of the potential for abuse by the patient, siblings, or members of the patient's peer group.

Nonetheless, CNS stimulants used in conjunction with counseling can be effective. Improvement for the ADHD patient means the ability to control behavior, to pay attention, and to learn. In short, these drugs give the adolescent an opportunity to succeed in school. The stimulant has a calming effect. This so-called paradoxic effect can be explained by the theory that low levels of these drugs stimulate inhibitory neurons in the CNS, thus producing an overall CNS "depression." Another view suggests that low doses of CNS stimulants, by stimulating the child's immature reticular activating system, enable the motor cortex to respond appropriately to external stimuli. The latter theory seems plausible for young children, but it loses some of its theoretic appeal when applied to adolescents. Presumably both effects are caused by the CNS stimulant's ability to increase the levels of dopamine, norepinephrine, and serotonin. Although many drugs used in the treatment of childhood behavior disorders simply make the child more "manageable," CNS stimulants directly affect the problem behavior. The box below provides a profile of drugs used in the treatment of ADHD.

Tricyclic antidepressants. Drugs other than CNS stimulants have been tried with varying degrees of success. Tricyclic antidepressants have been used to treat adolescent ADHD; they seem to have more side effects than do the CNS stimulants and, according to some clinicians, have short-lived results. On the other hand, TCAs have the following potential advantages over stimulants:

1. They have a longer duration of action.
2. They may be given as a single dose.

Drugs Used in the Treatment of Attention Deficit Hyperactivity Disorder*

Methylphenidate (Ritalin)
In children >6 yr, 5 mg qd or bid; optimum dose is 0.3 to 0.7 mg/kg bid or tid†; maximum dose is 60 mg/day; a sustained release form exists (Ritalin-SR); methylphenidate is a Controlled Substance Schedule II drug

Dextroamphetamine (Dexedrine)
Children >6 yr may be given 5 mg qd or bid with 5-mg increments once or twice weekly; usual optimum dose is between 0.15 and 0.5 mg/kg bid or tid†; maximum dose should not exceed 40 mg/day; amphetamines are Schedule II drugs; the American Academy of Pediatrics recommends that dextroamphetamine dosage should be approximately half the methylphenidate dosage

Pemoline (Cylert)
Usual maintenance dose is 56.25 to 75 mg per day; maximum daily dose is 112.5 mg

Side effects
Nervousness, insomnia, anorexia, stomachache, weight loss, and temporary growth retardation; long-term growth problems apparently do not occur; methylphenidate does not noticeably impair growth during early adolescence‡; Brown and Sexson§ reported a significant increase in diastolic blood pressure in adolescent boys receiving methylphenidate (see Chapters 13 and 15 of this text for further information)

Interactions
Other sympathomimetic agents, tricyclic antidepressants, antihypertensives, antipsychotics, monoamine oxidase inhibitors (see Chapter 13 of this text for further information)

*Dosages from *Physicians' Desk Reference*, Oradell, N J, 1992, Medical Economics, unless otherwise noted.
†Duncan MK: *J Child Adolescent Psychopharmacol* 1:7, 1990.
‡Vincent J, Carley CK, Leger P: *Am J Psychiatry* 147:501, 1990.
§Brown TR, Sexson SB: *J Adolescent Health Care* 10:179, 1989.

3. Plasma levels can be confirmed.
4. They have little potential for abuse (Gastfriend, Biederman, and Jillinek, 1984).

Dosages for ADHD are lower than those for depression. Gastfriend, Bierderman, and Jillinek (1984) found improvement in 11 of 12 adolescent patients using desipramine. Starting dosages were 10 to 25 mg per day; mean dosages after the fourth week of study were 1.57 mg/kg. Pliska (1987) found that, overall, TCAs were not as effective as CNS stimulants; however, TCAs were effective for highly anxious patients with ADHD. Bupropion (Wellbutrin), a new antidepressant, has also been prescribed in the treatment of ADHD with some success (Green, 1991).

Issues associated with tricyclic antidepressants in treating attention deficit hyperactivity disorder. Tricyclic antidepressants are toxic, and overdoses should be treated seriously (see Chapter 5). Gastfriend, Bierderman, and Jillinek (1984) reported the following significant side effects associated with desipramine in an adolescent population with ADHD: drowsiness (50%), postural dizziness (25%), weight loss and decreased appetite (25%), headache (16%), insomnia (8%), and racing thoughts (8%). Other common side effects of TCAs include dry mouth, sedation, and cognitive problems.

Other drugs used for treatment of attention deficit hyperactivity disorder. Phenothiazines and haloperidol have been studied, but these drugs seem less effective than stimulants for the treatment of ADHD. Lithium, diphenhydramine (Benadryl), phenobarbital, and benzodiazepines have also had less-than-satisfactory results. In addition, the amino acid phenylalanine has been found ineffective (Zametkin, Larpi, and Rapoport, 1987). Central nervous system stimulants remain the drugs of choice for ADHD; however, for the significant group of persons with ADHD who do not respond to stimulants or in other cases when stimulant abuse is suspected, alternate drugs remain a viable option.

Psychotic Disorders

Schizophrenia usually begins to emerge in adolescence or early adulthood. Symptoms include hallucination, delusions, disordered thoughts, anxiety, inappropriate affect, idiosyncratic speech, morbid thoughts, absence of friends, and concrete thinking. During childhood there is frequently some diagnostic confusion between schizophrenia and autism; however, that confusion is much less prominent during the adolescent years. Autism almost always has its onset before 30 months of age, and schizophrenia often has its onset during adolescence. Autism in most cases continues into adolescence, at which time the cardinal symptoms of social and language skills deficits may improve or worsen. A thorough history often minimizes misdiagnosis, but a significant level of false-positive results for autism cases by use of the *Diagnostic and Statistical Manual of Mental Disorders, Third Edition-Revised (DSM-III-R)* criteria has promoted work to change the criteria for *DSM-IV* (Volkmar, 1991).

A reactive depression, that is, a depression caused by the realization that one is "handicapped by autism," is not uncommon in late-adolescent autism. Schizophrenia, autism, and other psychotic processes share similar psychopharmacologic intervention strategies.

Indications. The goal of drug treatment for the schizophrenic adolescent is to decrease thought disorganization so that restoration to a previous normal level of functioning can occur. For the autistic individual the goal is to decrease biting, head banging, and anxiety. Antipsychotics are used in both groups of patients to manage aggressive, assaultive, or self-destructive behavior. Psychotropic drugs alone are never considered adequate in the treatment of these adolescents. Drugs are but one aspect of a treatment plan that includes therapeutic communication, milieu management, and parental educational involvement.

Drugs used to treat psychotic disorders. Phenothiazines are often the first drugs used to treat psychoses in adolescents (Wiener, 1977). There is little empiric evidence that one antipsychotic is more effective than another. An overview of drugs used in the treatment of psychotic disorders is found in the boxes on pp. 329 to 331. For general discussion of antipsychotic drugs see Chapter 4, and for information related to pediatric usage review Chapter 15.

Depression and Mania

Depression and mania in adolescents have emerged as significant problems in the 1990s. Adolescent suicide related to depression is the topic of many articles and a source of fear for many parents. In children depression is more easily recognized than is mania; however, as adolescence approaches, mania takes on the characteristics of the adult manic disorder and is readily detectable. It is important for the psychiatric professional to understand the psychopharmacologic treatment of these conditions.

Drugs used to treat depression. The two major antidepressant drug classes are the TCAs and the monoamine oxidase inhibitors (MAOIs). Monoamine oxidase inhibitors have potentially life-threatening side effects and are not recommended for children younger than the age of 16 years.

Indications. Tricyclic antidepressants listed in the box on p. 332 are indicated for the treatment of depression in adolescents and adults. Some TCAs and other non-MAOI antidepressants are restricted to adult usage.

Tricyclic antidepressants. Tricyclic antidepressants were developed in the late 1950s and gained acceptance for treatment of childhood depression in the 1960s. Although the clinical effectiveness of TCAs in the treatment of adult depression is clear, little evidence supports the assertion that TCAs are effective in treating major adolescent depression (Puig-Antich, Ryan, and Rabinovich, 1985). For general information about TCAs see Chapter 5. For signs of TCA toxicity see the box on p. 333.

Drugs used to treat bipolar disorder

Lithium. Lithium has been used to successfully treat adult bipolar illness for 30 years in the United States. Its effectiveness in adolescents with depression is not

Phenothiazines Used to Treat Psychotic Disorders

Chlorpromazine (Thorazine)

Begin with 10 mg tid to 25 mg tid; dosages can be titrated upward by 20 to 50 mg twice weekly; chlorpromazine is usually prescribed at 0.5 mg/kg q 4-6 hr and gradually increased up to an oral dosage of 50-200 mg per day for severely ill and hospitalized children; whether an adolescent (12 to 18 yr) is given a prescription based on an adult dosage or a child's dosage is related to his or her physical development

Continued.

Phenothiazines Used to Treat Psychotic Disorders—cont'd

Thioridazine (Mellaril)

Typically begin with 25-50 mg bid or tid, but higher doses can be given depending on the severity of the illness; as with adults, an absolute upper limit of 800 mg/day should be adhered to; Realmuto et al.* gave a mean dose of 178 mg/day to 21 adolescent patients (11 to 18 yr) with improvement in about half of the group

Trifluoperazine (Stelazine)

Usual starting dosage is 2-5 mg bid; Wolpert, Hagamen, and Merlis† gave 13-20 mg/day to autistic children (8 to 15 yr) and found improvement

Fluphenazine (Prolixin)

Werry‡ recommended a starting dosage of 0.025-0.05 mg/kg up to 0.3 mg/kg/day (3-6 mg per day); Joshi, Capozzoli, and Coyle§ found that low maintenance dosages of 0.05 mg/kg/day produced significant results

Effects

The neuroleptic effect of phenothiazines is characterized by sedation, emotional quieting, and psychomotor slowing. The antipsychotic effect is manifested by normalization of thought, mood, and behavior. The neuroleptic effect may be more significant for the autistic adolescent, and the antipsychotic effect may be more significant for the adolescent with a psychotic disorder.

Interactions

Phenothiazines interact with central nervous system depressants and anticholinergics (for example, cold or hay fever medications).

Side effects

Extrapyramidal side effects (EPSEs), anticholineric effects, sedation, and weight gain occur. Extrapyramidal side effects are prevalent among adolescents, and antiparkinson agents are sometimes used for prophylaxis among these patients. See Chapter 4 for more information.

Rules for administering antipsychotics

The following general rules regarding antipsychotic medication should be addressed by all clinicians:

1. Antipsychotic drugs should not be used for nonapproved indications.
2. Antipsychotic drugs should be given in lowest effective dose for maintenance therapy because of relationship between dose and EPSEs.
3. Adolescents should occasionally be placed on physician-approved drug-free "holidays."‖

*Realmuto GM et al: *Am J Psychiatry* 141:440, 1984.
†Wolpert A, Hagamen MB, Merlis S: *Curr Therapeutic Res* 9:482, 1967.
‡Werry J: *Pediatric psychopharmacology*, New York, 1978, Brunner-Mazel.
§Joshi PT, Capozzoli JA, Coyle JT: *Am J Psychiatry* 145:335, 1988.
‖Keltner NL. In Hogarth C, editor: *Adolescent psychiatric nursing*, St Louis, 1991, Mosby.

Other Antipsychotics Used to Treat Psychotic Disorders

Haloperidol (Haldol)
From 0.5 to 5 mg bid or tid; higher doses may be required for more rapid neurolepization; Pool et al.* found that a mean dosage of 9.8 mg per day of haloperidol was effective in reducing target symptoms; at somewhat lower dosages, haloperidol is also used to treat adolescent autism

Thiothixene (Navane)
For adults and children >12 yr, recommended dosage is 2 mg three times daily or 5 mg three times daily; optimum maintenance dosage is 20-30 mg per day for severe conditions

Chlorprothixene (Taractan)
For adolescents >12 yr and for adults, 25-50 mg three or four times daily is suggested

Molindone (Moban)
For adults and children >12 yr, 50-75 mg per day is recommended initially for psychotic episodes; maintenance dosages for mild symptoms are usually 5-15 mg three or four times daily

Loxapine (Loxitane)
Loxapine is not recommended for use in children <16 yr; however, Pool et al.* gave adolescent schizophrenics (13 to 18 yr) a mean dosage of 87.5 mg per day and found loxapine to be safe; hallucinations, delusions, and other symptoms improved

Pool D et al: *Curr Therapeutic Res* 19:99, 1976.

clearly demonstrated. See the box on p. 333, bottom, for a profile of lithium as used in adolescent bipolar disorders.

Of all bipolar patients, 20% to 30% first experience affective symptoms before the age of 20 years (Carroll, Jefferson, and Griest, 1987). Lithium, if effective, is therefore an important drug to consider for adolescent bipolar patients. Most research indicates that children tolerate lithium well (Carroll, Jefferson, and Griest, 1987). More detailed information concerning this drug can be found in Chapter 5.

Administration. Puig-Antich, Ryan, and Rabinovich, (1985) recommended that adolescents be started on a regimen of dosages of 300 mg per day (in divided doses), to be increased by 300 mg per day every 5 to 7 days until a favorable response is obtained. The effective lithium serum level range is 0.6 to 1.2 mEq/L. Carroll, Jefferson, and Griest (1987) found that a dosage of 30 mg/kg per day was sufficient for prepubertal children. Strober et al. (1990) found that adolescents who discontinue taking lithium relapsed three times more often than those who continued their treatment.

Other drugs used to treat bipolar disorder

Clonidine (Catapres). Clonidine has been used successfully in the treatment of

Tricyclic Antidepressants Used to Treat Depression

Imipramine (Tofranil)

A beginning dosage of 10 mg tid or qid is appropriate; dosage should not exceed 100 mg per day; therapeutic serum levels are 150 to 240 ng/ml*

Desipramine (Norpramin, Pertofrane)

Usual dosage is 25 mg, one to four times per day; dosage should be initiated at a lower level and increased according to tolerance and clinical response; Dosage should not exceed 150 mg per day; therapeutic serum levels are 115 ng/ml*

Amitriptyline (Elavil, Endep)

Recommended dosage is 10 mg three times per day plus 20 mg hs; this total dose of 50 mg is usually sufficient; research has shown use of as much as 200 mg per day with no appreciable reduction in symptoms; therapeutic serum levels are 100 to 300 ng/ml*

Effect

Tricyclic antidepressants decrease the level of depression and exert this effect by increasing central nervous system levels of norepinephrine, serotonin, and dopamine; it takes 3 to 4 weeks to achieve a full clinical effect

Interactions

Sympathomimetics and anticholinergic drugs can intensify the effects of TCAs

Side effects

Anticholinergic side effects, a blood pressure higher than 140/90 mm Hg, and a heart rate greater than 130 beats per minute are cause for alarm;* tricyclic antidepressants have a narrow therapeutic index; adolescents are thought to be more sensitive to overdoses than are adults

*From Martin JE, Agran M. In Matson JL, editor: *Handbook of treatment approaches in childhood psychopathology*, New York, 1988, Plenum; Puig-Antich J, Ryan ND, Rabinovich H. In Wiener JM, editor: *Diagnosis and psychopharmacology for childhood and adolescent disorders*, New York, 1985, John Wiley & Sons.

manic disorder. Zubenko et al. (1984) found that 0.2 mg of clonidine twice daily was effective in relieving manic symptoms after lithium had failed to do so.

Carbamazepine (Tegretol). Lithium is the drug of choice for bipolar disorder; however up to 40% of these patients do not respond (Wise, 1989). Carbamazepine can be used in the treatment of manic disorder when lithium is ineffective. Hematologic risks associated with carbamazepine include aplastic anemia and agranulocytosis (Olin, 1990); however, these adverse affects are rare (Wise, 1989) and the less significant side effects are typically transient and manageable (Pellock, 1987). Serum levels do not guide the clinician in prescribing carbamazepine as they do for lithium (Wise, 1989). Carbamazepine dosages vary from person to person.

Signs of Toxic Effects of Tricyclic Antidepressants

Tricyclic antidepressants are the most frequently used drugs in cases of overdose in the United States.* For this reason the prescribed dose must be carefully maintained and monitored. The potential for suicide or accidental overdose demands that these drugs be kept away from younger adolescents and children.

Peripheral effects
Tachycardia, tachyarrythmias, diarrhea or constipation, urinary retention

Motor effects
Muscle rigidity, hyperactive reflex, ataxia, convulsions

Central nervous system effects
Sedation, respiratory tract depression, disorientation, agitation, confusion, lethargy, poor memory and concentration

*Harsch HH, Holt RE: *Hosp Community Psychiatry* 39:990, 1988.

Profile of Lithium as Used in the Treatment of Adolescent Bipolar Disorders

Toxic effects
Lithium has a narrow therapeutic index; consequently, frequent lithium serum level measurements are needed. In some adolescent inpatient programs, daily blood lithium levels are obtained. Nausea and vomiting, slurred speech, and drowsiness may be early indications of intoxication.* If intoxication is suspected, withhold the lithium.

Side effects
Side effects include weakness, tremor, weight gain, stomachache, and blurred vision. If diarrhea occurs, the adolescent should be observed closely because a loss of sodium through extraurinary routes can lead to lithium intoxication.

Interactions
The most serious interactions are with drugs that increase lithium serum levels; these include most diuretics and salt substitutes, which can reduce the amount of sodium ingested, leading to increased levels of lithium. Lithium and haloperidol are reported to cause neurotoxic effects when used together.

*Puig-Antich J, Ryan ND, Rabinovich H. In Wiener JM, editor: *Diagnosis and psychopharmacology for childhood and adolescent disorders*, New York, 1985, John Wiley & Sons.

Other Disorders

Aggressive behavior. Aggressive behavior is a real issue on inpatient adolescent care units. Although persons under the age of 18 represent only 15% of the population, they account for 25% of serious crimes (i.e., murder, rape, robbery, etc.). About half of all children seen for emotional problems are brought in for evaluation because of aggressive behavior (Marohn, 1992). Aggressive behavior is associated with ADHD, schizophrenia, bipolar disorder, paranoid thinking, seizure disorders, and what are described as episodic dyscontrol disorders (Marohn, 1992).

Inability to control impulses has led to many serious injuries that could have been avoided. For older adolescents the information presented in Chapter 9 is appropriate for both dosage and other intervention approaches. For younger adolescents requiring immediate treatment, an intramuscular dosage of chlorpromazine 0.5 mg/kg every 6 to 8 hours, as needed, is appropriate. For severely agitated adolescents an intramuscular dose of 25 mg may be given and repeated in 1 hour. Thereafter injections should be spaced at least 4 to 6 hours apart. A 12-year-old child should not receive more than 75 mg intramuscularly per day. Other medications used to treat aggressive behavior include other neuroleptics, lithium, anticonvulsants, CNS stimulants, antidepressants, and beta blockers.

Tourette's syndrome. Tourette's syndrome (TS) is characterized by involuntary, repetitive, purposeless muscle movements such as gyrating, hopping, clapping, and kicking, accompanied by multiple verbal tics, including screaming and coprolalia (Adkins, 1989) and is discussed in Chapter 15. Social problems can be monumental for the patient and family. Haloperidol and pimozide are the drugs used most often. Shapiro et al. (1989) found haloperidol to be effective but also to have increased side effects.

Haloperidol (Haldol). The recommended dosage of haloperidol is 0.05 to 0.075 mg/kg per day for children with TS younger than 12 years of age. Shapiro et al. (1989) gave a group of adolescents up to 10 mg per day. Bruun (1988) gave 4 to 7 mg per day of haloperidol to patients. Weiden and Bruun (1987) used between 1 and 6 mg per day in their study. Young et al. (1985) recommended giving no more than 3 to 4 mg per day in divided dosages. Extrapyramidal symptoms are significant in adolescents. Weiden and Bruun (1987) found that neuroleptic drug-induced akathisia was responsible for suicide, violent outbursts, and a worsening of TS. About 80% of the patients treated with haloperidol are helped (Young et al., 1985). Therapeutic serum levels range between 1 and 3 ng/ml (Green, 1991).

Pimozide (Orap). Pimozide is an antipsychotic drug used for managing severe motor or vocal tics in patients with TS. It is not recommended in children younger than 12 years of age; however, pimozide is used widely with adolescents. Shapiro et al. (1989) gave dosages of up to 20 mg per day in their study, with significant results. They found that patients had fewer side effects with pimozide than with haloperidol. Brunn (1988) recommended that no more than 8 mg per day of pimozide be given. Weiden and Brunn (1987) gave between 2 and 6 mg per day of pimozide to adolescents with TS. The researchers thought that at higher dosages neuroleptic drug-induced side effects can be a serious treatment problem. Olin (1990) recommended an initial dosage of 1 to 2 mg per day in divided doses, increasing every other day. Maintenance dosages should be less than 0.2 mg/kg per day or 10 mg per day, whichever is less.

Clonidine (Catapres). Clonidine is an antihypertensive, and although it is not Food and Drug Administration (FDA)–approved for use in TS, it is used by many clinicians. It is an alpha-2 agonist that should be initiated at low dosages of 0.05 mg per day and slowly increased for several weeks to 0.15 to 0.30 mg per day. Dosages over 0.4 or 0.5 mg per day lead to side effects (Gallico, Burns, and Grob, 1988; Young et al., 1985). Clonidine has a slower onset of action than does haloperidol, taking 3 or more weeks before a therapeutic improvement is noted (Young et al., 1985). Side effects include sedation, dry mouth, and hypotension.

Other Drugs Used to Treat Mental Disorders

Carbamazepine (Tegretol). Carbamazepine, an anticonvulsant, is used in a variety of psychiatric diagnoses, including bipolar illness, schizo-affective illness, resistant schizophrenia, and impulse-control problems. Post et al. (1987) postulated that a kindling phenomenon, similar to what occurs with epilepsy, may occur in bipolar illness, thus explaining the efficacy of carbamazepine, an anticonvulsant. Carbamazepine is also used in the treatment of conduct disorders. The impulsive and angry outbursts associated with some conduct-disordered children may well respond to carbamazepine for reasons similar to (but not the same as) the reason bipolar patients are helped.

Benzodiazepines. Diazepam (Valium) is a benzodiazepine that has been used in the treatment of separation anxiety, alcohol withdrawal symptoms, panic attacks, and seizures. It may be used when excessive anxiety occurs; however, concerns related to initiating an early life-style of coping through drugs may overrule its use. The benzodiazepines used in adolescents are chlordiazepoxide (Librium) and alprazolam (Xanax). Side effects include sedation, disinhibition, and loss of coordination. A withdrawal reaction occurs when benzodiazepinens are withdrawn too fast. Withdrawal reactions can include severe anxiety and seizures. Santos and Morton (1989) have found clonazepam (Klonopin) and lorazepam (Ativan) to be effective for managing manic agitation, although the authors did not specifically mention adolescent cases.

Clomipramine (Anafranil). Clomipramine can be used in adolescents with obsessive-compulsive disorder. The maximum dosage for adolescents and children is 3 mg/kg per day, up to 200 mg, whichever is smaller. Somnolence, dizziness, dry mouth, and fatigue are the most frequently reported side effects in children and adolescents.

Clozapine (Clozaril). Clozapine is a new antipsychotic, which was released for public use in 1990. Clozapine use for adolescents 15 years of age and younger has not yet been established as safe and effective (Olin, 1990).

Remarks

Adolescent psychopharmacology is an increasingly important dimension of psychiatric care. However, as with children, these drugs are not the first avenue of help but rather are used when less intrusive approaches are ineffective. As the clinician carefully considers the implications of psychotropic drugs for adolescent patients including appropriate dosage, side effects, drug interactions, and toxic effects, a thorough treatment plan can be developed and implemented. Although the treatment of ADHD is the most carefully studied current pharmacologic approach, continuing research may enable us to treat psychosis, depression, bipolar disorder, and other disorders more confidently in the future.

REFERENCES

Adkins AS: Helping your patient cope with Tourette's syndrome, *Pediatr Nurs* 15:135, 1989.

American Psychiatric Association: *Diagnostic and statistical manual of mental disorders, third edition-revised,* Washington, DC, 1987, The Association.

Bruun RD: Subtle and underrecognized side effects of neuroleptic treatment in children with Tourette's disorder, *Am J Psychiatry* 145:621, 1988.

Cantwell DP: Psychopharmacologic treatment of the minimal brain dysfunction syndrome. In Wiener J, editor: *Psychopharmacology in childhood and adolescence,* New York, 1977, Basic Books.

Cantwell DP: Hyperactive children have grown up, *Arch Gen Psychiatry* 42:1026, 1985.

Carroll JA, Jefferson JW, Greist JH: Psychiatric uses of lithium for children and adolescents, *Hosp Community Psychiatry* 38:927, 1987.

Clampit MK, Pirkle JB: Stimulant medications and the hyperactive adolescent: myths and facts, *Adolescence* 18:811, 1983.

Esman AH: Treatment and services for adolescents: an introduction, *Hosp Community Psychiatry* 43(6):616, 1992.

Gallico RP, Burns TJ, Grob CS: *Emotional and behavioral problems in children with learning disabilities,* Boston, 1988, College-Hill.

Garfinkel BD, Amrami KK: A perspective on the attention-deficit disorders, *Hosp Community Psychiatry* 43(6):445, 1992.

Gastfriend DR, Biederman, J, Jillinek MS: Desipramine in the treatment of adolescents with attention deficit disorder, *Am J Psychiatry* 141:906, 1984.

Green WH: *Child and adolescent clinical psychopharmacology,* Baltimore, 1991, Williams & Wilkins.

Harsch HH, Holt RE: Use of antidepressants in attempted suicide, *Hosp Community Psychiatry* 39:990, 1988.

Hogarth C: *Adolescent psychiatric nursing,* St Louis, 1991, Mosby.

Kalogerakis MG: Emergency evaluation of adolescents, *Hosp Community Psychiatry* 43(6):617, 1992.

Keltner NL: Psychopharmacology. In Hogarth C: *Adolescent psychiatric nursing,* St Louis, 1991, Mosby.

Lerer RJ, Lerer P: Responses of adolescents with minimal brain dysfunction to methylphenidate, *J Learning Disabilities* 10:223, 1977.

Marohn RC: Management of the assaultive adolescent, *Hosp Community Psychiatry* 43(6):622, 1992.

Munoz-Millan RJ, Casteel CR: Attention-deficit hyperactivity disorder: recent literature, *Hosp Community Psychiatry* 40:699, 1989.

News & Notes: Almost 20 percent of American children have psychological, learning problems, survey finds, *Hosp Community Psychiatry* 42(4):438, 1991.

Olin BP: *Drug facts and comparisons,* Philadelphia, 1990, JB Lippincott.

Pellock JM: Carbamazepine side effects in children and adults, *Epilepsia* 28:564, 1987.

Physician's desk reference, 1992, Oradell, N J, Medical Economics.

Pliska SR: Tricyclic antidepressants in the treatment of children with attention deficit disorder, *J Am Acad Child Adolescent Psychiatry* 26:127, 1987.

Post RM et al: Correlates of antimanic response to carbamazepine, *Psychiatry Res* 21:71, 1987.

Puig-Antich J, Ryan ND, Rabinovich H: Affective disorders in children and adolescent. In Wiener JM, editor: *Diagnosis and psychopharmacology for childhood and adolescent disorders,* New York, 1985, John Wiley & Sons.

Realmuto GM et al: Clinical comparison of thiothixene and thioridazine in schizophrenic adolescents, *Am J Psychiatry* 141:440, 1984.

Safer DJ, Krager JM: A survey of medication treatments for hyperactive/inattentive students, *J Am Med Assoc* 260:2256, 1988.

Santos AB, Morton WA: Use of benzodiazepines to improve management of manic agitation, *Hosp Community Psychiatry* 40:1069, 1989.

Shapiro E et al: Controlled study of haloperidol, pimozide, and placebo for the treatment of Gilles de la Tourette's syndrome, *Arch Gen Psychiatry* 46:722, 1989.

Strober M et al: Relapse following discontinuation of lithium maintenance therapy in adolescents with bipolar-I illness: a naturalistic study, *Am J Psychiatry* 147:457, 1990.

Volkmar FR: Autism and the pervasive developmental disorders, *Hosp Community Psychiatry* 42(1):33, 1991.

Weiden P, Bruun R: Worsening of Tourette's disorder due to neuroleptic induced akathisia, *Am J Psychiatry* 144:504, 1987.

Wiener JM: *Psychopharmacology in childhood and adolescence,* New York, 1977, Basic Books.

Wise SS: Carbamazepine: treatment option for bipolar patients, *Hosp Community Psychiatry* 40:123, 1989.

Young JG et al: Tourette's syndrome and tic disorders. In Wiener JM, editor: *Diagnosis and psychopharmacology of childhood and adolescent disorders,* New York, 1985, John Wiley & Sons.

Zametkin AJ, Larpi F, Rapoport JL: Treatment of hyperactive children with D-phenylalanine, *Am J Psychiatry* 144:792, 1987.

Zubenko GS et al: Clonidine in the treatment of mania and mixed bipolar disorder, *Am J Psychiatry* 141:1617, 1984.

CHAPTER 17

Psychopharmacology for Elderly Persons

Psychotropics are the second most frequently prescribed class of drugs for older patients (Folks, 1990). Regarding single-drug prescriptions, more sedative-hypnotics are prescribed to older patients than any other single drug (Balter and Bauer, 1975). The segment of the population older than 65 years of age accounts for about 25% of the total drug expenditures in developed countries (Williams and Lowenthal, 1992). This figure is predicted to reach 40% by 2030 (Vestal, 1982).

Psychotropic drug therapy in an older patient can be complicated by many factors. Reduced life expectancy and functional capacity, the relative physiologic effects of aging, pharmacokinetic and pharmacodynamic influences, polypharmacy, drug interaction, treatment setting, coexisting medical conditions, cognitive impairment, and issues pertinent to compliance are all important considerations in the effective pharmacologic approach to the geriatric patient (Folks, 1990). When pharmacologic treatment is indicated for an older patient, specific knowledge of drug actions and effects are especially pertinent. Ultimately the primary goal of psychotropic drug therapy for a geriatric patient is to improve quality of life. By enhancing communication and understanding between an older patient and clinician, the overall quality of care can often be significantly improved.

The psychopharmacologic approach to treatment in a geriatric patient requires knowledge of psychiatric and nonpsychiatric conditions that are more prevalent in these patients. An appreciation of comorbid medical conditions is sometimes critical to safe and effective drug treatment. Also, the health care provider who is familiar with the bioepidemiologic differences among older adults will be better prepared to individualize treatment plans and evaluate the response to drug intervention (Montamat, Cusack, and Vestal, 1989).

SCOPE OF THE PROBLEM

The geriatric population is growing at a remarkable rate. Several factors account for disproportionate growth among the geriatric population; decreased infant mortality, declining birth rates, increased life expectancy, and declining death rates for those over 65 years of age are the factors mostly responsible. As depicted in Figure 17-1, the significant rate of growth among the elderly has occurred steadily since the turn of the century, when about 3.1 million persons, or 4% of the population in the United States, were over the age of 65 years. Currently approximately 13% of the population, or 30 million individuals, have reached their sixty-fifth birthday. As the "baby boomers" begin to reach their sixty-fifth birthdays, after 2010 and beyond, as many as 65 million people, or approximately 20% to 25% of the population in the United States, are estimated to account for those over the age of 65 years by the year 2030 (Gaitz, Niederehe, and Wilson, 1985). Declining death rates for those over 65 years of age are primarily responsible for the rapid growth of the "true elderly seg-

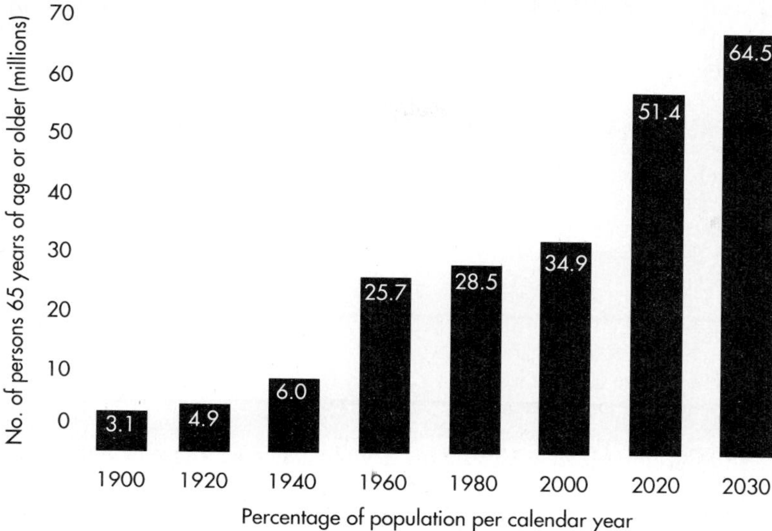

Figure 17-1 Geriatric population demographics through the year 2030. The disproportionate growth rate for the geriatric population in the United States is evident. (From Folks DG: *Drug Ther Suppl,* August 1990, p 72.)

ment," that is, those over 85 years of age. This subsegment is indeed the most rapidly growing of all age groups. It is staggering to realize that the "elderly" subsegment of the population will more than double in the next decade, with a growth rate approximately 22 times that of the adolescent subsegment of our population.

Psychiatric disorders are not generally encountered in isolation in geriatric patients (Masoro, 1987). Acute, life-threatening, serious illness and prevalent chronic conditions require careful consideration with respect to psychiatric intervention (see the boxes on p. 340). Multiple disease processes, common environmental influences, and genetic variation often combine with the physiologic or psychobiologic effects of aging, significantly influencing pharmacologic treatment outcome (see the boxes on p. 340). Of course, physiologic aging does not necessarily parallel chronologic aging; apart from the prominent effects of overt disease states, physiologic aging more often underlies the age-related differences in the action of psychotropic drugs (Rowe and Kahn, 1987). Thus, understanding the pharmacologic consequences of the physiologic effects of aging is also critical to safe and effective pharmacotherapeutics.

GENERAL FACTORS PERTINENT TO PSYCHOTROPIC DRUG THERAPY

This section outlines the pharmacokinetic, pharmacodynamic, and nontherapeutic effects of drugs as they relate to psychotropics used in the treatment of geriatric patients. Additionally, issues relating to compliance are outlined with respect to the clinical approach. These factors determine many of the general principles that are useful in the clinical approach to common psychiatric syndromes encountered in late life.

Diseases Causing Death in Individuals 65 Years of Age and Older

Heart disease
Cancer, malignant neoplasms
Stroke, cerebrovascular disease
Alzheimer's disease, related disorders
Influenza, pneumonia
Accidents: Falls and motor-pedestrian
Suicide

Chronic Medical Conditions in Individuals 65 Years of Age and Older

Arthritis and rheumatologic disease
Neurosensory loss: Hearing disturbance, visual disturbance
Cardiovascular disease: Congestive heart failure, ischemic heart disease, hypertension, peripheral vascular disease
Gastrointestinal disorders
Chronic sinusitis and upper respiratory disturbances
Genitourinary tract problems
Chronic obstructive pulmonary disease
Adult-onset diabetes mellitus
Thyroid disease, endocrinopathy
Dermatologic disturbances

Targets of Psychobiologic Effects of Aging

Autonomic nervous system
Behavioral and personality function
Bone density
Body composition
Cognitive function
Glucose tolerance
Hearing and vision
Immune function
Pulmonary function
Renal function
Skin
Systolic blood pressure

Pharmacokinetics

Pharmacokinetics refers to what the body does to a drug with respect to absorption, distribution, metabolism, and elimination. Altered pharmacokinetics in elderly individuals is due in part to physiologic changes that accompany aging. The predictable age-related changes in body composition and organ function in older adults also result in altered pharmacokinetics. These changes include diminished renal function, diminished hepatic blood flow, decreased serum albumin level and lean-muscle mass, decreased total body water, and increased alpha-1 acid glycoprotein (AGP). Thus age-related differences and drug disposition are multifactorial and are significantly influenced by environmental, genetic, physiologic, and pathologic factors.

Most studies of older populations and pharmacokinetics are cross-sectional and merely provide information about the "average" age-related differences. Because of the difficulties in design, administration, and cost of longitudinal studies, few studies have provided a precise picture of the changes in pharmacokinetics that occur within an aging cohort (William and Lowenthal, 1992). Whereas some age-related physiologic changes have a profound effect on drug kinetics, for example, renal function, others do not appear to alter pharmacokinetic values consistently, for example, gastrointestinal absorption.

Absorption. Despite several age-related alterations that occur with age in the gastrointestinal (GI) tract, such as increased gastric pH, delayed gastric emptying, diminished blood flow, and impaired intestinal motility, few psychotropic drugs actually show any delayed rates of GI tract absorption after oral administration (Montamat, Cusack, and Vestal, 1989). Thus the anatomic and physiologic changes that occur with aging in the GI tract have little effect on drug metabolism.

The term *bioavailability* refers to the relative amount of drug reaching the systemic circulation after absorption. The bioavailability of a drug is determined not only by the extent of absorption through the GI tract but also by the presystemic drug elimination in the liver as the drug passes from the portal circulation. The bioavailability of drugs is generally unchanged in older adults, except in the case of those drugs that are abstracted at a high rate by the liver (Cusack and Vestal, 1986). Decreased presystemic hepatic extraction leads to modest increases in the bioavailability of certain drugs, for example, beta blockers. However, these findings have no real clinical significance. By contrast, pathologic and surgical alterations in the GI tract and interactions between psychotropics and drugs such as laxatives, antacids, and agents that decrease gastric emptying may alter absorption.

Distribution. Changes in body composition (Figure 17-2) and blood flow may profoundly affect drug distribution in an older adult. A decrease in total body water and lean body mass with a proportional increase in body fat undoubtedly affects the volume of distribution of many drugs. Water soluble drugs, for example, ethanol and lithium, have a reduced volume of distribution in elderly individuals, with increased initial concentrations in the central compartment and resultant higher plasma concentrations. Lipid soluble drugs, for example, the benzodiazepines, tend to have a much greater distribution in older persons because of the average increase in body fat. Interestingly, some lipophilic drugs, most notably, lorazepam (Ativan) and amobarbital (Amytal), do not have significantly different volumes of distribution with increased age. When the volume of distribution is increased for an anxiolytic or another psychotropic, as is the case with diazepam, the result may be a prolonged action because of an even longer elimination half-life, as discussed in Chapter 6.

Free and unbound drug concentrations are important determinants of both drug

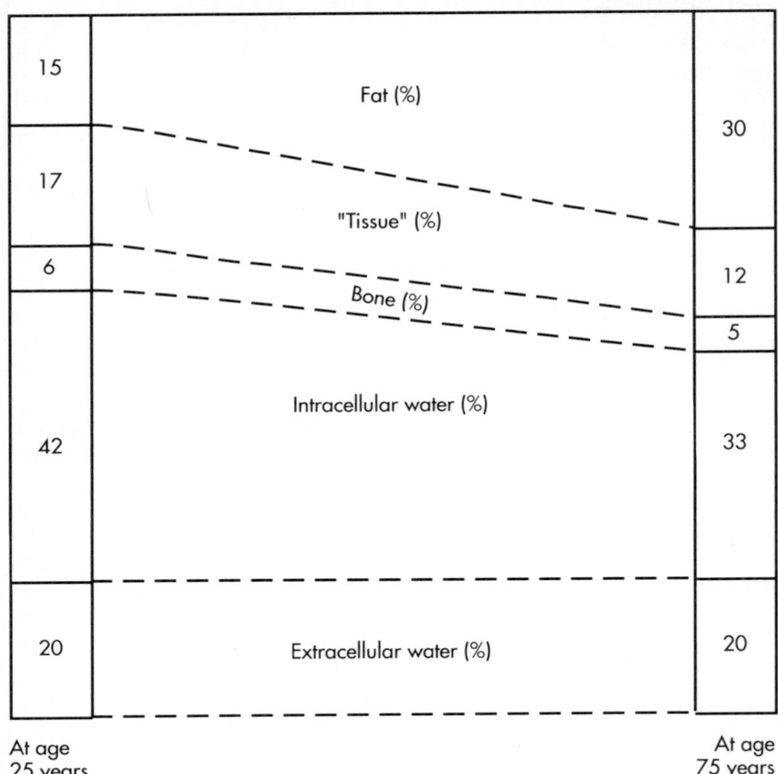

Figure 17-2 Representation of changes in body composition in the "average" individual, comparing body composition at 25 and 75 years of age. (From Folks DG: *Drug Ther Suppl*, August 1990, p 72.)

distribution and elimination. Thus alterations in binding of drugs to plasma proteins, red blood cells, and metabolic organs can and do alter pharmacokinetic properties in elderly persons. The tendency is toward lower protein binding of drugs related to the average decline in serum albumin concentration or alteration in albumin receptor configuration, or both, related to age and disease. In fact, however, epidemiologic studies indicate that decreases in albumin concentrations are minimal in healthy elderly persons and not likely to be of clinical significance (Folks & Fuller, in press; Greenblatt, 1979). In contrast, chronic diseases may be associated with substantial reductions in serum albumin levels. In this case it is important to note that weakly acidic drugs, for example, barbiturates and phenytoin, bind primarily to plasma albumin. Weak bases such as propranolol are bound basically to AGP; thus some degree of variability exists in the concentration of this specific agent, especially since the concentration of AGP tends to increase with age (Abernathy and Kerznel, 1984). Thus in elderly persons the decrease in albumin and the increase in AGP concentrations may be associated with both reduced and increased protein bindings of drugs, respectively (Wallace and Verbeeck, 1987).

Hepatic metabolism. Metabolism of drugs by the liver depends on the activity of enzymes, which carry out biotransformation and are influenced by the extent of hepatic blood flow that determines the rate of delivery of drugs to the liver. Drugs that are metabolized slowly with low intrinsic clearance are processed proportionately to the rate of hepatic metabolism. Since hepatic mass decreases with age in absolute terms and in proportion to body weight, the clearance of drugs with low intrinsic clearance is reduced. Generally this includes drugs that to a great extent depend on oxidation, that is, those that utilize oxidative pathways of drug metabolism (Wynne et al., 1989).

Drugs with a rapid rate of metabolism and high intrinsic clearance are extracted rapidly by the liver. The rate-limiting step in this case is hepatic blood flow. This relationship is particularly pertinent to drugs which are administered intravenously, for example, diazepam (Valium). Advancing age is associated with the reduction in the presystemic metabolism of drugs with a relatively higher rate of extraction (Castleden and George, 1979). Thus the bioavailability of certain drugs such as beta blockers is increased, and accordingly other drugs with high rates of hepatic extraction, for example, antipsychotics or tricyclic antidepressants (TCAs) should be administered with great caution and careful monitoring for side effects.

Liver metabolism can be classified on the basis of biotransformation reactions as phase 1 with oxidation, reduction, and hydrolysis and phase 2 with conjugation reactions that include glucuronidation, acetylation, and sulfation. Microsomal and nonmicrosomal enzymes are involved in both processes. Phase 1 pathways of metabolism are either reduced or unchanged in elderly persons, whereas phase 2 pathways are not altered and are more predictable. Benzodiazepines undergo both types of metabolism (Bellatuono et al., 1980). For example, chlordiazepoxide (Librium), diazepam, clorazepate (Tranxene), and prazepam (Centrax) all undergo oxidative metabolism and therefore have prolonged elimination in elderly persons. These drugs are converted to an active metabolite, for example, desmethyldiazepam, which in turn has other active metabolites for which half-life is substantially longer than in the parent compound, that is, up to 220 hours in elderly patients. Other benzodiazepines, oxazepam (Serax), lorazepam, and temazepam (Restoril), undergo conjugation reactions; the metabolism of these agents remains unaltered by age. Thus these compounds do not give rise to active metabolites and represent safer compounds within the benzodiazepine class for treatment in elderly persons (Folks, 1990).

Age is only one of many factors that potentially affect drug metabolism. For example, cigarette smoking, alcohol intake, dietary consideration, drugs, illness, and caffeine consumption may all affect the rate of drug metabolism. Enzyme induction through smoking and alcohol consumption and hepatic enzyme inhibition through decreased drug clearance by other drugs such as cimetidine (Tagamet) may also impact drug metabolism in older individuals. In short, hepatic metabolism is a complex process and psychotropic agents that are more easily metabolized, for example, the benzodiazepine lorazepam or the secondary amine TCA nortriptyline (Pamelor, Aventyl), are generally preferred for older patients.

Elimination. Perhaps the best documented and the most predictable alteration in pharmacokinetics with advancing age is the reduction in the rate of renal elimination or excretion (Rowe et al., 1976). This reduction is due to a decline in both the glomerular filtration rate (GFR) and the tubular secretion rate, which accounts for the decreased creatinine clearance resulting from the aging process. Beginning with the fourth decade of life a 6% to 10% reduction in GFR and renal plasma occurs every 10 years. Thus by 70 years of age an individual may have as much as a 50% decrease in renal function in the absence of renal disease.

Drug elimination in patients who have normal serum creatinine concentrations is affected because creatinine production decreases with age. Thus, measuring creatinine clearance is useful in determining a dosage. Direct measurement can be difficult to achieve, but an estimate may be derived from the following formula: Creatinine clearance equals 140 minus age (times the body weight in kilograms) divided by 72 times the serum creatinine (Cockcroft and Gault, 1976). For women this result should be multiplied by 0.85. As a caveat, this formula has been shown to be less than accurate in estimating creatinine clearance among nursing home patients (Drusano et al., 1988). Thus this method of assessment may provide only a crude estimate of dosage requirements.

Drugs that are eliminated predominantly by the kidney and therefore have untoward pharmacologic effects are even more potentially serious with respect to toxic effects in elderly persons. Amantadine (Symmetrel), lithium, beta blockers, clonidine (Catapres), and several nonpsychotropic drugs, that is, aminoglycosides, digoxin, antiarrhythmics, diuretics, nonsteroidal antiinflammatory drugs, and angiotensin-converting enzyme inhibitors are noteworthy examples (Williams and Lowenthal, 1992). The discussion of lithium excretion in kidney function, as noted in Chapter 5, is of particular concern in elderly persons.

Drug interaction. The pharmacokinetic effects outlined in this section prominently affect interactions with other drugs. Absorption may be affected significantly by antacids. Distribution of drugs may be affected by the competition for binding proteins among various drugs. Metabolism of drugs that utilize the oxidative, cytochrome P 450 enzyme system may induce drug metabolism, for example, barbiturates, anticonvulsants, and oral hypoglycemics. Other compounds may inhibit metabolism, for example, cimetidine, neuroleptics, TCAs, selective serotonin reuptake inhibitors, beta blockers, and methylphenidate (Ritalin). Excretion of psychotropic agents may be significantly affected by proximal-loop and potassium-sparing diuretics, especially lithium. Nonsteroidal antiinflammatory agents may also be responsible for disrupting excretions of lithium and other psychotropic agents. In short, GI tract diseases may affect absorption; diseases affecting volume of distribution may result from altered concentrations of binding protein; hepatic disease may affect metabolism; and renal disease may affect excretion.

Pharmacodynamics

Pharmacodynamics refers to what a drug does to the system and to the study of effects of drugs on the target site; more broadly, *pharmacodynamics* reflects the physiologic or psychologic response to a drug or combination of drugs. Pharmacodynamics have been examined less extensively in elderly persons than has pharmacokinetics, largely because of the difficulty of such investigation. In general, older patients are more responsive to the effects of psychotropic agents, perhaps because of changes in neurotransmitter systems or receptor site sensitivity.

Geriatric patients can be exquisitely sensitive to the effects of psychotrophics but less so to nonpsychotropic agents such as cardiovascular preparations. This is in part due to some changes with respect to the beta receptor functioning and resultant vulnerability to side effects, for example, orthostatic hypotension. Beta receptor density and affinity for antagonists on human lymphocytes are not altered with age (Abrass and Scarpace, 1981). Lower levels of cyclic adenosine monophosphate (AMP) and adenylate cyclase activity after beta adrenergic stimulation have been noted in the lymphocytes of elderly persons (Scarpace, 1986). Receptor affinity for antagonists is reduced in association with reduction in the ability to form a high affinity state for agonists, and this reduction may result in an age-related alteration in the interaction between the beta-adrenergic receptors and regulatory proteins. In contrast, studies of alpha-adrenergic receptors have revealed either no change or a decrease in the relative affinities for receptors with increasing age (Buckley et al., 1986). Thus receptor changes result in a differential (and sometimes exaggerated or diminished) response in the older individual.

Other significant age-related neurophysiologic changes include cholinergic degeneration that is known to occur in older adults and can affect memory function and presumably predispose patients to the effects of drugs that potentially exacerbate disorders of cognitive impairment. For example, the patient with Alzheimer's disease is vulnerable to drugs that exert anticholinergic effects. The degeneration of the nigrostriatal pathways may also result in an older individual's predisposition to extrapyramidal side effects (EPSEs) or to the development of tardive dyskinesia with use of a neuroleptic. Moreover, the sedation threshold and unfavorable effects on memory in response to benzodiazepines may be exaggerated in older patients. The effects of TCAs on cardiac conduction in cardiac patients and neuroleptics in patients with Parkinson's disease may also be accentuated. There is thought to be a greater potential for TCAs to interact with antihypertensive agents, antiarrhythmics, and other agents that possess anticholinergic properties. Similarly, low-potency neuroleptics may affect response to antihypertensives; specifically, alpha-receptor blockade may also be accentuated as a result of the pharmacodynamic interactions with the nonpsychiatric medication.

Drug Reactions

Nontherapeutic drug reactions are commonly encountered in older adults who receive psychotropic medications. As forementioned, many side effects are related to sedation, which can result in excessive drowsiness, cognitive impairment, or motor impairment or simply can compound the sedation resulting from other drugs, interacting with sedative-hypnotic agents, including alcohol. The high prevalence of dizziness reported in elderly persons in association with certain psychotropics, that is, benzodiazepines, TCAs, and antipsychotic agents, may also predispose these individuals to falls that may result in hip fracture (Ray et al., 1987; Sloane, Blazer, and George, 1989).

Many psychotropic agents used safely in younger patients require closer attention when prescribed for the elderly because of clinically important adverse drug reactions. Risk factors for adverse drug reactions include multiple medications, increased number of illnesses, severe illness, or increase in individual sensitivity to drug effects. The incidence of adverse drug reactions or nontherapeutic effects ranges between 10% and 20% among inpatients (Cusack, 1989). Patients taking nonsteroidal antiinflammatory drugs have an increased risk of hyperkalemia, renal failure, or death resulting from GI hemorrhage. Patients receiving diuretic therapy are more susceptible to fluid and electrolyte disorders, including volume depletion, hypokalemia, hyponatremia, and hypomagnesemia. As forementioned, disease states may also alter the disposition or effect of a drug, and because in geriatric patients more than one disease is often involved, careful attention should be given when prescribing any medication (Folks, 1990; Montamat, Cusack, and Vestal, 1989).

Compliance

Noncompliance with drug therapy is reported to occur in one third to one half of geriatric patients (Morrow, Leirer, and Sheikh, 1988). Causes of noncompliance include poor communication with the health care professional, decline in cognitive function, and complicated dosing regimens. Using the fewest possible drugs at low doses and convenient combinations usually enhances compliance. Once a therapeutic goal has been achieved, a dosage of a particular drug should be reduced and therapy discontinued whenever possible. Of course, continuation therapy should be followed by maintenance throughout the period in which the patient may be most susceptible to recurrence or relapse.

Dosage schedules should be kept simple and multiple drug regimens minimized. If a geriatric patient is unable to read or comprehend directions, family members or caregivers should be given simple written instructions. Containers that are easy to open should be provided. Liquid formulations should be used for those individuals who have difficulty with swallowing. Various aids and devices can be improvised or obtained to assist patients and their families with accurate self-administration.

Psychiatric Disturbances Prevalent in Late Life

Psychotropic drugs are prescribed for geriatric patients with disabling or debilitating target symptoms, clinically significant syndromes, or bona fide psychiatric disorders, as defined within the nomenclature. Symptoms that become a focus of treatment include anxiety, insomnia, agitation, and aggression. Syndromes commonly treated include mixed anxiety-depression, psychosis, and agitation or confusion complicating disorders of cognitive impairment, in particular, dementia and delirium. Psychiatric disorders that are commonly encountered in late life include anxiety disorders, mood disorders, sleep disorders, and disorders of cognitive impairment, in particular, Alzheimer's disease. Of course, chronic psychotic disorders, personality disorders, and other significant disturbances may also extend into later life. As with younger patients, these symptoms, syndromes, and disorders are ideally treated with a combination of primary interventions. Pharmacologic treatment is best combined with psychotherapeutic interventions, which may include counseling, patient education, or formal psychotherapy (for those patients with significant or core psychologic issues). Behavioral techniques may also be beneficial, particularly for patients with anxiety, insomnia, or agitation. Moreover, it would be unthinkable to prescribe a psychotropic drug to an older patient without first providing an adequate assessment that seeks to optimize the patient's medical and physiologic condition while providing some documentation of the patient's baseline mental and psychosocial status. Generally, this assessment should seek to answer the following questions:

1. What is the patient's medical status?
2. What is the patient's mental status?
3. What is the patient's functional status and capacity to carry out daily activities?
4. What is the patient's psychosocial status and ability to function socially and occupationally, and to maintain interpersonal and relationship functioning?
5. What is the patient's or caregiver's potential to comply with medical regimen, including any recommendations for nonpharmacologic interventions or adjunctive interventions that might serve to enhance compliance?

Mood Disorders

Mood disorders are frequently encountered among geriatric patients who require psychotropic intervention. Epidemiologic data suggest that about half of all major depression is encountered initially by an individual over 65 years of age (Kalayam and Shamoian, 1990). Thirteen percent of community-dwelling elderly persons are found to have clinically significant symptoms within the depressive spectrum (Blazer et al.,

1988). Medical illnesses are frequently associated with depression; for example, 20% to 35% of patients within medical-surgical settings are found to have coexisting symptoms of depression (Folks and Ford, 1985). Mortality rates are increased for geriatric patients with depression, and the suicide rate among elderly individuals is disproportionate (Folks, 1990). The current geriatric population accounts for at least 25% of all completed suicides, but elderly persons attempt suicide at least three times less frequently than do nongeriatric patients, that is, suicide attempts made by older adults are more often successfully completed (Folks and Ford, in press). Thus effective drug treatment of depression, careful monitoring of response, and an appreciation of potential suicide risk are imperative for depressed geriatric patients.

Depression. Among the antidepressants and mood stabilizers, the TCAs are frequently prescribed; newer agents, for example, fluoxetine (Prozac) are most frequently prescribed. Geriatric patients may require either significantly lower doses or standard doses of TCAs, as discussed in Chapter 5. The secondary amine tricyclics, desipramine (Norpramin) and nortriptyline, are generally preferred because of their more favorable side effect profile, as discussed in Chapter 5. Acute antidepressant drug treatment with resultant remission of symptoms and continuation for at least 6 to 12 months is recommended, since more than 50% of successfully treated patients have a relapse in the first year or have a recurrent episode (Rubin, Kinscherf, and Wehrman, 1991). Generally the nontherapeutic effects, as outlined in Chapter 5, are more likely to emerge or be problematic for older adults.

Regarding new-generation antidepressants, the selective serotonin reuptake inhibitors, including fluoxetine and sertraline (Zoloft), are well tolerated by geriatric patients and have fewer side effects than do the TCAs (as discussed in Chapter 5). Among the heterocyclic agents, trazodone (Desyrel) may be particularly beneficial in geriatric patients because of its sedative profile and virtual lack of anticholinergic effects. However, orthostatic symptoms may result with trazodone and should be assiduously monitored. Bupropion (Wellbutrin) may also be beneficial, particularly in those patients who are not responsive to other conventional antidepressants. Bupropion has been touted as having particular utility in patients with a history of bipolar disorder or in those who require maintenance antidepressant therapy after electroconvulsive therapy (Jenike, 1988).

Monoamine oxidase inhibitors may be found to be effective for those depressed elderly patients who are refractory to tricyclic or other antidepressant intervention (Jenike, 1989). Moreover, since monoamine oxidase enzyme activity increases with increasing age, a special niche for these agents in the geriatric population is implied, particularly for those individuals with dementia complicated by depression. However, orthostatic hypotension or other adverse reactions, as outlined in Chapter 5, may emerge; geriatric patients can also be potentially at risk for noncompliance with the necessary dietary precautions.

Although activating antidepressants, for example, desipramine, fluoxetine, or bupropion, are useful in geriatric patients who may be abulic, motor retarded, or cognitively impaired, psychostimulants have gained popularity as being useful in the initial or sustained treatment of depression among geriatric patients (Jenike, 1988). Psychostimulants can be used safely for the initial (or sustained) treatment of major depression, for the treatment of organic affective disorders, for the treatment of apathy, or for depressive symptoms in patients with Alzheimer's disease and related dementias. Surprisingly these agents have few adverse or nontherapeutic effects, as noted in Chapter 13. The use of methylphenidate in doses of 5 to 30 mg is generally preferred both as a short-term agent with or without concomitant administration of a conventional antidepressant and as an adjunct in the long-term treatment of treatment-refractory cases. The stimulant challenge test, in which a test dose of a stimulant is given before conventional antidepressant intervention is begun, has also been reported as a useful way of predicting potential responses to antidepressant drug therapy (Goff, 1986).

Bipolar disorder. The use of lithium carbonate in the treatment of bipolar disorder in geriatric patients is well documented. Lithium has also been useful for augmentation of antidepressant agents (Price, Charney, and Heninger, 1986). The dose-response relationship for the use of lithium in bipolar illness in geriatric cases can result in a response or maintenance prophylaxis with low therapeutic plasma levels, that is, 0.4 to 0.8 mEq/L. Low-dose treatment is preferred, since side effects and adverse reactions are much more commonly encountered among older adult patients, including a great potential for neurotoxic effects and dyskinesia. Lithium may also prove to be beneficial for patients with agitation, irritability, or mood instability, especially those with Alzheimer's disease or physiologic or medical causes of affective syndromes (Zimmer et al., 1991). Interestingly, many older patients who seek medical attention with an apparent agitated depression may actually have mixed bipolar disorder that is ultimately responsive to lithium or other mood-stabilizing agents in concert with antidepressant therapy (Folks and Ford, in press; Stone and Folks, in press). For the 30% to 50% of patients who are either nonresponders to lithium or intolerant of its side effects, carbamazepine (Tegretol), valproate (Depakote), or other mood stabilizers can be used alternatively. These antiepileptic drugs, carbamazepine and valproate, as discussed in Chapter 5, possess similar dose-response relationships for psychotropic uses in older patients (Keltner and Folks, 1991; Lerer et al., 1987). Because these alternative mood-stabilizing compounds do not lower the seizure threshold or significantly interfere with cognitive functioning, they may also be useful in cognitively impaired patients with prominent symptoms of mood instability or aggression.

Psychotic Disorders

Psychotic syndromes in older patients may include schizophrenia or other syndromes potentially treatable or maintained with antipsychotic or neuroleptic agents (as they are in younger patients). The choice of drug often entails selection of a high-potency agent or a low-potency agent, as discussed in Chapter 4. The relative efficacy versus the side-effect profile generally includes consideration of whether the patient has any preexisting conditions that might result in greater risk for side effects of the high-potency or low-potency agent. In general, high-potency agents in low doses, for example, haloperidol (Haldol), are preferred as initial drugs for the treatment of psychotic symptoms (Peabody et al., 1987). However, EPSEs, akinesia, and akathisia are frequent problems in the geriatric population, as is the emergence of tardive dyskinesia over time, which occurs with the highest frequency in elderly persons. For some patients sedation associated with a low-potency neuroleptic may represent a "therapeutic fringe benefit," and the relative risk is low for nontherapeutic effects using lower doses, that is, anticholinergic effects, orthostatic effects, or adverse influence on cardiac conduction time. In general, low doses of a compound such as thioridazine (Mellaril) 10 to 50 mg two to four times daily may be quite effective. Likewise, the low-potency novel antipsychotic agent clozapine may be beneficial for geriatric conditions that are treatment refractory, as discussed in Chapter 4 (Small et al., 1987). Clozapine (Clozaril) may be particularly beneficial in elderly persons with Parkinson's disease.

Older patients with schizophrenia, delusional disorder, or other psychoses constitute one of several groups for whom there is a special role for the use of depot neuroleptics. Both fluphenazine (Prolixin) decanoate and haloperidol decanoate have proven to be quite useful, particularly because elderly noncompliant patients in the community can be treated effectively with periodic home visits. Moreover, for patients in institutional settings lower doses of depot rather than oral neuroleptic agents may ultimately be required, to maintain the antipsychotic effect. Antipsychotic agents may also be generally useful for patients with sundowning, confusional episodes, delirium, transient psychosis, agitation, or behavioral disturbances secondary to dementia, as well as for patients who may be at risk for harm to themselves or others or for those individuals who are simply unable to carry out essential daily activities without some degree of tranquilzation.

Anxiety Disorders and Acute Insomnia

As forementioned, anxiety disorders represent one of the common syndromes encountered in later life and represent symptoms for which patients readily seek treatment. The use of anxiolytics primarily involves the choice of a benzodiazepine, an antidepressant for the treatment of specific anxiety subtypes, or buspirone (as noted in Chapter 6). Benzodiazepine, sedatives, trazodone, or a short-term regimen of chloral hydrate is also useful in the treatment of acute insomnia.

The pharmacology and pharmacologic properties of anxiolytics and sedatives have been discussed in preceding chapters with respect to neurobiology and basic science. Differential drug effects related to drug metabolism and pharmacokinetics in elderly persons may be exaggerated, as outlined generally in this chapter with respect to plasma protein binding, increased volume of distribution, diminished hepatic biotransformation, and impaired renal clearance. However, as forementioned, the clinical impact resulting from alteration of plasma proteins is not thought to be marked. In fact, the equilibrium between bound and unbound drug is not changed significantly in the vast majority of elderly patients. Thus the amount of psychotropic drug available to produce clinical effects often remains unchanged, although the total amount of protein binding is diminished.

Hepatic biotransformation and renal clearance are significant pharmacokinetic considerations that often do account for differences in drug response. For example, reduced hepatic biotransformation and reduced renal clearance in elderly persons lead to metabolic accumulation, diminished clearing of the drug, and a resultant higher blood level of drug or active metabolite, or both. This is, indeed, why short-acting benzodiazepines that undergo metabolism through conjugation pathways in the liver, that is, oxazepam, lorazepam, and temazepam, are preferred.

A number of treatment issues and guidelines must be considered with the use of anxiolytics (and sedatives) in the geriatric patient. These primarily relate to the potential for nontherapeutic effects of the drugs in relation to the effects of aging per se, as outlined in Chapter 8. Diazepam and other benzodiazepines, that is, alprazolam (Xanax), oxazepam, and lorazepam, are known to result in disinhibition; this phenomenon is characterized by an episode of violence or increasing agitation that is clearly drug induced (Hall and Zisook, 1981). The loss of behavioral control and explosive or violent behavior may also occur during the course of benzodiazepine treatment (Folks, 1990; Gardos et al., 1968). Triazolam occasionally has shown this effect but more often produces other significant side effects in older patients, for example, amnestic episodes. Benzodiazepines have well-known amnestic properties, which are prominent in elderly persons (Kumar et al., 1987; Wolkowitz et al., 1987). The potential for lorazepam, alprazolam, and triazolam (Halcion) to produce amnestic effects has been discussed in Chapter 8.

Drug accumulation with long-acting benzodiazepines is thought to explain the higher incidence of falls in elderly persons (Ray et al., 1987; Sloane, Blazer, and George, 1989). Moreover, the benzodiazepines with long half-lives have been demonstrated to pose the greatest risk for resultant falls that may be complicated by hip fracture or head injury, or both (Ray, Griffin, and Downey, 1989). The potential adverse effects of sedation and negative direct influence on cognition are also compounded in elderly patients with preexisting dementia, creating additional risk for accidents (Folks, 1990).

The clinical approach to sedative treatment of acute insomnia requires careful selection of a specific drug with the most suitable pharmacologic profile in relatively low doses. The dose should preserve normal sleep architecture to the extent possible during ingestion and after withdrawal. The pharmacokinetic profile should meet the clinical requirement to shorten sleep onset, to reduce nocturnal wakefulness, or to provide the anxiolytic effect required during the following day. This approach should result in the patient being as free as possible from untoward effects on daytime functioning. The utility and clinical appropriateness of any hypnotic must depend to some extent on whether the therapeutic profile solves the clinical problems.

Benzodiazepines used as hypnotics are likely to have some side effects. However, unnecessarily high doses for long periods are the major problem, essentially resulting in adverse effects. Impaired daytime performance, anterograde amnesia, and other adverse effects associated with several of the anxiolytics are especially problematic for elderly persons (Nicholson and Ward, 1984). Anterograde amnesia can also be associated with rage or psychosis. A 20% incidence of amnesia is associated with triazolam, but approximately 45% of patients with insomnia who do not receive treatment also complain of memory problems, making it difficult to establish the clinical significance of triazolam's effect on memory (Mendelson, 1992). Also, on cessation of sedative treatment, insomnia may arise as a "rebound" phenomenon, particularly when short-acting agents are withdrawn suddenly. Rebound insomnia occurs more often when a relatively high dose of a rapidly eliminated drug is prescribed and used nightly. Generally this phenomenon is not observed when these drugs are used in recommended doses for limited periods (Roehrs et al., 1986).

Benzodiazepine hypnotics remain effective as sleeping agents for approximately 6 months of continued use (Oswald et al., 1982); however, they do produce adaption and tolerance (Greenblatt and Shader, 1978). For example, the patient may have fewer sedating effects (tolerance) over time and achieve physiologic homeostasis with loss of hypnotic effect. Drug dependence is also a possible consequence with the use of hypnotics, as with the anxiolytics. The possibility of dependence can be minimized by intermittent use of low doses together with limited duration of prescription and gradual withdrawal in the event that continuous treatment has been given for more than 1 month (Ladewig, 1983). Indeed, withdrawal of hypnotics after long-term use may lead to a recrudescence of the original symptoms, as well as to rebound insomnia (Nicholson, 1980). Dependence on and addiction to sedatives are much more likely to occur in patients with coexisting psychiatric disturbance or a history of an addictive disorder, or in patients with personality or somatoform disorders (Folks and Houck, in press).

Mixed Anxiety-Depression

Mixed anxiety-depression is frequently assigned as a diagnosis in older adults who receive treatment in primary care settings. Clinical presentations may not meet the full syndromal criteria for a mood or anxiety disorder, and anxiety or depression may not always be distinguishable as the overriding disorder. Elderly individuals may also come to medical attention with clinical symptoms for which diagnostic criteria are not clearly identifiable or for which the clinical setting or brief nature of the assessment may not lend itself to a definitive diagnosis, for example, the nursing home or emergency department. Nonetheless, these patients come to medical attention with clinically significant symptoms that are potentially responsive to anxiolytics (Feigner, Merideth, and Hendrickson, 1982; Keltner and Folks, in press; Rakel, 1990; Rickels et al., 1982; Sussman, 1988).

The pharmacotherapy of mixed anxiety-depression is perhaps best accomplished with a broad-spectrum, first-line agent such as buspirone (Buspar) or alprazolam or with a sedating antidepressant such as trazodone or imipramine (Tofranil). Mixed anxiety-depression is perhaps better treated with a benzodiazepine when anxiety is associated with an acute stressor or overwhelming situational factors. Buspirone or, perhaps, trazodone represents an ideal drug in patients requiring long-term therapy and may ultimately alleviate several target symptoms of anxiety-depression, diminishing agitation, improving concentration, and enhancing functional ability (Folks, 1990; Preskorn, 1990).

Agitation and Aggression

Older patients, particularly those who may be cognitively impaired or institutionalized, often receive treatment with an anxiolytic (or sedative drug) for agitation or aggression. In many cases, when the agitation is the result of psychosis or delirium, the best treatment choice is an antipsychotic or neuroleptic, for example, haloperidol. However, the anxiolytics, particularly buspirone, or the benzodiazepines, for example, oxazepam and lorazepam, may offer certain advantages with reduced potential for side effects such as EPSEs and oversedation. Moreover, in long-term care settings the Omnibus Budget Reconciliation Act of 1987 (OBRA) guidelines restrict the prescription of antipsychotic medications and further restrictions are being developed for the "tranquilizing" anxiolytics. These guidelines require that nursing-home patients receive appropriate diagnosis. Patients can then receive treatment in adherence to the federal guidelines, which mandate that specific psychiatric conditions be appropriately treated with a selected psychotropic agent (Domantay and Napoliello, 1989; Keltner and Folks, in press).

The OBRA guidelines require both a rationale and a justification for the use of a psychotropic drug, including documentation and monitoring. Additionally, drug selection, dosage, duration of therapy, and discontinuation of prescription when potential dependency and addiction are present are addressed by OBRA guidelines. Thus, anxiolytic drug therapy, as well as antipsychotics, in long-term care settings will soon be subject to the OBRA guidelines. Also, as a result of the OBRA legislation the incidental use of anxiolytics in long-term care settings will be discouraged and may even be prohibited. Further discussion of this topic is found in Chapter 8.

Antipsychotic or neuroleptic drugs have been vigorously recommended and condemned in the treatment of chronically agitated (or anxious) elderly patients in any clinical setting. Although high-potency neuroleptics such as haloperidol are often used for this purpose, drugs with strongly sedating properties may be preferred. For example, thioridazine may be prescribed at low doses, as forementioned, in the range of 10 to 50 mg one to four times per day. Although use of a neuroleptic agent avoids the risk of drug dependency, the risk of tardive dyskinesia and the emergence of other equally problematic side effects are concerns. Thus the use of neuroleptics is *not* recommended for simple anxiety or agitation.

The availability of newly developed anxiolytics, for example, short-acting benzodiazepines or buspirone, should also be considered as therapeutic in the context of risks versus benefits for the treatment of agitation and aggression. Buspirone, low doses of short-acting benzodiazepines such as alprazolam, lorazepam, and oxazepam, and other agents may be useful alone or as adjuncts in the treatment of agitation; trazodone, lithium, carbamazepine, and the beta blockers, for example, propranolol (Inderal), have been reported to be most often potentially useful (Keltner and Folks, in press; Maletta, 1990). One or more of these alternative agents may be necessary in the long term when persistent agitation, aggression, or suicidality poses a significant risk.

Short-acting benzodiazepines have been useful primarily for the acute treatment of agitation associated with underlying anxiety or depression. Interestingly, severe agitation not amenable to a neuroleptic may sometimes be more likely to respond to a benzodiazepine. Lorazepam is particularly useful in this regard because it may be given intramuscularly. Lenox et al. (1992) have advocated the use of lorazepam as an adjunct to the neuroleptics in violent or aggressive patients at a ratio of 1 mg of lorazepam for every 5 mg of haloperidol. Similarly, clonazepam (Klonopin) is useful for agitated patients with mania (Rosenbaum, 1989). Buspirone is likely to reduce agitation and aggression in mentally retarded (Ratey et al., 1989) or cognitively impaired elderly persons (Eison, 1989). Moreover, the long-term use of buspirone avoids the problem of addiction or dependency and is not likely to impair the older patient's cognition or motor function. However, aggressive patients who do not respond or remit with neuroleptic or anxiolytic intervention may require the long-term use of lithium, carbamazepine, or a beta-adrenergic blocking agent, as outlined in Chapter 9.

Delirium, "Sundowning," and Confusion Associated with Dementia

A variety of psychotropic agents may be useful in the treatment of agitation, confusion, or aggression in patients with disturbed cognition. In many cases the patient has some degree of delirium. See the box below for diagnostic measures for delirium. Effective management of delirium may require any of three therapeutic tasks. The first, fundamental task requires assessment for the underlying physiologic or anatomic disturbance(s) thought to be causal. Generally this phase of treatment requires a diligent clinical evaluation using any or all of the diagnostic tests listed in the box below. Medications must also be assiduously evaluated, in particular, their accumulative doses and temporal relationship to the onset of the delirium. A high index of suspicion is warranted for any of the classes of medications depicted in the box on p. 353, top.

Delirium: Diagnostic Measures

Serum chemical survey
Complete blood cell count
Arterial blood gas levels
Urinalysis
Serum and urine drug screen
Serum B_{12} and folate levels
Thyroid functions
Serum test for syphilis
Chest radiograph
Electrocardiogram (Holter monitor)
Electroencephalogram
Computed tomography scan of head
Cerebral spinal fluid examination

Classes and Examples of Medications that Induce Delirium

Anticholinergics:	Benztropine, trihexyphenidyl
Anticonvulsants:	Barbiturates, phenytoin
Antidiabetics:	Insulin, oral hypoglycemics
Antihypertensives:	Clonidine, methyldopa
Antiparkinsons:	Levodopa, carbidopa
Cancer chemotherapeutics:	Procarbazine, nitrogen mustard
Cardiovascular agents:	Digoxin, lidocaine
Corticosteroids:	Prednisone, prednisolone
Gastrointestinal agents:	Cimetidine, belladona
Narcotic analgesics:	Opiates, synthetic narcotics
Nonnarcotic analgesics:	Salicylates, propoxyphene
Psychotropics:	Anxiolytics, antidepressants

The second therapeutic task is to provide general supportive measures, including both environmental manipulation and physiologic maintenance (see the box below). Ideally these therapeutic principles obviate the need for pharmacologic intervention or prolonged physical restraint. However, the effective use of psychotropic drugs is indicated when behavioral disturbances, psychomotor agitation, or psychosis predominates the clinical picture.

The third therapeutic task involves the selection of a pharmacologic agent(s) that will result in symptomatic relief or effectively treat the underlying cause, or both. The box on p. 354 outlines the pharmacologic considerations, and specific medications are listed for each of the three categories of delirium. Cases categorized as withdrawal from alcohol, sedative-hypnotic agents, or a similar agent are best treated with the judicious use of a benzodiazepine drug. However, delirium precipitated by an an-

Nonpharmacologic Treatment of Delirium

Environmental manipulation
Arrange consistent, supportive nursing care
Minimize personnel
Place family member or significant other at bedside
Utilize orienting remarks and devices such as calendar or clock
Place in well-lighted room with window
Provide familiar objects such as personal belongings and photos

Supportive measures
Effect fluid and electrolyte balance
Maintain nutritional and vitamin status
Obtain visual or hearing aids
Provide moderate sensory input
Encourage physical activity or ambulation
Apply physical restraints as necessary

Pharmacologic Treatment of Delirium

Sedative hypnotic, similar agent, or alcohol withdrawal

1. Careful maintenance of fluid and electrolyte balance
2. Careful replacement or provision of nutritional and vitamin requirements
3. Effective sedation with a benzodiazepine agent: Chlordiazepoxide (Librium) 25-50 mg orally or intramuscularly every 4-6 hr or lorazepam (Ativan) 1-2 mg orally or intramuscularly every 6-8 hr

Anticholinergic-induced delirium

1. Withdraw offending anticholinergic agent(s)
2. Counteract severe cases with physostigmine (Antilirium) 1-2 mg slowly intravenously; may be repeated every 30-60 min

Multifactorial or miscellaneous variables

1. Withdraw offending agent(s) or treat underlying cause(s)
2. Enhance sleep with short–half-life hypnotic*†: Triazolam (Halcion) 0.25-0.5 mg; oxazepam (Serax) 10-30 mg; temazepam (Restoril) 15-30 mg orally hs; or chloral hydrate 500-1000 mg orally hs
3. Treat "sundowning" or disruptive behavior with high-potency antipsychotic†: Haloperidol (Haldol) or fluphenazine (Prolixin) hydrochloride 1-2 mg orally (concentrate) or intramuscularly, two to four times daily

*Hypnotics can potentially worsen the clinical course and diminish cognition.
†Dosage must be adjusted individually; geriatric patients may be started on a regimen of half doses.

ticholinergic drug(s) requires withdrawal of the offending agent(s) and urgent cases may also benefit from the use of an anticholinesterase agent such as physostigmine (Antilirium). Antipsychotic drug treatment is to be avoided or minimized in cases of anticholinergic delirium because of the potential for additional anticholinergic effects and the possible lowering of the seizure threshold. Most cases that represent delirium either are multifactorial or result from a nonspecific cause and simply require a drug regimen that is designed to normalize sleep or control psychomotor agitation, psychosis, or disruptive behavior. Although the use of a short-acting sedative may be quite useful for sleep enhancement, behavioral symptoms of motor agitation, aggression, or psychosis are more effectively treated with a low-dose antipsychotic agent such as haloperidol, as discussed in Chapter 9. These potent antipsychotic medications possess minimal anticholinergic effects and rarely result in an adverse drug interaction or contribute to the delirium; furthermore, serious hypotension or cardiotoxic effects are unlikely to occur. However, EPSEs (dystonic reaction, akathisia, or parkinsonian symptoms) should be monitored and counteracted, preferably with amantadine (Symmetrel) 100 mg orally once or twice daily. As a corollary, psychotropic drugs are unnecessary in the absence of psychotic or behavioral disturbances, except in drug or alcohol withdrawal states, which notoriously intensify if the patient is not adequately sedated (Folks, 1988).

REMARKS

The primary goal of psychotropic drug therapy in elderly patients is an improvement in the quality of life. Often a psychiatric disturbance is not curable; this is particularly true for disorders of cognitive impairment such as Alzheimer's disease. Thus the goal of drug therapy can be alleviation of secondary psychiatric symptoms or maintenance. The therapeutic goal may sometimes be accomplished with simple behavioral or environmental measures, often without the use of drugs. The potential effects of aging and disease with respect to pharmacokinetics and pharmacodynamics and the possible ramifications of adverse drug reaction or interaction must be considered carefully. Increased knowledge of the action and effects of drugs in older patients and enhancement of communication between the patient and treatment team can significantly improve the overall quality of care.

The use of a psychotropic agent in a geriatric patient must be carefully planned. Psychotropics should not be used merely for the convenience of staff or family and should not be used without appropriate evaluation. Diagnostic uncertainty regarding symptoms of anxiety, insomnia, and agitation should lead to assessment for underlying psychiatric conditions such as major depression, delusional disorder, or dementia. Symptomatic treatment without diagnostic clarification should not be undertaken. A clear rationale for the use of a drug must be based on a sound risk-benefit analysis that should be carefully developed and documented, especially in settings where federal guidelines or reimbursement mechanisms are strict.

In general, the use of benzodiazepines and antipsychotic agents is justified when drug therapy results in improvement in the patient's functional status. Benzodiazepines and antipsychotics may be used as primary treatment for major psychiatric conditions, for example, panic, generalized anxiety, mood disorder, dementia, or delirium. In using anxiolytics, sedatives, or antipsychotic agents, frequent attempts should be made to reduce the dosage or discontinue the medication, or both. These efforts should take place at intervals no longer than 4 months. Alternative pharmacologic intervention should be considered when appropriate or indicated.

The geriatric patient is more sensitive to the nontherapeutic effects of anxiolytics, sedatives, and antipsychotics than is the younger patient; initial dose regulation should be low and titrated perhaps at one fourth to one half of the usual adult dosage. Short-acting benzodiazepines are preferred because of their pharmacokinetic properties and because of reduced potential for metabolic accumulation. Furthermore, drugs requiring only phase 2 hepatic metabolism have more predictable effects. Drugs that meet these criteria, that is, oxazepam, lorazepam, and temazepam, are preferred for older patients. High-potency antipsychotic agents in low doses may be better tolerated in geriatric patients, although the potential for EPSEs and oversedation exists. Subtle nontherapeutic effects of anxiolytics, sedatives, and antipsychotic agents may not be evident immediately after starting drug treatment. Thus geriatric patients receiving these drugs must be monitored carefully. Cognitive impairment, confusion, concentration difficulties, conceptual defects, and motor dysfunction, including incoordination and ataxia, should be identified promptly.

Alternative agents, that is, low-potency neuroleptics or antihistamines, are sometimes prescribed simply to sedate geriatric patients, but this practice is generally not effective and these drugs are not as well tolerated as are the benzodiazepines. Occasionally a barbiturate such as phenobarbital is used as an anxiolytic; again, however, these older agents are not as effective as a short-acting benzodiazepine or the newer anxiolytic agents. In abandoning older agents, it is important to recognize the potential risk of dependency associated with their long-term use, as well as the superior safety profile of benzodiazepines.

The use of conventional antidepressants or newer anxiolytic agents should be considered in the treatment of both anxiety and insomnia, as well as in cases involving depression. Low-dose antipsychotics, lithium, or carbamazepine may be indicated in the treatment of severely agitated elderly patients who do not respond to buspirone, trazodone, or a benzodiazepine. Patients with symptoms that are frankly psychotic, that is, delusions, hallucinations, or conceptual disorganization, are best treated with an antipsychotic drug.

Caution is the hallmark for drug treatment in elderly persons. Diagnosis, drug selection, and evaluation of the clinical effectiveness of the pharmacologic agent over time are important management considerations. Ideally drug treatment should be combined with other nonpharmacologic approaches, which may also serve to enhance compliance and improve the likelihood of an initial or sustained response.

REFERENCES

Abernathy DR, Kerznel L: Age effects on alpha-1 acid glycoprotein concentrations and imipramine plasma protein binding, *J Am Geriatr Soc* 32:705, 1984.

Abrass IB, Scarpace PJ: Human lymphocyte beta-adrenergic receptors are unaltered with age, *J Gerontol* 36:298, 1981.

Balter MB, Bauer ML: Patterns of prescribing and use of hypnotic drugs in the United States. In Clift AD, editor: *Sleep disturbances and hypnotic drug dependence*, Amsterdam, 1975, *Excerpta Medica.*

Bellatuono C et al: Benzodiazepines: clinical pharmacology and therapeutic use, *Drugs* 19:195, 1980.

Blazer D et al: Depressive symptoms and depressive diagnoses in a community population: use of a new procedure for analysis of psychiatric classification, *Arch Gen Psychiatry* 45:1078, 1988.

Buckley C et al: Ageing and platelet alpha$_2$-adrenoreceptors, *Br J Clin Pharmacol* 21:721, 1986.

Castleden CM, George CF: The effect of aging on the hepatic clearance of propranolol, *Br J Clin Pharmacol* 7:49, 1979.

Cockcroft DW, Gault MH: Prediction of creatinine clearance from serum creatinine, *Nephron* 16:31, 1976.

Cusack BJ: Polypharmacy and clinical pharmacology. In Beck J, editor: *Geriatrics review syllabus: a core in geriatric medicine*, New York, 1989, American Geriatrics Society.

Cusack B, Vestal RE: Clinical pharmacology: special considerations in the elderly. In Calkins E, editor: *The practice of geriatrics*, Philadelphia, 1986, WB Saunders.

Domantay AG, Napoliello MJ: Buspirone for elderly anxious patients, *Int Med Certif* 3:1, 1989.

Drusano GL et al: Commonly used methods of estimating creatinine clearance are inadequate for elderly debilitated nursing home patients, *J Am Geriatr Soc* 36:437, 1988.

Eison MS: The new generation of serotonergic anxiolytics: possible clinical roles, *Psychopathology* 22(suppl 1):13, 1989.

Feighner JP, Merideth CH, Hendrickson RM: A double-blind comparison of buspirone and diazepam in outpatients with generalized anxiety disorder, *J Clin Psychiatry* 43:102, 1982.

Folks DG: Delirium. In Rakel RE, editor: *Conn's current therapy*, Philadelphia, 1988, WB Saunders.

Folks DG: Clinical approaches to anxiety in the medically ill elderly, *Drug Ther Suppl* p 72, August 1990.

Folks DG, Ford CV: Psychiatric disorders in geriatric medical-surgical patient. Part I. Report of 195 consecutive consultations, *Southern Med J* 78:239, 1985.

Folks DG, Ford CV: Clinical features of depression and dysthymia in older adults. In Blazer D, editor: *The psychiatry of old age*, John Wiley & Sons (in press).

Folks DG, Fuller WC: Uses of anxiolytics and sedatives in geriatric practice: clinical selection and treatment considerations. In Smith DA, editor: *Psychotropic therapy in the elderly patient*, Marcel Dekker (in press).

Folks DG, Houck CA: Somatoform disorders, factitious disorders and malingering. In Stoudemire A, Fogel BS, editors: *Principles of medical psychiatry*, ed 2, Oxford University (in press).

Gaitz CM, Niederehe G, Wilson NL: *Aging 2000: our health care destiny: vol 2, psychosocial and policy issues*, New York, 1985, Springer-Verlag.

Gardos G et al: Differential actions of chlordiazepoxide and oxazepam on hostility, *Arch Gen Psychiatry* 18:757, 1968.

Goff DC: The stimulant challenge test in depression, *J Clin Psychiatry* 47:538, 1986.

Greenblatt DJ: Reduced serum albumin concentration in the elderly: a report from the Boston Collaborative Drug Surveillance Program, *J Am Geriatr Soc* 27:20, 1979.

Greenblatt DJ, Shader RI: Dependence, tolerance and addiction to benzodiazepines: clinical and pharmacokinetic considerations, *Drug Metab Rev* 8:13, 1978.

Hall RCW, Zisook S: Paradoxical reactions to benzodiazepines, *Br J Clin Pharmacol* 11:995, 1981.

Jenike MA: Assessment and treatment of affective illness in the elderly, *J Geriatr Psychiatry Neurol* 1:89, 1988.

Jenike MA: *Geriatric psychiatry and psychopharmacology: a clinical approach,* St Louis, 1989, Mosby.

Kalayam B, Shamoian CA: Geriatric psychiatry: an update, *J Clin Psychiatry* 51(5):177, 1990.

Keltner NL, Folks DG: Federal regulation: impact on psychotropic drug use in long-term care facilities, *Perspect Psychiatr Care* (in press).

Kumar R et al: Anxiolytics and memory: a comparison of lorazepam and alprazolam, *J Clin Psychiatry* 48:158, 1987.

Ladewig D: Abuse of benzodiazepines in Western European society: incidence and prevalence motives, drug acquisition, *Pharmacopsychiatry* 16:103, 1983.

Lenox RH et al: Adjunctive treatment of manic agitation with lorazepam versus haloperidol: a double-blind study, *J Clin Psychiatry* 53:47, 1992.

Lerer B et al: Carbamazepine versus lithium in mania: a double-blind study, *J Clin Psychiatry* 48(3):89, 1987.

Maletta GJ: Pharmacologic treatment and management of the aggressive demented patient, *Psychiatr Ann* 20(8):454, 1990.

Masoro EJ: Biology of aging: current state of knowledge, *Arch Intern Med* 147:166, 1987.

Mendelson W: Pharmacologic treatment of insomnia. In Pies R, editor: Advances in psychiatric medicine, *Psychiatric Times* (suppl), p 2, 1992.

Montamat S, Cusack B, Vestal RE: Management of drug therapy in the elderly, *New Engl J Med* 321:303, 1989.

Morrow D, Leirer V, Sheikh J: Adherence and medication instructions: review and recommendations, *J Am Geriatr Soc* 36:1147, 1988.

Nicholson AN: Hypnotics: rebound insomnia and residual sequelae, *Br J Clin Pharmacol* 9:223, 1980.

Nicholson AN, Ward J, editors: Psychomotor drugs and performance, *Br J Clin Pharmacol* 18(suppl 1):1S-139S, 1984.

Oswald I et al: Benzodiazepine hypnotics remain effective for 24 weeks, *Br Med J* 284:860, 1982.

Peabody CA et al: Neuroleptics and the elderly, *J Am Geriatr Soc* 35:233, 1987.

Preskorn SH: The future and psychopharmacology: potentials and needs, *Psychiatr Ann* 20(11):625, 1990.

Price LH, Charney DS, Heninger GR: Variability of response to lithium augmentation in refractory depression, *Am J Psychiatry* 143:1387, 1986.

Rakel RE: Mixed anxiety/depression, *Drug Ther Suppl* p 137, August 1990.

Ratey JJ et al: Buspirone therapy for maladaptive behavior and anxiety in developmentally disabled persons, *J Clin Psychiatry* 50:382, 1989.

Ray WA, Griffin MR, Downey W: Benzodiazepines of long and short elimination half-life and the risk of hip fracture, *JAMA* 262(23):3303, 1989.

Ray WA et al: Psychotropic drug use and the risk of hip fracture, *New Engl J Med* 316:363, 1987.

Rickels K et al: Buspirone and diazepam in anxiety: a controlled study, *J Clin Psychiatry* 43:81, 1982.

Roehrs TA et al: Dose determinants of rebound insomnia, *Br J Clin Pharmacol* 22:143, 1986.

Rosenbaum JF, editor: *Clonazepam update: a review of the literature,* vol 1, Bellemead, NJ, 1989, Excerpta Medica, Elsevier.

Rowe JW, Kahn RL: Human aging: usual and successful, *Science* 237:143, 1987.

Rowe JW et al: The effect of age on creatinine clearance in men: a cross-sectional and longitudinal study, *J Gerontol* 31:155, 1976.

Rubin EH, Kinscherf BA, Wehrman SA: Response to treatment of depression in the old and very old, *J Geriatr Psychiatry Neurol* 4:65, 1991.

Scarpace PJ: Decreased beta-adrenergic responsiveness during senescence, *Fed Proc* 45:51, 1986.

Sloane P, Blazer D, George LK: Dizziness in a community elderly population, *J Am Geriatr Soc* 37:101, 1989.

Small JG et al: Treatment outcome with clozapine in tardive dyskinesia, neuroleptic sensitivity, and treatment-resistant psychosis, *J Clin Psychiatry* 48:263, 1987.

Stone T, Folks DG: Somatization in the elderly. In Hall RCW, editor: *Psychiatric medicine* (in press).

Sussman N: Diagnosis and drug treatment of anxiety in the elderly, *Geriatr Med Today* 7(10):1, 1988.

Vestal RE: Pharmacology and aging, *J Am Geriatr Soc* 30:191, 1982.

Wallace SM, Verbeeck RK: Plasma protein binding of drugs in the elderly, *Clin Pharmacokinet* 12:41, 1987.

Williams L, Lowenthal DT: Drug therapy in the elderly, *Southern Med* 85(2):127, 1992.

Wolkowitz OM et al: Diazepam-induced amnesia: a neuropharmacological model of an "organic amnestic syndrome," *Am J Psychiatry* 144:25, 1987.

Wynne HA et al: The effect of age upon liver volume and apparent liver blood flow in healthy men, *Hepatology* 9:297, 1989.

Zimmer B et al: Adjunctive lithium carbonate in nortriptyline-resistant elderly depressed patients, *J Clin Psychol* 11:254, 1991.

PSYCHOTROPIC DRUG PROFILES

PART

TWO

A

Acetazolamide

DIAMOX, AK-ZOL, DAZAMIDE
(a-set-a-zole′ a-mide) (Chapter 7)

Functional classification: Diuretic, anticonvulsant
Chemical classification: Carbonic anhydrase inhibitor
FDA pregnancy category: C

Indications: *Diuretic* indications are not discussed here, e.g., edema related to CHF, glaucoma; *Anticonvulsant:* Especially petit mal and tonic-clonic seizures, particularly in children

Contraindications: Known hypersensitivity to acetazolamide; depressed sodium or potassium levels; kidney and liver disease or dysfunction; suprarenal gland failure

Pharmacologic Effects: Inhibition of carbonic anhydrase apparently slows abnormal firing of CNS neurons. However, anticonvulsant effect not truly understood

Pharmacokinetics: Absorbed from GI tract; distributed to body tissues and CNS; eliminated unchanged in urine

Side Effects: *CNS:* Convulsions, weakness, malaise, fatigue, nervousness, sedation, depression; *Peripheral:* Nausea, vomiting, constipation, hematuria, urinary frequency, hepatic insufficiency, blood dyscrasias, skin problems, weight loss, fever, acidosis

Interactions
- Amphetamines: Because it alkalinizes urine, may increase effect of amphetamines (and ephedrine, pseudoephedrine, flecainide, and quinidine)
- Digitalis: May sensitize patient to digitalis toxicity r/t hypokalemia
- Primidone: May delay primidone absorption
- Salicylates: Together may cause metabolic acidosis

Implications
Assess
- Weight, I&O for fluid loss, respirations, B/P
- Check potassium, sodium, and other electrolyte levels

Teaching
- To increase fluid, if indicated
- To rise slowly when orthostatic hypotension is a problem
- To notify clinician when symptoms of blood dyscrasias occur, i.e., sore throat, bruising, etc

Evaluate
- For seizure activity, CNS side effects, confusion in elderly, signs of metabolic acidosis, signs of hypokalemia

Lab Test Interference: May interfere with tests for urinary protein, i.e., false positive

Treatment of Overdose: Lavage for oral doses, monitor electrolytes and fluid profile, assess renal function, give dextrose in saline, give bicarbonate for acidosis

Administration
- Epilepsy: 8 to 30 mg/kg/day in divided doses; optimum range 375 to 1000 mg/day
- Concomitant antiepileptic dosage: start with 250 mg/day and increase to levels for epilepsy
- Available forms include: Tabs 125, 250 mg; caps sus rel 500 mg; inj 500 mg/vial

Acetophenazine*

TINDAL
(a-set-oh-fen′-a-zeen) (Chapter 4)

Functional classification: Antipsychotic
Chemical classification: Piperazine phenothiazine
FDA pregnancy category: C

Indications: Management of psychotic disorders

Contraindications: See trifluoperazine

Pharmacologic Effects: See trifluoperazine

Pharmacokinetics: See trifluoperazine

Side Effects: *CNS:* See trifluoperazine; *Peripheral:* See trifluoperazine

Interactions: See trifluoperazine

Implications: See trifluoperazine

*Infrequently used.

Treatment of Overdose: See trifluoperazine

Administration
- 20 mg tid; if insommia present, give last tablet 1 hr before bedtime; usual daily dosage 40 to 80 mg
- Hospitalized patients: Optimally 80 to 120 mg/day in divided doses
- Severe schizophrenia: Up to 400 to 600 mg/day
- Available forms: Tabs 20 mg

Alprazolam
XANAX
(al-pray'zoe-lam) (Chapter 6)

Functional classification: Antianxiety
Chemical classification: Benzodiazepine
Controlled substance schedule IV
FDA pregnancy category: D

Indications: Anxiety, panic disorders

Contraindications: Hypersensitivity to benzodiazepines; narrow-angle glaucoma; psychosis; nursing women; child <18 yr
Cautious use: Elderly or debilitated patients; hepatic disease, renal disease

Pharmacologic Effects: Apparently potentiates effects of GABA and other inhibitory transmitters by binding to specific benzodiazepine receptor sites; depresses subcortical levels of CNS, including limbic system and reticular formation

Pharmacokinetics
- Speed of onset: intermediate
- PO: Onset 30 min, peak 1-2 hr, duration 4-6 hr, therapeutic response 2-3 days; metabolized by liver; excreted by kidneys; crosses placenta, breast milk; half-life 12-15 hr

Side Effects: *CNS:* **Drowsiness, dizziness, confusion, headache,** anxiety, tremor, stimulation, fatigue, **depression, insomnia**; paradoxic agitation can occur
Peripheral: Photophobia due to mydriasis, **blurred vision** due to cyclopegia; sleeplike slowing of respirations with therapeutic doses; cough; **orthostatic hypotension; tachycardia;** hypotension; **constipation, dry mouth**

Interactions
- Alcohol and other CNS depressants: Increased risk of excessive CNS depression
- Cimetidine: Potentiation of CNS depression
- Digoxin: Increased risk of cardiac side effects
- Levodopa: Decreased antiparkinson effect
- Phenytoin: Increased phenytoin serum levels

Implications
Assess
- Patient's level of anxiety and method of coping
- B/P, VS
- Establish baseline physical assessment data before medications are started
- Periodically perform CBC, UA
- Reassess need for treatment q4mo

Planning/Implementation
- Monitor patient's response to medication
- Observe elderly, very young, and debilitated patients for paradoxic excitement
- Reduce dose of other depressant drugs
- Observe for signs of withdrawal when discontinuing antianxiety medication; discontinue by decreasing daily dose no more than 0.5 mg q3days

Teaching
- To avoid operating dangerous machinery and other tasks requiring good reflexes
- To report ocular pain at once, and any other visual disturbances
- Drug may be taken with food

Evaluate
- Whether patient achieves lower levels of anxiety without undue sedation
- Whether patient can follow prescribed regimen
- For physical dependence: withdrawal symptoms include headache, nausea, vomiting, muscle pain, and weakness after long-term use

Lab Test Interferences
- Increase: AST/ALT, serum bilirubin
- False increase: 17-OHCS
- Decrease: RAIU

Treatment of Overdose: Lavage, VS, supportive care. There have been few deaths, if any, from benzodiazepine overdose alone. Deaths occur when benzodiazepines are mixed with other drugs, i.e., alcohol

Administration
Adult: PO 0.25-0.5 mg tid, not to exceed 4 mg/day in divided doses; *geriatric:* PO 0.25 mg bid-tid

- Available forms include: Tabs 0.25, 0.5, 1 mg

Amantadine HCl

SYMMETREL

(a-man'ta-deen) (Chapter 14)

Functional classification: Antiparkinson agent, antiviral
Chemical classification: Tricyclic amine
FDA pregnancy category: C

Indications: Extrapyramidal reactions, parkinsonism, antiviral (A)

Contraindications: Hypersensitivity, lactation, child <1 yr
Cautious use: Epilepsy, CHF, orthostatic hypotension, psychiatric disorders, hepatic disease and renal diseases

Pharmacologic Effect: Causes release of dopamine from neurons

Pharmacokinetics: PO: Onset 48 hr, peak 4 hr, half-life 18-24 hr in normal renal function, not metabolized, excreted in urine (90%) unchanged, crosses placenta, excreted in breast milk

Side effects: *CNS:* **Confusion,** headache, **dizziness, drowsiness,** fatigue, anxiety, psychosis, depression, **hallucinations,** tremors, convulsions, insomnia; *Peripheral:* **Orthosatic hypotension,** CHF, photosensitivity, dermatitis, livedo reticularis, **blurred vision,** leukopenia, **nausea, vomiting,** constipation, **dry mouth,** urinary frequency, retention

Interactions

- Atropine, other anticholinergics: Increased anticholinergic responses
- CNS stimulants: Increased CNS stimulation

Implications
Assess

- EPSEs; urinary frequency
- Mental alertness
- History of seizure activity; may increase seizure activity

Planning/Implementation

- Give at least 4 hr before bedtime to prevent insomnia
- Give after meals for better absorption to decrease GI symptoms
- Give in divided doses to prevent CNS disturbances: headache, dizziness, fatigue, drowsiness

Teaching

- Change body position slowly to prevent orthostatic hypotension
- To report dyspnea, weight gain, dizziness, poor concentration, behavioral changes
- To avoid hazardous activities when dizziness occurs
- To take drug exactly as prescribed; if drug is discontinued abruptly, parkinsonian crisis may occur

Evaluate

- Therapeutic response: Decrease in EPSE
- Bowel pattern before and during treatment
- Skin eruptions, photosensitivity after administration of drugs
- Respiratory status: Breathing rate and character, wheezing, tightness in chest

Treatment of Overdose: Withdraw drug, empty stomach, maintain airway, administer O_2, IV corticosteroids; use appropriate antiarrhythmic and vasopressor therapy as needed

Administration

- Extrapyramidal reaction and parkinsonism: *Adult:* PO 100 mg bid, up to 400 mg/day for EPSEs in divided doses; *geriatric:* 100 mg/day
- Influenza type A: Not addressed here
- Available forms include: Caps 100 mg; syr 50 mg/5 ml
- A suggested dosing guideline for patients with impaired renal function is available

Amitriptyline HCl

ELAVIL, ENDEP, ENOVIL, LEVATE,† MERAVIL,† NOVOTRIPTYN,† ROLAVIL†
(a-mee-trip'ti-leen) (Chapter 5)

Functional classification: TCA
Chemical classification: Dibenzocycloheptadiene, tertiary amine
FDA pregnancy category: C

Indications: Depression

Contraindications: Hypersensitivity to TCAs, recovery phase of myocardial infarction
Cautious use: Suicidal patients, convulsive disorders, prostatic hypertrophy, schizophrenia, psychosis, severe depression, increased intraocular pressure, narrow-angle glaucoma, urinary retention, cardiac disease, hepatic disease or renal disease, hyperthyroidism, ECT, elective surgery, child <12 yr, MAOI therapy

Pharmacologic Effects: Blocks reuptake of norepinephrine, serotonin into nerve endings, increasing action of norepinephrine, serotonin in nerve cells; also r/t changes in receptor sensitivity; therapeutic plasma levels 110-250 ng/ml

Pharmacokinetics: PO/IM onset 45 min, peak 2-12 hr, therapeutic response 2-3 wk; metabolized by liver, excreted in urine and feces, crosses placenta, excreted in breast milk, half-life 31-46 hr

Side Effects: *CNS:* **Sedation,** ataxia; confusion, delirium; *Peripheral:* **Blurred vision,** photophobia, increased intraocular pressure, decreased tearing, orthostatic hypotension, arrhythmias, tachycardia, palpitations, dry mouth, constipation, diarrhea, decreased sweating, **urinary retention, hesitancy**

Interactions
- Anticholinergic agents: Additive anticholinergic effects
  - Atropine
  - Antihistamines (H_1 blocker)
  - Antiparkinson drugs
  - Antipsychotics
  - OTC cold and allergy drugs
- CNS depressants: Additive depressant effect
- Guanethidine, clonidine: Decreased antihypertensive effect
- MAOIs: Hypertensive crisis; atropine-like poisoning
- Oral contraceptives: Inhibit metabolism of TCAs
- Phenothiazines: May increase TCA serum level
- Quinidine: Additive effect, heart block possible
- Sympathomimetics: Potentiates sympathomimetic effects
- Thyroid preparations: Tachycardia, arrhythmias; may increase TCA effect

Implications
Assess
- Establish baseline data to aid recognition of adverse responses to medication, e.g., liver enzyme levels, VS, renal function, mental status, speech patterns, affect, weight
- Assess for signs of noncompliance, e.g., poor therapeutic response
- Observe for major symptoms of depression: apathy, sadness, sleep disturbances, hopelessness, guilt, decreased libido, spontaneous crying
- Review history for contraindicated conditions, e.g., glaucoma, CV disease, GI conditions, urologic conditions, seizures, pregnancy

Planning/Implementation
- Monitor for "cheeking" or hoarding; check drug dosage carefully—a small overdose may cause toxicity
- Monitor for suicidal ideations; suicidal thought content may increase as antidepressants begin to "energize" patient
- Monitor vital signs; withhold TCAs when hypotension, tachycardia, or arrhythmias occur
- Give most TCAs in a single dose hs
- Observe for early signs of toxicity, e.g., drowsiness, tachycardia, mydriasis, hypotension, agitation, vomiting, confusion, fever, restlessness, sweating
- Discontinue drug when CNS overstimulation occurs, e.g., hypomania, delirium

Teaching
- That these drugs have a lag time of up to 1 month

†Available in Canada only.

- To adhere to drug regimen
- To avoid OTC drugs, particularly those containing sympathomimetics or anticholinergics
- To avoid drugs listed in section on interactions
- About ways to deal with minor side effects, as follows: dry mouth: with hard candies, sips of water, mouth rinses; visual disturbances: with artificial tears, sunglasses, assistance with ambulation; constipation: with bulk-forming foods, increased fluids; urinary hesitancy: with adequate fluids, privacy; decreased perspiration: with appropriate clothing, avoidance of unnecessary exercise; orthostatic hypotension: with slow positional changes, avoidance of hot baths and showers; drowsiness: take single dose hs with physician approval, avoid driving
- That abrupt discontinuance may result in cholinergic rebound, e.g., nausea, vomiting, insomnia, headache

Evaluate
- Desired therapeutic serum level
- Verbalize decrease in subjective symptoms
- Observe decrease in objective symptoms
- Minimal to no adverse drug effects
- Stable VS
- Less anxiety; sleep, talk, and feel better

Lab Test Interferences
- Increase: Serum bilirubin, blood glucose, and alkaline phosphatase levels
- Decrease: VMA, 5-HIAA
- False increase: Urinary catecholamines

Treatment of Overdose: ECG monitoring, induce emesis, lavage, activated charcoal, treat anticholinergic effects, administer anticonvulsants if needed

Administration
Adult: PO 40-100 mg hs, may increase to 200 mg qd, not to exceed 300 mg/day; IM 20-30 mg qid
Adolescent/geriatric: PO 30 mg/day in divided doses, may add 20 mg hs
- Available forms include: Tabs 10, 25, 50, 75, 100, 150 mg; IM 10 mg/ml

Amobarbital/ Amobarbital Sodium

AMYTAL, ISOBEC, AMYTAL SODIUM
(am-oh-bar′ bi-tal) (Chapter 8)

Functional classifications: Sedative, hypnotic
Chemical classification: Amylobarbitone
Controlled substance schedule II
FDA pregnancy category: B

Indications: Sedation, preanesthetic sedation, anticonvulsant

Contraindications: Hypersensitivity to barbiturates, respiratory depression, addiction to barbiturates, severe liver dysfunction, porphyria

Pharmacologic Effects: Depresses activity in reticular activating system; when used as anticonvulsant, inhibits CNS neural firing.

Pharmacokinetics: Onset within 45-60 min after PO dose with duration of action of 6-8 hr; metabolized by liver, excreted by kidneys; highly protein bound; Half-life 16-40 hrs; excreted in breast milk; onset in 5 min when given IV (e.g., for seizures)

Side Effects: *CNS:* Lethargy, drowsiness, barbiturate hangover, dizziness, paradoxic stimulation of children and elderly patients on occasion, CNS depression, slurred speech, physical dependence; *Peripheral:* Nausea, vomiting, diarrhea, constipation, skin eruptions (e.g., rashes), hypotension, bradycardia, respiratory depression, apnea, blood dyscrasias

Interactions
- CNS depressants: Increased CNS depression
- MAOIs: CNS depression
- Valproic acid: decreased half-life of valproic acid
- Oral anticoagulants, corticosteroids, quinidine, oral contraceptives: Decreased effect of these drugs
- Phenytoin: Unpredictable effect

Implications
Assess
- If given parenterally, check VS q 30 min for 2 hr
- Assess blood values because of potential for blood dyscrasias
- Check prothrombin time when patient is on anticoagulant regimen
- Hepatic studies to determine liver status

Planning/Implementation
- Have staff assist patient in walking after dose is given, to prevent falls
- Maintain safety

Teaching
- Physical dependence potential with long-term use
- To avoid alcohol and other CNS depressants
- To notify other prescribers about amobarbital

Evaluate
- Therapeutic responses
- Mental status
- Tendencies toward dependence
- Toxic effects
- Respiratory depression
- Blood dyscrasias

Treatment of Overdose: In general, 1 g causes serious poisoning in adults; lavage if taken orally, alkalinize urine; warm with blankets if needed; supportive measures, including monitoring VS; hemodialysis may be required

Administration
- Sedation: *Adult:* PO 30-50 mg bid or tid; range from 15 to 120 mg bid-qid; *child:* PO 2 mg/kg/day in four divided doses
- Anticonvulsant: *Adult:* Give IV 65-500 mg over several minutes, should not exceed 100 mg/min, do not exceed 1 g; *child:* < 6 yr: IV/IM 3-5 mg/kg over several minutes
- Available forms: Tabs 30, 50, 100 mg; caps 65, 200 mg; powder for inj IM, IV 250, 500 mg/vial

Amoxapine

ASENDIN

(a-mox'a-peen) (Chapter 5)

Functional classification: TCA
Chemical classification: Dibenzoxazepine-derivative secondary amine
FDA pregnancy category: C

Indications: Depression

Contraindications: Hypersensitivity to TCAs, recovery phase of myocardial infarction
Cautious use: Seizure disorders, suicidal patients, severe depression, increased intraocular pressure, narrow-angle glaucoma, urinary retention, CV disease, hepatic disease, hyperthyroidism, ECT, elective surgery, elderly patients, patients receiving MAOI therapy, NMS, child < 16 yr

Pharmacologic Effects: Blocks reuptake of norepinephrine, serotonin into nerve endings, increasing action of norepinephrine, serotonin in nerve cells; also blocks dopamine receptors and can produce EPSEs; therapeutic plasma levels 200-500 ng/ml

Pharmacokinetics: PO: Steady state 2-7 days, metabolized by liver, excreted by kidneys, crosses placenta, half-life 8 hr

Side Effects: *CNS:* **Sedation,** ataxia; confusion, delirium, tardive dyskinesia, NMS; *Peripheral effects:* **Blurred vision,** photophobia, increased intraocular pressure; decreased tearing; orthostatic hypotension, potension, arrhythmias, tachycardia, palpitations, **dry mouth, constipation,** diarrhea, decreased sweating, **urinary retention, hesitancy, nausea**

Interactions
- Anticholinergic agents: Additive anticholinergic effects with atropine, antihistamines (H_1 blockers), antiparkinson drugs, antipsychotics, OTC cold and allergy drugs
- CNS depressants: Additive depressant effect
- Guanethidine, clonidine: Decreased antihypertensive effect;
- MAOIs: Hypertensive crisis, atropine-like poisoning

- Oral contraceptives: Inhibits effects of TCAs
- Phenothiazines: May increase TCA serum level, EPSEs
- Quinidine: Additive effect, heart block possible
- Sympathomimetics: Potentiates sympathomimetic effects
- Thyroid preparations: Tachycardia, arrhythmias; may increase TCA effect

Implications

Assess

- Establish baseline data to aid recognition of adverse responses to medication, e.g., liver enzyme levels, VS, renal function, mental status, speech patterns, affect, weight
- Assess for signs of noncompliance, e.g., poor therapeutic response
- Observe for major symptoms of depression: apathy, sadness, sleep disturbances, hopelessness, guilt, decreased libido, spontaneous crying
- Review history for contraindicated conditions, e.g., glaucoma, CV disease, GI conditions, urologic conditions, seizures, pregnancy

Planning/Implementation

- Monitor for "cheeking" or hoarding; check drug dosage carefully, since a small overdose may cause toxicity
- Monitor for suicidal ideations; suicidal thought content may increase as antidepressants begin to "energize" patient
- Monitor VS; withhold TCAs when hypotension, tachycardia, or arrhythmias occur
- Give most TCAs in a single dose hs
- Observe for early signs of toxicity, e.g., drowsiness, tachycardia, mydriasis, hypotension, agitation, vomiting, confusion, fever, restlessness, sweating
- Discontinue drug when CNS overstimulation occurs, e.g., hypomania, delirium

Teaching

- That amoxapine has a shorter lag time (4-7 days) than other TCAs
- To adhere to drug regimen
- To avoid OTC drugs, particularly those containing sympathomimetics or anticholinergics
- To avoid drugs listed in section on interactions
- About ways to deal with minor side effects, as follows: dry mouth: with sugarless hard candies, sips of water, mouth rinses; visual disturbances: with artificial tears, sunglasses, assistance with ambulation; constipation: with bulk-forming foods, increased fluids; urinary hesitancy: with adequate fluids, privacy; decreased perspiration: with appropriate clothing, avoidance of unnecessary exercise; orthostatic hypotension: with slow positional changes, avoidance of hot baths and showers; for drowsiness, take single dose hs with physician approval, avoid driving
- That abrupt discontinuance may result in cholinergic rebound, e.g., nausea, vomiting, insomnia

Evaluate

- Desired therapeutic serum level
- Verbalize decrease in subjective symptoms
- Observe decrease in objective symptoms
- Minimal to no adverse drug effects
- Stable VS
- Less anxiety: sleep, talk, and feel better
- For EPSEs

Lab Test Interferences

- Increase: Serum bilirubin, blood glucose, alkaline phosphatase levels
- False increase: Urinary catecholamines
- Decrease: VMA, 5-HIAA

Treatment of Overdose: ECG monitoring, induce emesis, lavage; consider prophylactic antiepileptics; support respirations

Administration

Adult >16 yr: PO 100-150 mg/day in divided doses, may increase to 300 mg/day or may give daily dose hs

Geriatric: PO 50-75 mg/day, may increase to 150 mg/day

- Available forms include: Tabs 25, 50, 100, 150 mg

Amphetamine Sulfate

AMPHETAMINE SULFATE
(am-fet'a-meen) (Chapters 12, 13, 15, 16)

Functional classification: Cerebral stimulant
Chemical classification: Amphetamine
Controlled substance schedule II
FDA pregnancy category: X

Indications: Narcolepsy, exogenous obesity, ADHD

Contraindications: Hypersensitive to sympathomimetic amines, hyperthyroidism, hypertension, glaucoma, severe arteriosclerosis, nephritis, angina pectoris, parkinsonism, drug abuse, CV disease, anxiety, MAOI use
Cautious use: Tourette's disorder, lactation, child <3 yr, diabetes mellitus, elderly patients

Pharmacologic Effects: Stimulates release of norepinephrine in cerebral cortex, brain stem, and reticular activating system and dopamine in the mesolimbic system; therapeutic plasma levels 5-10 μg/dl

Pharmacokinetics: PO: Onset 30 min, peak 1-3 hr, duration 4-20 hr, metabolized by liver, excreted by kidneys, crosses placenta, enters breast milk, half-life 10-30 hr

Side Effects: *CNS:* **Hyperactivity, insomnia, restlessness, talkativeness,** dizziness, headache, chills, stimulation, dysphoria, irritability, aggressiveness; *Peripheral:* Nausea, vomiting, anorexia, dry mouth, diarrhea, constipation, weight loss, metallic taste, cramps, impotence, change in libido, **palpitations, tachycardia,** hypertension, hypotension

Interactions
- MAOIs or within 14 days of MAOIs: Hypertensive crisis
- Acetazolamide, antacids, sodium bicarbonate, ascorbic acid, ammonium chloride, phenothiazines, haloperidol: Increases half-life of amphetamine
- Urinary acidifiers: decreased half-life of amphetamines
- Guanethidine, other antihypertensives: Decreased effects of these drugs

Implications
Assess
- VS, B/P because this drug may reverse antihypertensives; check patients with cardiac disease more often
- CBC, urinalysis; in diabetes: Blood and urine sugar levels, insulin changes may need to be made because eating decreases
- **Height, growth rate in children, growth rate may be decreased**

Planning/Implementation
- Give at least 6 hr before bedtime to avoid sleeplessness
- For obesity only when patient is on weight reduction program that includes dietary changes, exercise; tolerance develops, and weight loss will not occur without additional methods
- Sugarless gum, hard candy, frequent sips of water for dry mouth
- If drug is for obesity, 30-60 min before meals
- Dispense lease amount feasible to minimize risk of overdose

Teaching
- To decrease caffeine consumption (coffee, tea, cola, chocolate), which may increase irritability, stimulation
- Avoid OTC preparations unless approved by physician
- To taper off drug over several weeks, or depression, increased sleeping, lethargy may occur
- To avoid alcohol ingestion
- To avoid hazardous activities until patient's condition is stabilized on medication regimen
- To get needed rest; patients feel more tired than usual at end of day
- Check to see that PO medication has been swallowed

Evaluate
- Mental status: mood, sensorium, affect, stimulation, insomnia; aggressiveness may occur
- Physical dependency; should not be used for extended time; drug should be discontinued gradually
- **Withdrawal symptoms: headache, nausea, vomiting, muscle pain, weakness**

- Drug tolerance develops after long-term use
- If tolerance develops, dosage should not be increased

Treatment of Overdose: Gastric evacuation if overdose < 4 hr old; otherwise, acidify urine, administer fluids until urine flow is 3-6 ml/kg/hr; hemodialysis, peritoneal dialysis may be helpful; antihypertensives for increased B/P; ammonium chloride for increased excretion; chlorpromazine for CNS stimulation

Administration
- Narcolepsy: PO 5-60 mg qd in divided doses; *adult and adolescent >12 yr*: PO 10 mg qd, increasing by 10 mg/day at weekly intervals; *child* 6-12 yr: PO 5 mg qd, increasing by 5 mg/wk, maximum dose, 60 mg/day
- ADHD: *Child >6 yr*: PO 5 mg qd-bid, increasing by 5 mg/wk; *child 3-6 yr:* PO 2.5 mg qd, increasing by 2.5 mg/day at weekly intervals
- Obesity in adult: PO 5-30 mg in divided doses 30-60 min before meals
- Available forms include: Tabs 5, 10 mg

Benztropine

COGENTIN

(Benz'-troe-peen) (Chapter 14)

Functional classification: Anticholinergic
Chemical classification: Tertiary amine
FDA pregnancy category: C

Indications: Parkinsonism, EPSEs

Contraindications: Hypersensitivity, narrow-angle glaucoma, duodenal obstruction, peptic ulcer, prostatic hypertrophy, myasthenia gravis, megacolon

Pharmacological Effects: Block cholinergic receptors, may inhibit the reuptake and storage of dopamine

Pharmacokinetics: Little pharmacokinetic information is known

Side Effects: *CNS:* Depression develops in 19% to 30% of patients; disorientation, confusion, memory loss, hallucinations, psychoses, agitation, delusion, nervousness; *Peripheral:* **Tachycardia,** palpitations, hypotension, **orthostatic hypotension, dry mouth,** nausea, vomiting, constipation, paralytic ileus, **blurred vision,** mydriasis, diplopia, urinary retention and hesitancy, elevated temperature

Interactions
- Amantadine: Increased anticholinergic effect
- Digoxin: Digoxin serum levels increased
- Haloperidol: Worsening of schizophrenia, decreased haloperidol serum levels
- Levodopa: Possible reduction of levodopa efficacy
- Phenothiazines: increased anticholinergic effect, decreased antipsychotic effect

Implications

Assess
- VS, B/P
- For glaucoma
- Mental status

Planning/Implementation
- Provide instructions for anticholinergic responses, i.e., dry mouth, constipation, urinary hesitancy, decreased sweating, and the like

Teaching
- Give with meals
- May cause drowsiness, blurred vision, dizziness: Emphasize safety
- Avoidance of alcohol and other CNS depressants
- Notify physician for rapid or pounding heartbeat
- Use caution in hot weather

Evaluate
- EPSE improvement
- For adverse effects
- Mental status: Confusion, delirium, memory

Treatment of Overdose: Emesis, lavage, activated charcoal, treat respiratory depression, hyperpyrexia

Administration
- EPSEs: *Adult:* PO/IM 1-4 mg qd-bid
- Acute EPSEs: *Adult:* IM/IV 1-2 mg, followed by 1-2 mg PO, taken twice to prevent recurrences
- Prophylactic: *Adult* PO 1-2 mg bid-tid

Biperiden
AKINETON
(bye-per′-i-den) (Chapter 14)

Functional classification: Anticholinergic
FDA pregnancy category: C

Indications: Parkinsonism, EPSEs

Contraindications: Hypersensitivity, narrow-angle glaucoma, duodenal obstruction, peptic ulcer, prostatic hypertrophy, myasthenia gravis, megacolon

Pharmacologic Effects: Block cholinergic receptors, may inhibit reuptake and storage of dopamine

Pharmacokinetics: Peak 1-1.5 hr, half-life 18.4-24.3 hr; little pharmacokinetic information is known

Side Effects: *CNS:* Depression develops in 19% to 30% of patients; disorientation, confusion, memory loss, hallucinations, psychoses, agitation, delusions, nervousness; *Peripheral:* **Tachycardia,** palpitations, hypotension, **orthostatic hypotension, dry mouth,** nausea, vomiting, constipation, paralytic ileus, **blurred vision,** mydriasis, diplopia, urinary retention and hesitancy, elevated temperature

Interactions
- Amantadine: Increased anticholinergic effect
- Digoxin: Digoxin serum levels increased
- Haloperidol: Worsening of schizophrenia, decreased haloperidol serum levels
- Levodopa: Possible reduction of levodopa efficacy
- Phenothiazines: Increased anticholingergic effect, decreased antipsychotic effect

Implications
Assess
- VS, B/P
- For glaucoma
- Mental status

Planning/Implementation
- Provide instructions for anticholinergic responses, i.e., dry mouth, constipation, urinary hesitancy, decreased sweating, and the like

Teaching
- Give with meals
- May cause drowsiness, blurred vision, dizziness: Emphasize safety
- Avoidance of alcohol and other CNS depressants
- Notify physician for rapid or pounding heartbeat
- Use caution in hot weather

Evaluate
- EPSE improvement
- For adverse effects
- Mental status: Confusion, delirium, memory

Treatment of Overdose: Emesis, lavage, activated charcoal, treat respiratory depression, hyperpyrexia

Administration
- EPSEs: *Adult*: PO 2 mg qd-tid
- Acute EPSEs: *Adult*: IM/IV 2 mg q 30 min prn, up to four doses in 24 hr

Bromocriptine Mesylate
PARLODEL
(broe-moe-krip′teen) (Chapter 14)

Functional classification: Dopamine receptor agonist
Chemical classification: Ergot alkaloid derivative
FDA pregnancy category: C

Indications: Female infertility, Parkinson's disease, prevention of postpartum lactation, amenorrhea, galactorrhea caused by hyperprolactinemia, acromegaly
Unlabeled use: Treatment of NMS; cocaine withdrawal and craving

Contraindications: Hypersensitivity to ergot, severe ischemic disease, pregnancy
Cautious use: Lactation, hepatic disease, renal disease, hypotension, acromegalic patients

Pharmacologic Effects: Stimulates prolactin release by activating postsynaptic dopamine receptors; activation of dopamine receptors is reason for improvement in Parkinson's disease and NMS (symptom of primary interest in this text)

Pharmacokinetics: PO: Peak 1-3 hr, duration 4-8 hr, 90% to 96% protein bound, half-life 3-8 hr, metabolized by liver (inactive metabolites), excreted in feces (85% to 98%) and urine (2.5% to 5.5%)

Side Effects: *CNS:* **Headache, abnormal involuntary movements,** depression, restlessness, anxiety, nervousness, confusion, **convulsions,** hallucinations; *Peripheral:* Frequency, retention, incontinence, diuresis, blurred vision, diplopia, burning eyes, **nausea, vomiting, anorexia,** cramps, constipation, diarrhea, dry mouth, rash on face or arms, alopecia, orthostatic hypotension, decreased B/P, palpitation, shock, arrhythmias, **shortness of breath**

Interactions:
- Phenothiazines, haloperidol, droperidol, oral contraceptives: Decrease action of bromocriptine, thus increasing likelihood of conception in women taking birth control pills
- Antihypertensives, levodopa: Increase effect of these drugs

Implications (for NMS treatment only)
Assess
- B/P; this drug decreases B/P

Planning/Implementation
- With meals to prevent GI symptoms
- Administer hs so that dizziness, orthostatic hypotension are not problems

Teaching
- To prevent orthostatic hypotension, change position slowly
- To use barrier contraceptives during treatment with this drug; pregnancy may occur
- To avoid hazardous activity when dizziness occurs

Evaluate
- Therapeutic response (NMS): Decreased fever, sweating, rigidity, decreased slow movements, drooling

Lab Test Interferences: Increase: BUN, SGOT, CPK, alkaline phosphatase

Administration:
- Parkinson's disease: *Adult:* PO 1.25 mg bid with meals, may increase q2-4 wk, not to exceed 100 mg qd
- NMS: Although standardized dose not established for this unlabeled use, 2.5-20 mg q8h *have been reported* to be effective (for other uses see *PDR*)
- Cocaine withdrawal: 1.25 mg tid for 7 days, then discontinue
- Available forms include: caps 5 mg; tabs 2.5 mg (must be cut in half for 1.25-mg dose)

B

Bupropion HCl

WELLBUTRIN

(byoo-proe′ pee on) (Chapter 5)

Functional classification: Unicyclic antidepressant
Chemical classification: Aminoketone
FDA pregnancy category: B

Indications: Depression

Contraindications: Hypersensitivity, concomitant use of MAOIs, seizure history, children <18 yr, patients with prior diagnosis of bulimia or anorexia (high incidence of seizures in these patients)
Cautious use: Psychoses, suicidal patients, CV disorders, hepatic or renal disorders, elderly patients

Pharmacologic Effects: Not clear; *does not* block reuptake of serotonin or norepinephrine well; *does not* inhibit monoamine oxidase

Pharmacokinetics: Peak levels 2 hr; metabolized in liver, excreted in urine (87%) and feces (10%), half-life 8-24 hr, average half-life 14 hr

Side Effects: *CNS:* **Seizures** that are dose related (doses below 450 mg/day reduce risk of seizures); **agitation, confusion,** insomnia, **headache, sedation,** tremor; *Peripheral:* Blurred vision, **dizziness, tachycardia,** arrhythmias, **dry mouth, constipation, weight loss or gain, nausea and vomiting,** anorexia; **excessive sweating,** menstrual complaints, **rash,** impotence, upper respiratory tract complaints

Interactions
- Carbamazepine, phenytoin, cimetidine, phenobarbital: Slow metabolism of bupropion
- Levodopa: Increased incidence of adverse effects of bupropion
- MAOIs and alcohol: Increased toxicity of bupropion and seizures (alcohol)

- Drugs that lower seizure threshold (phenothiazines, TCAs): Increased risk of seizures

Implications

Assess

- Blood studies: CBC, leukocyte count, cardiac enzyme levels
- Liver function tests before and during, therapy: bilirubin level, AST, ALT
- ECG: Flattening of T wave; bundle branch block; AV block; arrhythmias in cardiac patients

Planning/Implementation

- Treat constipation and dry mouth
- Give with food or milk for GI upset
- Assist with ambulation
- Give last dose no later than 4 PM to minimize effects on sleep

Teaching

- Therapeutic effects take 2-4 weeks
- Use caution in driving or other hazardous activities
- To avoid alcohol; when alcohol is consumed, to wait until next morning to take bupropion
- Not to discontinue use abruptly

Evaluate

- Therapeutic response: Level of depression; ability to perform activities of daily living, ability to sleep
- Mental status: Mood, suicidal ideation

Treatment of Overdose: Hospitalization; give emetic, if patient is conscious; activated charcoal, provide adequate fluids, treat seizures with IV benzodiazepines

Administration

Adult: 100 mg bid to start (morning and evening); based on clinical response, may be increased to 300 mg/day in divided doses no sooner than 3 days after beginning therapy; maximum dose 450 mg/day, with never more than 150 mg given in single dose

- Available forms: Tabs 75, 100 mg

Buspirone HCl

BUSPAR

(byoo-spear'-own) (Chapter 6)

Functional classification: Antianxiety agent

Chemical classification: Azaspirodecanedione

FDA pregnancy category: B

Indications: Management and short-term relief of anxiety disorders

Contraindications: Hypersensitivity, psychosis

Cautious use: Lactation, child <18 yr, elderly patients, impaired hepatic or renal function

Pharmacologic Effects: Unknown; not related to benzodiazepines; may act by binding to serotonin receptors in brain

Pharmacokinetics: Rapidly absorbed and undergoes extensive first-pass metabolism, peak serum levels within 90 min, excreted in urine and feces, half-life 2-11 hr

Side Effects: *CNS:* **Dizziness, headache,** depression, **stimulation,** insomnia, nervousness, lightheadedness, numbness, paresthesia, incoordination, tremors, excitment, involuntary movements, confusion, akathisia; *Peripheral:* **Nausea, dry mouth,** diarrhea, constipation; tachycardia, palpitations, hypotension; sore throat, tinnitus, blurred vision, nasal congestion; frequency, hesitancy; muscle cramps; hyperventilation, chest congestion, shortness of breath; rash, edema, pruritus, alopecia, dry skin

Interactions

- MAOIs: Increase B/P
- Alcohol: Do not mix, even though serious interactions have not been documented
- Trazodone: Increases ALT
- Haloperidol: Increased haloperidol serum levels

Implications

Assess

- B/P, pulse; if systolic B/P drops 20 mm Hg, withhold drug

- Hepatic studies: AST, ALT, bilirubin, creatinine, LDH, alkaline phosphatase levels
- Mental status
- Give with food or milk for GI symptoms; food may decrease absorption but increase bioavailability

Planning/Implementation
- Assistance with ambulation during beginning of therapy; drowsiness, dizziness occur
- Safety measures, including side rails, when drowsiness occurs

Teaching
- Optimum results may take 3 to 6 weeks; some improvement within 7 to 10 days
- That drug may be taken with food
- To avoid driving and activities requiring alertness because drowsiness may occur
- To avoid alcohol or other CNS depressant medications, unless prescribed by physician
- Not to discontinue medication abruptly after long-term use
- To rise slowly, or fainting may occur
- To notify physician if chronic abnormal movements occur (restlessness, involuntary movements)

Evaluate
- Therapeutic response: Decreased anxiety
- Physical dependency, withdrawal symptoms, headache, nausea, vomiting, muscle pain, weakness after long-term use
- Suicidal tendencies

Treatment of Overdose: Gastic lavage, VS, supportive care; no deaths from overdose have been reported

Administration
Adult: PO 5 mg tid, may increase 5 mg/day q2-3 days, not to exceed 60 mg/day
- Available forms include: Tabs 5, 10 mg

Butabarbital/ Butabarbital Sodium*

BUTISOL, MEDARSED, BUTATRAN, BUTICAPS, BUTISOL SODIUM
(byoo-ta-bar'bi-tal) (Chapter 8)

Functional classifications: Sedative, hypnotic
Chemical classification: Barbitone
Controlled substance schedule II
FDA pregnancy category: D

Indications: Sedation, insomnia

Contraindications: See amobarbital

Pharmacologic Effects: See amobarbital

Pharmacokinetics: Onset 45-60 min, duration 6-8 hr; metabolized by liver, excreted in urine; half-life 66-140 hr

Side Effects: *CNS:* See amobarbital; *Peripheral:* See amobarbital

Interactions: See amobarbital

Implications: See amobarbital

Treatment of Overdose: See amobarbital

Administration
- Insomnia: PO 50-100 mg hs
- Available forms: Tabs 15, 30, 50, 100 mg; caps 15, 30 mg; elix 30, 33.3 mg/5 ml

Caffeine

NO DOZ, TIREND, VIVARIN
(kaf-een) (Chapter 13)

Functional classification: Cerebral stimulant
Chemical classification: Xanthine
FDA pregnancy category: C

Indications: Mild CNS stimulation to stay awake or increase mental alertness, used with analgesics

*Infrequently used.

Contraindications: Gastric or duodenal hypersensitivity
Cautious use: Arrthythmias, lactation

Pharmacologic Effects: Promotes accumulation of cyclic AMP by increasing calcium permeability and causes CNS stimulation; constricts cerebral blood vessels and relaxes smooth muscles in blood vessels to bronchi

Pharmacokinetics: PO: Readily absorbed, onset 15 min, peak½ -1 hr, metabolized by liver, excreted by kidneys, crosses placenta, enters breast milk, half-life 3-4 hr

Side Effects: *CNS:* **Hyperactivity, insomnia, restlessness, talkativeness,** dizziness, headache, **stimulation,** irritability, aggressiveness, tremors, twitching; *Peripheral:* Nausea, vomiting, anorexia, diuresis, **tachycardia**

Interactions: Oral contraceptives, cimetidine: Increased effects of caffeine
Smoking: Enhances caffeine elimination

Implications
Assess
- VS, B/P

Planning/Implementation
- Do not give to patient with peptic ulcer disease

Teaching
- To decrease other caffeine consumption (coffee, tea, cola, chocolate), which may increase irritability, stimulation
- To taper off drug over several weeks after long-term use
- To not use as a substitute for regular sleep

Evaluate
- Therapeutic response; increased CNS stimulation, decreased drowsiness
- Mental status; stimulation, insomnia, irritability
- Tolerance or dependency; an increased amount may be used to get same effect
- Overdose: Pain, fever, dehydration, insomnia, hyperactivity

Treatment of Overdose: Lavage, activated charcoal, monitor electrolyte levels, VS, administer anticonvulsants if needed

Administration
Adult: PO 100-200 mg q4h prn
Infant or child: 8 mg/kg, not to exceed 500 mg
- Available forms include: Tabs 100, 200 mg; time rel caps 200, 250 mg

Carbamazepine

MAZEPINE,† TEGRETOL
(kar-ba-maz'e-peen) (Chapters 4, 5, 7, 15, 16)

Functional classification: Antiepileptic
Chemical classification: Iminostilbene derivative
FDA pregnancy category: C

Indications: Tonic-clonic, psychomotor, mixed seizures; pain-associated trigeminal neuralgia; *unlabeled uses:* bipolar illness, schizoaffective illness, resistant schizophrenia; PTSD

Contraindications: History of bone marrow depression; hypersensitivity to carbamazepine and TCAs; concomitant use of MAOIs; *Cautious use:* History of hematologic reaction to any drug, glaucoma, psychosis history, child <6 yr, lactation

Pharmacologic Effects: Unrelated to other antiepileptics; mechanism of action unknown but might act by reducing polysynaptic responses and blocking posttetanic potentiation; therapeutic serum levels 4-12 μg/ml

Pharmacokinetics: PO peak serum in 4-5 hr, metabolized in liver, excreted in urine (72%) and feces (28%), half-life 12-17 hr with repeated doses

Side Effects: *CNS:* **Drowsiness, dizziness, unsteadiness,** confusion, fatigue, paralysis, headache, hallucinations; *Peripheral:* **Nausea, vomiting, diarrhea,** blood dyscrasias that lead to fatalities, i.e., aplastic anemia, leukopenia, agranulocytosis, thrombocytopenia, bone marrow depression; hepatitis; urinary frequency and retention; pulmonary hypersensitivity; fever, dyspnea; CHF, **hypertension,** hypotension, transient diplopia, fever and chills; rash

Interactions
- Cimetidine, danazol, diltiazem, erythromycin, isoniazid, nicotinamide, propoxyphene, verapamil: Drugs that elevate carbamazepine serum levels

†Available in Canada only.

- Carbamazepine: Increases the metabolism of acetaminophen and oral anticoagulants
- Barbiturates; primidone: Lower serum level of carbamazepine
- Doxycycline: Reduces half-life of doxycycline
- Haloperidol: Decreases effect of haloperidol
- Hydantoins: Decreases carbamazepine levels; both increases and decreases hydantoin serum levels
- Lithium: Increases CNS intoxication or enhanced antimanic effects
- Nondepolarizing muscle relaxants: Resist or reverse muscle relaxants
- Succinimides: Reduces succinimide levels
- Theophylline: Both drugs decrease effects
- Valproic acid: Decreases serum levels of valproic acid

Implications

Assess
- Renal studies, blood studies, hepatic studies for baseline data and to determine whether carbamazepine therapy is appropriate

Planning/Implementation
- Give with food or milk to decrease GI upset (may enhance absorption)
- Chewable tabs to be chewed, not swallowed
- Assist with ambulation, if patient is dizzy

Teaching
- To avoid driving or operating hazardous machinery when dizzy, drowsy, or having blurred vision
- To notify physician of unusual bleeding or bruising, jaundice, abdominal pain, pale stools, darkened urine, impotence, CNS disturbances, edema, fever, chills, sore throat, or ulcer in mouth
- MedicAlert* identification bracelet
- That abrupt discontinuation can cause seizures

Evaluate
- Therapeutic responses, decreased seizure activity, decreased flashbacks, and the like
- Mental status

*MedicAlert, Turlock, Calif.

- Blood dyscrasias: Fever, sore throat, rash, bruising
- Toxic effects: Bone marrow depression, nausea and vomiting

Treatment of Overdose

Symptoms: Neuromuscular disturbances, irregular breathing, hypotension or hypertension, respiratory depression; treat symptoms with lavage, charcoal; maintain airway; elevate legs and administer plasma volume expander for hypotension; monitor breathing, heart rate (ECG), B/P, kidney function

Administration
- Seizures: *Adults and children >12 yr:* Initially 200 mg bid; increase at weekly intervals by up to 200 mg/day in three to four doses; not to exceed 1000 mg/day in children 12-15 yr; not to exceed 1200 mg/day in children >15 yr; maintenance usually 800 to 1200 mg/day *Children 6-12 yr:* Initially 100 mg bid; increase at weekly intervals by adding 100 mg/day in three to four doses; do not exceed 1000 mg/day; maintenance dose usually 400-800 mg/day
- Available forms: Tabs, chewable 100 mg; tabs 200 mg, suspension 100 mg/5 ml

Carbidopa-levodopa

SINEMET

(kar-bi-doé/pa lee-voe-doé/pa)

(Chapter 14)

Functional classification: Antiparkinson drug

Chemical classification: Catecholamine

FDA pregnancy category: C

Indications: Parkinsonism

Contraindications: Narrow-angle glaucoma, hypersensitivity, undiagnosed skin lesions, MAOI therapy

Pharmacologic Effects: Carbidopa prevents metabolism of levodopa to dopamine (dopamine cannot cross blood-brain barrier in significant amounts), so more levodopa enters CNS

Pharmacokinetics: Peak blood level 1-3 hr; excreted in urine

Side Effects: *CNS:* Tremors of hand, fatigue, involuntary movements, headache, anxiety, twitching, anxiety, confusion, agitation, insomnia, nightmares, hallucinations; *Peripheral:* **Nausea,** vomiting, GI symptoms, gas, dysphagia, skin eruptions, orthostatic hypotension, tachycardia, palpitations, blurred vision, dilated pupils, dark urine, urinary retention

Interactions
- MAOIs: Hypertensive crisis
- Anticholinergics, hydantoins, papaverine, pyridoxine, haloperidol: Decreased effect of levodopa
- Antihypertensives: Orthostatic hypotension
- Antacids, metoclopramide: Increased effects of levodopa
- TCAs: Hypertension
- Consult *PDR* for the many other interactions

Implications
Assess
- B/P, respirations, mental status

Planning/Implementation
- Assist patient with ambulation until condition is stabilized on drug regimen

Teaching
- Change positions slowly
- To not discontinue use abruptly, since parkinsonian crisis can occur
- To not be alarmed by dark urine or sweat
- That a therapeutic effect may take 3 to 4 mo

Evaluate
- Mental status, therapeutic response

Lab Test Interferences
- False positive: urine ketones
- False negative: urine glucose
- False increase: uric acid, urine protein
- Decrease: VMA, BUN, creatinine levels

Treatment of Overdose: There are no reports of overdosage with carbidopa; for levodopa, provide supportive care with immediate gastric lavage; monitor for airway, development of arrhythmias

Administration
Adult: PO 3-6 tabs of 25 mg carbidopa/250 mg levodopa per day in divided doses; maximum dose should not exceed 8 tabs/day
- Available forms: Tabs 10 mg (carbidopa)/100 mg (levodopa), 25/100, 25/250 mg

Chloral Hydrate

AQUACHLORAL SUPPRETTES, COHIDRATE, NOTEC, NOVOCHLORHYDRATE†
(klor-al hye′drate) (Chapter 8)

Functional classifications: Sedative, hypnotic
Chemical classification: Chloral derivative
Controlled substance schedule IV
FDA pregnancy category: C

Indications: Sedation, insomnia

Contraindications: Hypersensitivity to chloral hydrate, severe renal and hepatic disease, GI problems

Pharmacologic Effects: Mechanism of action not clear; hypnotic dose causes mild CNS depression

Pharmacokinetics: Metabolized to trichloroethanol, an active metabolite that has a half-life of 7-10 hr; protein binding is 35% to 41%; trichloroethanol is metabolized to trichloroacetic acid, an inactive metabolite; trichloroacetic acid is excreted in urine and bile and has a protein binding capacity of 71% to 88%; it can displace other acidic drugs from protein binding sites

Side Effects: *CNS:* Somnabulism, disorientation, incoherence, paradoxic excitement, delirium, drowsiness, ataxia; *Peripheral:* Nausea and vomiting; other GI disturbances; blood dyscrasias; skin disruptions (e.g., rashes, hives)

Interactions
- Alcohol: Synergistic effect with a disulfiram-like reactions (i.e., tachycardia, flushing)
- CNS depressants: Additive effect
- Oral anticoagulants: Slight increased effect
- Furosemide: Sweating, hot flashes, tachycardia
- Hydantoins: Reduced effect of hydantoin

†Available in Canada only.

Implications

Assess

- Blood studies

Planning/Implementation

- Maintain safety, e.g., prevent falls, keep side rails up, etc.
- Give ½ -1 hr before bedtime for insomnia
- Give after meals to decrease GI effect

Teaching

- To **avoid driving and use of alcohol** and other CNS depressants
- Potential for dependence
- Do not discontinue use abruptly
- Do not chew capsules

Evaluate

- Therapeutic response, mental status, respiratory difficulties, monitor for blood dyscrasias

Lab Test Interferences: Interferes with urine catecholamines and urinary 17-OHCS determinations; false-positive result for urinary glucose when using copper sulfate test

Treatment of Overdose: Symptoms are similar to those for barbiturate overdose; doses >2 g may produce intoxication; deaths have occurred with doses as low as 1.25 to 3 g; doses as high as 36 g have been tolerated; treatment is gastric lavage or induced emesis; activated charcoal may retard absorption; hemodialysis may be helpful; other supportive care as needed

Administration

- Insomnia: *Adult:* PO/rec 500 mg-1 g ½ -1 hr before bedtime; *child:* PO/rec 25-50 mg/kg in one dose, up to 1 g (hypnotic) or 500 mg (sedative)
- Available forms: Caps 250, 500 mg; syr 250, 500 mg/5ml, supp 324, 500, 648 mg

Chlordiazepoxide HCl

A-POXIDE, CHLORDIAZEPOXIDE HCL, LIBRITABS, LIBRIUM, MEDILIUM,† NOVOPOXIDE,† SOLIUM†

(klor-dye-az-e-pox'ide) (Chapters 6 and 10)

C

Functional classification: Antianxiety
Chemical classification: Benzodiazepine
Controlled substance schedule IV
FDA pregnancy category: D

Indications: Short-term management of anxiety, acute alcohol withdrawal, preoperatively for relaxation

Contraindications: Hypersensitivity to benzodiazepines, narrow-angle glaucoma, psychosis, child <6 yr (oral), child <12 yr (inj)

Cautious use: Elderly or debilitated patients, hepatic disease, renal disease

Pharmacologic Effects: Apparently potentiate effects of GABA and other inhibitory transmitters by binding to specific benzodiazepine receptor sites; depresses subcortical levels of CNS, including limbic system and reticular formation

Pharmacokinetics

- Speed of onset: Intermediate
- PO: Onset 30 min, peak ½ hr, duration 4-6 hr, metabolized by liver, excreted by kidneys, crosses placenta, enters breast milk, half-life 5-30 hr

Side Effects: *CNS:* **Drowsiness, dizziness,** confusion, headache, anxiety, tremor, stimulation, fatigue, depression, insomnia; *Peripheral:* Photophobia due to mydriasis, **blurred vision** due to cyclopegia; sleep-like slowing of respirations with therapeutic doses, cough; **orthostatic hypotension, tachycardia,** hypotension; constipation, dry mouth

Interactions

- Alcohol and other CNS depressants: Increased risk of excessive CNS depression
- Cimetidine: Potentiation of CNS depression

†Available in Canada only.

- Digoxin: Increased risk of cardiac side effects from digoxin
- Levodopa: Decreased antiparkinson effect
- Phenytoin: Increased phenytoin serum levels
- Oral anticoagulants: Increases or decreases anticoagulant effect

Implications
Assess
- Patient's level of anxiety and method of coping
- B/P, VS
- Establish baseline physical assessment data before medications are started

Planning/Implementation
- Monitor patient's response to medication
- Observe elderly, very young, and debilitated patients for paradoxic excitement
- Reduce dose of other depressant drugs
- Observe for signs of withdrawal when discontinuing antianxiety drug regimen

Teaching
- To avoid operating dangerous machinery and performing other tasks requiring good reflexes
- To report ocular pain at once, as well as other visual disturbances
- That drug may be taken with food

Evaluate
- Whether patient achieves lower levels of anxiety without undue sedation
- Whether patient can follow prescribed regimen
- For physical dependence: withdrawal symptoms of headache, nausea, vomiting, muscle pain, weakness after long-term use.

Lab Test Interferences
Increase: AST/ALT, serum bilirubin level
False increase: 17-OHCS
Decrease: RAIU

Treatment of Overdose: Lavage, VS, supportive care; there have been few deaths, if any, resulting from benzodiazepine overdose alone; deaths occur when benzodiazepines are mixed with other drugs, especially alcohol

Administration
- Mild anxiety: *Adult:* PO 5-10 mg tid or qid; *child* >6 yr: 5 mg bid-qid, not to exceed 10 mg bid-tid
- Severe anxiety: *Adult:* PO 20-25 mg tid-qid
- Alcohol withdrawal: *Adult:* PO/IM/IV 50-100 mg, not to exceed 300 mg/day; is poorly absorbed
- Available forms include: Caps 5, 10, 25 mg; tabs 5, 10, 25 mg; powder for IM inj 100-mg ampule

Chlorpromazine HCl

THORAZINE, CHLORPROMANYL, ORMAZINE
(klor-proe'ma'zeen) (Chapter 4)

Functional classifications: Antipsychotic neuroleptic
Chemical classification: Phenothiazine, aliphatic
FDA pregnancy category: D

Indications: Psychiatric psychotic disorders, mania, schizophrenia; *other:* Intractable hiccups, nausea, vomiting, preoperatively for relaxation, acute intermittent porphyria

Contraindications: Hypersensitivity, liver damage, cerebral arteriosclerosis, coronary disease, severe hypertension or hypotension, blood dyscrasias, coma, child <6 mo, brain damage, bone marrow depression, presence of alcohol and barbiturate
Cautious use: Lactation, seizure disorders, hypertension, hepatic disease, cardiac disease, respiratory impairment, especially in children

Pharmacologic Effects: Antipsychotic drugs produce a neuroleptic effect characterized by sedation, emotional quieting, psychomotor slowing, and affective indifference; exact mode of action is not fully understood; antipsychotics block dopamine receptors in the basal ganglia, hypothalamus, limbic system, brain stem, and medulla; they are also thought to depress certain components of the reticular activating system, which partially control body temperature, wakefulness, vasomotor tone, emesis, and hormonal balance; additionally, antipsychotics have significant anticholinergic and alpha-adrenergic blocking effects. Therapeutic plasma levels are 30-500 ng/ml.

Pharmacokinetics

- PO: Onset erratic, peak 2-4 hr, duration may be detected for up to 6 mo after last dose
- IM: Onset 15-30 min, peak 15-20 min, duration may be detected for up to 6 mo after last dose; IM provides 4 to 10 times more active drug than do oral doses
- IV: Onset 5 min, peak 10 min, duration may be detected for up to 6 mo after last dose
- REC: Onset erratic, peak 3 hr
- Metabolized by liver, excreted in urine (metabolites), crosses placenta, enters breast milk; 95% bound to plasma proteins; elimination half-life 10-30 hr

Side Effects: *CNS:* Parkinsonism, akathisias, dystonias, tardive dyskinesias, oculogyric crisis *Peripheral:* Blurred vision (cycloplegia or paralysis of accommodation), ocular pain, photophobia, mydriasis, impaired vision; intolerance of extreme heat or cold, possible heat stroke or fatal hyperthermia; nasal congestion, wheezing, dyspnea; **hypotension, especially orthostatic,** leading to dizziness, syncope, **tachycardia,** irregular pulse, arrhythmias; **dry mouth, constipation,** jaundice, abdominal pain, urinary retention; urinary hesitancy, galactorrhea, gynecomastia, impaired ejaculation, amenorrhea

Interactions

- Alcohol and other CNS depressants (barbiturates, antihistamines, antianxiety or antidepressant drugs): Increased CNS depression; increased risk of EPSEs
- Amphetamines: Possible decreased antipsychotic effect
- Antacids (magnesium and aluminum products): Possible decreased antipsychotic effect
- Anticholinergics (atropine, H_1-type antihistamines, antidepressants, etc.): Increased risk of excessive atropine-like side effects or toxic effects
- Benztropine: Possible decreased antipsychotic effect, increased risk of severity of peripheral anticholinergic side effects
- Diazoxide: Possible severe hyperglycemia, prediabetic coma
- Guanethidine: Poor control of hypertension by guanethidine
- Hypoglycemia drugs (insulin, oral hypoglycemia agents): Poor diabetic control
- Lithium: Poor control of psychosis with combined therapy; can mask lithium intoxication; neurotoxic effects with confusion, delirium, seizures, encephalopathy
- Meperidine, morphine: Increased risk of severe CNS depression, respiratory depression, hypotension
- Propranolol: Increased pharmacologic effects of either drug

C

Implications

Assess

- Establish baseline VS, laboratory values to aid in assessing side effects, allergic or hypersensitivity reactions
- Physiologic and psychologic status before therapy, to determine needs and evaluate progress
- For early stages of tardive dyskinesia, use abnormal involuntary movement scale
- Identify concurrent symptoms that may be aggravated by antipsychotics, e.g., glaucoma, diabetes

Planning/Implementation

- Ensure that drug has been taken; check mouth for "cheeking"
- When giving liquid antipsychotics, use at least 60 ml of compatible beverage to mask taste; dilute and give immediately; take drug with food to minimize GI upset; give IM injections in lateral thigh
- Keep patient quiet after injection to prevent falls associated with postural hypotension
- For dry mouth, give chewing gum, hard candies, lip balm, monitor urinary output, check for bladder distention in inactive patients, older men, and patients receiving high doses
- Assist patient with ambulation when blurred vision occurs; dim room lights for photosensitivity
- Ensure safety with hypotension; sit on side of bed before rising, head-low position for dizziness, avoid hot showers, wear elastic stockings
- Check B/P (supine, sitting, standing) and pulse before and after each dose when possible; observe for side effects

- Monitor body temperature for indications of muscle rigidity, fever, depressed neurologic status; ensure adequate hydration, nutrition, and ventilation
- Protect patient from exposure to extreme hot or cold
- Recognize impending hypersensitivity: pruritus or jaundice with hepatitis, flu or coldlike symptoms, evidence of bleeding with blood dyscrasia
- Observe for involuntary movements

Teaching
- About benefits and potential harm of antipsychotic drugs; weigh need to know against causing apprehension
- To comply with drug treatment
- To avoid activities requiring clear vision for a few weeks after treatment starts; to report eye pain immediately
- About importance of exercise, fluids, and fiber in the diet
- To watch for symptoms of heart failure: weight gain, dyspnea, distended neck veins, tachycardia
- Possible male sexual performance failure; suggest relaxed, stress-free environment
- To avoid conception; women should practice effective contraception; phenothiazines may cause false-positive results in pregnancy tests
- To avoid exposure to sunlight; keep skin covered but with temperature-appropriate clothing
- That patient cannot become addicted to antipsychotic drugs

Evaluate
- Follows prescribed regimen, takes medications as ordered
- Avoids injury; reports dizziness or need for assistance
- Verbalizes reduced anxiety
- Experiences minimal or no adverse responses
- Uses appropriate interventions to minimize side effects
- Achieves improved mental status; most problems occur during first 2 weeks of therapy
- For agranulocytosis, especially within 4 to 10 weeks after initiation of chlorpromazine therapy

Lab Test Interferences
Increase: Liver function tests; determinations of cardiac enzymes, cholesterol, blood glucose, prolactin, bilirubin, PBI, cholinesterase, I-131
Decrease: Hormones (blood and urine)
False positive: Pregnancy tests, PKU
False negative: Urinary steroids, 17-OHCS

Treatment of Overdose: Lavage, if orally ingested; provide an airway; do not induce vomiting; control EPSEs and hypotension

Administration: (Psychiatric Indications)
- Psychiatry: *Adult:* PO 10-50 mg q1-4h initially, then increase up to 2000 mg/day if necessary; *Adult:* IM 10-50 mg q1-4h; *Child:* PO 0.25 mg/lb q4-6h or 0.5 mg/kg; *Child:* IM 0.25 mg/lb q6-8h or 0.5 mg/kg; *Child:* REC 0.5 mg/lb q6-8h or 1 mg/kg; *Other uses:* See *PDR*
- Available forms include: Tabs 10, 25, 50, 100, 200 mg; time-rel caps 30, 75, 150, 200, 300 mg; syr 10 mg/5ml; conc 30, 100 mg/ml; supp 25, 100 mg; inj IM, IV 25 mg/ml

Chlorprothixene

TARACTAN

(klor-proe-thix′een) (Chapter 4)

Functional classifications: Antipsychotic neuroleptic
Chemical classification: Thioxanthene
FDA pregnancy category: C

Indications: Psychotic disorders, schizophrenia

Contraindications: Hypersensitivity, liver damage, cerebral arteriosclerosis, coronary disease, severe hypertension or hypotension, blood dyscrasias, coma, child <6 yr (PO), child <12 yr (IM), brain damage, bone marrow depression, alcohol and barbiturate withdrawal states
Cautious use: Lactation, seizure disorders, hypertension, hepatic disease, cardiac disease

Pharmacologic Effects: Antipsychotic drugs produce a neuroleptic effect characterized by sedation, emotional quieting, psychomotor slowing, and affective indifference; exact mode of action is not fully understood; antipsychotics block dopamine receptors in the basal ganglia, hypothalamus, limbic system, brain stem, and medulla; antipsychotics are also thought to depress certain components of the reticular activating system that partially control body temperature, wakefulness, vasomotor tone, emesis, and hormonal balance; additionally, antipsychotics have significant anticholinergic and alpha-adrenergic blocking effects

Pharmacokinetics: PO: Onset erratic, peak 2-4 hr; duration may be detected for up to 6 mo after last dose; metabolized by liver, excreted in urine (metabolites), crosses placenta, enters breast milk

Side Effects: *CNS:* Parkinsonism, akathisias, dystonias, tardive dyskinesia, oculogyric crisis; *Peripheral:* Blurred vision (cycloplegia or paralysis of accommodation); ocular pain, photophobia, mydriasis, impaired vision; intolerance of extreme heat or cold, possible heat stroke or fatal hyperthermia; nasal congestion, wheezing, dyspnea; **hypotension, especially orthostatic,** leading to dizziness, syncope; **tachycardia,** irregular pulse, arrhythmias; **dry mouth, constipation,** jaundice, abdominal pain; urinary retention, urinary hesitancy, galactorrhea, gynecomastia, impaired ejaculation, amenorrhea

Interactions

- Alcohol and other CNS depressants (barbiturates, antihistamines, antianxiety or antidepressant drugs): Increased CNS depression; increased risk of EPSEs
- Amphetamines: Possible decreased antipsychotic effect
- Antacids (magnesium and aluminum products): Possible decreased antipsychotic effect
- Anticholinergics (atropine, H_1-type antihistamines, antidepressants, etc.): Increased risk of excessive atropine-like side effects or toxic effects
- Benztropine: Possible decreased antipsychotic effect, increased risk of severity of peripheral anticholinergic side effects
- Diazoxide: Possible severe hyperglycemia, prediabetic coma
- Guanethidine: Poor control of hypertension by guanethidine
- Hypoglycemia drugs (insulin, oral hypoglycemia agents): Poor diabetic control
- Lithium: Poor control of psychosis with combined therapy; can mask lithium intoxication; neurotoxic effects with confusion, delirium, seizures, encephalopathy
- Meperidine, morphine: Increased risk of severe CNS depression, respiratory depression, hypotension
- Propranolol: Increased pharmacologic effects of either drug

Implications

Assess

- Establish baseline VS, laboratory values, to aid recognition of side effects, allergic or hypersensitivity reactions
- Assess physiologic and psychologic status before therapy, to determine needs and evaluate progress
- Assess for early stages of tardive dyskinesia by use of abnormal involuntary movement scale
- Identify concurrent symptoms that may be aggravated by antipsychotics, e.g., glaucoma, diabetes

Planning/Implementation

- Ensure that drug has been taken; check mouth for "cheeking"
- When giving liquid, dilute in milk, water, fruit juice, coffee, or soft drink; take drug with food to minimize GI upset; give IM injections in lateral thigh
- Keep patient quiet after injection to prevent falls associated with postural hypotension
- For dry mouth, give chewing gum, hard candies, lip balm, monitor urinary output; check for bladder distention in inactive patients, older men, and patients receiving high doses
- Assist with ambulation when patient has blurred vision; dim room lights for photosensitivity
- Ensure safety with hypotension; sit on side of bed before rising, head-low position for dizziness, avoid hot showers, wear elastic stockings
- Check B/P (supine, sitting, standing) and pulse before and after each dose when possible; observe for side effects
- Monitor body temperature for indications of NMS, e.g., muscle rigidity, fever, depressed neurologic status; ensure adequate hydration, nutrition, and ventilation

C

Bold = Most common side effects.

- Protect patient from exposure to extreme hot or cold
- Recognize impending hypersensitivity: pruritus or jaundice with hepatitis, flu or coldlike symptoms, evidence of bleeding with blood dyscrasia
- Observe for involuntary movements

Teaching
- About benefits and potential harm of antipsychotic drugs; weigh need to know against causing apprehension
- To comply with drug treatment
- To avoid activities requiring clear vision for a few weeks after treatment starts; to report eye pain immediately
- About importance of exercise, fluids, and fiber in diet
- To watch for symptoms of heart failure: weight gain, dyspnea, distended neck veins, tachycardia
- Possible male sexual performance failure; suggest relaxed, stress-free environment
- To avoid conception; women should practice effective contraception
- To avoid exposure to sunlight; keep skin covered but with temperature-appropriate clothing
- That patient cannot become addicted to antipsychotic drugs

Evaluate
- Follows prescribed regimen, takes medications as ordered
- Avoids injury; reports dizziness or need for assistance
- Verbalizes reduced anxiety
- Experiences minimal or no adverse responses
- Uses appropriate interventions to minimize side effects
- Achieves improved mental status

Lab Test Interferences
- Increase: Liver function tests; determinations of cardiac enzymes, cholesterol, blood glucose, prolactin, bilrubin, PBI, cholinesterase, I-131
- Decrease: Hormones (blood and urine)
- False positive: Pregnancy tests, PKU
- False negative: Urinary steroids, 17-OHCS

Treatment of Overdose: Lavage, if orally ingested; provide an airway; do not induce vomiting

Administration
Adult: PO 25-50 mg tid or qid, increased to desired response, maximum dosage 600 mg/qd
Geriatric: Start at 10-25 mg tid or qid; IM 25-50 mg tid or qid
Child >6 yr: PO 10-25 mg tid or qid; IM not recommended for children <12 yr
- Available forms include: Tabs* 10, 25, 50, 100 mg; conc 100 mg/5 ml; inj IM 12.5 mg/ml

Clomipramine

ANAFRANIL
(kloe-mi'pra-meen) **(Chapter 5)**

Functional classification: TCA
Chemical classification: Tertiary amine
FDA pregnancy category: C

Indications: Obsessive-compulsive disorder

Contraindications: Hypersensitivity to TCAs; acute recovery phase following MI; concomitant use with MAOIs; children <10 yr
Cautious use: Seizure disorders, glaucoma, urinary retention, hepatic and renal disorders, psychosis, ECT, elective surgery

Pharmacologic Effects: Blocks serotonin reuptake while the active metabolite desmethylclomipramine blocks norepinephrine reuptake; therapeutic plasma level 150-300 ng/ml

Pharmacokinetics: Metabolized by liver, excreted in urine; half-life 19-37 hr

Side Effects: *CNS:* **Sedation, headache** (52%), **insomnia** (25%), **libido change** (21%), **nervousness** (18%), **myoclonus** (13%), **increased appetite** (11%), ataxia; confusion, delirium; *Peripheral:* **Blurred vision,** photophobia, increased intraocular pressure; decreased tearing; **orthostatic hypotension;** arrythmias, tachycardia, palpitations; **dry mouth** (84%), **constipation**

*Roche Laboratories (Nutley, New Jersey) is making change in tablet color for this product in 1991 to 1992.

(47%), **diarrhea; increased sweating; urinary retention, hesitancy, ejaculation failure** (42%), **impotence** (20%), **fatigue** (39%), **weight gain** (18%)

Interactions

- Alcohol and other CNS depressants: Increased CNS depression
- Anticholinergics: Increased anticholinergic effect
- Sympathomimetics: Increased risk of sympathomimetic effect
- Haloperidol, cimetidine: Toxic effects r/t increased plasma levels of clomipramine
- Estrogens: Decreased or increased effects of clomipramine
- MAOIs: Hypertensive crisis, convulsions
- Phenytoin, phenobarbital: Decreased seizure threshold
- Ethchlorvynol: Delirium

Implications

Assess

- Establish baseline data, to aid recognition of adverse responses to medication, e.g., liver enzyme levels, VS, renal function, mental status, speech patterns, affect, weight
- Assess for signs of noncompliance, e.g., poor therapeutic response
- Observe for major symptoms of depression: apathy, sadness, sleep disturbances, hopelessness, guilt, decreased libido, spontaneous crying
- Review history for contraindicated conditions, e.g., glaucoma, CV disease, GI conditions, urologic conditions, seizures, pregnancy

Planning/Implementation

- Monitor for "cheeking" or hoarding; check drug dosage carefully, since a small overdose may cause toxic effects
- Monitor for suicidal ideations; suicidal thought content is associated with obsessive-compulsive disorder
- Monitor VS; withold when hypotension, tachycardia, or arrhythmias occur
- After titration, may give in a single dose hs
- Observe for early signs of toxicity, e.g., drowsiness, tachycardia, mydriasis, hypotension, agitation, vomiting, confusion, fever, restlessness, sweating
- Discontinue drug when CNS overstimulation occurs, e.g., hypomania, delirium

Teaching

- That these drugs have a lag time of up to 1 month
- Warn males of high incidence of sexual dysfunction
- To adhere to drug regimen
- To avoid OTC drugs, particularly those containing sympathomimetics or anticholinergics
- To avoid drugs listed in section on interactions
- About ways to deal with minor side effects, as follows: dry mouth: with sugarless hard candies, sips of water, mouth rinse; visual disturbances: with artificial tears, sunglasses, assistance with ambulation; constipation: with bulk-forming foods, increased fluids; urinary hesitancy: with adequate fluids, privacy; decreased perspiration: with appropriate clothing, avoidance of unnecessary exercise; orthostatic hypotension: with slow positional changes, avoidance of hot baths and showers; for drowsiness, take large dose at bedtime with physician approval, avoid driving
- That abrupt discontinuance may result in dizziness, nausea, vomiting, insomnia

Evaluate

- For therapeutic serum level
- For decrease in subjective symptoms
- For decrease in objective symptoms
- For mental impairment
- Stable VS
- Level of anxiety; should sleep, talk, and feel better

Administration

Adult: 25 mg/day to start, gradually increase to 100-150 mg/day during first 2 weeks; give in divided doses and with food to reduce GI upset; maximum dose is 250 mg/day; eventually total doses can be given hs

Children and adolescents: 25 mg/day to start, gradually increase in first 2 weeks to 3 mg/kg or 200 mg, whichever is smaller; can be given once a day hs

- Available forms include: Caps 25, 50, 75 mg

C

Clonazepam

KLONOPIN

(kloe-na'zi-pam) (Chapters 6, 7)

Functional classification: Anticonvulsant
Chemical classification: Benzodiazepine
Controlled substance schedule IV
FDA pregnancy category: C

Indications: Absence, Lennox-Gastaut, atypical absence, akinetic, myoclonic seizures; *unlabeled use:* panic attacks, benzodiazepine withdrawal

Contraindications: Hypersensitivity to benzodiazepines, acute narrow-angle glaucoma

Cautious use: Open-angle glaucoma, chronic respiratory disease, impaired hepatic and renal function

Pharmacologic Effects: Inhibits spike, wave formation in absence seizures (petit mal), decreases amplitude, frequency, duration, and spread of discharge in minor motor seizures

Pharmacokinetics: PO: Peak 1-2 hr, metabolized by liver, excreted in urine, half-life 18-50 hr; therapeutic plasma level is 20 to 80 ng/ml

Side Effects: *CNS:* **Drowsiness** (50%), **ataxia** (30%), dizziness, confusion, **behavioral changes,** tremors, insomnia, headache, suicidal tendencies; *Peripheral:* Nausea, constipation, polyphagia, anorexia, xerostomia, diarrhea, rash, alopecia, hirsutism, increased salivation, nystagmus, diplopia, abnormal eye movements, sore gums, respiratory depression, dyspnea, congestion (from increased salivation), palpitations, bradycardia, thrombocytopenia, leukocytosis, eosinophilia

Interactions

- Alcohol, CNS depressants, and other anticonvulsants: Increased CNS depression
- Carbamazepine: Increased carbamazepine serum level
- Valproic acid: Increased potential for seizures

Implications

Assess

- Renal studies: urinalysis, BUN and urine creatinine levels
- Blood studies: RBC, hematocrit, hemoglobin level, reticulocyte counts q wk for 4 wk, then q mo
- Hepatic studies: ALT, AST, bilirubin and creatinine levels
- Drug serum levels during initial treatment

Planning/Implementation

- Give with milk or food, to decrease GI symptoms
- Hard candy, frequent rinsing of mouth, gums for dry mouth
- Assistance with ambulation during early part of treatment; dizziness occurs

Teaching

- To carry MedicAlert identification bracelet
- To avoid driving, other activities that require alertness
- To avoid ingestion of alcohol or CNS depressants; increased sedation may occur
- Not to discontinue medication quickly after long-term use; taper off over several weeks (can precipitate status epilepticus)

Evaluate

- Therapeutic response: Decreased seizure activity, document on patient's chart
- Mental status
- Eye problems: Need for ophthalmic examinations before, during, and after treatment
- Allergic reaction: Red raised rash; if rash occurs, drug should be discontinued
- Blood dyscrasias: Fever, sore throat, bruising, rash, jaundice
- Toxic effects: Ataxia, hypotension, hypotonia

Lab Test Interferences: Increase: AST, alkaline phosphatase

Treatment of Overdose: Lavage, activated charcoal, monitor electrolyte levels, VS, administer vasopressors

Administration

Adult: PO not to exceed 1.5 mg/day in three divided doses; may be increased 0.5-1 mg q3 days until desired response, not to exceed 20 mg/day; *infant or child <10 yr or 30 kg:* PO 0.01-0.03 mg/kg/day in divided doses q8h, not to exceed 0.05 mg/kg/day; may be increased 0.25-0.5 mg q3 days until desired response, not to exceed 0.1.-0.2 mg/kg/day

- Available forms include: Tabs 0.5, 1, 2 mg

Clorazepate Dipotassium

TRANXENE

(klor-az′-pate) (Chapter 6)

Functional classification: Antianxiety
Chemical classification: Benzodiazepine
Controlled substance schedule IV
FDA pregnancy category: D

Indications: Anxiety, acute alcohol withdrawal, adjunct in partial seizure treatment

Contraindications: Hypersensitivity to benzodiazepines, narrow-angle glaucoma, psychosis, child <9 yr
Cautious use: Elderly or debilitated patients, hepatic disease, renal disease, lactation

Pharmacologic Effects: Apparently potentiates effects of GABA and other inhibitory transmitters by binding to specific benzodiazepine receptor sites; depresses subcortical levels of CNS, including limbic system and reticular formation

Pharmacokinetics: Speed of onset: Fast
PO: Onset 15 min, peak 1-2 hr, duration 4-6 hr, metabolized by liver, excreted by kidneys, crosses placenta, enters breast milk, half-life 30-100 hr

Side Effects: *CNS:* **Drowsiness, dizziness,** confusion, headache, anxiety, tremor, stimulation, fatigue, depression, insomnia; *Peripheral:* Photophobia due to mydriasis, blurred vision due to cycloplegia; sleeplike slowing of respirations with therapeutic doses, cough; orthostatic hypotension, tachycardia, hypotension; constipation, dry mouth, decreased hematocrit, transient skin rash

Interactions
- Alcohol and other CNS depressants: Increased risk of excessive CNS depression
- Cimetidine: Decreased clearance of clorazepate
- Digoxin: Increased risk of cardiac side effects from digoxin
- Levodopa: Decreased antiparkinson effect
- Phenytoin: Increased phenytoin serum levels

Implications
Assess
- Patient's level of anxiety and method of coping
- B/P, VS
- Establish baseline physical assessment data before medications are started

Planning/Implementation
- Monitor patient's response to medication
- Observe elderly, very young, and debilitated patients for paradoxic excitement
- Reduce dose of other depressant drugs
- Observe for signs of withdrawal when discontinuing antianxiety medication

Teaching
- To avoid operating dangerous machinery and other tasks requiring good reflexes
- To report ocular pain at once, as well as other visual disturbances
- Drug may be taken with food

Evaluate
- Whether patient achieves lower levels of anxiety without undue sedation
- Whether patient can follow prescribed regimen
- For physical dependence: withdrawal symptoms of headache, nausea, vomiting, muscle pain, weakness after long-term use.

Lab Test Interferences
Increase: AST/ALT, serum bilirubin level
Decrease: RAIU
False increase: 17-OHCS

Treatment of Overdose: Lavage, VS, supportive care; there have been few deaths, if any, from benzodiazepine overdose alone; deaths occur when benzodiazepines are mixed with other drugs, especially alcohol

Administration
- Anxiety: *Adult:* PO 15-60 mg/day; *geriatric:* 7.5-15 mg/day
- Alcohol withdrawal: *Adult:* PO 30 mg, then 30-60 mg in divided doses; day 2, 45-90 mg in divided doses; day 3, 22.5-45 mg in divided doses; day 4, 15-30 mg in divided doses; then reduce daily dose to 7.5-15 mg
- Seizure disorders: *Adult and child >12 yr:* PO 7.5 mg tid, may increase by 7.5 mg/wk or less, not to exceed 90 mg/day

Children (9-12 yr): PO 7.5 bid; increase by 7.5 mg/week, not to exceed 60 mg/day

- Available forms: Caps 3.75, 7.5, 15 mg; tabs 3.75 7.5, 11.25, 15, 22.5 mg

Clozapine

CLOZARIL

(kloź-a-peen) (Chapter 4)

Functional classifications: Antipsychotic neuroleptic

Chemical classification: Dibenzodiazepine

FDA pregnancy category: B

Indications: Management of schizophrenia refractory to other antipsychotics

Contraindications: History of clozapine-induced agranulocytosis; myeloproliferative disorders; concomitant use with other agents that can depress bone marrow function, severe CNS depression, coma, child <16 yr, lactation

Cautious use: Patients with hepatic, renal, or cardiac disease

Pharmacologic Effects: Interferes with binding of dopamine at D_1 and D_2 receptors; preferentially more active at limbic than at striatal dopamine receptors, probably accounting for the relative lack of EPSEs

Pharmacokinetics: Metabolized in liver, excreted in urine (50%) and feces (30%), half-life 4-12 hr

Side Effects: Clozapine has relatively few EPSEs; *CNS:* Drowsiness (39%), dizziness or vertigo (19%), headache (7%), tremor (6%), syncope (6%), disturbed sleep or nightmares (4%), restlessness (4%), akinesia (4%), agitation (4%), dose-related seizures (3%), ridigity (3%), akathisia (3%), confusion (3%); *Peripheral:* Salivation (31%), sweating (6%), dry mouth (6%), visual disturbances (5%), tachycardia (25%), hypotension (9%), hypertension (4%), constipation (14%), nausea (5%), fever (5%), agranulcytosis (1%); fatalities have occurred often enough to necessitate a special monitoring system

Interactions

- Anticholinergics: Increased anticholinergic effect
- Antihypertensives: Increased hypotensive effect
- CNS depressants: Additive effect
- Agents that suppress bone marrow function: Agranulocytosis
- Protein binding drugs: Potentiation of clozapine or the other drug
- Epinephrine: Severe hypotension

Implications

Assess

- Blood studies
- Concomitant illness
- Fever; flulike symptoms may indicate agranulocytosis

Planning/Implementation

- Monitor WBC and granulocyte count weekly
- Monitor ECG
- Monitor B/P (standing and sitting) for hypotension

Teaching

- Warn patient about risk of agranulocytosis and need to submit to weekly blood tests
- Inform about significant risk of seizures
- To avoid driving or operating hazardous machinery
- Advise about risk of orthostatic hypotension
- Not to become pregnant
- Not to breast feed

Evaluate

- Blood values
- Mental status
- Seizure activity

Treatment of Overdose: Symptoms of altered states of consciousness, i.e., drowsiness, delirium, coma, tachycardia, respiratory depression: Establish and maintain airway, ensure adequate ventilation and oxygenation; activated charcoal; supportive care: **Do not use epinephrine or its derivatives for hypotension**

Administration

Adult: PO: 25 mg qd or bid, then increase by 25 to 50 mg/day; target dose is 300 to 450 mg/day by the end of 2 weeks, if tolerated; some patients may require 600 to 900 mg/day

- Available forms: Tabs 25, 100 mg

Dantrolene Sodium

DANTRIUM, DANTRIUM IV
(dan'troe-leen) (Chapter 14)

Functional classifications: Skeletal muscle relaxant, direct acting
Chemical classification: Hydantoin
FDA pregnancy category: C

Indications: Spasticity caused by upper motor neuron disorders, **malignant hyperthermia** and NMS

Contraindications: Hypersensitivity, active hepatic disease, impaired myocardial function, lactation, children < 5 yr
Cautious use: Peptic ulcer disease, renal disease, hepatic disease, stroke, seizure disorder, diabetes mellitus, impaired pulmonary function

Pharmacologic Effect: Produces skeletal muscle relaxation by affecting the muscle directly. Probably this effect is associated with interference with the release of calcium

Pharmacokinetics: PO: Peak 5 hr, half-life 8 hr, metabolized in liver, excreted in urine (metabolites)

Side Effects: *CNS:* **Dizziness, weakness, fatigue, drowsiness,** headache, disorientation, insomnia, paresthesias, tremors, decreased seizure threshold; *Peripheral:* Nasal congestion, blurred vision, mydriasis, eosinophilia, hypotension, chest pain, palpitations, **nausea,** constipation, vomiting, abdominal pain, dry mouth, anorexia, urinary frequency, rash, pruritus

Interactions
- Alcohol and CNS depressants: CNS depression
- Warfarin and clofibrate: Reduce plasma protein binding of dantrolene

Implications (for Treatment of Neuroleptic Malignant Syndrome)
Assess
- For increased seizure activity in patient with epilepsy
- Hepatic function by frequent determination of AST, ALT

Planning/Implementation
- With meals for GI symptoms
- Sugarless gum, frequent sips of water for dry mouth
- Assistance with ambulation when dizziness or drowsiness occurs

Teaching
- Not to discontinue medication quickly, since hallucinations, spasticity, tachycardia may occur; drug should be tapered off over 1-2 wk
- Not to take with alcohol or other CNS depressants
- To avoid altering activities while taking this drug
- To avoid hazardous activities when drowsiness or dizziness occurs
- To avoid using OTC medication such as cough preparations and antihistamines unless directed by physician

Evaluate
- Therapeutic response: For neuroleptic malignant syndrome, decreased fever, sweating, rigidity
- Allergic reactions: Rash, fever, respiratory distress
- Severe weakness, numbness in extremities
- CNS depression: Dizziness, drowsiness, psychiatric symptoms

Treatment of Overdose: Induce emesis in conscious patient, lavage, dialysis

Administration
- Spasticity: *Adult:* PO 25 mg/day; may increase by 25-100 mg bid-qid, not to exceed 400 mg/day; *child:* PO 0.5 mg/kg/day bid; may increase gradually, not to exceed 100 mg qid
- Malignant hyperthermia: *Adult and child:* IV 1 mg/kg, may repeat to total dose of 10 mg/kg; PO 4-8 mg/kg/day in four divided doses for 1-3 days to prevent further hyperthermia
- NMS: 4-10 mg/kg/day
- Available forms include: Caps 25, 50, 100 mg; powder for inj IV 20 mg/vial

D

Desipramine HCl

NORPRAMIN, PERTOFRANE
(dess-ip'ra-meen) (Chapter 5)

Functional classification: TCA
Chemical classifications: Dibenzazepine, secondary amine
FDA pregnancy category: C

Indications: Depression; unlabeled use: Cocaine withdrawal

Contraindications: Hypersensitivity to TCAs, recovery phase of myocardial infarction, narrow-angle glaucoma
Cautious use: Convulsive disorders, prostatic hypertrophy, child < 12 yr; suicidal patients, severe depression, increased intraocular pressure, narrow-angle glaucoma, elderly patients, thyroid disease, MAOI therapy, ECT

Pharmacologic Effects: Blocks uptake of norepinephrine, serotonin in nerve cells; therapeutic plasma level 125-300 ng/ml

Pharmacokinetics: PO: Steady state 2-11 days; metabolized by liver, excreted by kidneys, crosses placenta, half-life 12-24 hr

Side Effects: *CNS:* **Sedation,** ataxia; confusion, delirium; *Peripheral:* **Blurred vision,** photophobia, increased intraocular pressure, decreased tearing, orthostatic hypotension, arrhythmias, tachycardia, palpitations, dry mouth, constipation, diarrhea, decreased sweating, **urinary retention, hesitancy**

Interactions
- Anticholinergic agents: Additive anticholinergic effects with atropine, antihistamines (H_1 blocker), antiparkinson drugs, antipsychotics, OTC cold and allergy drugs
- CNS depressants: Additive depressant effect
- Guanethidine, clonidine: Decreases antihypertensive effect
- MAOIs: Hypertensive crisis, atropine-like poisoning
- Oral contraceptives: Inhibit metabolism of TCAs
- Phenothiazines: May increase tricyclic serum level
- Quinidine: Additive effect, heart block possible
- Sympathomimetics: Potentiates sympathomimetic effects
- Thyroid preparations: Tachycardia, arrhythmias; may increase TCA effect

Implications
Assess
- Establish baseline data to aid recognition of adverse responses to medication, e.g., liver enzyme levels, VS, renal function, mental status, speech patterns, affect, weight
- For signs of noncompliance, e.g., poor therapeutic response
- Observe for major symptoms of depression: apathy, sadness, sleep disturbances, hopelessness, guilt, decreased libido, spontaneous crying
- Review history for contraindicated conditions, e.g., glaucoma, CV disease, GI conditions, urologic conditions, seizures, pregnancy

Planning/Implementation
- Monitor for "cheeking" or hoarding; check drug dosage carefully, since a small overdose may cause toxic effects
- Monitor for suicidal ideations; suicidal thought content may increase as antidepressants begin to "energize" patient
- Monitor VS, withold TCAs when hypotension, tachycardia, or arrhythmias occur
- Give most TCAs in a single dose hs
- Observe for early signs of toxic effects, e.g., drowsiness, tachycardia, mydriasis, hypotension, agitation, vomiting, confusion, fever, restlessness, sweating
- Discontinue drug when CNS overstimulation occurs, e.g., hypomania, delirium

Teaching
- That these drugs have a lag time of up to 1 month
- To adhere to drug regimen
- To avoid OTC drugs, particularly those containing sympathomimetics or anticholinergics
- To avoid drugs listed in section on interactions
- About ways to deal with minor side effects, as follows: dry mouth, with sugarless hard candies, sips of water, mouth rinses; visual disturbances, with artificial tears, sunglasses, assistance with ambu-

lation; constipation, with bulk-forming foods, increased fluids; urinary hesitancy, with adequate fluids, privacy; decreased perspiration, with appropriate clothing, avoidance of unnecessary exercise; orthostatic hypotension, with slow positional changes, avoidance of hot baths and showers; for drowsiness, take single dose hs with physician approval, avoid driving

- That abrupt discontinuance may result in cholinergic rebound, e.g., nausea, vomiting, insomnia, headache

Evaluate

- Desired therapeutic serum level
- Verbalize decrease in subjective symptoms
- Observe decrease in objective symptoms
- Minimal to no adverse drug effects
- Stable VS
- Less anxiety: sleep, talk, and feel better

Lab Test Interferences

- Increase: Serum bilirubin, blood glucose, alkaline phosphatase levels
- False increase: Urinary catecholamines
- Decrease: VMA, 5-HIAA

Treatment of Overdose: Hospitalization, ECG monitoring, monitor cardiac function for at least 5 days, induce emesis, lavage, support airway

Administration

Adult: PO 100-200 mg/day in divided doses, may increase to 300 mg/day or may give daily dose; *Adolescent/geriatric:* PO 25-100 mg/day, may increase to 150 mg/day

- Available forms include: Tabs 10, 25, 50, 75, 100, 150 mg; caps 25, 50 mg

Dextroamphetamine Sulfate

DEXEDRINE, FERNDEX, OXYDESS II, SPANCAP NO. 1
(dex-troe-am-fet'a-meen) (Chapters 12, 13, 15, 16)

Functional classification: Cerebral stimulant
Chemical classification: Amphetamine
Controlled substance schedule II
FDA pregnancy category: C

D

Indications: Narcolepsy, exogenous obesity, ADHD

Contraindications: Hypersensitivity to sympathomimetic amines, glaucoma, severe arteriosclerosis, drug abuse, CV disease, anxiety, hyperthyroidism, MAOI use *Cautious use:* Tourette's disorder, lactation, child <3 yr

Pharmacologic Effects: Increases release of norepinephrine, dopamine in cerebral cortex, brain stem, and reticular activating system; therapeutic plasma level 5-10 μg/dl

Pharmacokinetics: PO: Onset 30 min, peak 1-3 hr, duration 4-20 hr, metabolized by liver, excreted by kidneys, crosses placenta, enters breast milk, half-life 10-30 hr

Side Effects: *CNS:* **Hyperactivity, insomnia, restlessness, talkativeness,** dizziness, headache, chills, stimulation, dysphoria, irritability, aggressiveness; *Peripheral:* Nausea, vomiting, anorexia, dry mouth, diarrhea, constipation, weight loss, metallic taste, cramps, impotence, change in libido, **palpitations, tachycardia,** hypertension, hypotension

Interactions

- MAOIs or within 14 days of MAOIs: Hypertensive crisis
- Acetazolamide, antacids, sodium bicarbonate, ascorbic acid, ammonium chloride, phenothiazines, haloperidol: Increases half-life of amphetamine
- Barbiturates: Decreased effects of this drug
- Guanethidine, other antihypertensives: Decreased effects of these drugs

Implications
Assess
- VS B/P because this drug may reverse antihypertensives; check patients with cardiac disease more often
- CBC, urinalysis; in diabetes, blood and urine sugar levels, insulin changes may be necessary because eating decreases
- **Height, growth rate in children, growth rate may be decreased**

Planning/Implementation
- Give at least 6 hr before bedtime to avoid sleeplessness
- For obesity, only when patient is on weight reduction program that includes dietary changes, exercise; patient tolerance develops, and weight loss will not occur without additional methods
- Gum, hard candy, frequent sips of water for dry mouth
- If drug is for obesity, 30-60 min before meals
- Dispense least amount feasible, to minimize risk of overdose

Teaching
- To decrease caffeine consumption (coffee, tea, cola, chocolate) that may increase irritability, stimulation
- Avoid OTC preparations unless approved by physician
- To taper off drug over several weeks, or depression, increased sleeping, lethargy may occur
- To avoid alcohol ingestion
- To avoid hazardous activities until condition is stabilized on medication
- To get needed rest; patients feel more tired at end of day
- Check to see that PO medication has been swallowed

Evaluate
- Mental status: mood, sensorium, affect, stimulation, insomnia; aggressiveness may occur
- Physical dependency; should not be used for extended time; dosage should be discontinued gradually
- **Withdrawal symptoms: headache, nausea, vomiting, muscle pain, weakness**
- Drug tolerance develops after long-term use
- If tolerance develops, dosage should not be increased

Treatment of Overdose: Administer fluids, hemodialysis or peritoneal dialysis; antihypertensive for increased B/P, ammonium chloride for increased excretion, chlorpromazine for CNS stimulation

Administration
- Narcolepsy: PO 5-60 mg qd in divided doses; *adult and adolescents* >*12 yr:* PO 10 mg qd, increasing by 10 mg/day at weekly intervals; *child 6-12 yr:* PO 5 mg qd, increasing by 5 mg/day at weekly intervals, up to 60 mg/day
- ADHD: *Child* >*6 yr:* PO 5 mg qd-bid, increasing by 5 mg/wk; *Child 3-6 yr:* PO 2.5 mg qd, increasing by 2.5 mg/wk
- Obesity: *Adult:* PO 5-30 mg qd in divided doses 30-60 min before meals
- Available forms: Tabs 5, 10 mg; caps time-rel 5, 10, 15 mg; elix 5 mg/5 ml

Diazepam

D-TRAN,† E-PAM,† MEVAL,† NOVODIPAM,† STRESS-PAM,† VALIUM, VALRELEASE, VIVOL†
(dye-az′-e-pam) (Chapters 6, 7, 9, 14)

Functional classification: Antianxiety
Chemical classification: Benzodiazepine
Controlled substance schedule IV
FDA pregnancy category: D

Indications: Anxiety, acute alcohol withdrawal, status epilepticus

Contraindications: Hypersensitivity to benzodiazepines, narrow-angle glaucoma, psychosis, child <6 months (oral)
Cautious use: Elderly or debilitated patients, hepatic disease, renal disease

Pharmacologic Effects: Apparently potentiates effects of GABA and other inhibitory transmitters by binding to specific benzodiazepine receptor sites; depresses subcortical levels of CNS, including limbic system and reticular formation

Pharmacokinetics: Speed of onset: Very fast
PO: Onset ½ hr, duration 2-3 hr; IM: Onset 15-30 min, duration 1-1½ hr; IV: Onset 1-5 min, duration 15 min; metabolized

†Available in Canada only.

by liver, excreted by kidneys, crosses placenta, enters breast milk, half-life 20-80 hr

Side Effects: *CNS:* **Drowsiness, dizziness,** confusion, headache, anxiety, tremor, stimulation, fatigue, depression, insomnia; *Peripheral:* Photophobia due to mydriasis, **blurred vision** due to cycloplegia; sleeplike slowing of respirations with therapeutic doses, cough; **orthostatic hypotension, tachycardia,** hypotension; constipation, dry mouth

Interactions

- Alcohol and other CNS depressants: Increased risk of excessive CNS depression;
- Cimetidine: Potentiation of CNS depression
- Digoxin: Increased risk of cardiac side effects from digoxin
- Levodopa: Decreased antiparkinson effect
- Phenytoin: Increased phenytoin serum levels
- Oral anticoagulants: Increases or decreases anticoagulant effect

Implications

Assess

- Patient's level of anxiety and method of coping
- B/P, VS
- Establish baseline physical assessment data before medications are started

Planning/Implementation

- Monitor patient's response to medication
- Observe elderly, very young, and debilitated patients for paradoxic excitement
- Reduce dose of other depressant drugs
- Observe for signs of withdrawal when discontinuing antianxiety agent

Teaching

- To avoid operating dangerous machinery and performing other tasks requiring good reflexes
- To report ocular pain at once, as well as other visual disturbances
- Drug may be taken with food

Evaluate

- Whether patient achieves lower levels of anxiety without undue sedation
- Whether patient can follow prescribed regimen
- For physical dependence: withdrawal symptoms of headache, nausea, vomiting, muscle pain, weakness after long-term use

Lab Test Interferences

Increase: AST/ALT, serum bilirubin levels
False increase: 17-OHCS
Decrease: RAIU

Treatment of Overdose: Lavage, VS, supportive care; there have been few deaths, if any, from benzodiazepine overdose alone; deaths occur when benzodiazepines are mixed with other drugs, especially alcohol

Administration

- Anxiety: *Adult:* PO 2-10 mg tid-qid or time-rel 15-30 mg qd; *child >6 mo:* PO 1-2.5 mg tid-qid
- Acute alcohol withdrawal: 10 mg tid-qid during first 24 hr; then reduce to 5 mg tid-qid PRN
- Status epilepticus: *Adult:* IV bolus 5-10 mg, 5 mg/min, may repeat q5-10 min, not to exceed 30 mg, may repeat in 2-4 hr, if seizures reappear; *child > 5 yr:* IV bolus 0.1-0.3 mg/kg (1 mg/min q 2-5 min), up to a maximum of 10 mg; repeat in 2-4 hr if necessary; *child 30 days to 5 yr:* 0.2-0.5 mg slowly q 2-5 min, up to a maximum of 5 mg
- Available forms include: Tabs 2, 5, 10 mg; caps time-rel 15 mg, IM/IV inj 5 mg/ml; oral solution 5 mg/5ml, 5 mg/ml

D

Diphenhydramine

ALLERDRYL, BARAMINE, BAX, BENACHLOR, BENADRYL, BENAHIST, BENTRACT, COMPOZ, DIPHENACEN, FENYLHIST, NORDRYL, ROHYORA, SPAN-LANIN, VAIDRENE, WEHDRYL

(dye-fen-hye′dra-meen) (Chapter 14)

Functional classification: Antihistamine
Chemical classifications: H_1-receptor antagonist, ethanolamine
FDA pregnancy category: C

Indications: Parkinsonism, EPSEs, motion sickness, allergies and allergic reactions, sedation, other nonpsychiatric uses

Contraindications: Hypersensitivity, acute asthma attacks, lower respiratory tract disease

Pharmacologic Effects: Competes with histamine for H_1-receptor sites; blocks allergic responses by blocking histamine

Pharmacokinetics: Absorbed readily in GI tract; PO peaks in 1-3 hr; duration of action 4-7 hr; IM onset ½ hr, peak 1-4 hr, duration 4-7 hr; IV onset immediate, duration 4-7 hr; metabolized in liver, excreted in urine, crosses placenta, excreted in breast milk, half-life 2-7 hr

Side Effects: *CNS:* Drowsiness (usually transient), sedation, dizziness, disturbed coordination; *Less frequent:* Fatigue, confusion, restlessness, nervousness; *Peripheral:* Nausea and vomiting; dry mouth, blood dyscrasias, urinary retention, blurred vision, nasal stuffiness, dry throat and nose

Interactions
- CNS depressants: Increased depression
- Heparin: Decreased effect of heparin
- MAOIs: Increased anticholinergic effect

Implications
Assess
- For urinary retention
- Blood studies with long-term use

Planning/Implementation
- Give with meals to decrease GI upset
- Give IV at 25 mg/min
- Give IM in large muscle

Teaching
- Hard candies, gum for dry mouth
- To avoid driving
- To avoid CNS depressants, e.g., alcohol

Evaluate
- For EPSEs: Therapeutic responses
- For congestion: Ability to breathe
- Insomnia: Sleep
- For wheezing and chest tightness

Lab Test Interference
False negative: Skin allergy tests

Treatment of Overdose: Anticholinergic toxicity includes flushing, dry mouth, hyperthermia (up to 107° F), gastric lavage or induced emesis, diazepam, vasopressors, and short-acting barbiturates

Administration
- Parkinsonism and EPSEs: *PO Adults:* 25-50 mg tid to qid daily; *PO Children >20 lb:* 12.5 to 25 mg tid or qid daily or 5 mg/kg/day, not to exceed 300 mg/day; *IM or IV Adult:* 10-50 mg, 100 mg if required, maximum daily dosage is 400 mg; *Children:* 5 mg/kg/day divided into four doses, maximum daily dosage is 300 mg
- Available forms: Caps 25, 50 mg; tabs 25, 50 mg; elixir 12.5 mg/5 ml; syr 12.5 mg/5 ml; IM, IV 10, 50 mg/ml

Disulfiram

ANTABUSE

(dye-sul'fi-ram) (Chapter 10)

Functional classification: Alcohol deterrent
Chemical classification: Aldehyde dehydrogenase inhibitor
FDA pregnancy category: X

Indications: Treatment of chronic alcoholism

Contraindications: Hypersensitivity, patients who have received paraldehyde, alcohol intoxication, psychoses, CV disease *Cautious use:* Hypothyroidism, hepatic disease, diabetes mellitus, seizure disorders, nephritis

Pharmacologic Effects: Blocks oxidation of alcohol at acetaldehyde stage by inhibiting aldehyde dehydrogenase

Pharmacokinetics: PO: Onset 12 hr, oxidized by liver, excreted in urine

Side Effects: *CNS:* **Headache, drowsiness,** restlessness, dizziness, fatigue, tremors, psychosis, neuritis, **sweating, convulsions, death;** *Peripheral:* Nausea, vomiting, anorexia, severe thirst, hepatoxicity; rash, dermatitis, urticaria; respiratory depression, hyperventilation; tachycardia, chest pain, hypotension, arrhythmia

Interactions
- Alcohol: Violent symptoms of sweating, throbbing headache, nausea and profuse vomiting, flushed face and neck, palpitations, tightness of chest, tremor, dyspnea

- TCAs, diazepam, hydantoins, oral anticoagulants, paraldehyde, phenytoin, chlordiazepoxide: Increased effects of these drugs
  Metronidazole, isoniazid: Psychosis

Implications

Assess

- Liver function studies q2 wk during therapy; AST, ALT, CBC, SMA-12 q3-6 mo to detect any abnormality

Planning/Implementation

- If drowsiness occurs, give once per day in morning or hs
- Give only after patient has not been drinking for >12 hr

Teaching

- Effect of this drug when alcohol is taken; written consent for disulfiram therapy should be obtained
- That shaving lotions, creams, cough preparations, skin products must be checked for alcohol content; even in small amount, alcohol can produce a reaction
- That tolerance does not develop when treatment is prolonged
- That reaction may occur for 14 days after last dose
- That tabs can be crushed, mixed with liquid beverage
- To carry identification that lists disulfiram therapy and physician phone number
- To avoid driving or hazardous tasks when drowsiness occurs
- That disulfiram reaction can be fatal and occurs 15 min after drinking

Evaluate

- Mental status: Ability to abstain from alcohol

Treatment of Overdose: IV vitamin C, ephedrine sulfate, antihistamines, O_2

Administration

Adult: PO 250-500 mg qd for 1-2 wk, then 125-500 mg qd until desired response

- Available forms include: Tabs 250, 500 mg

Doxepin HCl

ADAPIN, SINEQUAN

(dox′e-pin) (Chapter 5)

Functional classification: TCA
Chemical classification: Dibenzoxepin, tertiary amine
FDA pregnancy category: C

Indications: Depression, anxiety

Contraindications: Hypersensitivity to TCAs, urinary retention, narrow-angle glaucoma, prostatic hypertrophy
Cautious use: Suicidal or elderly patients, lactation, MAOI therapy, children < 12 yr

Pharmacologic Effects: Blocks reuptake of norepinephrine, serotonin into nerve endings, increasing action of norepinephrine, serotonin in nerve cells; also r/t changes in receptor sensitivity; therapeutic plasma levels 100-200 ng/ml

Pharmacokinetics: PO: Steady state 2-8 days; metabolized by liver, excreted in kidneys, crosses placenta, excreted in breast milk, half-life 8-24 hr

Side Effects: *CNS:* **Sedation,** ataxia; confusion, delirium; *Peripheral:* **Blurred vision,** photophobia, increased intraocular pressure, decreased tearing, orthostatic hypotension, arrhythmias, tachycardia, palpitations, dry mouth, constipation, diarrhea, decreased sweating, **urinary retention, hesitancy**

Interactions

- Anticholinergic agents: Additive anticholinergic effects with atropine, antihistamines (H_1 blocker), antiparkinson drugs, antipsychotics, OTC cold and allergy drugs
- CNS depressants: Additive depressant effect
- Guanethidine, clonidine: Decreased antihypertensive effect
- MAOIs: Hypertensive crisis, atropine-like poisoning
- Oral contraceptives: Inhibits metabolism of tricyclics
- Phenothiazines: May increase TCA serum level
- Quinidine: Additive effect, heart block possible

D

- Sympathomimetics: Potentiates sympathomimetic effects
- Thyroid preparations: Tachycardia, arrhythmias; may increase TCA effect

Implications

Assess

- Establish baseline data to aid recognition of adverse responses to medication, e.g., liver enzyme levels, VS, renal function, mental status, speech patterns, affect, weight
- For signs of noncompliance, e.g., poor therapeutic response
- For major symptoms of depression: Apathy, sadness, sleep disturbances, hopelessness, guilt, decreased libido, spontaneous crying
- History for contraindicated conditions, e.g., glaucoma, CV disease, GI conditions, urologic conditions, seizures, pregnancy

Planning/Implementation

- Monitor for "cheeking" or hoarding; check drug dosage carefully, since a small overdose may cause toxic effects
- Monitor for suicidal ideations; suicidal thought content may increase as antidepressants begin to "energize" patient
- Monitor VS; if hypotension, tachycardia, or arrhythmias occur, withhold TCAs
- Give most TCAs in a single dose hs
- Observe for early signs of toxic effects, e.g., drowsiness, tachycardia, mydriasis, hypotension, agitation, vomiting, confusion, fever, restlessness, sweating
- If CNS overstimulation occurs, e.g., hypomania, delirium, discontinue drug
- Dilute oral concentrate with 120 ml water, milk, or fruit juice

Teaching

- That these drugs have a lag time of up to 1 month
- To adhere to drug regimen
- To avoid OTC drugs, particularly those containing sympathomimetics or anticholinergics
- To avoid drugs listed in section on interactions
- About ways to deal with minor side effects, as follows: dry mouth, with hard candies, sips of water, mouth rinses; visual disturbances, with artificial tears, sunglasses, assistance with ambulation; constipation, with bulk-forming foods, increased fluids; urinary hesitancy, with adequate fluids, privacy; decreased perspiration, with appropriate clothing, avoidance of unnecessary exercise; orthostatic hypotension, with slow positional changes, avoidance of hot baths and showers; for drowsiness, take single dose hs with physician approval, avoid driving
- That abrupt discontinuance may result in cholinergic rebound, e.g., nausea, vomiting, insomnia, headache

Evaluate

- Desired therapeutic serum level
- Verbalize decrease in subjective symptoms
- Observe decrease in objective symptoms
- Minimal to no adverse drug effects
- Stable VS
- Less anxiety; sleep, talk, and feel better

Lab Test Interferences

Increase: Serum bilirubin, blood glucose, alkaline phosphatase levels
False increase: Urinary catecholamines
Decrease: VMA, 5-HIAA

Treatment of Overdose: ECG monitoring, induce emesis, lavage, activated charcoal, administer anticonvulsant

Administration

Adult: PO 10-25 mg tid to start, may increase to 300 mg/day or may give daily dose hs

- Available forms include: Caps 10, 25, 50, 75, 100, 150 mg; oral conc 10 mg/ml

Estazolam

PROSOM

(esś-ta-zoe-lam) (Chapter 8)

Functional classification: Sedative, hypnotic
Chemical classification: Benzodiazepine
Controlled substance schedule IV
FDA pregnancy category: X

Indications: Insomnia

Contraindications: Hypersensitivity, sleep apenea

Pharmacologic Effects: Believed to potentiate GABA receptors, which are inhibitory, causing CNS depression; may affect BZ_1 (sleep) receptors

Pharmacokinetics: Peak levels 2 hr, half-life 10-24 hr, protein binding 93%, less than 5% excreted unchanged in urine, metabolized in liver

Side Effects: *CNS:* Somnolence (42%), asthenia (11%), hypokinesia (8%), hangover (3%), headache, nervousness, talkativeness, drowsiness, dizziness, confusion; see diazepam for other benzodiazepine side effects; *Peripheral:* Nausea and vomiting, other GI upsets, constipation, skin eruptions, blood dyscrasias

Interactions
- Cimetidine, disulfiram, isoniazid, probenecid: Estazolam effects increased
- CNS depressants and alcohol: Additive CNS depression
- Theophylline, rifampin: Decreased effect of estazolam

Implications
Assess
- B/P
- Blood studies, if indicated

Planning/Implementation
- Give ½ -1 hr before bedtime
- Give with food for GI upset
- Maintain safety

Teaching
- To avoid driving
- To avoid alcohol

Evaluate
- Therapeutic response, sleeping
- Mental status

Lab Test Interference
Increase: AST, ALT

Treatment of Overdose: Deaths due to benzodiazepine overdose alone have not been recorded; lavage, monitor VS, provide supportive care

Administration
- Insomnia: *Adult:* 1 mg hs, up to 2 mg; *Elderly:* If healthy, 1 mg hs; if small or debilitated, 0.5 mg hs (effectiveness not clear)
- Available forms: Tabs 1, 2 mg

Ethchlorvynol*
PLACIDYL
(eth-klor-vi'nole) (Chapter 8)

Functional classifications: Sedative, hypnotic
Chemical classification: Tertiary acetylenic alcohol
Controlled substance schedule IV
FDA pregnancy category: C

Indications: Sedation, insomnia

Contraindications: Hypersensitivity, severe pain, porphyria, lactation
Cautious use: Pain

Pharmacologic Effects: Mechanism of action not known, produces CNS depression

Pharmacokinetics: Rapidly absorbed from GI tract; onset 15-30 min, peak level 2 hr, duration 5 hr, metabolized in liver, excreted in urine, half-life 10-20 hr for parent compound

Side Effects: *CNS:* Dizziness, facial numbness, giddiness; *Peripheral:* Nausea and vomiting; GI upset, blood dyscrasias, blurred vision, hypotension, rash

Interactions
- Alcohol and other CNS depressants: Additive depressive effect
- Oral anticoagulants: Decreased thrombin time
- TCAs: Transient delirium
- MAOIs: Increased CNS depression

Implications
Assess
- Blood studies may be indicated

Planning/Implementation
- Give with food ½-1 hr before bedtime for sleeplessness, to decrease dizziness and giddiness; maintain safety, i.e., protect from falls, keep bed rails up, etc.

Teaching
- To avoid driving
- To avoid alcohol and other CNS depressants

Evaluate
- Ability to sleep through night
- Mental status

*Infrequently used.

E

- Decreased respiration (if below 10/min, withhold drug)

Lab Test Interference: Interferes with Clinitest

Treatment of Overdose: Overdose is characterized by deep coma, severe respiratory depression, hypothermia, hypotension, bradycardia; death has been reported at doses of 6 g but doses as high as 50 g have been survived; lavage or other approaches to gastric evacuation should be performed immediately; provide supportive care; forced diuresis with high urinary output is helpful

Administration
- Do not prescribe for more than 1 week
- Sedation: *Adult:* PO 100-200 mg bid or tid
- Insomnia: *Adult* PO 500-1000 mg ½ hr before bedtime, may repeat 200 mg, if original dose was 500-750 mg
- Available forms: Caps 200, 500, 750 mg

Ethopropazine HCl*

HCL PARSIDOL
(eth-oh-proé-pa-zeen) (Chapter 14)

Functional classification: Anticholinergic
Chemical classification: Phenothiazine
FDA pregnancy category: C

Indications: For parkinsonism and EPSEs but not frequently prescribed

Contraindications: See trihexyphenidyl

Pharmacologic Effects: See trihexyphenidyl

Pharmacokinetics: See trihexyphenidyl

Side Effects: *CNS:* See trihexyphenidyl; *Peripheral:* See trihexyphenidyl

Interactions: See trihexyphenidyl

Implications: See trihexyphenidyl

Lab Test Interference: See trihexyphenidyl

Treatment of Overdose: See trihexyphenidyl

Administration
- Parkinsonism and EPSEs: PO *adult:* Begin with 50 mg qd or bid, increase gradually, if necessary; *for mild to moderate symptoms:* 100 to 400 mg/day; *severe cases:* Gradually increase to 500 to 600 mg/day or more
- Available forms: Tabs 10, 50 mg

Ethosuximide

ZARONTIN
(eth-oh-sux'i-mide) (Chapter 7)

Functional classification: Antiepileptic
Chemical classification: Succinimide
FDA pregnancy category: C

Indications: Absence seizures (petit mal)

Contraindications: Hypersensitivity to succinimide derivatives
Cautious use: Lactation, hepatic disease, renal disease

Pharmacologic Effect: Inhibits spike and wave formation in absence seizures; therapeutic serum level 40-100 μg/ml

Pharmacokinetics: PO peak 3-7 hr; steady state 5-10 days; metabolized by liver; excreted in urine, bile, feces; half-life 60 hr (adult), 30 hr (child)

Side Effects: *CNS:* **Drowsiness, dizziness, fatigue, euphoria, lethargy;** anxiety, aggressiveness, irritability, depression, insomnia; *Peripheral:* **Nausea, vomiting, heartburn, anorexia, diarrhea, abdominal pain, cramps, constipation,** vaginal bleeding, hematuria, renal damage, urticaria, pruritic erythema, hirsutism, Stevens-Johnson syndrome, myopia, gum hypertrophy, tongue swelling, blurred vision, agranulocytosis, aplastic anemia, thrombocytopenia, leukocytosis, eosinophilia, pancytopenia (some blood dyscrasias have been fatal)

Interactions
- TCAs: Antagonist effect (imipramine, doxepin); also, lower seizure threshold
- Estrogens: Decreased effects of oral contraceptives
- CNS depressants: Increased CNS depression

*Infrequently used.

Implications

Assess

- Renal studies: Urinalysis, BUN and urine creatinine levels
- Blood studies: CBC, hematocrit, hemoglobin level
- Hepatic studies: AST, ALT, bilirubin and creatinine levels
- Drug levels during initial treatment, therapeutic range (40-100 μg/ml)

Planning/Implementation

- Take with milk or food, to decrease GI symptoms
- Assistance with ambulation during early part of treatment; dizziness occurs

Teaching

- To carry identification card or Medic-Alert bracelet stating drugs taken, condition, physician's name and phone number
- To avoid driving, other activities that require alertness
- To avoid alcohol ingestion, CNS depressants; increased sedation may occur
- Not to discontinue medication quickly after long-term use

Evaluate

- Therapeutic response: decreased seizure activity, document on patient's chart
- Mental status
- Allergic reaction: red raised rash, exfoliative dermatitis; if these occur, drug should be discontinued
- Blood dyscrasias: fever, sore throat, bruising, rash, jaundice
- Toxic effects: Bone marrow depression, lupus have been reported

Lab Test Interferences

- Increase: Coomb's test

Treatment of Overdose: Lavage, activated charcoal, monitor electrolyte levels, VS

Administration

Adult and child >6 yr: PO 500 mg/day or 250 mg bid initially; may increase by 250 mg q4-7 days, not to exceed 1.5 g/day

Child 3-6 yr: PO 250 mg/day or 125 mg bid; may increase by 250 mg q4-7 days, not to exceed 1.5g/day; optimal dose 20 mg/kg/day

- Available forms include: Caps 250 mg, syr 250 mg/5ml

Ethotoin*

PEGANONE

(eth′-oh-toyin) (Chapter 7)

Functional classification: Antiepileptic
Chemical classification: Hydantoin derivative
FDA pregnancy category: D

Indications: Generalized tonic-clonic or psychomotor seizures

Contraindications: Hypersensitivity to hydantoins, blood dyscrasias, hematologic disease, **hepatic disease,** lactation
Cautious use: Renal disorders

Pharmacologic Effect: Inhibits spread of seizure activity in motor cortex; therapeutic plasma level 15-50 μg/ml

Pharmacokinetics: Metabolized by liver, excreted in urine, half-life 3-9 hr

Side Effects: *CNS:* Drowsiness, dizziness, insomnia, paresthesias, depression, suicidal tendencies, aggression, headache; *Peripheral:* **Nausea, vomiting, constipation,** anorexia, weight loss, hepatitis, jaundice, nephritis, albuminuria, rash, agranulocytosis, leukopenia, aplastic anemia

Interactions

- Allopurinol, cimetidine, diazepam, disulfiram, alcohol (acute ingestion) phenacemide, succinimides, valproic acid: Increased effect of hydantoins
- Barbiturates, carbamazepine, alcohol (chronic use) theophylline, antacids, dietary calcium: Decreased effects of hydantoins
- Corticosteroids, dicumarol, digitoxin, doxycycline, haloperidol, methadone, oral contraceptives, dopamine, furosemide, levodopa: Decreased effects of these drugs

Implications

Assess

- Blood studies: CBC, platelets q mo until stabilized, discontinue if marked depression of blood cell count occurs

Planning/Implementation

- Describe seizures accurately

*Infrequently used.

E

Teaching

- All aspects of drug administration, i.e., route, action, dose
- To report side effects
- To avoid driving or operating dangerous equipment
- To practice good oral hygiene
- Not to discontinue abruptly
- To wear MedicAlert identification bracelet

Evaluate

- Mental status: mood, sensorium, affect, memory (long-term, short-term)
- Respiratory depression
- Blood dyscrasias: Fever, sore throat, bruising, rash, jaundice

Treatment of Overdose: Mean lethal dose in adults is thought to be 2-5 g; initial symptoms are nystagmus, ataxia; death is due to respiratory and circulatory depression; lavage, emesis, activated charcoal

Administration

Adult: PO 250 mg qid (1000 mg/day) or less initially, may increase over several days to 3 g/day in divided doses; *Child:* PO 250 mg bid, may increase to 250 mg qid (1000 mg/day)

- Available forms: Tabs 250, 500 mg

Fluoxetine

PROZAC

(floo-ox'e-teen) (Chapter 5)

Functional classification: Selective serotonin reuptake inhibitor, antidepressant

FDA pregnancy category: B

Indications: Depression

Contraindications: Hypersensitivity
Cautious use: Anxiety, insomnia, lactation, children, elderly patients, MAOI therapy

Pharmacologic Effects: Inhibits CNS neuron uptake of serotonin, but only slightly inhibits that of norepinephrine

Pharmacokinetics: PO: Peak 6-8 hr; metabolized in liver, excreted in urine; half-life 7-9 days

Side Effects: *CNS:* Anxiety (9.4%), nervousness (14.9%), insomnia (13.8%), drowsiness, headache (20.3%) tremor, dizziness, fatigue; *Peripheral:* Nausea (21.1%), diarrhea (12.3%), dry mouth (9.5%), anorexia (8.7%), dyspepsia, constipation, cramps, vomiting, taste changes, flatulence, sweating (8.4%), rash, pruritus, acne, alopecia, urticaria, infection (7.6%), nasal congestion, hot flashes (1.8%), palpitations, dysmenorrhea (2%), decreased libido, urinary frequency, urinary tract infection, visual changes (2.8%), ear or eye pain, photophobia, tinnitus, asthenia (4.4%), viral infection (3.4%)

Interactions

- Do not use with MAOIs
- L-tryptophan: agitation
- Highly protein bound drugs (i.e., digitoxin): Increased side effects
- Diazepam: Half-life of diazepam increases
- TCAs: Toxic effects of tricyclics increased

Implications

Assess

- Mental status: mood, sensorium, affect, suicidal tendencies, increase in psychiatric symptoms, depression, panic
- B/P (lying, standing), pulse q4h; if systolic B/P drops 20 mm Hg, withhold drug, notify physician; VS q4h in patients with CV disease
- Blood studies: CBC, leukocyte count, differential blood cell count; cardiac enzyme level when patient is receiving long-term therapy
- Hepatic studies: AST, ALT, bilirubin and creatinine levels
- Weight q wk, appetite may increase
- ECG for flattening of T wave, bundle branch or AV block, arrhythmias in cardiac disease

Planning/Implementation

- If constipation, urinary retention occur, increase fluids, bulk in diet
- With food or milk for GI symptoms
- Empty pulvule if patient is unable to swallow medication whole
- Dosage hs if oversedation occurs during day; may take entire dose hs; elderly patients may not tolerate once-per-day dosage
- Sugarless gum, hard candy, frequent sips of water for dry mouth
- Store at room temperature, do not freeze

- Assistance with ambulation during therapy because drowsiness, dizziness occur
- Safety measures, including side rails, primarily with elderly patients
- Check to see that PO medication is swallowed

Teaching
- That therapeutic effect may take several days to weeks
- Use caution when driving or performing other activities requiring alertness because of drowsiness, dizziness, or blurred vision
- Not to discontinue medication suddenly after long-term use, since abrupt discontinuance may cause nausea, headache, malaise
- To avoid ingesting alcohol or other CNS depressants
- To notify physician when pregnant or when planning to become pregnant or to breast feed

Evaluate
- EPSEs, primarily in elderly; rigidity, dystonia, akathisia
- Urinary retention, constipation
- Withdrawal symptoms: Headache, nausea, vomiting, muscle pain, weakness; do not usually occur unless drug is discontinued abruptly
- Alcohol consumption: If alcohol is consumed, withhold dose until morning

Lab Test Interferences
- Increase: Serum bilirubin, blood glucose, alkaline phosphatase levels
- Decrease: VMA, 5-HIAA
- False increase: Urinary catecholamines

Treatment of Overdose: There are no antidotes; establish and maintain airway; ensure adequate oxygenation and ventilation; activated charcoal may be more effective than emesis or lavage

Administration

Adult: PO 20 mg qd in morning; after several weeks, if no clinical improvement is noted, dose may be increased to 20 mg bid in morning, noon, not to exceed 80 mg/day
- Available forms include: Pulvules 20 mg

Fluphenazine Decanoate, Fluphenazine Enanthate, Fluphenazine HCl

MODECATE DECANOATE,† PROLIXIN DECANOATE/MODITEN ENANTHATE,† PROXLIN ENANTHATE/MODITEN HCL,† PERMITIL HCL, PROLIXIN HCL†
(floo-fen′-a-zeen) (Chapter 4)

Functional classifications: Antipsychotic, neuroleptic
Chemical classifications: Phenothiazine, piperazine
FDA pregnancy category: C

Indications: Psychotic disorders, schizophrenia

Contraindications: Hypersensitivity to sesame seeds or fluphenazine, liver damage, CV disease, severe hypertension or hypotension, blood dyscrasias, coma, child <12 yr, brain damage, bone marrow depression, alcohol and barbiturate withdrawal states
Cautious use: Lactation, seizure disorders, hypertension, hepatic disease, cardiac disease, extreme heat

Pharmacologic Effects: Antipsychotic drugs produce a neuroleptic effect characterized by sedation, emotional quieting, psychomotor slowing, and affective indifference; exact mode of action is not fully understood; antipsychotics block dopamine receptors in the basal ganglia, hypothalamus, limbic system, brain stem, and medulla; antipsychotics are also thought to depress certain components of the reticular activating system that partially control body temperature, wakefulness, vasomotor tone, emesis, and hormonal balance; additionally, antipsychotics have significant anticholinergic and alpha-adrenergic blocking effects; therapeutic plasma levels 0.13-2.8 ng/ml

†Available in Canada only.

F

Pharmacokinetics: PO/IM (HCl): Onset 1 hr, peak 2-4 hr, duration 6-8 hr; SC (enanthate): Onset 1-3 days, peak 2-3 days, duration 1-3 wk, half-life 3½-4 days; decanoate: onset 1-3 days, peak 1-2 days, duration over 4 wk, half-life (single dose) 6.8-9.6 days, (multiple dose) 14.3 days; metabolized by liver, excreted in urine (metabolites), crosses placenta, enters breast milk

Side Effects: *CNS:* Parkinsonism, akathisias, dystonias, tardive dyskinesias, oculogyric crisis; neuroleptic malignant syndrome; *Peripheral:* Blurred vision (cycloplegia or paralysis of accommodation); ocular pain, photophobia, mydriasis, impaired vision; intolerance of extreme heat or cold, possible heat stroke or fatal hyperthermia; nasal congestion, wheezing, dyspnea; **hypotension, especially orthostatic,** leading to dizziness, syncope; **tachycardia,** irregular pulse, arrhythmias; **dry mouth, constipation,** jaundice, abdominal pain; urinary retention, urinary hesitancy, galactorrhea, gynecomastia, impaired ejaculation, amenorrhea

Interactions
- Alcohol and other CNS depressants (barbiturates, antihistamines, antianxiety, or antidepressant drugs): Increased CNS depression, increased risk of EPSEs
- Amphetamines: Possible decreased antipsychotic effect
- Antacids (magnesium and aluminum products): Possible decreased antipsychotic effect
- Anticholinergics (atropine, H_1-type antihistamines, antidepressants, etc.): Increased risk of excessive atropine-like side effects or toxic effects
- Anticonvulsants: Increased risk of seizures
- Benztropine: Possible decreased antipsychotic effect, increased risk of severity of peripheral anticholinergic side effects
- Diazoxide: Possible severe hyperglycemia, prediabetic coma
- Guanethidine: Poor control of hypertension by guanethidine
- Hypoglycemia drugs (insulin, oral hypoglycemia agents): Poor diabetic control
- Lithium: Poor control of psychosis with combined therapy, encephalopathy
- Meperidine, morphine: Increased risk of severe CNS depression, respiratory depression, hypotension
- Propranolol: Increased pharmacologic effects of either drug

Implications

Assess
- Establish baseline VS, laboratory values, to assess side effects, allergic or hypersensitivity reactions
- Use test dose SC to check for hypersensitivity
- Physiologic and psychologic status before therapy, to determine needs and evaluate progress
- For early stages of tardive dyskinesia by use of abnormal involuntary movement scale
- Identify concurrent symptoms that may be aggravated by antipsychotics, e.g., glaucoma, diabetes

Planning/Implementation
- Ensure that drug has been taken; check mouth for "cheeking"
- If giving liquid, use water, clear soda, milk, fruit juice; *do not* mix with caffeine, tannics (tea), or pectinates (apple juice); take drug with food to minimize GI upset; give IM injections in lateral thigh
- Keep patient quiet after injection to prevent falls associated with postural hypotension
- For dry mouth, give chewing gum, hard candies, lip balm
- Monitor urinary output; check for bladder distention in inactive patients, older men, and patients on high doses
- Assist with ambulation, if patient is having blurred vision; dim room lights for photosensitivity
- Ensure safety with hypotension; sit on side of bed before rising, head-low position for dizziness, avoid hot showers, wear elastic stockings
- Check B/P (supine, sitting, standing) and pulse before and after each dose when possible; observe for side effects
- Monitor body temperature for indications of neuroleptic malignant syndrome, e.g., muscle rigidity, fever, depressed neurologic status; ensure adequate hydration, nutrition, and ventilation

- Protect patient from exposure to extreme hot or cold
- Recognize impending hypersensitivity: pruritus or jaundice with hepatitis; flu or coldlike symptoms, evidence of bleeding with blood dyscrasia
- Observe for involuntary movements

Teaching

- About benefits and potential harm of antipsychotic drugs; weigh need to know against causing apprehension
- To comply with drug treatment
- To avoid activities requiring clear vision for a few weeks after treatment starts; to report eye pain immediately
- About the importance of exercise, fluids, and fiber in diet
- To watch for symptoms of heart failure: weight gain, dyspnea, distended neck veins, tachycardia
- Possible male sexual performance failure; suggest relaxed, stress-free environment
- To avoid conception; women should practice effective contraception; phenothiazines may cause false-positive result in pregnancy tests
- To avoid exposure to sunlight; keep skin covered but with temperature-appropriate clothing
- That patient cannot become addicted to antipsychotic drugs

Evaluate

- Follows prescribed regimen, takes medications as ordered
- Avoids injury; reports dizziness or need for assistance
- Verbalizes reduced anxiety
- Experiences minimal or no adverse responses
- Uses appropriate interventions to minimize side effects
- Achieves improved mental status

Lab Test Interferences

- Increase: Liver function tests, determinations of cardiac enzymes, cholesterol, blood glucose, prolactin, bilirubin, PBI, cholinesterase, I-131
- Decrease: Hormones (blood and urine)
- False positive: Pregnancy test, PKU
- False negative: Urinary steroids, 17-OHCS

Treatment of Overdose: Lavage; if orally ingested, provide an airway, do not induce vomiting, control EPSEs and hypotension

Administration

- Enanthate, decanoate: *Adult and child >12 yr:* IM or SC 12.5-25 mg q1-3 wk HCl; *Adult:* PO 0.5-10 mg in divided doses q6-8h, typically not to exceed 20 mg qd; *geriatrics:* Start with 1-2.5 mg/day, adjust according to response; IM initially 1.25 mg, then 2.5-10 mg in divided doses q6-8h
- Concentrate *should not* be mixed with caffeine, tannics, or pectinates
- Available forms include: HCl tabs 1, 2.5, 5, 10 mg; elixir 2.5 mg/5 ml; concentrate 5 mg/ml; inj IM, 2.5 mg/ml; enanthate, decanoate, inj SC, IM 25 mg/ml

Flurazepam

DALMANE, SOMNOL†

(flure-az′e-pam) (Chapter 8)

F

Functional classifications: Sedative, hypnotic

Chemical classification: Benzodiazepine derivative

Controlled substance schedule IV

FDA pregnancy category: NR

Indications: Insomnia

Contraindications: Hypersensitivity to benzodiazepines, pregnancy, lactation, intermittent porphyria

Cautious use: Anemia, hepatic disease, renal disease, suicidal patients, drug abuse, elderly patients, child <15 yr, psychosis

Pharmacologic Effects: Produces CNS depression

Pharmacokinetics: PO onset 15-45 min, duration 7-8 hr; active metabolite peak plasma level 1-3 hr; metabolized by liver, excreted by kidneys, crosses placenta, excreted in breast milk; half-life 47-100 hr

Side Effects: *CNS:* Lethargy, drowsiness, daytime sedation, dizziness, confusion, lightheadedness, headache, anxiety, irritability; *Peripheral:* Nausea, vomiting, diar-

†Available in Canada only.

rhea, heartburn, abdominal pain, constipation, chest pain, pulse changes palpitations

Interactions
- Cimetidine, disulfiram: Prolong half-life of flurazepam
- Alcohol, CNS depressants: CNS depression
- Antacids: Decrease effects of flurazepam

Implications
Assess
- Blood studies: Hematocrit, hemoglobin level, RBCs (if on long-term therapy regimen)
- Suicide potential: Use with caution in suicidal patients

Planning/Implementation
- ½-1 hr before bedtime for sleeplessness
- Fast onset on empty stomach, but if GI symptoms occur, may be taken with food
- Assistance with ambulation after receiving dose
- Safety measure: siderails, night light, call bell within easy reach
- Checking to see that PO medication has been swallowed

Teaching
- To avoid driving or other activities requiring alertness until drug regimen is stabilized
- To avoid alcohol ingestion or CNS depressants because serious CNS depression may result
- That may take 2 nights for clinical effect
- Alternate measures to improve sleep: reading, exercise several hours before bedtime, warm bath, warm milk, television, self-hypnosis, deep breathing
- That hangover is common in elderly patients but less common than with barbiturates

Evaluate
- Therapeutic response: Ability to sleep at night, decreased amount of early-morning awakening when taking drug for insomnia
- Mental status: Mood, sensorium, affect, memory (long-term, short-term)
- Blood dyscrasias (rare): Fever, sore throat, bruising, rash, jaundice, epistaxis
- Type of sleep problem: Falling asleep, staying asleep

Lab Test Interferences
- Increase: ALT/AST, serum bilirubin level
- Decrease: RAIU
- False increase: Urinary 17-OHCS

Treatment of Overdose: Lavage, activated charcoal, monitor electrolyte levels, VS

Administration
Adult: PO 15-30 mg hs, may repeat dose once, if needed; *Geriatric:* PO 15 mg hs, may increase, if needed;
- Available forms include: Caps 15, 30 mg

Glutethimide*

DORIDEN
(gloo-teth′i-mide) (Chapter 8)

Functional classifications: Sedative, hypnotic
Chemical classification: Piperidine derivative
Controlled substance schedule III
FDA pregnancy category: C

Indications: Insomnia

Contraindications: Hypersensitivity, porphyria

Pharmacologic Effects: Produces CNS depression

Pharmacokinetics: Is erratically absorbed from GI tract; average half-life 10-12 hr; 50% bound to plasma proteins; conjugant excreted in urine

Side Effects: *CNS:* Hangover (1.1%), drowsiness (1%); *Peripheral:* Skin rash (8.6%), nausea (2.7%), blood dyscrasias are rare

Interactions
- Alcohol and CNS depressants: Additive depressant effect
- Oral anticoagulants: Decreased effect of anticoagulant

Implications
Assess
- Blood studies for rare individual with blood dyscrasias

*Infrequently used.

Planning/Implementation
- Give ½ -1 hr before bedtime
- Maintain safety

Teaching
- To avoid driving
- To avoid alcohol and other CNS depressants
- To taper drug discontinuance, to avoid withdrawal syndrome

Evaluate
- Ability to sleep through night
- Mental status
- Blood dyscrasias (rare)

Lab Test Interference
Interferes with 17-OHCS

Treatment of Overdose: Lethal dose ranges from 10 to 20 g; a low dose of 5 g has killed a patient and a high dose of 35 g has been survived; symptoms same as barbiturate intoxication; maintain airway, monitor VS, gastric lavage (induce emesis only in alert patient); lavage in all cases, regardless of elapsed time, with a 1:1 mixture of castor oil and water; charcoal delays absorption

Administration
- Insomnia: *Adult* PO 250-500 mg hs, may repeat dose if over 4 hr before usual awakening; *do not* exceed 1 g
- Available forms: Tablets 250, 500 mg, caps 500 mg

Halazepam

PAXIPAM
(hal-az′e-pam) (Chapter 6)

Functional classification: Antianxiety
Chemical classification: Benzodiazepine
Controlled substance schedule IV
FDA pregnancy category: D

Indications: Anxiety

Contraindications: Hypersensitivity, psychosis, narrow-angle glaucoma, child <18 yr

Pharmacologic Effects: Depresses CNS, i.e., limbic and reticular formation

Pharmacokinetics: Speed of onset: Intermediate to slow; PO peak level 1-3 hr, duration 3-6 hr, metabolized by liver, excreted by kidneys, crosses placenta and breast milk, half-life 14 hr

Side Effects: *CNS:* See diazepam; *Peripheral:* See diazepam

Interactions: See diazepam

Implications: See diazepam

Lab Test Interference: See diazepam

Treatment of Overdose: See diazepam

Administration
Adult: PO 60-160 mg/day in divided doses; *geriatric:* PO 20 mg qd to bid
- Available forms: Tabs 20, 40 mg

Haloperidol, Haloperidol Decanoate

HALDOL, HALDOL DECANOATE
(ha-loe-per′idole) (Chapter 4)

Functional classifications: Antipsychotic, neuroleptic
Chemical classification: Butyrophenone
FDA pregnancy category: C

Indications: Psychotic disorders, control of tics and vocal utterances in Tourette's syndrome, short-term treatment of hyperactive children showing excessive motor activity, severe behavioral problems in children

Contraindications: Hypersensitivity, blood dyscrasias, coma, child <3 yr, brain damage, bone marrow depression, alcohol and barbiturate withdrawal states, parkinsonism
Cautious use: Lactation, seizure disorders, hypertension, hepatic disease, cardiac disease, breast cancer

Pharmacologic Effects: Antipsychotic drugs produce a neuroleptic effect characterized by sedation, emotional quieting, psychomotor slowing, and affective indifference; exact mode of action is not fully understood; antipsychotics block dopamine receptors in the basal ganglia, hypothalamus, limbic system, brain stem, and medulla; antipsychotics are also thought to depress certain components of the reticular activating system that partially control body temperature, wakefulness, vasomotor tone, emesis, and hormonal balance; additionally, antipsychotics have significant anticholinergic and alpha-adrenergic blocking effects; therapeutic plasma levels 5-20 ng/ml

Pharmacokinetics: PO: Onset erratic, peak 3-5 hr, half-life 24 hr; IM: Onset 15-30 min, peak 15-20 min, half-life 21 hr; IM (decanoate): Peak 4-11 days, half-life 3 wk; metabolized by liver, excreted in urine (40%) and bile (15%), crosses placenta, enters breast milk

Side Effects: *CNS:* **Parkinsonism, akathisias, dystonias,** tardive dyskinesia, oculogyric crisis, neuroleptic malignant syndrome; *Peripheral:* Blurred vision (cycloplegia or paralysis of accommodation), ocular pain, photophobia, mydriasis, impaired vision; intolerance of extreme heat or cold, possible heat stroke or fatal hyperthermia; nasal congestion; wheezing, dyspnea; hypotension, especially orthostatic, leading to dizziness, syncope; **tachycardia,** irregular pulse, arrhythmias; dry mouth, constipation, jaundice, abdominal pain; urinary retention, urinary hesitancy, galactorrhea, gynecomastia, impaired ejaculation, amenorrhea

Interactions

- Alcohol and other CNS depressants (barbiturates, antihistamines, antianxiety, or antidepressant drugs): Increased CNS depression, increased risk of EPSEs
- Amphetamines: Possible decreased antipsychotic effect
- Antacids (magnesium and aluminum products): Possible decreased antipsychotic effect
- Anticholinergics (atropine, H_1-type antihistamines, antidepressants, etc.): Increased risk of excessive atropine-like side effects or toxic effects
- Benztropine: Possible decreased antipsychotic effect, increased risk of severity of peripheral anticholinergic side effects
- Diazoxide: Possible severe hyperglycemia, prediabetic coma
- Fluoxetine: EPSEs
- Guanethidine: poor control of hypertension by guanethidine
- Hypoglycemia drugs (insulin, oral hypoglycemia agents): Poor diabetic control
- Lithium: Disorientation, unconsciousness, EPSEs, and potentially neurotoxic effects
- Meperidine, morphine: Increased risk of severe CNS depression, respiratory depression, hypotension
- Propranolol: Increased pharmacologic effects of either drug

Implications

Assess

- Establish baseline VS, laboratory values, to assess side effects, allergic or hypersensitivity reactions
- Physiologic and psychologic status before therapy, to determine needs and evaluate progress
- For early stages of tardive dyskinesia—use abnormal involuntary movement scale
- Identify concurrent symptoms that may be aggravated by antipsychotics, e.g., glaucoma, diabetes

Planning/Implementation

- Ensure that drug has been taken; check mouth for "cheeking"
- If giving liquid haloperidol, use at least 60 ml of compatible beverage to mask taste; dilute and give immediately; take drug with food to minimize GI upset; give IM injections in lateral thigh
- Keep patient quiet after injection to prevent falls associated with postural hypotension
- For dry mouth, give chewing gum, hard candies, lip balm; monitor urinary output; check for bladder distention in inactive patients, older men, and patients on high doses
- Assist with ambulation, if patient is having blurred vision; dim room lights for photosensitivity
- Ensure safety with hypotension; sit on side of bed before rising, head-low position for dizziness, avoid hot showers, wear elastic stockings
- Check B/P (supine, sitting, standing) and pulse before and after each dose when possible; observe for side effects
- Monitor body temperature for indications of neuroleptic malignant syndrome, e.g., muscle rigidity, fever, depressed neurologic status; ensure adequate hydration, nutrition, and ventilation
- Protect patient from exposure to extreme hot or cold

- Recognize impending hypersensitivity, i.e., to pruritus or jaundice with hepatitis; flu or coldlike symptoms, evidence of bleeding with blood dyscrasia
- Observe for involuntary movements

Teaching

- About benefits and potential harm of antipsychotic drugs; weigh need to know against causing apprehension
- To comply with drug treatment
- To avoid activities requiring clear vision for a few weeks after treatment starts; to report eye pain immediately
- About importance of exercise, fluids, and fiber in diet
- To watch for symptoms of heart failure: weigh gain, dyspnea, distended neck veins, tachycardia
- Possible male sexual performance failure; suggest relaxed, stress-free environment
- To avoid conception; women should practice effective contraception
- To avoid exposure to sunlight; keep skin covered but with temperature-appropriate clothing
- That patient cannot become addicted to antipsychotic drugs

Evaluate

- Follows prescribed regimen, takes medications as ordered
- Avoids injury; reports dizziness or need for assistance
- Verbalizes reduced anxiety
- Experiences minimal or no adverse responses
- Uses appropriate interventions to minimize side effects
- Achieves improved mental status.

Lab Test Interferences
Increase: Liver function test, determinations of cardiac enzymes, cholesterol, blood glucose, prolactin, bilirubin, PBI, cholinesterase, I-131
Decrease: Hormones (blood urine)
False positive: Pregnancy tests, PKU
False negative: Urinary steroids

Treatment of Overdose: Lavage; if orally ingested, provide an airway; do not induce vomiting

Administration

- Psychosis; *Adult:* PO 0.5-5 mg bid or tid initially depending on severity of condition; dose is increased to desired dose, max 100 mg/day; IM 2-5 mg q1-8h; *child 3-12 yr:* PO/IM 0.05-0.15 mg/kg/day; decanoate: Initial dose IM is 10-15 times the daily oral dose at 4-wk interval; do not administer IV
- Tourette's disorder: *Adult:* PO 0.5-5 mg bid or tid, increased until desired response occurs; *child 3-12 yr:* PO 0.05-0.075 mg/kg/day
- Hyperactive children: *child 3-12 yr:* PO 0.05-0.075 mg/kg/day
- Available forms include: Tabs 0.5, 1, 2, 5, 10, 20 mg; conc 2 mg/ml; inj IM 5 mg/ml; decanoate IM 50, 100 mg/ml

Hydroxyzine*

ATARAX QUIESS, VISTARIL/ VISTARIL IM
(hye-drox'-i-zeen) (Chapter 6)

Functional classification: Antianxiety
Chemical classification: Piperazine
FDA pregnancy category: C

Indications: Anxiety, often used preoperatively to prevent nausea; IM form for hysterical patients

Contraindications: Hypersensitivity, early pregnancy

Pharmacologic Effects: Depresses subcortical CNS, i.e., limbic and reticular areas

Pharmacokinetics: Rapidly absorbed from gut; clinical effect in 15-30 min; half-life 3 hr. but longer in elderly patients; metabolized by liver

Side Effects: *CNS:* Drowsiness (transient); rarely reported: tremor and seizures; *Peripheral:* Dry mouth; respiratory problems have occurred

Interactions

- CNS depressants: Additive effect
- Phenothiazines: Decreased antipsychotic effect

Implications

Assess

- B/P

*Infrequently used.

Planning/Implementation
- Give with food or milk
- Assist with ambulation
- Maintain safety

Teaching
- To take hard candies, gum, etc. for dry mouth
- To avoid alcohol, CNS depressants
- To avoid driving

Evaluate
- Mental status

Lab Test Interference
False increase: 17-OHCS

Treatment of Overdose: Oversedation most common problem; induce vomiting, gastric lavage; if hypotension occurs, give IV fluids and norepinephrine (do not use epinephrine)

Administration
- Anxiety: *Adult:* PO 50-100 mg qid; *child >6 yr:* 50-100 mg/day in divided doses; *child <6 yr:* 50 mg/day in divided doses
- Available forms: Tabs 10, 25, 50, 100 mg; caps 25, 50, 100 mg; syr 10 mg/5 ml; oral suspension 25 mg/5 ml; IM inj 25, 50 mg/ml

Imipramine HCl

JANIMINE, NOVOPRAMINE,† TOFRANIL
(im-ip′ra-meen) (Chapter 5)

Functional classification: TCA
Chemical classifications: Dibenzazepine, tertiary amine
FDA pregnancy category: C

Indications: Depression, enuresis in children
Unlabeled use: Panic disorder

Contraindications: Hypersensitivity to TCAs, recovery phase of myocardial infarction; *Cautious use:* Suicidal patients, severe depression, increased intraocular pressure, narrow-angle glaucoma, urinary retention, cardiac disease, hepatic disease, hyperthyroidism, ECT, elective surgery, elderly patients, MAOI therapy, convulsive disorders, prostatic hypertrophy

†Available in Canada only.

Pharmacologic Effects: Blocks reuptake of norepinephrine, serotonin into nerve endings, increasing action of norepinephrine, serotonin in nerve cells; also r/t changes in receptor sensitivity; therapeutic plasma levels 200-350 ng/ml

Pharmacokinetics: PO: Steady state 2-5 days, metabolized by liver, excreted by kidneys and feces, crosses placenta, excreted in breast milk, half-life 11-25 hr; desipramine is a metabolite

Side Effects: *CNS:* **Sedation,** ataxia, confusion, delirium; *Peripheral:* **Blurred vision,** photophobia, increased intraocular pressure, decreased tearing, orthostatic hypotension, arrhythmias, tachycardia, palpitations, dry mouth, constipation, diarrhea, decreased sweating, **urinary retention, hesitancy**

Interactions
- Anticholinergic agents: Additive anticholinergic effects with atropine, antihistamines (H_1 blocker), antiparkinson drugs, antipsychotics, OTC cold and allergy drugs
- CNS depressants: Additive depressant effect
- Guanethidine, clonidine: Decreased antihypertensive effect
- MAOIs: Hypertensive crisis, atropine-like poisoning
- Oral contraceptives: Inhibit effects of TCAs
- Haloperidol: May increase TCA serum level
- Quinidine: Additive effect, heart block possible
- Sympathomimetics: Potentiates sympathomimetic effects
- Thyroid preparations: Tachycardia, arrhythmias; may increase TCA effect

Implications

Assess
- Establish baseline data to aid recognition of adverse responses to medication, e.g., liver enzyme levels, VS, renal function, mental status, speech patterns, affect, weight
- For signs of noncompliance, e.g., poor therapeutic response
- For major symptoms of depression: apathy, sadness, sleep disturbances, hopelessness, guilt, decreased libido, spontaneous crying

- Review history for contraindicated conditions, e.g., glaucoma, CV disease, GI conditions, urologic conditions, seizures, pregnancy

Planning/Implementation

- Monitor for "cheeking" or hoarding; check drug dosage carefully, since a small overdose may cause toxic effects
- Monitor for suicidal ideations; suicidal thought content may increase as antidepressants begin to "energize" patient
- Monitor vital signs; if hypotension tachycardia or arrhythmias occur, withhold TCAs
- Give most TCAs in a single dose hs
- Observe for early signs of toxic effects, e.g., drowsiness, tachycardia, mydriasis, hypotension, agitation, vomiting, confusion, fever, restlessness, sweating
- If CNS overstimulation occurs, e.g., hypomania, delirium, discontinue drug

Teaching

- That these drugs have a lag time of up to 1 month
- To adhere to drug regimen
- To avoid OTC drugs, particularly those containing sympathomimetics or anticholinergics
- To avoid drugs listed in section on interactions
- About ways to deal with minor side effects, as follows: dry mouth, with sugarless hard candies, sips of water, mouth rinse; visual disturbances, with artificial tears, sunglasses, assistance with ambulation; constipation, with bulk-forming foods, increased fluids; urinary hesitancy, with adequate fluids, privacy; decreased perspiration; with appropriate clothing, avoidance of unnecessary exercise; orthostatic hypotension, with slow positional changes, avoid hot baths and showers; for drowsiness, take single dose hs with physician approval, avoid driving
- That abrupt discontinuance may result in cholinergic rebound, e.g., nausea, vomiting, insomnia, headache

Evaluate

- Desired therapeutic serum level
- Verbalize decrease in subjective symptoms
- Observe decrease in objective symptoms
- Minimal to no adverse drug effects
- Stable VS
- Less anxiety; sleep, talk, and feel better

Lab Test Interferences

Increase: Serum bilirubin, alkaline phosphatase, blood glucose levels

Decrease: 5-HIAA, VMA, urinary catecholamines

Treatment of Overdose: ECG monitoring, induce emesis, lavage, activated charcoal, administer anticonvulsant, if needed; treat anticholinergic effects

Administration

- Depression: *Adult:* PO/IM 75-100 mg/day in divided doses, may gradually increase to 200 mg, not to exceed 300 mg/day; may give daily dose hs; *child:* 1.5 mg/kg/day in three divided doses to start; may increase by 1-1.5 mg/kg/day q 3-5 days; maximum dose 5 mg/kg/day; *adolescent and geriatric:* 10 mg tid-qid, typically not necessary to exceed 100 mg/day
- Enuresis: *Child 6-12 yr:* 25 mg/day 1 hr before bedtime; if no improvement in 1 week, may increase to 50 mg/night; *adolescent:* may give up to 75 mg/night
- Available forms: Tabs 10, 25, 50, mg; inj IM 25 mg/2 ml; Pamoate salt (slow-release capsules) 75, 100, 125, 150 mg

Isocarboxazid

MARPLAN

(eye-soe-kar-box'a-zid) (Chapter 5)

Functional classifications: Antidepressant, MAOI

Chemical classification: Hydrazine

FDA pregnancy category: C

Indications: Depression in patients refractory to TCAs and ECT

Contraindications: Hypersensitivity to MAOIs, elderly patients (>60 yr), children <16 yr, hypertension, CHF, severe hepatic disease, pheochromocytoma, severe renal disease, severe cardiac disease, paranoid schizophrenia

Cautious use: Suicidal patients, convulsive disorders, schizophrenia, hyperactivity, diabetes mellitus, hypomania, agitation, hyperthyroidism, lactation

Pharmacologic Effect: Inhibits monoamine oxidase, thus increasing the concentration of endogenous epinephrine, norepinephrine, serotonin, dopamine in storage sites in CNS

Pharmacokinetics: PO: Metabolized by liver, excreted in kidneys, half-life not established

Side Effects: *CNS:* Dizziness, drowsiness, confusion, **headache,** anxiety, **tremors,** stimulation, weakness, **hyperreflexia,** mania, **insomnia, fatigue,** weight gain; *Peripheral:* Change in libido; **constipation, dry mouth,** nausea and vomiting, **anorexia,** diarrhea, rash, flushing, increased perspiration, jaundice, **orthostatic hypotension, hypertension, dysrhythmias,** hypertensive crisis, **blurred vision**

Interactions
- Drug-drug: *Sympathomimetics (indirect or mixed acting)*: Severe headache, hypertension, hyperpyrexia, and hypertensive crisis; sympathomimetic drugs include amphetamines, levodopa, tryptophan, methylphenidate, OTC compounds containing phenylpropanolamine, ephedrine, and pseudoephedrine, TCAs, other MAOIs, guanethidine, methyldopa, guanadrel, reserpine; *Anticholingeric drugs*: Additive effect; *Antihypertensives (diuretics, beta blockers, hydralazine, nitroglycerin, prazosin)*: Hypotension
- Drug-food: *Tyramine-rich foods* (see text): Hypertensive crisis

Implications
Assess
- B/P (lying, standing), pulse; if systolic B/P drops 20 mm Hg, withhold drug, notify physician
- Blood studies: CBC, leukocyte count, cardiac enzyme levels (if patient is receiving long-term therapy)
- Hepatic studies: Hepatotoxicity may occur

Planning/Implementation
- Increased fluids, bulk in diet when constipation, urinary retention occur
- With food or milk for GI symptoms
- Gum, hard candy, or frequent sips of water for dry mouth
- Phentolamine for severe hypertension
- Storage in tight container in cool environment
- Assistance with ambulation during beginning of therapy because drowsiness or dizziness occurs
- Safety measures, including use of side rails
- Checking to see that PO medication is swallowed

Teaching
- That therapeutic effects may take 1-4 wk
- To avoid driving or other activities that require alertness
- To avoid ingesting alcohol, CNS depressants, or OTC medications for cold, weight control, hay fever; to avoid cough syrups
- Not to discontinue medication quickly after long-term use
- To avoid high-tyramine foods, e.g., cheese (aged), caviar, dried fish, game meat, beer, wine, pickled products, liver, raisins, bananas, figs, avocados, meat tenderizers, chocolate, yogurt, increased caffeine, soy sauce
- Report headache, palpitations, neck stiffness

Evaluate
- Toxic effects: Increased headache, palpitation; discontinue drug immediately
- Mental status
- Urinary retention, constipation
- Withdrawal symptoms: Headache, nausea, vomiting, muscle pain, weakness

Treatment of Overdose: Lavage, activated charcoal, monitor electrolyte levels, VS, treat hypotension

Administration
Adult: PO 30 mg/day in divided doses, reduce to maintenance dose of 10-20 mg/day, if feasible
- Available forms include: Tabs 10 mg

Lithium Carbonate

CIBALITH-S, LITHANE, ESKALITH, LITHONATE, LITHOTABS, LITHOBID, LITHIUM CITRATE, LITHONATE-S
(li'thee-um) (Chapter 5)

Functional classification: Antimanic
Chemical classification: Alkali metal ion salt
FDA pregnancy category: D

Indications: Manic-depressive illness (manic phase), prevention of bipolar manic depressive psychosis

Contraindications: Children <12 yr, hepatic disease, renal disease, brain trauma, lactation, schizophrenia, severe cardiac disease, severe dehydration, organic mental syndrome, sodium depletion
Cautious use: Concomitant neuroleptic therapy, elderly patients, hypothyroidism, seizure disorders, diabetes mellitus, systemic infection, urinary retention

Pharmacologic Effects: Alters sodium ion transport in nerve, muscle cells; effects norepinephrine reuptake and increases serotonin receptor sensitivity

Pharmacokinetics: PO: Onset rapid, peak 1-4 hr, half-life 17-36 hr, depending on age; crosses blood-brain barrier, excreted in urine, crosses placenta, enters breast milk, well absorbed by oral method; sodium loading increases lithium excretion

Side Effects: *CNS:* Headache, drowsiness, dizziness, tremors, twitching, ataxia, seizure, slurred speech, restlessness, confusion, stupor, memory loss, clonic movements; *Peripheral:* Dry mouth, anorexia, nausea, vomiting, diarrhea, hypotension, leukocytosis, blurred vision, hypothyroidism, hyponatremia, muscle weakness

Interactions
- Haloperidol: Encephalopathy
- Neuromuscular blocking agents, phenothiazines: Increased effects of these drugs
- Sodium bicarbonate, acetazolamide, mannitol, aminophylline: Increased renal clearance
- Indomethacin, thiazide diuretics, NSAIs: Increased toxic effects
- Theophyllines, urinary alkalinizers: Decreased effects of lithium
- Carbamazepine: Neurotoxic effects
- Captopril, lisinopril (ACE inhibitors): Reported to produce a three- to four-fold increase in serum lithium levels (a potentially fatal combination)

Implications
Assess
- Initiate serum creatinine and thyroid function studies before starting lithium regimen
- Weight daily, check for edema in legs, ankles, wrists, if present, report
- Sodium intake; decreased sodium intake with decreased fluid intake may lead to lithium retention; increased sodium and fluids may decrease lithium retention
- Skin turgor at least daily
- Urine for albuminuria, glycosuria, uric acid during beginning of treatment, q 2 mo thereafter
- Neurologic status: Gait, motor reflexes, hand tremors
- Serum lithium levels weekly initially, then obtain lithium levels 8-12 hr after previous dose (therapeutic serum level 0.6-1.2 mEq/L)

Planning/Implementation
- With meals to avoid GI upset
- Adequate fluids (2-3 L/day) to prevent dehydration during initial treatment, 1-2 L/day during maintenance

Teaching
- Symptoms of minor toxic effects, i.e., vomiting, diarrhea, poor coordination, fine motor tremors, weakness, lassitude; major toxic effects, i.e., coarse tremors, severe thirst, tinnitus, dilute urine
- Action, dosage, side effects; when to notify physician
- To monitor urine specific gravity
- That contraception is necessary because lithium may harm fetus
- Not to operate machinery until lithium serum levels are stable

Evaluate
- Reduction in manic symptoms
- Patient verbalizes understanding of side effects, symptoms of toxic effects, and need for compliance

Lab Test Interferences
Increase: Potassium excretion, urine glucose, blood glucose, protein, BUN levels
Decrease: VMA, T_3, T_4, PBI, I-131

Treatment of Overdose: Lavage, maintain airway, respiratory function; dialysis for severe intoxication

- Lithium levels <2 mEq/L: Diarrhea, vomiting, nausea, drowsiness, weakness
- Lithium levels 2 to 3 mEq/L: Giddiness, ataxia, blurred vision, tinnitus, slurred speech, blackouts, fasciculations, incontinence
- Lithium levels >3 mEq/L: Multiple organs and organ systems failure, seizures, vascular collapse, coma

Administration
Adult: PO 600 mg tid, maintenance 300 mg tid or qid; slow rel tabs 450 mg bid, dose should be individualized to maintain blood levels at 0.5-1.5 mEq/L; maintenance serum concentrations are 0.6-1.2 mEq/L

- Available forms include: Caps 150, 300, 600 mg; tabs 300 mg; tabs slow rel 300, 450 mg; syrup 8 mEq/5 ml (as citrate)

Lorazepam

ATIVAN
(lor-a′-ze-pam) (Chapter 6)

Functional classification: Antianxiety
Chemical classification: Benzodiazepine
Controlled substance schedule IV
FDA pregnancy category: D

Indications: Anxiety

Contraindications: Hypersensitivity to benzodiazepines, narrow-angle glaucoma, psychosis, child <18 yr (inj), child 12 yr (oral)
Cautious use: Elderly or debilitated patients, hepatic disease, renal disease

Pharmacologic Effects: Apparently potentiates effects of GABA and other inhibitory transmitters by binding to specific benzodiazepine receptor sites; depresses subcortical levels of CNS, including limbic system and reticular formation

Pharmacokinetics: Speed of onset: Intermediate
PO peak 1-6 hr, duration 3-6 hr, metabolized by liver, excreted by kidneys, crosses placenta, enters breast milk, half-life 10-20 hr

Side Effects: *CNS:* **Drowsiness, dizziness,** confusion, headache, anxiety, tremor, stimulation, fatigue, depression, insomnia; *Peripheral:* Photophobia due to mydriasis, **blurred vision** due to cycloplegia; sleeplike slowing of respirations with therapeutic doses, cough; **orthostatic hypotension, tachycardia,** hypotension; constipation, dry mouth

Interactions

- Alcohol and other CNS depressants: Increased risk of excessive CNS depression
- Cimetidine: Potentiation of CNS depression
- Digoxin: Increased risk of cardiac side effects from digoxin
- Levodopa: Decreased antiparkinson effect
- Phenytoin: Increased phenytoin serum levels

Implications
Assess

- Patient's level of anxiety and method of coping
- B/P, VS
- Establish baseline physical assessment data before medications are started

Planning/Implementation

- Monitor patient's response to medication
- Observe elderly, very young, and debilitated patients for paradoxic excitement
- Reduce dose of other depressant drugs
- Observe for signs of withdrawal when discontinuing antianxiety agent

Teaching

- To avoid operating dangerous machinery and performing other tasks requiring good reflexes
- To report ocular pain at once, as well as other visual disturbances
- Drug may be taken with food

Evaluate

- Whether patient achieves lower levels of anxiety without undue sedations
- Whether patient can follow prescribed regimen
- For physical dependence: withdrawal symptoms of headache, nausea, vomiting, muscle pain, weakness after long-term use

Lab Test Interferences
Increase: AST, ALT, serum bilirubin level
Decrease: RAIU
False increase: 17-OHCS

Treatment of Overdose: Lavage, VS, supportive care; there have been few deaths, if any, from benzodiazepine overdose alone; deaths occur when benzodiazepines are mixed with other drugs

Administration

- Anxiety: *Adult:* PO 2-6 mg/day in divided doses, not to exceed 10 mg/day; take largest dose before bedtime; *geriatric:* Initially 1-2 mg/day in divided doses, adjust as needed or tolerated
- Insomnia: *Adult:* PO 2-4 mg hs
- IM: 0.05 mg/kg up to a maximum of 4 mg
- IV: Initially 2 mg or 0.044 mg/kg, whichever is smaller, not to exceed 2 mg/min
- Available forms include: Tabs 0.5, 1, 2 mg; IM/IV inj 2-4 mg/ml: must refrigerate

Loxapine Succinate/ Loxapine HCl

LOXAPAX,† LOXITANE, LOXITANE-C
(lox-a'peen) (Chapter 4)

Functional classifications: Antipsychotic, neuroleptic
Chemical classification: Dibenzoxazepine
FDA pregnancy category: C

Indications: Psychotic disorders

Contraindications: Hypersensitivity, blood dyscrasias, coma, child <16 yr, brain damage, bone marrow depression, alcohol and barbiturate withdrawal states
Cautious use: Lactation, seizure disorders, hypertension, hepatic disease, cardiac disease, glaucoma, urinary retention

Pharmacologic Effects: Antipsychotic drugs produce a neuroleptic effect characterized by sedation, emotional quieting, psychomotor slowing, and affective indifference; exact mode of action is not fully understood; antipsychotics block dopamine receptors in the basal ganglia, hypothalamus, limbic system, brain stem, and medulla; antipsychotics are also thought to depress certain components of the reticular activating system, which partially controls body temperature, wakefulness, vasomotor tone, emesis, and hormonal balance; additionally, antipsychotics have significant anticholinergic and alpha-adrenergic blocking effects

Pharmacokinetics: PO: Onset 20-30 min, peak 2-4 hr, duration 12 hr; IM: Onset 15-30 min, peak 15-20 min, duration 12 hr; metabolized by liver, excreted in urine, crosses placenta, enters breast milk, initial half-life 5 hr, terminal half-life 19 hr

Side Effects: *CNS:* Parkinsonism, akathisias, dystonias, tardive dyskinesia, oculogyric crisis; *Peripheral:* Blurred vision (cycloplegia or paralysis of accommodation); ocular pain, photophobia, mydriasis, impaired vision; intolerance of extreme heat or cold, possible heat stroke or fatal hyperthermia; nasal congestion, wheezing, dyspnea; **hypotension, especially orthostatic,** leading to dizziness, syncope; **tachycardia,** irregular pulse, arrhythmias; **dry mouth, constipation,** jaundice, abdominal pain; urinary retention, urinary hesitancy, galactorrhea, gynecomastia, impaired ejaculation, amenorrhea

Interactions

- Alcohol and other CNS depressants (barbiturates, antihistamines, antianxiety or antidepressant drugs): Increased CNS depression; increased risk of EPSEs
- Amphetamines: Possible decreased antipsychotic effect
- Antacids (magnesium and aluminum products): Possible decreased antipsychotic effect
- Anticholinergics (atropine, H_1-type antihistamines, antidepressants, etc.): Increased risk of excessive atropine-like side effects or toxic effects
- Benztropine: Possible decreased antipsychotic effect, increased risk of severity of peripheral anticholinergic side effects
- Diazoxide: Possible severe hyperglycemia, prediabetic coma
- Guanethidine: Poor control of hypertension by guanethidine

†Available in Canada only.

K L

- Hypoglycemia drugs (insulin, oral hypoglycemia agents): Poor diabetic control
- Lithium: Poor control of psychosis with combined therapy; can mask lithium toxic effects; neurotoxic effects with confusion, delirium, seizures, encephalopathy
- Meperidine, morphine: Increased risk of severe CNS depression, respiratory depression, hypotension
- Propranolol: Increased pharmacologic effects of either drug

Implications

Assess

- Establish baseline VS, laboratory values to assess side effects, allergic or hypersensitivity reactions
- Physiologic and psychologic status before therapy, to determine needs and evaluate progress
- For early stages of tardive dyskinesia—use abnormal involuntary movement scale
- Identify concurrent symptoms that may be aggravated by antipsychotics, e.g., glaucoma, diabetes

Planning/Implementation

- Ensure that drug has been taken; check mouth for "cheeking"
- If giving liquid antipsychotics, use at least 60 ml of compatible beverage to mask taste; dilute and give immediately; take drug with food to minimize GI upset; give IM injections in lateral thigh
- Keep patient quiet after injection, to prevent falls associated with postural hypotension
- For dry mouth, give chewing gum, hard candies, lip balm
- Monitor urinary output; check for bladder distention in inactive patients, older men, and patients on high doses
- Assist with ambulation, if patient is having blurred vision; dim room lights for photosensitivity
- Ensure safety with hypotension; sit on side of bed before rising, head-low position for dizziness, avoid hot showers, wear elastic stockings
- Check B/P (supine, sitting, standing) and pulse before and after each dose when possible; observe for side effects
- Monitor body temperature for indications of neuroleptic malignant syndrome, e.g., muscle rigidity, fever, depressed neurologic status; ensure adequate hydration, nutrition, and ventilation
- Protect patient from exposure to extreme hot or cold
- Recognize impending hypersensitivity: pruritus or jaundice with hepatitis; flu or coldlike symptoms, evidence of bleeding with blood dyscrasia
- Observe for involuntary movements

Teaching

- About benefits and potential harm of antipsychotic drugs; weigh need to know against causing apprehension
- To comply with drug treatment
- To avoid activities requiring clear vision for a few weeks after treatment starts; to report eye pain immediately
- About the importance of exercise, fluids, and fiber in diet
- To watch for symptoms of heart failure, i.e., weight gain, dyspnea, distended neck veins, tachycardia
- Possible male sexual performance failure; suggest relaxed, stress-free environment
- To avoid conception; women should practice effective contraception
- To avoid exposure to sunlight; keep skin covered but with temperature-appropriate clothing
- That patient cannot become addicted to antipsychotic drugs

Evaluate

- Follows prescribed regimen, takes medications as ordered
- Avoids injury; reports dizziness or need for assistance
- Verbalizes reduced anxiety
- Experiences minimal or no adverse responses
- Uses appropriate interventions to minimize side effects
- Achieves improved mental status

Treatment of Overdose: Lavage, if orally ingested; provide an airway; do not induce vomiting

Administration

Adult >15 yr: PO 10 mg bid initially, may be rapidly increased depending on severity of condition, maintenance 20-60 mg/day; IM 12.5-50 mg q4-6h or more until desired response, then start PO form

- Mix concentrate in orange or grapefruit juice
- Available forms: Caps 5, 10, 25, 50 mg; conc 25 mg/ml; inj IM 50 mg/ml

Maprotiline HCl

LUDIOMIL

(ma-proe′ti-leen) (Chapter 5)

Functional classification: Antidepressant
Chemical classification: Tetracyclic
FDA pregnancy category: B

Indications: Depression, dysthymic disorder, bipolar–depressed, anxiety associated with depression

Contraindications: Hypersensitivity to TCAs, CV disease, convulsive disorders
Cautious use: Suicidal patients, severe depression, increased intraocular pressure, narrow-angle glaucoma, urinary retention, cardiac disease, hepatic disease, hypothyroidism, hyperthyroidism, ECT, elective surgery, elderly patients, lactation, child <18 yr, prostatic hypertrophy

Pharmacologic Effect: Blocks reuptake of norepinephrine, serotonin into nerve endings, increasing action of norepinephrine, serotonin in nerve cells; also r/t receptor sensitivity; therapeutic plasma levels 200-300 ng/ml

Pharmacokinetics: PO: Onset 15-30 min, peak 12 hr, duration up to 3 wk, steady state 6-10 days; metabolized by liver, excreted by kidneys and feces; crosses placenta, half-life 21-25 hr

Side Effects: *CNS:* **Sedation,** ataxia; confusion, delirium; *Peripheral:* **Blurred vision,** photophobia, increased intraocular pressure; decreased tearing, orthostatic hypotension; arrhythmias, tachycardia, palpitations, dry mouth, constipation, diarrhea, decreased sweating, **urinary retention, hesitancy**

Interactions

- Anticholinergic agents: Additive anticholinergic effects with atropine, antihistamines (H_1 blocker), antiparkinson drugs, antipsychotics, OTC cold and allergy drugs
- CNS depressants: Additive depressant effect
- Guanethidine, clonidine: Decreased antihypertensive effect
- MAOIs: Hypertensive crisis, atropine-like poisoning
- Oral contraceptives: Inhibit metabolism of TCAs
- Phenothiazines: May increase tricyclic serum level
- Quinidine: Additive effect, heart block possible
- Sympathomimetics: Potentiate sympathomimetic effects
- Thyroid preparations: Tachycardia, arrhythmias; may increase TCA effect

Implications

Assess

- Establish baseline data to aid recognition of adverse responses to medication, e.g., liver enzyme levels, VS, renal function, mental status, speech patterns, affect, weight
- For signs of noncompliance, e.g., poor therapeutic response
- Observe for major symptoms of depression, i.e., apathy, sadness, sleep disturbances, hopelessness, guilt, decreased libido, spontaneous crying
- Review history for contraindicated conditions, e.g., glaucoma, CV disease, GI conditions, urologic conditions, seizures, pregnancy

Planning/Implementation

- Monitor for "cheeking" or hoarding; check drug dosage carefully, since a small overdose may cause toxic effects
- Monitor for suicidal ideations; suicidal thought content may increase as antidepressants begin to "energize" patient
- Monitor VS; if hypotension, tachycardia, or arrhythmias occur, withhold TCAs
- Give most TCAs in a single dose hs
- Observe for early signs of toxic effects, e.g., drowsiness, tachycardia, mydriasis, hypotension, agitation, vomiting, confusion, fever, restlessness, sweating
- If CNS overstimulation occurs, e.g., hypomania, delirium, discontinue drug

Teaching

- Maprotiline may produce clinical effects faster than TCAs do, sometimes within 3 to 7 days; however, a lag time of 2 to 3 weeks occurs in many patients
- To adhere to drug regimen

- To avoid OTC drugs, particularly those containing sympathomimetics or anticholinergics
- To avoid drugs listed in section on interactions
- About ways to deal with minor side effects, as follows: dry mouth, with hard candies, sips of water, mouth rinse; visual disturbances, with artificial tears, sunglasses, assistance with ambulation; constipation, with bulk-forming foods, increased fluids; urinary hesitancy, with adequate fluids, privacy; decreased perspiration, with appropriate clothing, avoidance of unnecessary exercise; orthostatic hypotension, with slow positional changes, avoidance of hot baths and showers; for drowsiness, take single dose hs with physician approval, avoid driving
- That abrupt discontinuance may result in cholinergic rebound, e.g., nausea, vomiting, insomnia, headache

Evaluate
- Desired therapeutic serum level
- Verbalize decrease in subjective symptoms
- Observe decrease in objective symptoms
- Minimal to no adverse drug effects
- Stable VS
- Less anxiety; sleep, talk, and feel better

Lab Test Interferences
- Increase: Serum bilirubin, blood glucose, alkaline phosphatase levels
- False increase: Urinary cathecholamines
- Decrease: VMA, 5-HIAA

Treatment of Overdose: ECG, monitoring, induce emesis, lavage, activated charcoal, rapid digitalization for CV failure, reduce tendency for convulsions, control hyperexia

Administration

Adult: PO 75 mg/day in moderate depression, may increase to 150 mg/day; not to exceed 225 mg in hospitalized patients; severely depressed patients who are hospitalized may be given 300 mg/day; *geriatrics:* 50-75 mg/day

- Available forms include: Tabs 25, 50, 75 mg

Mephenytoin*

MESANTOIN
(me-fen′i-toyn) (Chapter 7)

Functional classification: Antiepileptic
Chemical classification: Hydantoin derivative
FDA pregnancy category: C

Indications: Generalized tonic-clonic, psychomotor, focal seizures refractory to other agents

Contraindications: Hypersensitivity to hydantoins, sinus bradycardia, heart block, Adams-Stokes syndrome

Cautious use: Alcoholism, hepatic disease, renal disease, blood dyscrasias, CHF, elderly patients, respiratory depression, diabetes mellitus, lactation

Pharmacologic Effects: Inhibits spread of seizure activity in motor cortex

Pharmacokinetics: PO: Onset 30 min, duration 24-48 hr, metabolized by liver, excreted by kidneys, half-life unknown

Side Effects: *CNS:* Drowsiness, dizziness, insomnia, paresthesias, depression, suicidal tendencies, aggression, headache; *Peripheral:* **Nausea, vomiting, constipation,** anorexia, weight loss, hepatitis, jaundice, nephritis, albuminuria, rash, agranulocytosis, leukopenia, aplastic anemia

Interactions
- Allopurinol, cimetidine, diazepam, disulfiram, alcohol (acute ingestion) phenacemide, succinimides, valproic acid: Increased effect of hydantoins
- Barbiturates, carbamazepine, alcohol (chronic use) theophylline, antacids, dietary calcium: Decreased effects of hydantoins
- Corticosteroids, dicumarol, digitoxin, doxycycline, haloperidol, methadone, oral contraceptives, dopamine, furosemide, levodopa: Decreased effects of these drugs

Implications

Assess
- Blood studies: CBC, platelet count q2 wk until stabilized, then q mo for 12

*Infrequently used.

mo, then q 3 mo; if neutrophils are <1600 cells/mm^3 discontinue drug

Planning/Implementation

- Describe seizures accurately

Teaching

- All aspects of drug administration: route, action, dose
- To report side effects
- To avoid driving or operating dangerous equipment
- To practice good oral hygiene
- Not to discontinue abruptly
- To wear MedicAlert identification bracelet

Evaluate

- Mental status: Mood, sensorium, affect, memory (long-term, short-term)
- Respiratory depression
- Blood dyscrasias: Fever, sore throat, bruising, rash, jaundice
- Dilute with normal saline, never with water

Treatment of Overdose: Mean lethal dose in adults is thought to be 2-5 g; initial symptoms are nystagmus, ataxia; death is due to respiratory and circulatory depression; lavage, emesis, activated charcoal

Administration

Adult: PO 50-100 mg/day, may increase by 50-100 mg q 7 days, up to 200 mg tid (600 mg/day); *child:* Usually require 100-400 mg/day

- Available forms include: Tabs, 100 mg

Mephobarbital

MEBARAL

(me-foe-bar'bi-tal) (Chapter 7)

Functional classification: Antiepileptic (long-acting)

Chemical classification: Barbiturate

Controlled substance schedule IV

FDA pregnancy category: D

Indications: Generalized tonic-clonic, absence seizures

Contraindications: Hypersensitivity to barbiturates

Cautious use: Hepatic disease, renal disease, lactation, alcoholism, drug abuse, hyperthyroidism, myasthenia gravis, myxedema

Pharmacologic Effects: Depresses sensory cortex, motor activity

Pharmacokinetics: PO: Onset 30-60 min, duration 10-12 hr; metabolized by liver, excreted by kidneys, half-life 34 hr (mean)

Side Effects: *CNS:* **Somnolence, drowsiness,** lethargy, hangover headache, flushing, hallucinations, coma, **dizziness;** *Peripheral:* Nausea, vomiting, hypoventilation, bradycardia, hypotension, rash, urticaria, angioedema, local pain, swelling, necrosis, thrombophebitis, blood dyscrasias

Interactions

- CNS depressants, other antiepileptics: Drugs that increase the effects of barbiturates (toxic effects)
- Acetaminophen, digitoxin, oral anticoagulants, oral contraceptives, TCAs, possibly phenytoin, griseofulvin, doxycycline: Drugs whose effects are decreased by barbiturates

Implications

Assess

- Blood studies, liver function tests during long-term therapy
- Check VS, neurologic values regularly

Planning/Implementation

- Describe seizure accurately
- Offer consistent emotional support
- Monitor for early signs of toxic effects (slurred speech, ataxia, respiratory and CNS depression)

Teaching

- To report any side effects or adverse reactions
- To avoid driving or operating dangerous equipment
- To change position slowly
- To take drugs as prescribed because mephobarbital is habit forming
- Not to discontinue drug abruptly
- To wear MedicAlert identification bracelet
- To consult physician before becoming pregnant

Evaluate

- Mental status
- Respiratory depression
- Blood dyscrasias: Fever, sore throat, bruising, rash, jaundice

Treatment of Overdose: One g can cause serious poisoning in an adult; 2-10 g can be fatal; toxic effects can be confused with drunkenness. Emesis, if feasible; gastric lavage, if conscious; 30 g activated charcoal, maintain airway, good nursing care to prevent pneumonia

Administration
- Epilepsy: *Adult:* PO 400-600 mg/day or in divided doses; *child (under 5 yr):* 16-32 mg tid or qid; *Child (over 5 yr):* 32-64 mg tid or qid
- Available forms include: Tabs 32, 50, 100 mg

Methadone HCl

DOLOPHINE, METHADONE HCL
(meth'a-done) (Chapter 10)

Functional classification: Narcotic analgesic
Chemical classifications: Opiate, synthetic diphenylheptane derivative
Controlled substance schedule II
FDA pregnancy category: C

Indications: Narcotic withdrawal, severe pain

Contraindications: Hypersensitivity, addiction (narcotic)
Cautious use: Addictive personality, lactation, increased intracranial pressure, asthma, hypotension, acute abdominal condition, respiratory depression, hepatic disease, renal disease, child <18 yr

Pharmacologic Effects: Acts on mu and kappa opiate receptors

Pharmacokinetics: PO: Onset 30-60 min, duration 4-6 hr; peak 2-6 hr, metabolized by liver, excreted by kidneys, crosses placenta, excreted in breast milk, half-life 15-30 hr

Side Effects: *CNS:* **Drowsiness, dizziness, confusion, headache, sedation, euphoria;** *Peripheral:* **Nausea, vomiting, anorexia, constipation, cramps,** increased urinary output, dysuria, rash, urticaria, bruising, flushing, diaphoresis, pruritus, **respiratory depression,** tinnitus, blurred vision, miosis, diplopia, palpitations, bradycardia, change in B/P

Interactions
- Alcohol, narcotics, sedative hypnotics, antipsychotics, skeletal muscle relaxants, rifampin, phenytoin: Increased CNS depression
- Droperidol: Hypotension
- Hydantoins: Increase effects of methadone
- MAOIs: Unpredictable, have caused fatalities when used with related drugs

Implications
Assess
- I&O ratio: Check for decreasing output; may indicate urinary retention

Planning/Implementation
- If nausea, vomiting occurs, give with antiemetic
- Rotate injection sites
- Assist with ambulation
- Safety measures: Side rails, night light, call bell within easy reach

Teaching
- To report any symptoms of CNS changes
- That dependency may result
- Withdrawal symptoms may occur, e.g., Nausea, vomiting, cramps, fever, faintness, anorexia

Evaluate
- Therapeutic response
- CNS changes: Dizziness, drowsiness, hallucinations, euphoria, pupil reaction
- Respiratory dysfunction: Respiratory depression; if respirations are <12/min, notify physician
- Physical dependence

Lab Test Interferences: Increased amylase and lipase levels

Treatment of Overdose: Naloxone 0.2-0.8 mg IV, O_2, IV fluids, vasopressors

Administration
- Pain: *Adult:* PO/SC/IM 2.5-10 mg q3-4h prn
- Narcotic withdrawal: *Adult:* PO 15-40 mg/day individualized initially, then 20-120 mg/day as patient response indicates
- Available forms: Inj SC, IM 10 mg/ml; tabs 5, 10 mg; oral solution 5, 10 mg/5 ml, 10 mg/10 ml; dispersible tabs 40 mg, oral conc 10 mg/ml

Methamphetamine HCl

DESOXYN, DESOXYN GRADUMETS

(meth-am-fet′a-meen) (Chapters 12, 13, 15, 16)

Functional classification: Cerebral stimulant
Chemical classification: Amphetamine
Controlled substance schedule II
FDA pregnancy category: C

Indications: ADHD, Exogenous obesity

Contraindications: Hypersensitivity to sympathomimetic amines, hyperthyroidism, hypertension, glaucoma, severe arteriosclerosis, parkinsonism, drug abuse, anxiety, MAOI use
Cautious use: Tourette's disorder, lactation, child <3 yr

Pharmacologic Effect: Stimulates release of norepinephrine in cerebral cortex, brain stem, and reticular activating system and dopamine in the mesolimbic system; therapeutic plasma levels 5-10 μg/dl

Pharmacokinetics: PO: Duration 3-6 hr, metabolized by liver, excreted by kidneys, crosses blood-brain barrier, half-life 4-5 hr

Side Effects: *CNS:* **Hyperactivity, insomnia, restlessness, talkativeness,** dizziness, headache, chills, stimulation, dysphoria, irritability, aggressiveness; *Peripheral:* Nausea, vomiting, anorexia, dry mouth, diarrhea, constipation, weight loss, metallic taste, cramps; impotence, change in libido; **palpitations, tachycardia,** hypertension, hypotension

Interactions
- MAOIs or within 14 days of MAOIs: Hypertensive crisis
- Acetazolamide, antacids, sodium bicarbonate, ascorbic acid, ammonium chloride, phenothiazines, haloperidol: Increases half-life of amphetamine
- Barbiturates: Decreased effects of this drug
- Guanethidine, other antihypertensives: Decreased hypotensive effect
- Phenothiazines: Antogonize amphetamines

Implications
Assess:
- VS, B/P because this drug may reverse antihypertensives; check patients with cardiac disease more often
- CBC, urinalysis; in diabetes, blood and urine sugar levels, insulin changes may need to be made, since eating may decrease
- **Height, growth rate in children, growth rate may be decreased**

Planning/Implementation
- Give at least 6 hr before bedtime to avoid sleeplessness
- For obesity, only when patient is on weight reduction program that includes dietary changes, exercise; tolerance develops, and weight loss will not occur without additional methods
- Gum, hard candy, frequent sips of water for dry mouth
- If drug is for obesity, 30-60 min before meals
- Dispense least amount feasible, to minimize risk of overdose

Teaching
- To decrease caffeine consumption (coffee, tea, cola, chocolate), which may increase irritability, stimulation
- Avoid OTC preparations unless approved by physician
- To taper off drug over several weeks, or depression, increased sleeping, lethargy may occur
- To avoid alcohol ingestion
- To avoid hazardous activities until condition is stabilized on medication
- To get needed rest; patients feel more tired at end of day
- Check to see that PO medication has been swallowed

Evaluate
- Mental status: Mood, sensorium, affect, stimulation, insomnia; aggressiveness may occur
- Physical dependency; Should not be used for extended time; dose should be discontinued gradually
- **Withdrawal symptoms: Headache, nausea, vomiting, muscle pain, weakness**

M

- Drug tolerance develops after long-term use
- If tolerance develops, dosage should not be increased

Treatment of Overdose: Gastric evacuation if overdose occurred in preceding 24 hr; otherwise, acidify urine; administer fluids until urine flow is 3-6 ml/kg/hr; hemodialysis or peritoneal dialysis; antihypertensives for increased B/P; ammonium chloride for increased excretion; chlorpromazine for CNS stimulation

Administration
- ADHD: *Child* >6 yr: 2.5-5 mg qd or bid, increasing by 5 mg/wk; usual effective dose 20-25 mg/day
- Obesity: *Adult:* PO 5 mg 30 min ac or 10-15 mg long-acting qd in morning
- Available forms: Tabs 5 mg, long-acting tabs 5, 10, 15 mg

Metharbital*

GEMONIL

(meth-ar'bi-tal) (Chapter 7)

Functional classification: Antiepileptic
Chemical classification: Barbiturate derivative
Controlled substance schedule III
FDA pregnancy category: D

Indications: Generalized tonic-clonic, absence seizures

Contraindications: Hypersensitivity to barbiturates
Cautious use: Hepatic disease, renal disease, lactation, alcoholism, drug abuse, hyperthyroidism

Pharmacologic Effects: Depresses sensory cortex, motor activity

Pharmacokinetics: PO: Onset ≥1 hr, duration 10-12 hr; metabolized by liver, excreted by kidneys, half-life unknown

Side Effects: *CNS:* **Somnolence, drowsiness,** lethargy, hangover headache, flushing, hallucinations, coma; *Peripheral:* **Nausea, vomiting,** hypoventilation, bradycardia, hypotension, rash, urticaria, angioedema, local pain, swelling, necrosis, thrombophlebitis, blood dyscrasias

Interactions
- CNS depressants, other antiepileptics: Drugs that increase the effects of barbiturates (toxic effects)
- Acetaminophen, digitoxin, oral anticoagulants, oral contraceptives, TCAs, possibly phenytoin griseofulvin, doxycycline: Drugs whose effects are decreased by barbiturates

Implications

Assess
- Blood studies, liver function tests during long-term therapy
- Check VS, neurologic values regularly

Planning/Implementation
- Describe seizure accurately
- Offer consistent emotional support
- Monitor for early signs of toxic effects (slurred speech, ataxia, respiratory and CNS depression)

Teaching
- To report any side effects or adverse reactions
- To avoid driving or operating dangerous equipment
- To change position slowly
- To take drugs as prescribed because metharbital is habit forming
- Not to discontinue abruptly
- To wear MedicAlert identification bracelet
- To consult physician before becoming pregnant

Evaluate
- Mental status
- Respiratory depression
- Blood dyscrasias: Fever, sore throat, bruising, rash, jaundice

Treatment of Overdose: One g can cause serious poisoning in an adult; 2-10 g can be fatal. Toxic effects can be confused with drunkenness. Emesis, gastric lavage, if conscious; 30 g activated charcoal, maintain airway, good nursing care to prevent pneumonia

Administration

Adult: PO 100 mg qd-tid, may increase to 800 mg/day in divided doses; *child:* PO 5-15 mg/kg/day in divided doses
- Available forms include: Tabs 100 mg

*Infrequently used.

Methohexital

BREVITAL SODIUM, BRIETAL SODIUM†
(meth-oh-hex'i-tal) (Chapter 11)

Functional classification: General anesthetic
Chemical classification: Barbiturate
Controlled substance schedule IV
FDA pregnancy category: D

Indications: General anesthesia for ECT

Contraindications: Hypersensitivity, status asthmaticus, porphyria

Pharmacologic Effect: Ultrashort-acting barbiturate depresses CNS to produce anesthesia

Pharmacokinetics: Highly lipophilic; onset rapid but of brief duration; produces anesthesia in 1 min; plasma half-life 3 to 8 hr

Side Effects: *CNS:* Delirium, headache, prolonged somnolence and recovery; *Peripheral:* Circulatory depression, arrhythmias, respiratory depression, apnea, laryngospasm, bronchospasm, nausea, vomiting

Interactions
- CNS depressants including alcohol: Additive effect
- Furosemide: Aggravates orthostatic hypertension

Implications
Assess
- VS q 3-5 min until recovered from ECT

Planning/Implementation
- Have emergency drugs and resuscitation equipment available

Evaluate
- Cardiac status
- Respirations
- Mental status

Treatment of Overdose: Usually occurs due to rapid injection, resulting in apnea and respiratory difficulties; discontinue drug, maintain airway, give oxygen prn; ventilatory assistance prn

Administration
Adult and child: IV 50-120 mg (5-12 ml of 1% solution); this amount provides anesthesia for 5-7 min
- Available forms include: Powder for IV inj; ampules 2.5, 5 g; vials 500 mg/50 ml, 2.5 g/250 ml, 5 g/500 ml

†Available in Canada only.

Methsuximide*

CELONTIN
(meth-sux'i mide) (Chapter 7)

Functional classification: Antiepileptic
Chemical classification: Succinimide
FDA pregnancy category: C

Indications: Second-choice drug for absence seizures

Contraindications: Hypersensitivity

Pharmacologic Effects: See ethosuximide

Pharmacokinetics: Onset in 15-30 min, peak level 1-4 hr, duration of effect 3-4 hr, excreted in urine, half-life 2.6-4 hr

Side Effects: *CNS:* Drowsiness, ataxia, and dizziness most common side effect; see ethosuximide for other CNS effects; *Peripheral:* See ethosuximide

Interactions: See ethosuximide

Implications: See ethosuximide

Lab Test Interference: See ethosuximide

Treatment of Overdose: See ethosuximide

Administration
Adult and child: 300 mg/day at first, increase by 300 mg/day at weekly intervals as needed; do *not* exceed 1.2 g/day in divided doses
- Available forms: Caps half-strength 150 mg, caps 300 mg

*Infrequently used.

Methylphenidate HCl

RITALIN, RITALIN SR
(meth-ill-fen'i-date) (Chapters 12, 13, 15, 16)

Functional classification: Cerebral stimulant
Chemical classification: Piperidine derivative
Controlled substance schedule II
FDA pregnancy category: C

Indications: ADHD, narcolepsy

Contraindications: Hypersensitivity to sympathomimetic amines, anxiety, Tourette's disorder, history of seizures
Cautious use: Hypertension, severe depression, seizures, drug abuse, lactation

Pharmacologic Effect: Mild CNS stimulant, mechanism unknown

Pharmacokinetics: PO: Onset½ -1 hr, duration 4-6 hr, metabolized by liver, excreted by kidneys, half-life 1-3 hr

Side Effects: *CNS:* **Hyperactivity, insomnia, restlessness, talkativeness,** dizziness, headache, chills, stimulation, dysphoria, irritability, aggressiveness; *Peripheral:* Nausea, vomiting, anorexia, dry mouth, diarrhea, constipation, weight loss, metallic taste, cramps, impotence, change in libido, **palpitations, tachycardia,** hypertension, hypotension

Interactions
- MAOIs or within 14 days of MAOIs: Hypertensive crisis
- Acetazolamide, antacids, sodium bicarbonate, ascorbic acid, ammonium chloride, phenothiazines, haloperidol: Increases effects of amphetamine
- Barbiturates: Decreased effects of this drug
- Guanethidine, other antihypertensives: Decreased effects of this drug

Implications
Assess:
- VS, B/P
- Appetite: May be decreased
- Height, growth rate in children may be decreased (see Chapters 15 and 16)

Planning/Implementation
- Give at least 6 hr before bedtime to avoid sleeplessness

Teaching
- To decrease caffeine consumption (coffee, tea, cola, chocolate), which may increase irritability, stimulation
- Avoid OTC preparations unless approved by physician
- To taper off drug over several weeks, or depression, increased sleeping, lethargy may occur
- To avoid alcohol ingestion
- To avoid hazardous activities until condition is stabilized on medication
- To get needed rest; patients feel more tired at end of day
- Check to see that PO medication has been swallowed

Evaluate
- Mental status: Mood, sensorium, affect, stimulation, insomnia; aggressiveness may occur
- Physical dependency; should not be used for extended time; drug should be discontinued gradually
- **Withdrawal symptoms: Headache, nausea, vomiting, muscle pain, weakness**
- Drug tolerance can develop
- If tolerance develops, dosage should not be increased

Treatment of Overdose: Supportive measures; protect against self-injury; evacuate gastric contents, if possible; maintain circulation; external cooling, if hyperpyrexia occurs

Administration
- ADHD: *Child >6 yr:* 5 mg before breakfast and lunch, increasing by 5-10 mg/wk, not to exceed 60 mg/day
- Narcolepsy: *Adult:* PO 10 mg bid-tid, 30-45 min before meals, may increase to 40-60 mg/day
- Available forms: Tabs 5, 10, 20 mg; tabs time-rel 20 mg

Molindone HCl

MOBAN

(moe-lin'done) (Chapter 4)

Functional classifications: Antipsychotic, neuroleptic

Chemical classification: Dihydroindolone

FDA pregnancy category: C

Indications: Psychotic disorders

Contraindications: Hypersensitivity, coma, child <12 yr, brain damage, bone marrow depression, alcohol and barbiturate withdrawal states

Cautious use: Lactation, hypertension, hepatic disease, cardiac disease

Pharmacologic Effects: Antipsychotic drugs produce a neuroleptic effect characterized by sedation, emotional quieting, psychomotor slowing, and affective indifference; exact mode of action is not fully understood; antipsychotics block dopamine receptors in the basal ganglia, hypothalamus, limbic system, brain stem, and medulla; antipsychotics are also thought to depress certain components of the reticular activating system that partially control body temperature, wakefulness, vasomotor tone, emesis, and hormonal balance; additionally, antipsychotics have significant anticholinergic and alpha-adrenergic blocking effects

Pharmacokinetics: PO: Onset erratic, peak 1½ hr, duration 24-36 hr; metabolized by liver, excreted in urine and feces, may cross placenta, enters breast milk, half-life 10-20 hr

Side Effects: *CNS:* Parkinsonism, akathisias, dystonias, tardive dyskinesia, oculogyric crisis; *Peripheral:* Blurred vision (cycloplegia or paralysis of accommodation); ocular pain, photophobia, mydriasis, impaired vision; intolerance of extreme heat or cold, possible heat stroke or fatal hyperthermia; nasal congestion, wheezing, dyspnea; **hypotension, especially orthostatic,** leading to dizziness, syncope; **tachycardia,** irregular pulse, arrhythmias; **dry mouth, constipation,** jaundice, abdominal pain; urinary retention, urinary hesitancy, galactorrhea, gynecomastia, menses in previously amenorrheic women

Interactions

- Alcohol and other CNS depressants (barbiturates, antihistamines, antianxiety or antidepressant drugs): Increased CNS depression; increased risk of EPSEs
- Amphetamines: Possible decreased antipsychotic effect
- Antacids (magnesium and aluminum products): Possible decreased antipsychotic effect
- Anticholinergics (atropine, H_1-type antihistamines, antidepressants, etc.): Increased risk of excessive atropine-like side effects or toxic effects
- Benztropine: Possible decreased antipsychotic effect, increased risk of severity of peripheral anticholinergic side effects
- Diazoxide: Possible severe hyperglycemia, prediabetic coma
- Guanethidine: Poor control of hypertension by guanethidine
- Hypoglycemia drugs (insulin, oral hypoglycemia agents): Poor diabetic control
- Lithium: Poor control of psychosis with combined therapy; can mask lithium intoxication, neurotoxic effects with confusion, delirium, seizures, encephalopathy
- Meperidine, morphine: Increased risk of severe CNS depression, respiratory depression, hypotension
- Propranolol: Increased pharmacologic effects of either drug

Implications

Assess

- Establish baseline VS, laboratory values, to assess side effects, allergic or hypersensitivity reactions
- Physiologic and psychologic status before therapy, to determine needs and evaluate progress
- For early stages of tardive dyskinesia, use abnormal involuntary movement scale
- Identify concurrent symptoms that may be aggravated by antipsychotics, e.g., glaucoma, diabetes

Planning/Implementation

- Ensure that drug has been taken; check mouth for "cheeking"
- If giving liquid antipsychotics, use at least 60 ml of compatible beverage to mask taste; dilute and give immediately; take drug with food to minimize GI upset

M

- Keep patient quiet after injection, to prevent falls associated with postural hypotension
- For dry mouth, give chewing gum, hard candies, lip balm; monitor urinary output; check for bladder distention in inactive patients, older men, and patients on high doses
- Assist with ambulation, if patient is experiencing blurred vision; dim room lights for photosensitivity
- Ensure safety with hypotension; sit on side of bed before rising, head-low position for dizziness, avoid hot showers, wear elastic stockings
- Check B/P (supine, sitting, standing) and pulse before and after each dose, when possible; observe for side effects
- Monitor body temperature for indications of neuroleptic malignant syndrome, e.g., muscle rigidity, fever, depressed neurologic status; ensure adequate hydration, nutrition, and ventilation
- Protect patient from exposure to extreme heat or cold
- Recognize impending hypersensitivity: pruritus or jaundice with hepatitis, flu or coldlike symptoms, evidence of bleeding with blood dyscrasia
- Observe for involuntary movements

Teaching

- About benefits and potential harm of antipsychotic drugs; weigh need to know against causing apprehension
- To comply with drug treatment
- To avoid activities requiring clear vision for a few weeks after treatment starts; to report eye pain immediately
- About the importance of exercise, fluids, and fiber in diet
- To watch for symptoms of heart failure: weight gain, dyspnea, distended neck veins, tachycardia
- To avoid conception; women should practice effective contraception
- To avoid exposure to sunlight; keep skin covered but with temperature-appropriate clothing
- That patient cannot become addicted to antipsychotic drugs

Evaluate

- Follows prescribed regimen, takes medications as ordered
- Avoids injury; reports dizziness or need for assistance
- Experiences minimal or no adverse responses
- Uses appropriate interventions to minimize side effects
- Achieves improved mental status

Lab Test Interferences: Alterations in blood glucose and BUN levels and RBC are not clinically significant

Treatment of Overdose: If orally ingested, lavage, providing an airway; do not induce vomiting; symptomatic, supportive care

Administration

Adult >12 yr: PO 50-75 mg/day, increasing to 225 mg/day, if needed; maintenance dosage for mild condition is 5-15 mg tid-qid

- Concentrate mixed with orange or grapefruit juice
- Available forms include: Tabs 5, 10, 25, 50, 100 mg; conc 20 mg/ml

Naloxone HCl

NARCAN

(Nay-locks-own) (Chapter 10)

Functional classification: Narcotic antagonist

Chemical classification: Thebaine derivative

FDA pregnancy category: B

Indications: Narcotic-induced respiratory depression

Contraindications: Hypersensitivity

Cautious use: Children

Pharmacologic Effects: Competes with narcotics at opioid receptor sites

Pharmacokinetics: PO: Onset 2 min (IV), half-life 30-81 min; duration 1-4 hr; metabolized by liver, excreted by kidneys, crosses placenta

Side Effects: *CNS:* Stimulation, **drowsiness,** nervousness; *Peripheral:* Hypotension, hypertension, ventricular tachycardia, hyperpnea; withdrawal symptoms, e.g., nausea, vomiting, sweating, increased blood pressure, tremulousness

Interactions
- Potentially cardiotoxic drugs: Hypotension, hypertension, ventricular tachycardia
- Opioids: Loss of analgesia

Implications
Assess
- VS q 3-5 min

Planning/Implementation
- Remember that naloxone does not improve respiratory depression caused by nonnarcotic drugs
- Have resuscitative equipment nearby
- Give solutions prepared within 24 hr

Evaluate
- Signs of withdrawal in drug-dependent individuals
- Cardiac status: Tachycardia, hypertension
- Respiratory dysfunction: Respiratory depression, character, rate, and rhythm; if respirations are <10/min, respiratory stimulant should be administered

Lab Test Interferences: Urine VMA, 5-HIAA, urine glucose levels, pregnancy test

Administration
- Narcotic-induced respiratory depression: *Adult:* IV/SC/IM 0.4-2 mg; repeat q 2-3 min, if needed
- Postoperative respiratory depression: *Adult:* IV 0.1-0.2 mg q 2-3 min prn; *child:* IV/IM/SC 0.01 mg/kg q 2-3 min prn
- Available forms include: Inj IV, IM, SC 0.02, 0.4, 1 mg/ml

Naltrexone HCl

TREXAN

(nal-trex'one) (Chapter 10)

Functional classification: Narcotic antagonist
Chemical classification: Thebaine derivative
FDA pregnancy category: C

Indications: Blockage of opioid analgesics, narcotic addiction; longer-acting than naloxone; prevention of readdiction

Contraindications: Hypersensitivity, patients receiving opioid analgesics, opioid-dependent patients, hepatic failure, child <18 yr, hepatitis, patients who fail naloxone challenge test
Cautious use: Anemia, hepatic disease, renal disease, Hodgkin's disease

Pharmacologic Effect: Competes with narcotics at opioid receptor sites; blocks subjective effects of IV narcotics

Pharmacokinetics: PO: Onset 15-30 min, peak 1-2 hr, duration 4-6 hr; REC: Onset slow, duration 4-6 hr; metabolized by liver, excreted by kidneys, crosses placenta, excreted in breast milk, half-life 4 hr

Side Effects: *CNS:* Stimulation, drowsiness, dizziness, confusion, convulsion, headache, flushing, hallucinations, coma; *Peripheral:* **Nausea, vomiting, diarrhea,** anorexia, hepatitis; **rash,** urticaria, bruising, tinnitus, hearing loss, rapid pulse, pulmonary edema, wheezing, hyperpnea, hypoglycemia, hyponatremia, hypokalemia

Interactions
- Potentially cardiotoxic drugs: Hypotension, hypertension, ventricular tachycardia
- Opioids: Loss of analgesia

Implications
Assess
- VS q 3-5 min

Planning/Implementation
- Remember that naltrexone may precipitate an abstinence syndrome

Teaching
- Naltrexone is part of the treatment plan
- Carry MedicAlert bracelet to alert health care provider
- That large doses of heroin might kill the patient

Evaluate
- Cardiac status: Tachycardia, hypertension
- Respiratory dysfunction: Respiratory depression, character, rate, and rhythm; if respirations are <10/min, respiratory stimulant should be administered

Lab Test Interferences: Liver test abnormalities

Treatment of Overdose: Treat symptoms

N

Administration

Adult: PO 25 mg, may be given 25 mg after 1 hr, if there are no withdrawal symptoms; 50-150 mg may be given qd, depending on patient need

- Available forms: Tabs 50 mg

Nortriptyline HCl

AVENTYL, PAMELOR

(nor-trip'ti-leen) (Chapter 5)

Functional classification: TCA
Chemical classification: Dibenzocycloheptene, secondary amine
FDA pregnancy category: C

Indications: Depression
Unlabeled use: Panic disorder

Contraindications: Hypersensitivity to TCAs, recovery phase of myocardial infarction; *Cautious use:* Convulsive disorders, prostatic hypertrophy, suicidal patients, severe depression, increased intraocular pressure, narrow-angle glaucoma, urinary retention, cardiac disease, hepatic disease, hyperthyroidism, ECT, elective surgery, children

Pharmacologic Effect: Blocks reuptake of norepinephrine, serotonin into nerve endings, increasing action of norepinephrine, serotonin in nerve cells; also r/t changes in receptor sensitivity; therapeutic plasma levels 50-150 ng/ml

Pharmacokinetics: PO: Steady state 4-19 days; metabolized by liver, excreted by kidneys, crosses placenta, excreted in breast milk, half-life 18-44 hr

Side Effects: *CNS:* **Sedation,** ataxia; confusion, delirium; *Peripheral:* **Blurred vision,** photophobia, increased intraocular pressure; decreased tearing, orthostatic hypotension, arrhythmias, tachycardia, palpitations, dry mouth, constipation, diarrhea, decreased sweating, **urinary retention, hesitancy**

Interactions

- Anticholinergic agents: Additive anticholinergic effects with atropine, antihistamines (H_1 blocker), antiparkinson drugs, antipsychotics, OTC cold and allergy drugs
- CNS depressants: Additive depressant effect
- Guanethidine, clonidine: Decreased antihypertensive effect
- MAOIs: Hypertensive crisis, atropine-like poisoning
- Oral contraceptives: Inhibits effects of TCAs
- Phenothiazines, methylphenidates: May increase tricyclic serum level
- Quinidine: Additive effect, heart block possible
- Sympathomimetics: Potentiate sympathomimetic effects
- Thyroid preparations: Tachycardia, arrhythmias; may increase TCA effect

Implications

Assess

- Establish baseline data, to aid recognition of adverse responses to medication, e.g., liver enzyme levels, VS, renal function, mental status, speech patterns, affect, weight
- For signs of noncompliance, e.g., poor therapeutic response
- Observe for major symptoms of depression e.g., apathy, sadness, sleep disturbances, hopelessness, guilt, decreased libido, spontaneous crying
- Review history for contraindicated conditions, e.g., glaucoma, CV disease, GI conditions, urologic conditions, seizures, pregnancy

Planning/Implementation

- Monitor for "cheeking" or hoarding; check drug dosage carefully, since a small overdose may cause toxic effects
- Monitor for suicidal ideations; suicidal thought content may increase as antidepressants begin to "energize" patient
- Monitor VS; if hypotension tachycardia or arrhythmias occur, withhold TCAs
- Give most TCAs in a single dose hs
- Observe for early signs of toxic effects, e.g., drowsiness, tachycardia, mydriasis, hypotension, agitation, vomiting, confusion, fever, restlessness, sweating
- If CNS overstimulation occurs, e.g., hypomania, delirium, discontinue drug

Teaching

- That these drugs have a lag time of up to 1 month
- To adhere to drug regimen

- To avoid OTC drugs, particularly those containing sympathomimetics or anticholinergics
- To avoid drugs listed in section on interactions
- About ways to deal with minor side effects, as follows: dry mouth, with sugarless hard candies, sips of water, mouth rinses; visual disturbances, with artificial tears, sunglasses, assistance with ambulation; constipation, with bulk-forming foods, increased fluids; urinary hesitancy, with adequate fluids, privacy; decreased perspiration, with appropriate clothing, avoidance of unnecessary exercise; orthostatic hypotension, with slow positional changes, avoidance of hot baths and showers; for drowsiness, take single dose hs with physician approval, avoid driving
- That abrupt discontinuance may result in cholinergic rebound, e.g., nausea, vomiting, insomnia, headache

Evaluate

- Desired therapeutic serum level
- Verbalize decrease in subjective symptoms
- Observe decrease in objective symptoms
- Minimal to no adverse drug effects
- Stable VS
- Less anxiety; sleep, talk, and feel better

Lab Test Interferences

- Increase: Serum bilirubin, blood glucose, alkaline phosphatase levels
- False increase: Urinary catecholamines
- Decrease: VMA, 5-HIAA

Treatment of Overdose: ECG monitoring, induce emesis, lavage, activated charcoal, administer anticonvulsant, treat anticholinergic response, if needed

Administration

Adult: PO 25 mg tid or qid, may increase to 100 mg/day; may give daily dose hs

Adolescent and geriatric: 30-50 mg/day in divided doses

- Available forms include: Caps 10, 25, 50, 75 mg; solution 10 mg/5 ml

Oxazepam

SERAX

(ox-a′ze-pam) (Chapter 6)

Functional classification: Antianxiety
Chemical classification: Benzodiazepine
Controlled substance schedule IV
FDA pregnancy category: D

Indications: Anxiety, alcohol withdrawal, anxiety and tension in elderly

Contraindications: Hypersensitivity to benzodiazepines, psychoses, narrow-angle glaucoma, psychosis, child <12 yr

Cautious use: Elderly or debilitated patients, hepatic disease, renal disease

Pharmacologic Effects: Apparently potentiates effects of GABA and other inhibitory transmitters by binding to specific benzodiazepine receptor sites; depresses subcortical levels of CNS, including limbic system and reticular formation

Pharmacokinetics: Speed of onset: Intermediate to slow

PO: Peak 2-4 hr, metabolized by liver, excreted by kidneys, half-life 5-20 hr

Side Effects: *CNS:* **Drowsiness, dizziness,** confusion, headache, anxiety, tremor, stimulation, fatigue, depression, insomnia; *Peripheral:* Photophobia due to mydriasis, **blurred vision** due to cycloplegia; sleeplike slowing of respirations with therapeutic doses, cough; **orthostatic hypotension, tachycardia,** hypotension; constipation, dry mouth

Interactions

- Alcohol and other CNS depressants: Increased CNS depression
- Cimetidine: Potentiation of CNS depression
- Digoxin: Increased risk of cardiac side effects from digoxin
- Levodopa: Decreased antiparkinson effect
- Phenytoin: Increased phenytoin serum levels

Implications

Assess

- Patient's level of anxiety and method of coping
- B/P, VS

- Establish baseline physical assessment data before medications are started

Planning/Implementation

- Monitor patient's response to medication
- Observe elderly, very young, and debilitated patients for paradoxic excitement
- Reduce dose of other depressant drugs
- Observe for signs of withdrawal when discontinuing antianxiety drug

Teaching

- To avoid operating dangerous machinery and performing other tasks requiring good reflexes
- To report ocular pain at once, as well as other visual disturbances
- Drug may be taken with food

Evaluate

- Whether patient achieves lower levels of anxiety without undue sedation
- Whether patient can follow prescribed regimen
- For physical dependence: Withdrawal symptoms of headache, nausea, vomiting, muscle pain, weakness after long-term use.

Lab Test Interferences
Increase: AST/ALT, serum bilirubin level
Decrease: RAIU
False increase: 17-OHSC

Treatment of Overdose: Lavage, VS, supportive care; there have been few deaths, if any, resulting from benzodiazepine overdose alone; deaths occur when benzodiazepines are mixed with other drugs, especially alcohol

Administration

- Anxiety: *Adult:* PO 10-30 mg tid-qid; *geriatric:* 10 mg tid, up to 15 mg tid-qid (use cautiously)
- Alcohol withdrawal: *Adult:* PO 15-30 mg tid-qid
- Available forms include: Caps, 10, 15, 30 mg; tabs 15 mg

Paraldehyde

PARAL

(par-al'de-hyde) (Chapter 7)

Functional classification: Anticonvulsant
Chemical classification: Cyclic ether
Controlled substance schedule IV
FDA pregnancy category: C

Indications: Refractory seizures, status epilepticus, alcohol withdrawal, tetanus, eclampsia, sedation

Contraindications: Hypersensitivity, gastroenteritis, asthma, hepatic disease, pulmonary disease; *cautious use:* Labor, children

Pharmacologic Effects: CNS depressant; mechanism of action unknown

Pharmacokinetics: PO: Onset 10-15 min, peak 1 hr, duration 8-12 hr; REC: Onset slow, duration 4-6 hr; metabolized by liver, excreted by kidneys and lungs, crosses placenta, half-life 3.4-9.8 hr

Side Effects: *CNS:* **Stimulation, drowsiness,** dizziness, confusion, convulsions, headache, flushing, hallucinations, coma; *Peripheral:* **Foul breath,** irritation, nephrosis, **rash, erythema,** local pain, esophagitis, yellowing of eyes

Interactions

- Alcohol, CNS depressants, general anesthetics, disulfiram: increased paraldehyde blood levels
- Sulfonamides: Increased crystallization in kidneys
- Disulfiram: Blocks metabolism of paraldehyde; avoid use

Implications

Assess

- VS q 30 min after parenteral route
- Hepatic studies: AST, ALT, bilirubin and creatinine levels

Planning/Implementation

- IM inj in deep large muscle (Z-track) mass to prevent tissue sloughing; maximum, 5 ml at one site
- Give rectally, after diluting in cottonseed oil or olive oil, as retention enema or 200 ml NS for enema

- Give orally with juice or milk to cover taste and smell and decrease GI symptoms (orally)
- Ventilate room
- Use glass containers; not compatible with plastics
- Do not use if brownish or if vinegar odor is evident

Teaching
- That physical dependency may result when used for extended periods of time
- To avoid driving, other activities that require alertness
- Not to discontinue medication quickly after long-term use, taper over several weeks

Evaluate
- Mental status
- Respiratory dysfunction

Treatment of Overdose: Do not lavage; support respirations, treat acidosis

Administration
- Seizures: *Adult:* IM 5-10 ml; IV 0.2-0.4 ml/kg in NS inj; *child:* IM 0.15 ml/kg; REC 0.3 ml/kg q4-6h; IV 0.1-0.15 ml/kg ml NS inj
- For other uses see *PDR*
- Available forms include: Inj IM/IV, oral and rectal liquids 1g/ml

Paramethadione*

PARADIONE

(par-a-meth-a-dye'one) (Chapter 7)

Functional classification: Antiepileptic
Chemical classification: Oxazolidinedione
FDA pregnancy category: D

Indications: Refractory absence seizures

Contraindications: Hypersensitivity, blood dyscrasias
Cautious use: Hepatic disease, renal disease

Pharmacologic Effects: Increases seizure threshold in cortex and basal ganglia

Pharmacokinetics: PO: Onset 15-30 min, peak 1-2 hr, duration 4-6 hr; metabolized by the liver, excreted by the kidneys, crosses placenta, excreted in breast milk, half-life 1-3½ hr

Side Effects: *CNS:* **Drowsiness,** dizziness, fatigue, paresthesia, irritability, headache; *Peripheral:* Vaginal bleeding, albuminuria, nephrosis, abdominal pain, weight loss, nausea, vomiting, bleeding gums, abnormal liver function test, **exfoliative dermatitis,** rash, alopecia, petechiae, erythema, photophobia, diplopia, epistaxis, retinal hemorrhage, hypertension, hypotension, thrombocytopenia, agranulocytosis, leukopenia, neutropenia, hemolytic anemia

Interactions: None known

Implications

Assess
- Blood studies: Hematocrit, hemoglobin level, RBCs, serum folate level, vitamin D, if on long-term therapy
- Hepatic studies: ALT, AST, bilirubin and creatinine levels
- Skin: If rash occurs, withhold drug

Planning/Implementation
- Dilute oral solution with water
- Take orally with juice or milk to cover taste and smell and to decrease GI symptoms

Teaching
- To take with food, if GI upset
- To carry MedicAlert identification bracelet
- To notify physician, if visual disturbances, sore throat, etc., occur
- To avoid driving and other activities that require alertness
- Not to discontinue medication quickly after long-term use, since convulsions may result

Evaluate
- Mental status
- Renal and hematologic problems

Treatment of Overdose: Symptoms include nausea, drowsiness, dizziness, ataxia, visual disturbances; coma, if massive overdose; emesis, lavage, supportive care

Administration

Adult: PO 300 mg tid (900 mg/day), may increase by 300 mg/wk, not to exceed 600 mg qid (2400 mg/day); *child:* 300 to 900 mg/day in three or four equally divided doses; dilute with water because of high alcohol content
- Available forms include: Caps 150, 300 mg; sol 300 mg/ml (65% alcohol)

*Infrequently used.

Pemoline

CYLERT
(pem′oh-leen) (Chapters 13, 15, 16)

Functional classification: Cerebral stimulant
Chemical classification: Oxazolidinone derivative
Controlled substance schedule IV
FDA pregnancy category: B

Indications: ADHD

Contraindications: Hypersensitivity
Cautious use: Renal disease, child <6 yr

Pharmacologic Effects: Exact mechanism not known; may work through dopaminergic pathways

Pharmacokinetics: PO peak 2-4 hr, duration 8 hr, metabolized by liver, excreted by kidneys, half-life 12 hr

Side Effects: *CNS:* Hyperactivity, insomnia, restlessness, dizziness, depression, headache, stimulation, irritability, aggressiveness, hallucinations, seizures; *Peripheral:* Nausea, anorexia, diarrhea, abdominal pain, increased liver enzyme levels, hepatitis, growth suppression in children, rashes

Interactions: None known

Implications
Assess:
- Hepatic function studies: ALT, AST, bilirubin and creatinine levels
- Growth rate because retardation may occur (see Chapters 15 and 16)

Planning/Implementation
- Give at least 6 hr before bedtime
- Gum, hard candy, frequent sips of water for dry mouth

Teaching
- To decrease caffeine consumption (coffee, tea, cola, chocolate) because caffeine may increase irritability
- To avoid OTC preparations unless approved by physician
- To taper off drug over several weeks
- To avoid alcohol ingestion
- To avoid hazardous activities until condition is stabilized on medication
- Therapeutic effect may take 3-4 wk

Evaluate
- Mental status

Treatment of Overdose: *Symptoms:* CNS overstimulation and excessive sympathomimetic effect; vomiting, agitation, tremors, twitching, convulsions; *Treatment:* Supportive measures, if not too severe; Gastric contents may be evacuated; chlorpromazine may decrease CNS stimulation

Administration
Child >6 yr: 37.5 mg in morning, increasing by 18.75 mg/wk, not to exceed 112.5 mg/day; maintenance dose usually 56.25-75 mg/day
- Available forms include: Tabs 18.75, 37.5, 75 mg; chewable tabs 37.5 mg

Pentobarbital, Pentobarbital Sodium

NEMBUTAL SODIUM, NOVA-RECTAL,† PENTOGEN†
(pen-toe-bar′bi-tal) (Chapter 8)

Functional classifications: Sedative, hypnotic
Chemical classification: Barbiturate
Controlled substance schedule II
FDA pregnancy category: D

Indications: Insomnia, sedation, emergency control of seizures

Contraindications: Hypersensitivity, respiratory depression, barbiturate dependence, marked liver dysfunction, acute pain; *cautious use:* Seizure disorders, elderly patients, lactation, children

Pharmacologic Effects: Short-acting barbiturate: depresses sensory cortex to produces drowsiness, sedation, and sleep

Pharmacokinetics: PO Onset 10-15 minutes, duration 3-4 hr, half-life 15-50 hr

Side Effects: *CNS:* See secobarbital; *Peripheral:* See secobarbital

Interactions: See secobarbital

Implications: See secobarbital

†Available in Canada only.

Lab Test Interference: False increase: Sulfobromophthalein

Treatment of Overdose: Gastric lavage, activated charcoal, warm the patient; monitor VS, I&O; hemodialysis may be effective; roll patient from side to side q 30 min

Administration
- Insomnia: *Adult:* PO 100 mg hs
- Available forms: Caps 50, 100 mg; elix 18.2 mg/5 ml; rectal supp 30, 60, 120, 200 mg; IM inj, IV 50 mg/ml

Perphenazine

PHENAZINE, TRILAFON
(per-fen'a-zeen) (Chapter 4)

Functional classifications: Antipsychotic, neuroleptic
Chemical classifications: Phenothiazine, piperidine
FDA pregnancy category: C

Indications: Psychotic disorders, nausea, vomiting

Contraindications: Hypersensitivity, blood dyscrasias, coma, child <12 yr, brain damage, bone marrow depression, adynamic ileus
Cautious use: Lactation, seizure disorders, hypertension, hepatic disease, cardiac disease, glaucoma, renal impairment, ECT

Pharmacologic Effects: Antipsychotic drugs produce a neuroleptic effect characterized by sedation, emotional quieting, psychomotor slowing, and affective indifference; exact mode of action is not fully understood; antipsychotics block dopamine receptors in the basal ganglia, hypothalamus, limbic system, brain stem, and medulla; antipsychotics are also thought to depress certain components of the reticular activating system that partially control body temperature, wakefulness, vasomotor tone, emesis, and hormonal balance; additionally, antipsychotics have significant anticholinergic and alpha-adrenergic blocking effects; antiemetic effect r/t inhibition of chemoreceptor trigger zone

Pharmacokinetics: PO onset erratic, peak 2-4 hr; IM onset 10 min, peak 1-2 hr, duration 6 hr, occassionally 12-24 hr; metabolized by liver, excreted in urine, crosses placenta, enters breast milk; therapeutic plasma levels 0.8-1.2 ng/ml

Side Effects: *CNS:* Parkinsonism, akathisias, dystonias, tardive dyskinesia, oculogyric crisis; *Peripheral:* Blurred vision (cycloplegia or paralysis of accommodation), ocular pain, photophobia, mydriasis, impaired vision; intolerance of extreme heat or cold, possible heat stroke or fatal hyperthermia; nasal congestion, wheezing, dyspnea; **hypotension, especially orthostatic,** leading to dizziness, syncope; **tachycardia,** irregular pulse, arrhythmias; **dry mouth, constipation,** jaundice, abdominal pain; urinary retention, urinary hesitancy, galactorrhea, gynecomastia, impaired ejaculation, amenorrhea

Interactions
- Alcohol and other CNS depressants (barbiturates, antihistamines, antianxiety or antidepressant drugs): Increased CNS depression, increased risk of EPSEs
- Amphetamines: Possible decreased antipsychotic effect
- Antacids (magnesium and aluminum products): Possible decreased antipsychotic effect
- Anticholinergics (atropine, H_1-type antihistamines, antidepressants, etc.): Increased risk of excessive atropine-like side effects or toxic effects
- Benztropine: Possible decreased antipsychotic effect, increased risk of severity of peripheral anticholinergic side effects
- Diazoxide: Possible severe hyperglycemia, prediabetic coma
- Guanethidine: Poor control of hypertension by guanethidine
- Hypoglycemia drugs (insulin, oral hypoglycemia agents): Poor diabetic control
- Lithium: Poor control of psychosis with combined therapy; can mask lithium toxicity; neurotoxicity with confusion, delirium, seizures, encephalopathy
- Meperidine, morphine: Increased risk of severe CNS depression, respiratory depression, hypotension
- Propranolol: Increased pharmacologic effects of either drug

Implications
Assess
- Establish baseline VS, laboratory values, to assess side effects, allergic or hypersensitivity reactions

- Assess physiologic and psychologic status before therapy to determine needs and evaluate progress
- Assess for early stages of tardive dyskinesia by use of abnormal involuntary movement scale
- Identify concurrent symptoms that may be aggravated by antipsychotics, e.g., glaucoma, diabetes

Planning/Implementation
- Ensure that drug has been taken; check mouth for "cheeking"
- If giving liquid, use only water, fruit juices, and the like; do not use caffeinated drinks or tea; take drug with food to minimize GI upset; give IM injections in lateral thigh
- Keep patient quiet after injection, to prevent falls associated with postural hypotension
- For dry mouth, give chewing gum, hard candies, lip balm; monitor urinary output; check for bladder distention in inactive patients, older men, and patients on high doses
- Assist with ambulation, if patient is having blurred vision; dim room lights for photosensitivity
- Ensure safety with hypotension; sit on side of bed before rising, head-low position for dizziness, avoid hot showers, wear elastic stockings
- Check B/P (supine, sitting, standing) and pulse before and after each dose when possible; observe for side effects
- Monitor body temperature for indications of neuroleptic malignant syndrome, e.g., muscle rigidity, fever, depressed neurologic status; ensure adequate hydration, nutrition, and ventilation
- Protect patient from exposure to extreme hot or cold
- Recognize impending hypersensitivity: pruritus or jaundice with hepatitis; flu or coldlike symptoms, evidence of bleeding with blood dyscrasia
- Observe for involuntary movements

Teaching
- About benefits and potential harm of antipsychotic drugs; weigh need to know against causing apprehension
- To comply with drug treatment
- To avoid activities requiring clear vision for a few weeks after treatment starts; to report eye pain immediately
- About the importance of exercise, fluids, and fiber in diet
- To watch for symptoms of heart failure, e.g., weight gain, dyspnea, distended neck veins, tachycardia
- Possible male sexual performance failure; suggest relaxed, stress-free environment
- To avoid conception; women should practice effective contraception; phenothiazines may cause false positive result in pregnancy tests
- To avoid exposure to sunlight; keep skin covered but with temperature-appropriate clothing
- That patient cannot become addicted to antipsychotic drugs

Evaluate
- Follows prescribed regimen, takes medications as ordered
- Avoids injury
- Verbalizes reduced anxiety
- Experiences minimal or no adverse responses
- Uses appropriate interventions to minimize side effects
- Achieves improved mental status

Lab Test Interferences

Increase: Liver function tests, cardiac enzyme levels, cholesterol, blood glucose, prolactin, bilirubin, cholinesterase, I-131 levels

Decrease: Hormones (blood, urine)

False positive: Pregnancy tests, PKU

Treatment of Overdose: Lavage, if orally ingested; provide an airway; do not induce vomiting, control EPSEs and hypotension

Administration
- Psychiatric indications: Psychiatric use in hospitalized patients: *Adults:* PO 8-16 bid-qid, gradually increased to desired dose, not to exceed 64 mg/day; IM 5 mg q6h, not to exceed 30 mg/day; *child >12 yr;* PO 8 mg in divided doses; *geriatric:* one half to one third of adult dose
- Nonhospitalized patients: *Adult:* PO 4-8 mg tid; IM 5 mg q6h
- Do not mix concentrate with liquids containing caffeine, tannics, or pectinates

- Available forms include: Tabs 2, 4, 8, 16; conc 16 mg/5 ml; inj IM 5 mg/ml;

Phenacemide*

PHENURONE

(fe-nass′e-mide) (Chapter 7)

Functional classification: Antiepileptic
Chemical classification: Acetylurea derivative
FDA pregnancy category: D

Indications: Refractory psychomotor seizures

Contraindications: Hypersensitivity, personality disorders
Cautious use: Hepatic disease, renal disease; use with other antiepileptics, blood dyscrasias, child <5 yr

Pharmacologic Effect: Increases seizure threshold

Pharmacokinetics: Metabolized by liver, excreted by kidneys, half-life not known

Side Effects: *CNS:* **Drowsiness** (4%), dizziness, insomnia, paresthesias, **psychiatric** (17%), depression, suicidal tendencies, aggression, headache; *Peripheral:* **Anorexia** (5%), weight loss, hepatitis, jaundice, nausea, nephritis, albuminuria, blood dyscrasias (primarily leukopenia) (2%), **rash** (5%), agranulocytosis, leukopenia, aplastic anemia

Interactions: Extreme caution if used with other antiepileptics, particularly ethotoin

Implications

Assess
- Blood, **liver function,** renal function studies
- Drug level: Drug is extremely toxic

Planning/Implementation
- Food decreases GI symptoms

Teaching
- All aspects of drug therapy: Action, dosage, side effects
- To notify physician when sore throat, fever, rash, fatigue, bleeding, bruising occur (blood dyscrasia)

Evaluate
- Mental status: Psychosis not uncommon
- Liver function, renal function
- Blood dyscrasias: Fever, sore throat, bruising, rash, jaundice

Treatment of Overdose: *Symptoms:* Excitement or mania, followed by drowsiness, ataxia, and coma; *Treatment:* Emesis, lavage, supportive care, careful evaluation of liver and kidney function

Administration
Adult: PO 250-500 mg tid, may increase by 500 mg/wk, not to exceed 5 g/day, usual maintenance dose 2-3 g/day; *child 5-10 yr:* ½ of adult dose at same intervals
- Available forms include: Tabs 500 mg

*Infrequently used.

Phenelzine Sulfate

NARDIL

(fen′el-zeen) (Chapter 5)

Functional classifications: Antidepressant, MAOI
Chemical classification: Hydrazine
FDA pregnancy category: C

Indications: Depression in treatment-resistant patients, patients with mixed anxiety-depression
Unlabeled uses: Bulimia, cocaine deterrent

Contraindications: Hypersensitivity to MAOIs, elderly patients (>60 yr), children <16 yr, hypertension, CHF, severe hepatic disease, pheochromocytoma, severe renal disease, severe cardiac disease
Cautious use: Suicidal patients, convulsive disorders, hyperactivity, diabetes mellitus, hypomania, agitation, hyperthyroidism

Pharmacologic Effect: Inhibits monoamine oxidase, thus increasing the concentration of endogenous epinephrine, norepinephrine, serotonin, dopamine in storage sites in CNS

Pharmacokinetics: Metabolized by liver, excreted by kidneys, half-life not established

Side Effects: *CNS:* **Dizziness,** drowsiness, confusion, **headache,** anxiety, **tremors,** stimulation, weakness, **hyperreflexia,** mania, **insomnia, fatigue,** weight gain; *Peripheral:* Change in libido; **constipation, dry mouth,** nausea and vomiting, **anorexia,** diarrhea, rash, flushing, increased perspiration, jaundice, **orthostatic hypotension, hypertension, arrhythmias,** hypertensive crisis, blurred vision

Interactions

- Drug-drug: *Sympathomimetics (indirect or mixed acting)*: Severe headache, hypertension, hyperpyrexia, and hypertensive crisis; sympathomimetic drugs include amphetamines; levodopa; tryptophan; methylphenidate; OTC compounds containing phenylpropanolamine, ephedrine, and pseudoephedrine; TCAs, other MAOIs, guanethidine, methyldopa, guanadrel, reserpine; *Anticholingeric drugs:* Additive effect; *Antihypertensives (diuretics, beta blockers, hydralazine, nitroglycerin, prazosin)*: Hypotension
- Drug-food: *Tyramine-rich foods* (see text): Hypertensive crisis

Implications

Assess

- B/P (lying, standing), pulse; if systolic B/P drops 20 mm Hg, withhold drug, notify physician
- Blood studies: CBC, leukocyte counts, cardiac enzyme levels (if patient is receiving long-term therapy)
- Hepatic studies: Hepatotoxic effects may occur

Planning/Implementation

- Increased fluids, bulk in diet, if constipation, urinary retention occur
- With food or milk for GI symptoms
- Sugarless gum, hard candy, or frequent sips of water for dry mouth
- Phentolamine for severe hypertension
- Storage in tight container in cool environment
- Assistance with ambulation during beginning of therapy because drowsiness or dizziness occurs
- Safety measures, including side rails
- Checking to see that PO medication is swallowed

Teaching

- That therapeutic effects may take 1-4 wk
- To avoid driving or other activities that require alertness
- To avoid ingesting alcohol and CNS depressants, or OTC medications for cold, weight loss, hay fever, cough
- Not to discontinue medication abruptly after long-term use
- To avoid high-tyramine foods, e.g., cheese (aged), caviar, dried fish, game meat, beer, wine, pickled products, liver, raisins, bananas, figs, avocados, meat tenderizers, chocolate, yogurt, increased caffeine, soy sauce
- Report headache, palpitations, neck stiffness

Evaluate

- Toxic effects: Increased headache, palpitation; discontinue drug immediately
- Mental status
- Urinary retention, constipation
- Withdrawal symptoms, e.g., Headache, nausea, vomiting, muscle pain, weakness

Treatment of Overdose: Lavage, activated charcoal, monitor electrolyte levels, VS, treat hypotension

Administration

Adult: PO 15 mg tid, may increase to 60 mg/day, dose should be reduced to 15 mg/day, not to exceed 90 mg/day

- Available forms include: Tabs 15 mg

Phenobarbital, Phenobarbital Sodium

BARBITA, LUMINAL SODIUM, SOLFOTON

(fee-noe-bar'bi-tal) (Chapter 7)

Functional classification: Antiepileptic (long-acting)

Chemical classification: Barbiturate

Controlled substance schedule IV

FDA pregnancy category: D

Indications: Tonic-clonic, simple partial, complex partial, status epilepticus

Contraindications: Hypersensitivity to barbiturates, porphyria, hepatic disease, respiratory disease, nephritis, diabetes mellitus, elderly, lactation, barbiturate addiction

Cautious use: Anemia, cardiac disease, children, fever, hyperthyroidism

Pharmacologic Effects: Decreases impulse transmission, works at level of thalamus, increases seizure threshold at cerebral cortex level; therapeutic serum level 15-40 μg/ml

Pharmacokinetics: PO onset 20-60 min, peak 8-12 hr, duration 10-12 hr, metabolized by liver, excreted by kidneys, crosses placenta, excreted in breast milk, half-life 53-118 hr

Side Effects: *CNS:* **Somnolence, drowsiness,** lethargy, hangover headache, flushing, hallucinations, coma; *Peripheral:* **Nausea, vomiting,** hypoventilation, bradycardia, hypotension, rash, urticaria, angioedema, local pain, swelling, necrosis, thrombophlebitis, blood dyscrasias

Interactions
- CNS depressants, other antiepileptics: Drugs that increase the effects of barbiturates (toxic effects)
- Acetaminophen, digitoxin, oral anticoagulants, oral contraceptives, TCAs, possibly phenytoin: Drugs whose effects are decreased by barbiturates

Implications
Assess
- Blood studies, liver function tests during long-term therapy
- Check VS, neurologic values regularly

Planning/Implementation
- Describe seizure accurately
- Offer consistent emotional support
- Monitor for early signs of toxic effects (slurred speech, ataxia, respiratory and CNS depression)

Teaching
- To report any side effects or adverse reactions
- To avoid driving or operating dangerous equipment
- To change position slowly
- To take drugs as prescribed
- Not to discontinue drug abruptly
- To wear MedicAlert identification bracelet
- To consult physician before becoming pregnant

Evaluate
- Mental status
- Respiratory depression
- Blood dyscrasias: Fever, sore throat, bruising, rash, jaundice

Treatment of Overdose: One g can cause serious poisoning in an adult; 2-10 g can be fatal. Toxic effects can be confused with drunkeness. Emesis, gastric lavage, if conscious; 30 g activated charcoal, maintain airway, good nursing care to prevent pneumonia

Administration
- Seizures: *Adult:* PO 50-100 mg bid-tid or total dose hs; *child:* PO 3-5 mg/kg/day in three divided doses; may be given as single dose hs
- Status epilepticus: *Adult:* IV 200-300 mg, repeat in 6 hr if necessary, run no faster than 50 mg/min, may give up to 20 mg/kg; *child:* IV 15-20 mg/kg over 10-15 min, then 6 mg/kg q 20 min prn, maximum dose 40 mg/kg/24 hr, run no faster then 50 mg/min
- Available forms: Caps 16 mg; elix 15, 20 mg/5 ml; tabs 8, 16, 32, 65, 100 mg; inj 30, 60, 65, 130 mg/ml

Phensuximide*
MILONTIN
(fen-sux'i-mide) (Chapter 7)

Functional classification: Antiepileptic
Chemical classification: Succinimide
FDA pregnancy category: D

Indications: Absence seizures (petit mal) refractory to other drugs

Contraindications: Hypersensitivity to succinimide derivatives
Cautious use: Lactation, hepatic disease, renal disease

Pharmacologic Effect: Inhibits spike and wave formation in absence seizures, depresses motor cortex

Pharmacokinetics: PO peak 1-4 hr, metabolized by liver, excreted by kidneys, half-life 4 hr

Side Effects: *CNS:* **Drowsiness, dizziness, fatigue, euphoria, lethargy;** anxiety, aggressiveness, irritability, depression, insomnia; *Peripheral:* **Nausea, vomiting,** heartburn, **anorexia, diarrhea, abdominal pain, cramps, constipation,** vaginal bleeding, hematuria, renal damage, urticaria, pruritic erythema, hirsutism, Stevens-Johnson syndrome, myopia, gum hypertrophy, tongue swelling, blurred vision,

*Infrequently used.

agranulocytosis, aplastic anemia, thrombocytopenia, leukocytosis, eosinophilia, pancytopenia (some blood dyscrasias have been fatal); urinary frequency

Interactions
- TCAs: Antagonist effect (imipramine, doxepin); also, lower seizure threshold
- Estrogens: Decreased effects of oral contraceptives
- CNS depressants: Increased CNS depression

Implications
Assess
- Renal studies: Urinalysis; BUN, urine creatinine levels
- Blood studies: CBC, hematocrit, hemoglobin level, reticulocyte counts
- Hepatic studies: AST, ALT, bilirubin and creatinine levels
- Drug levels during initial treatment

Planning/Implementation
- With food or milk, to decease GI symptoms
- Hard candy, frequent rinsing of mouth and gums, for dry mouth
- Assistance with ambulation during early part of treatment; dizziness occurs

Teaching
- To carry identification card or Medic-Alert bracelet, stating drugs taken, condition, physician's name and phone number
- To avoid driving and other activities that require alertness
- To avoid ingestion of alcohol and CNS depressants, since increased sedation may occur
- Not to discontinue medication suddenly after long-term use

Evaluate
- Therapeutic response: Decreased seizure activity; document on patient's chart
- Mental status
- Allergic reaction: Red raised rash, exfoliative dermatitis; if these occur, drug should be discontinued; blood dyscrasias: Fever, sore throat, bruising, rash, jaundice
- Toxic effects: Bone marrow depression, lupus have been reported

Administration
Adult and child: PO 500 mg-1 g bid or tid
- Available forms include: Caps 500 mg

Phenytoin, Phenytoin Sodium Extended, Phenytoin Sodium Prompt

DILANTIN, DILANTIN CAPSULES, DIPHENYLAN
(fen'i-toy-in) (Chapter 7)

Functional classification: Anticonvulsant
Chemical classification: Hydantoin
FDA pregnancy category: D

Indications: Drug of choice for tonic-clonic seizures; status epilepticus, psychomotor seizures; simple partial seizures

Contraindications: Hypersensitivity, psychiatric disease, sinus bradycardia (IV use), lactation
Cautious use: Allergies, hepatic disease, renal disease, hypotension, myocardial insufficiency

Pharmacologic Effect: Inhibits spread of seizure activity in motor cortex; therapeutic serum levels, 10-20 μg/ml

Pharmacokinetics: PO slowly absorbed, peak 4-12 hr (extended), 1½-3 hr (prompt); duration 5 hr; time to steady-state, 7-10 days; average half-life 22 hr, but dose dependent and has little clinical importance, metabolized by liver, excreted by kidneys

Side Effects: *CNS:* Nystagmus, ataxia, drowsiness, dizziness, insomnia, paresthesias, depression, suicidal tendencies, aggression, headache; *Peripheral:* effects: **Nausea, vomiting, constipation,** anorexia, weight loss, hepatitis, jaundice, nephritis, albuminuria, rash, gingival hyperplasia, agranulocytosis, leukopenia, aplastic anemia

Interactions
- Allopurinol, cimetidine, diazepam, disulfiram, alcohol (acute ingestion) phenacemide, succinimides, valproic acid, others: Increased effect of hydantoins

- Barbiturates, carbamazepine, alcohol (chronic use) theophylline, antacids, dietary calcium: Decreased effects of hydantoins
- Corticosteroids, dicumarol, digitoxin, doxycycline, haloperidol, methadone, oral contraceptives, dopamine, furosemide, levodopa: Decreased effects of these drugs

Implications

Assess

- Blood studies: CBC, platelet count q mo until stabilized, discontinue drug, if marked depression of the blood cell count occurs

Planning/Implementation

- Observe for gingival hyperplasia
- Describe seizures accurately

Teaching

- All aspects of drug administration: Route, action, dose
- To report side effects
- To avoid driving or operating dangerous equipment
- To practice good oral hygiene
- Not to discontinue abruptly
- To wear MedicAlert identification bracelet

Evaluate

- Mental status
- Respiratory depression
- Blood dyscrasias: Fever, sore throat, bruising, rash, jaundice

Treatment of Overdose: Mean lethal dose in adults is thought to be 2-5 g; initial symptoms are nystagmus, ataxia; death is due to respiratory and circulatory depression; lavage, emesis, activated charcoal

Administration

- Seizures: *Adult:* IV loading dose 10-15 mg/kg, run at 50 mg/min; PO loading dose 1 g in three divided doses, then after 24 hr, 300 mg/day (extended) or divided tid (prompt); *child:* IV 15-20 mg/kg, run at 50 mg/min; PO 4-8 mg/kg/day in divided doses
- Available forms include: Suspension 30, 125 mg/5 ml; tabs, chewable 50 mg; inj 50 mg/ml; caps ext rel 30, 100 mg; caps, prompt 30, 100 mg

Pimozide

ORAP

(pi′moe-zide) (Chapters 4, 15, 16)

Functional classifications: Antipsychotic, neuroleptic
Chemical classification: Diphenylbutylpiperidine
FDA pregnancy category: C

Indications: Tourette's disorder

Contraindications: Hypersensitivity, CNS depression, coma, tics other than those of Tourette's disorder, cardiac arrhythmias, long-QT interval
Cautious use: Child <12 yr, lactation, seizure disorders, hypertension, hepatic disease, cardiac disease, renal disease, hypokalemia

Pharmacologic Effects: Blocks CNS dopamine receptors

Pharmacokinetics: PO peak 6-8 hr; metabolized by liver, excreted in urine, half-life 55 hr

Side Effects: *CNS:* Parkinsonism, akathisias, dystonias, tardive dyskinesia, oculogyric crisis; *Peripheral:* Blurred vision (cycloplegia or paralysis of accommodation), ocular pain, photophobia, mydriasis, impaired vision; intolerance of extreme heat or cold, cold, possible heat stroke or fatal hyperthermia; nasal congestion, wheezing, dyspnea; **hypotension, especially orthostatic,** leading to dizziness, syncope; **tachycardia,** irregular pulse, arrhythmias; **dry mouth, constipation,** jaundice, abdominal pain; urinary frequency, galactorrhea, gynecomastia, impaired ejaculation, amenorrhea; prolonged QT interval, sudden death has occurred at doses >20 mg/day

Interactions

- Anticonvulsants: Decreased convulsive threshold
- Antiarrhythmics, phenothiazines: Increased QT interval
- Increased CNS depression: Alcohol and other CNS depressants
- Other antipsychotics: Increased EPSEs

Implications

Assess

- For prolonged QT interval
- Establish baseline VS, laboratory values, to assess side effects, allergic or hypersensitivity reactions
- Physiologic and psychologic status before therapy, to determine needs and evaluate progress
- For early stages of tardive dyskinesia by using abnormal involuntary movement scale
- Identify concurrent symptoms that may be aggravated by antipsychotics, e.g., glaucoma, diabetes

Planning/Implementation

- Ensure that drug has been taken; check mouth for "cheeking"
- Keep patient quiet after injection, to prevent falls associated with postural hypotension
- For dry mouth, give chewing gum, hard candies, lip balm, monitor urinary output; check for bladder distention in inactive patients, older men, and patients on high doses
- Assist with ambulation, if patient is having blurred vision; dim room lights for photosensitivity
- Ensure safety with hypotension; sit on side of bed before rising, head-low position for dizziness, avoid hot showers, wear elastic stockings
- Check B/P (supine, sitting, standing) and pulse before and after each dose when possible; observe for side effects
- Monitor body temperature for indications of neuroleptic malignant syndrome, e.g., muscle rigidity, fever, depressed neurologic status; ensure adequate hydration, nutrition, and ventilation
- Protect patient from exposure to extreme heat or cold
- Recognize impending hypersensitivity to pruritus or jaundice with hepatitis; flu or coldlike symptoms, evidence of bleeding with blood dyscrasia
- Observe for involuntary movements

Teaching:

- To comply with drug treatment
- To avoid activities requiring clear vision for a few weeks after treatment starts; to report eye pain immediately
- About the importance of exercise, fluids, and fiber in diet
- To watch for symptoms of heart failure, e.g., weight gain, dyspnea, distended neck veins, tachycardia
- Possible male sexual performance failure; suggest relaxed, stress-free environment
- To avoid conception; women should practice effective contraception
- To avoid exposure to sunlight; keep skin covered but with temperature-appropriate clothing
- That they cannot become addicted to antipsychotic drugs

Evaluate

- Follows prescribed regimen, takes medications as ordered
- Avoids injury; reports dizziness or need for assistance
- Verbalizes reduced anxiety
- Experiences minimal or no adverse responses
- Uses appropriate interventions to minimize side effects
- Achieves improved mental status

Treatment of Overdose: Lavage, if orally ingested; provide an airway; monitor ECG; do not induce vomiting; *do not* use epinephrine for hypotension; observe patient for at least 4 days

Administration

Adult and child >12 yr: PO 1-2 mg qd in divided doses; increase dose qod, if needed; maintenance <0.2 mg/kg/day or 10 mg/day, whichever is less, not to exceed 0.2 mg/kg/day or 10 mg/day

- Available forms include: Tabs 2 mg

Prazepam

CENTRAX

(pra'ze-pam) (Chapter 6)

Functional classification: Antianxiety
Chemical classification: Benzodiazepine
Controlled substance schedule IV
FDA pregnancy category: D

Indications: Anxiety

Contraindications: Hypersensitivity, narrow-angle glaucoma, psychosis, children <18 yr

Pharmacologic Effects: Depresses CNS, including limbic and reticular areas by potentiating GABA inhibitory neurotransmitters

Pharmacokinetics: Speed of onset: Slow PO peak levels 6 hr, half-life 30-100 hr, metabolized by liver, excreted in urine

Side Effects: *CNS:* Dizziness, drowsiness are main effects; see diazepam for other side effects; *Peripheral:* GI effects, i.e., dry mouth, nausea, vomiting; blurred vision, orthostatic hypotension; see diazepam for other side effects

Interactions
- Valproic acid: Increased effect of prazepam
- CNS depressants, alcohol, disulfiram: Increased CNS depression

Implications
Assess
- B/P

Planning/Implementation
- Give with food or milk to decrease GI upset
- Provide gum, hard candies for dry mouth
- Maintain safety

Teaching
- To avoid driving
- To avoid alcohol
- To check with clinician before taking OTC drugs

Evaluate
- Mental status
- Therapeutic response: Level of anxiety

Lab Test Interference
Increase: AST, ALT, serum bilirubin level, LDH
Decrease: RAIU
False increase: 17-OHCS

Treatment of Overdose: Lavage, monitor VS, provide supportive care as indicated; there are no recorded deaths with benzodiazepines alone; death occurs when these drugs are mixed with other CNS depressants

Administration
Adult: PO 30 mg/day in divided doses, range is 20 to 60 mg/day; *geriatric:* 10-15 mg/day in divided doses, can be given as single dose hs
- Available forms: Caps 5, 10, 20 mg; tabs 10 mg

Primidone

MYSOLINE, SERTAN†
(prí-mi-done) (Chapter 7)

Functional classification: Antiepileptic
Chemical classification: Barbiturate derivative
FDA pregnancy category: D

Indications: Generalized tonic-clonic, complex-partial seizures

Contraindications: Hypersensitivity, porphyria
Cautious use: Lactation

Pharmacologic Effects: Raises seizure threshold; metabolites (phenobaritol is one) have anticonvulsant properties; therapeutic serum level 5-12 μg/ml

Pharmacokinetics: PO peak 3 hr, excreted in breast milk, half-life 3-12 hr, but active metabolites are longer PEMA (24-48 hr); phenobarbital (53-118 hr)

Side Effects: *CNS:* Ataxia, vertigo, fatigue, drowsiness, nystagmus; *Peripheral:* **Nausea, vomiting, anorexia; rash,** alopecia, lupuslike syndrome, diplopia, nystagmus, impotence, thrombocytopenia, leukopenia, megaloblastic anemia

Interactions
- Alcohol, heparin, carbamazepine CNS depressants, isoniazid, phenytoin, phenobarbital: Increased levels of primidone
- Acetazolamide: Decreased effect of primidone

Implications
Assess
- Establish baseline data

Planning/Implementation
- Monitor for early signs of toxic effects

Teaching
- All aspects of drug administration: action, route, dose
- Not to withdraw drug quickly; withdrawal symptoms may occur
- Not to drive
- Notify physician if rash or blood dyscrasia symptoms occur
- Wear MedicAlert identification bracelet

†Available in Canada only.

Evaluate
- Mental status
- Respiratory depression
- Blood dyscrasias: Fever, sore throat, bruising, rash, jaundice

Administration
Adult and child >8 yr: Day 1-3, 100-125 mg hs; day 4-6, 100-125 mg bid; day 7-9, 100-125 mg tid; day 10 and maintenance, 250 mg tid or qid; do not exceed 500 mg/day; *child <8 yr:* Day 1-3, 50 mg hs; day 4-6, 50 mg bid; day 7-9, 100 mg bid; day 10 and maintenance, 125-250 mg tid or 10-25 mg/kg/day
- Available forms include: Tabs 50, 250 mg; susp 250 mg/5 ml

Procyclidine
KEMADRIN
(proe-sye′-kli-deen)

Functional classification: Anticholingergic
Chemical classification: Tertiary amine
FDA pregnancy category: C

Indications: Parkinsonism, EPSEs

Contraindications: Hypersensitivity, narrow-angle glaucoma, duodenal obstruction, peptic ulcer, prostatic hypertrophy, myasthenia gravis, megacolon

Pharmacologic Effects: Blocks cholinergic receptors; may inhibit the reuptake and storage of dopamine

Pharmacokinetics: Peak 1.1-2 hr, half-life 11.5-12.6 hr; little pharmacokinetic information is known

Side Effects: *CNS:* Depression develops in 19% to 30% of patients; disorientation, confusion, memory loss, hallucinations, psychoses, agitation, delusions, nervousness; *Peripheral:* **Tachycardia,** palpitations, hypotension, **orthostatic hypotension, dry mouth,** nausea, vomiting, constipation, paralytic ileus, **blurred vision,** mydriasis, diplopia, urinary retention and hesitancy, elevated temperature

Interactions
- Amantadine: Increased anticholinergic effect
- Digoxin: Increased digoxin serum levels
- Haloperidol: Worsening of schizophrenia, decreased haloperidol serum levels
- Levodopa: Possible reduction of levodopa efficacy
- Phenothiazines: Increased anticholingergic effect, decreased antipsychotic effect

Implications
Assess
- VS, B/P
- For glaucoma
- Mental status

Planning/Implementation
- Provide instructions for anticholinergic responses, i.e., dry mouth, constipation, urinary hesitancy, decreased sweating

Teaching
- Give with meals
- May cause drowsiness, blurred vision, dizziness: emphasize safety
- Avoid alcohol and other CNS depressants
- For rapid or pounding heartbeat, notify physician
- Use caution in hot weather

Evaluate
- EPSE improvement
- For adverse effects
- Mental status: Confusion, delirium, memory

Treatment of Overdose: Emesis, lavage, activated charcoal, treat respiratory depression, hyperpyrexia

Administration
- EPSE: ***Adult:*** PO 2.5 mg tid, up to 10-20 mg/day

Promazine*
PROMANYL,† PROZINE, SPARINE
(proe′ma-zeen) (Chapter 4)

Functional classification: Antipsychotic
Chemical classification: Aliphatic phenothiazine
FDA pregnancy category: C

Indications: Psychosis; *infrequently used* as antipsychotic

Contraindications: Hypersensitivity, blood dyscrasias, coma, children <12 yr, bone

*Infrequently used.
†Available in Canada only.

marrow depression; see chlorpromazine

Pharmacologic Effects: Provides antipsychotic effect by antagonizing dopamine receptors; also antiadrenergic, anticholinergic, and antiemetic; see chlorpromazine for more extensive explanation

Pharmacokinetics: PO peak level 2-4 hr; IM onset 15 min, peak level 1 hr, duration 4-6 hr; metabolized by liver, excreted in urine, crosses placenta, enters breast milk

Side Effects: *CNS:* See chlorpromazine; *Peripheral:* See chlorpromazine

Interactions: See chlorpromazine

Implications: See chlorpromazine

Lab Test Interference: See chlorpromazine

Treatment of Overdose: Do *not* induce vomiting; lavage for oral dose; maintain airway and provide supportive care prn

Administration

- Psychosis: *Adult:* PO 10-200 mg q 4-6 hr; range 40-1200 mg/day; however, recommended to not exceed 1000 mg/day; *severe agitation:* 50-150 mg IM; if not effective in 30 min, give additional doses up to total dose of 300 mg; *child* >12 yr: PO 10-25 mg q 4-6 hr
- Available forms: Tabs 25, 50, 100 mg; inj IM, IV, 25, 50 mg/ml

Propranolol HCl

INDERAL

(proe-pran'oh-lole) (Chapter 6)

Functional classifications: Antihypertensive, antianginal
Chemical classification: Beta-adrenergic blocker
FDA pregnancy category: C

Indications: Chronic stable angina pectoris, prophylaxis of angina pain; *unapproved use* for "stage fright" (use is controversial), anxiety, acute panic

Contraindications: Hypersensitivity to this drug, cardiac failure, cardiogenic shock, second- or third-degree heart block, asthma, sinus bradycardia

Cautious use: Diabetes mellitus, pheochromocytoma, hypotension, renal disease, lactation, CHF, hyperthroidism, cardiopulmonary distress, peripheral vascular disease

Pharmacologic Effects: Nonselective beta-blockers; reduces major symptoms of anxiety, e.g., Tachycardia, palpitations, muscle tremors

Pharmacokinetics: PO onset 30 min, peak 1-1½ hr, duration 6 hr; IV onset 2 min, peak 15 min, duration 3-6 hr; half-life 3-5 hr, metabolized by liver, crosses placenta and blood-brain barrier, excreted in breast milk

Side Effects: *CNS:* Depression, hallucinations, dizziness, fatigue, lethargy, paresthesias; *Peripheral:* Dyspnea, respiratory dysfunction, bronchospasm; **bradycardia, hypotension,** CHF, palpitations, agranulocytosis, thrombocytopenia, nausea, vomiting, diarrhea, colitis, constipation, cramps, dry mouth, rash, pruritus, fever, sore throat, laryngospasm

Interactions

- Verapamil, disopyramide: Increased propranolol effect
- Reserpine: Increased effects
- Norepinephrine, isoproterenol, barbiturates, rifampin, dopamine: Reduced beta-blocking effects
- Cimetidine, morphine: Increased beta-blocking effect
- Quinidine, haloperidol: Increased hypotension

Implications

Assess

- B/P, pulse, respirations during beginning of therapy

Teaching

- That drug may be taken before stressful activity, e.g., exercise, sexual activity
- To avoid hazardous activities, if dizziness occurs
- Emphasize patient compliance with complete medical regimen
- To make position changes slowly, to prevent fainting

Evaluate

- Headache, lightheadedness, decreased B/P; may indicate need for decreased dosage

Administration

Adult: Dose for stage fright is low, i.e., 10 mg before appearances

- Dysrythmia, hypertension, angina, myocardial infarction, pheochromocytoma, migraines: See *PDR*
- Available forms include: Caps ext rel 60, 80, 120, 160 mg; tabs 10, 20, 40, 60, 80, 90 mg; inj 1 mg/ml, oral solution 4, 8, 80 mg/ml

Protriptyline HCl

VIVACTIL

(proe-trip'te-leen) (Chapter 5)

Functional classification: TCA

Chemical classification: Dibenzocycloheptene, secondary amine

FDA pregnancy category: C

Indications: Depression

Contraindications: Hypersensitivity to TCAs, recovery phase of myocardial infarction, convulsive disorders, prostatic hypertrophy

Cautious use: Suicidal patients, severe depression, increased intraocular pressure, narrow-angle glaucoma, urinary retention, cardiac disease, hyperthyroidism, ECT, elective surgery, children, MAOI therapy

Pharmacologic Effect: Blocks reuptake of norepinephrine, serotonin into nerve endings, therapeutic serum levels 100-200 ng/ml

Pharmacokinetics: PO onset 15-30 min, peak 24-30 hr, duration 4-6 hr; therapeutic effect 2-3 wk; metabolized by liver, excreted by kidneys, crosses placenta, half-life 67-89 hr

Side Effects: *CNS:* **Sedation,** ataxia; confusion, delirium; *Peripheral:* **Blurred vision,** photophobia, increased intraocular pressure; decreased tearing, orthostatic hypotension, arrhythmias, tachycardia, palpitations, dry mouth, constipation, diarrhea, decreased sweating, **urinary retention, hesitancy**

Interactions

- Anticholinergic agents: Additive anticholinergic effects with atropine, antihistamines (H_1 blocker), antiparkinson drugs, antipsychotics, OTC cold and allergy drugs
- CNS depressants: Additive depressant effect
- Guanethidine, clonidine: Decreased antihypertensive effect
- MAOIs: Hypertensive crisis, atropine-like poisoning
- Oral contraceptives: Inhibits metabolism of TCAs
- Phenothiazines: May increase TCA serum level
- Quinidine: Additive effect, heart block possible
- Sympathomimetics: Potentiates sympathomimetic effects
- Thyroid preparations: Tachycardia, arrhythmias; may increase TCA effect

Implications

Assess

- Establish baseline data, to aid recognition of adverse responses to medication, e.g., liver enzyme levels, VS, renal function, mental status, speech patterns, affect, weight
- For signs of noncompliance, e.g., poor therapeutic response
- Observe for major symptoms of depression, e.g., apathy, sadness, sleep disturbances, hopelessness, guilt, decreased libido, spontaneous crying
- Review history for contraindicated conditions, e.g., glaucoma, CV disease, GI conditions, urologic conditions, seizures, pregnancy

Planning/Implementation

- Monitor for "cheeking" or hoarding; check drug dosage carefully, since a small overdose may cause toxic effects
- Monitor for suicidal ideations; suicidal thought content may increase as antidepressants begin to "energize" patient
- Monitor VS; if hypotension, tachycardia, or arrhythmias occur, withhold TCAs
- Give most TCAs in a single dose hs
- Observe for early signs of toxic effects, e.g., drowsiness, tachycardia, mydriasis, hypotension, agitation, vomiting, confusion, fever, restlessness, sweating
- If CNS overstimulation occurs, e.g., hypomania, delirium, discontinue drug

Teaching

- That these drugs may have faster onset (1 wk) than other TCAs

- To adhere to drug regimen
- To avoid OTC drugs, particularly those containing sympathomimetics or anticholinergics
- To avoid drugs listed in section on interactions
- About ways to deal with minor side effects, as follows: dry mouth, with hard candies, sips of water, mouth rinses; visual disturbances, with artificial tears, sunglasses, assistance with ambulation; constipation, with bulk-forming foods, increased fluids; urinary hesitancy, with adequate fluids, privacy; decreased perspiration, with appropriate clothing, avoidance of unnecessary exercise; orthostatic hypotension, with slow positional changes, avoidance of hot baths and showers; for drowsiness, take single dose hs with physician approval, avoid driving
- That abrupt discontinuance may result in cholinergic rebound, e.g., nausea, vomiting, insomnia, headache

Evaluate

- Desired therapeutic serum level
- Verbalize decrease in subjective symptoms
- Observe decrease in objective symptoms
- Minimal to no adverse drug effects
- Stable VS
- Less anxiety; sleep, talk, and feel better

Lab Test Interferences

- Increase: Serum bilirubin, blood glucose, alkaline phosphatase levels
- False increase: Urinary catecholamines
- Decrease: VMA, 5-HIAA

Treatment of Overdose: ECG monitoring, induce emesis, lavage, activated charcoal, administer anticonvulsant, treat anticholinergic effects, if needed

Administration

Adult: PO 15-40 mg/day in divided doses, may increase to 60 mg/day

Adolescent and geriatric: 5 mg tid, increase gradually if needed; CV monitoring is necessary for elderly patient receiving dosages over 20 mg/day

- Available forms include: Tabs 5, 10 mg

Secobarbital, Secobarbital Sodium

SECONAL, SECOGEN SODIUM,† SECONAL SODIUM, SERAL†
(see-koe-bar′bi-tal) (Chapter 8)

Functional classifications: Sedative, hypnotic
Chemical classification: Barbitone
Controlled substance schedule II
FDA pregnancy category: D

Indications: Insomnia, status epilepticus, other uses

Contraindications: Hypersensitivity, respiratory depression, barbiturate dependency, liver impairment, blood dyscrasias

Pharmacologic Effects: Short-acting barbiturate, causing CNS depression in limbic and reticular areas

Pharmacokinetics: Onset 10-15 min, duration 3-4 hr, half-life 15-40 hr, metabolized by liver, excreted in urine; of barbiturates, secobarbital is the most lipophilic and has highest protein binding

Side Effects: *CNS:* Drowsiness, lethargy, hangover are primary CNS side effects; see phenobarbital for general barbiturate effects; *Peripheral:* Respiratory depression, laryngospasm, brochospasm, GI upset, blood dyscrasias; see phenobarbital

Interactions

- CNS depressants and alcohol: Additive CNS depression
- MAOIs: CNS depression
- Oral anticoagulants, corticosteroids: Decreased effects of these drugs
- Doxycycline: Decreased half-life

Implications

Assess

- B/P; blood studies, if indicated

Planning/Implementation

- IM in large muscles
- If given IV, have emergency equipment nearby
- Give ½ hr before bedtime
- Maintain safety

†Available in Canada only.

Teaching
- To avoid driving
- To avoid alcohol
- To avoid discontinuing drug abruptly (withdrawal)

Evaluate
- Therapeutic response, i.e., sleeping
- Mental status
- Dependence?
- Toxic effects

Lab Test Interference: False increase: Sulfobromophthalein

Treatment of Overdose: Gastric lavage, charcoal to absorb drug, monitor B/P, VS, I&O; warm patient; hemodialysis may be effective

Administration
- Insomnia: *Adult:* PO/IM 100-200 mg hs
- REC: 4-5 mg/kg
- Status epilepticus: *Adult and child:* IM/IV 5.5 mg/kg; repeat q3-4h; rate not to exceed 50 mg/15 sec
- Available forms: Caps 50, 100 mg; tabs 100 mg; inj IM, IV 50 mg/ml; rec inj 50 mg/ml

Selegiline HCl

ELDEPRYL

(sel-ee-gilĺ-ene) (Chapter 14)

Functional classification: Antiparkinson
Chemical classification: MAOI
FDA pregnancy category: C

Indications: Parkinsonism adjunct to carbidopa/levodopa

Contraindications: Hypersensitivity

Pharmacologic Effect: Inhibits monoamine oxidase type B, increasing dopamine

Pharmacokinetics: Rapidly absorbed, peak ½ -2 hr; three active metabolites, including amphetamine (half-life 18 hr) and methamphetamine (half-life 20 hr); excreted in urine

Side Effects: *CNS:* Dizziness and lightheadedness (7%); parkinson-like symptoms; confusion (3%); hallucinations (3%); dyskinesias (2%); headache (2%), anxiety; *Peripheral:* **Nausea** (10%); abdominal pain (4%); dry mouth (3%); generalized aches, diarrhea, leg and back pain; urinary retention; weight loss

Interactions
- Meperidine: Fatalities have been reported with this combination

Implications

Assess
- B/P, respirations

Planning/Implementation
- Give with meals; limit protein taken with drug
- Keep doses <10 mg/day because monoamine oxidase inhibition may not be selective (may also inhibit monoamine oxidase type A, which could precipitate hypertensive crisis)

Teaching
- Patient may need to reduce levodopa
- Not to exceed 10 mg/day

Evaluate
- Therapeutic response: Decrease in symptoms of parkinsonism

Lab Test Interference
False positive: Urine ketones, urine glucose
False negative: Urine glucose
False increase: Uric acid, urine protein
Decrease: VMA

Treatment of Overdose: *Symptoms:* If selegiline nonselectively inhibits monoamine oxidase, look for symptoms similar to those found with MAOI overdose; see isocarboxazid

Administration
Adult: PO 5 mg at breakfast and at lunch (10 mg total); after 2-3 days, begin reducing carbidopa/levodopa by 10% to 30%
- Available forms: Tabs 5 mg

Sertraline

ZOLOFT

(sér-tra-leen) (Chapter 5)

Functional classification: Antidepressant
Chemical classification: Selective serotonin reuptake inhibitor
FDA pregnancy category: B

Indications: Depression

Contraindications: Hepatic dysfunction, renal impairment, lactation

Pharmacologic Effect: Inhibits CNS neuronal uptake of serotonin

Pharmacokinetics: Peak levels 4.5-8.4 hr; half-life 26 hr; sertraline undergoes extensive first-pass metabolism; excreted in urine; protein binding 98%

Side Effects: *CNS* (from premarketing trials): Headache (20%), dizziness (11%), tremor (10%), paresthesia (2%), insomnia (16%), somnolence (13%), agitation (5.6%); *Peripheral* (from premarketing trials): Dry mouth (16%), increased sweating (8%), palpitations (3.5%), rash (2%), diarrhea (17%), constipation (8%), dyspepsia (6%), vomiting (4%), gas (3%), anorexia (3%), abdominal pain (2.4%), sexual dysfunction (15.5%), abnormal vision (4%)

Interactions
- MAOIs: Fatal hypertensive crises have resulted from combining MAOIs and another selective serotonin reuptake inhibitor
- Drugs highly bound to plasma proteins: Displacement of sertraline or one of these drugs could result in adverse responses
- Alcohol: CNS depression
- Diazepam: Decreased clearance of diazepam

Implications
Assess
- B/P, VS
- Hepatic studies because of sertraline's extensive liver metabolism
- Weight loss
- Activation of mania

Planning/Implementation
- Maintain safety
- Closely supervise patients at high risk for suicide because some professionals believe that a relationship exists between suicide and alterations in serotonin levels
- Give with food to minimize first-pass metabolism

Teaching
- Caution about driving (no impairment in driving ability has been recorded with use of sertraline)
- To avoid alcohol (no impairment resulting from this combination has been recorded)
- Caution about use of OTC products

Evaluate
- Therapeutic effect: Depression
- Mental status

Lab Test Interference
Increase: AST, ALT; small increase in cholesterol, triglyceride, and serum uric acid levels

Treatment of Overdose: Three cases (no deaths) have been reported as of 1992; establish and maintain airway; administer oxygen prn; charcoal may inhibit absorption and may be more effective than induced vomiting

Administration
Adult: PO 50 mg initially, once daily (morning or evening); increases can be made weekly (because of long half-life); maximum dose, 200 mg/day
- Available forms: Tabs 50, 100 mg

Succinylcholine Chloride

ANECTINE, ANECTINE FLO-PACK, QUELICIN, SCALINE,† SUCOSTRIN†
(suk-sin-ill-koe'leen) (Chapter 11)

Functional classification: Neuromuscular blocker (depolarizing, ultrashort)
FDA pregnancy category: C

Indications: Facilitates endotracheal intubation during ECT; reduces intensity of convulsions during ECT; other indications for use with general anesthesia are given in *PDR*

Contraindications: Hypersensitivity, malignant hyperthermia, **decreased plasma pseudocholinesterase**, elevated CPK
Cautious use: Cardiac disease, severe burns, fractures, lactation, children <2 yr, electrolyte imbalances, dehydration, neuromuscular disease, respiratory disease, collagen diseases, glaucoma, eye surgery, penetrating eye wounds, elderly or debilitated patients

Pharmacologic Effect: Inhibits transmission of nerve impulses by binding with cholinergic receptors at motor endplate; muscle depolarizes and can be seen as fa-

†Available in Canada only.

Bold = Most common side effects.

R S

siculations head to foot; recovery follows a reverse process

Pharmacokinetics: IV onset 30-60 sec, peak 2-3 min, duration 4-6 min; IM onset 1-3 min; hydrolyzed by pseudocholinesterase to active and inactive metabolites

Side Effects: *Peripheral:* Bradycardia, tachycardia, increased, decreased B/P, sinus arrest, arrhythmias, **prolonged apnea,** bronchospasm, cyanosis, **respiratory depression,** increased secretions, increased intraocular pressure, weakness, muscle pain, **fasciculations,** prolonged relaxation, myoglobulinemia, rash, flushing, pruritus, urticaria, malignant hyperthermia

Interactions
- Phenelzine, promazine, oxytocin, beta blockers, procainamide, anticholinesterases; quinidine, local anesthetics, polymyxin antibiotics, lithium, thiazides, enflurane, isoflurane: Increased neuromuscular blockade
- Theophylline: Arrhythmias
- Diazepam: Reduction of neuromuscular block
- Narcotic analgesics: Bradycardia
- Do not mix with barbiturates in solution or syringe

Implications
Assess
- For electrolyte imbalances (K, Mg); may lead to increased action of this drug
- VS until fully recovered from ECT; rate, depth, pattern of respirations, strength of hand grip

Planning/Implementation
- Anticholinesterase to reverse neuromuscular blockade
- If communication is difficult during recovery from neuromuscular blockade, offer reassurance

Evaluate
- Therapeutic response: Paralysis
- Recovery
- Prolonged apnea, allergic reactions, i.e., rash, fever, respiratory distress, pruritus: Drug should be discontinued

Treatment of Overdose: Use peripheral nerve stimulator to determine whether in phase I or phase II block; if phase II, give anticholinesterase, monitor VS; may require mechanical ventilation

Administration
Adult: IV 25-75 mg (average dose 0.6 mg/kg), then 2.5 mg/min prn; IM 2.5 mg/kg, not to exceed 150 mg; *child:* IV 1-2 mg/kg, IM 3-4 mg/kg, not to exceed 150 mg IM
- Available forms include: Inj IM IV 20, 50, 100 mg/ml; powder for inj 100, 500 mg/vial, 1 g/vial

Temazepam

RESTORIL

(te-maz'e-pam) (Chapter 8)

Functional classifications: Sedative, hypnotic
Chemical classification: Benzodiazepine
Controlled substance schedule IV
FDA pregnancy category: X

Indications: Insomnia

Contraindications: Hypersensitivity to benzodiazepines, lactation
Cautious use: Sleep apnea, hepatic disease, renal disease, suicidal individuals, drug abuse, elderly patients, depression, child <18 yr

Pharmacologic Effect: Produces CNS depression

Pharmacokinetics: PO onset 30-45 min, duration 6-8 hr, half-life 9.5-12.4 hr; metabolized by liver, excreted by kidneys, crosses placenta, excreted in breast milk

Side Effects: *CNS:* Euphoria, drowsiness, daytime sedation, dizziness, confusion, lightheadedness, headache, depression, irritability; *Peripheral:* Nausea, vomiting, diarrhea, heartburn, abdominal pain, constipation, chest pain, palpitations

Interactions
- Cimetidine, disulfiram: Prolong half-life of benzodiazepines
- Alcohol, CNS depressants: CNS depression
- Antacids: Decrease effects of benzodiazepines
- Digoxin: Digoxin intoxication

Implications
Assess
- VS

Planning/Implementation
- For sleeplessness, ½ -1 hr before bedtime
- If GI symptoms occur, may be taken with food
- Assistance with ambulation
- Side rails, night light, call bell within easy reach
- Checking to see that medication has been swallowed

Teaching
- To avoid driving or other activities requiring alertness until drug regimen is stabilized
- To avoid ingestion of alcohol or CNS depressants
- That it may take two nights for benefits to be noticed
- That hangover is common in elderly persons but less common than with barbiturates

Evaluate
- Therapeutic response: Ability to sleep at night, decreased amount of early morning awakening when taking drug for insomnia
- Mental status
- Type of sleep problem, falling asleep, staying asleep

Lab Test Interferences
Increase: ALT/AST, serum bilirubin level
Decrease: RAIU
False increase: Urinary 17-OHCS

Treatment of Overdose: Lavage, monitor electrolytes, VS, supportive care

Administration
Adult: PO 15-30 mg hs
Geriatric, debilitated: 15 mg until individual response is determined
- Available forms include: Caps 15, 30 mg

Thioridazine HCl

MELLARIL, NOVORIDAZINE,† THIORIDAZINE
(thyr-or-rid'a-zeen) (Chapters 4, 17)

Functional classifications: Antipsychotic, neuroleptic
Chemical classifications: Phenothiazine, piperidine
FDA pregnancy category: C

Indications: Psychotic disorders, behavioral problems in children, anxiety, major depressive disorders

Contraindications: Hypersensitivity, blood dyscrasias, coma, child <2 yr, brain damage, bone marrow depression, parkinsonism
Cautious use: Lactation, seizure disorders, hypertension, hepatic disease, cardiac disease

Pharmacologic Effects: Antipsychotic drugs produce a neuroleptic effect characterized by sedation, emotional quieting, psychomotor slowing, and affective indifference; exact mode of action is not fully understood; antipsychotics block dopamine receptors in the basal ganglia, hypothalamus, limbic system, brain stem, and medulla; antipsychotics are also thought to depress certain components of the reticular activating system that partially control body temperature, wakefulness, vasomotor tone, emesis, and hormonal balance; additionally, antipsychotics have significant anticholinergic and alpha-adrenergic blocking effects; least antiemetic of all phenothiazines

Pharmacokinetics: PO onset erratic, peak 2-4 hr; metabolized by liver, excreted in urine, crosses placenta, enters breast milk, half-life 26-36 hr

Side Effects: *CNS:* Parkinsonism, akathisias, dystonias, tardive dyskinesias, oculogyric crisis; *Peripheral:* Blurred vision (cycloplegia or paralysis of accommodation); ocular pain, photophobia, mydriasis, impaired vision; intolerance of extreme heat or cold, possible heat stroke or fatal hyperthermia; nasal congestion, wheezing, dys-

†Available in Canada only.

pnea; **hypotension, especially orthostatic,** leading to dizziness, syncope; **tachycardia,** irregular pulse, arrhythmias; **dry mouth, constipation,** jaundice, abdominal pain; urinary retention, urinary hesitancy, galactorrhea, gynecomastia, impaired ejaculation, amenorrhea

Interactions

- Alcohol and other CNS depressants (barbiturates, antihistamines, antianxiety or antidepressant drugs): Increased CNS depression, increased risk of EPSEs
- Amphetamines: Possible decreased antipsychotic effect
- Antacids (magnesium and aluminum products): Possible decreased antipsychotic effect
- Anticholinergics (atropine, H_1-type antihistamines, antidepressants, etc.): Increased risk of excessive atropine-like side effects or toxic effects
- Benztropine: Possible decreased antipsychotic effect, increased risk of severity of peripheral anticholinergic side effects
- Diazoxide: Possible severe hyperglycemia, prediabetic coma
- Guanethidine: Poor control of hypertension by guanethidine
- Hypoglycemia drugs (insulin, oral hypoglycemia agents): Poor diabetic control
- Lithium: Poor control of psychosis with combined therapy; can mask lithium intoxication; neurotoxic effects with confusion, delirium, seizures, encephalopathy
- Meperidine, morphine: Increased risk of severe CNS depression, respiratory depression, hypotension
- Propranolol: Increased pharmacologic effects of either drug

Implications

Assess

- Establish baseline VS, laboratory values, to assess side effects, allergic or hypersensitivity reactions
- Physiologic and psychologic status before therapy, to determine needs and evaluate progress
- For early stages of tardive dyskinesia by use of abnormal involuntary movement scale
- Identify concurrent symptoms that may be aggravated by antipsychotics, e.g., glaucoma, diabetes

Planning/Implementation

- Ensure that drug has been taken; check mouth for "cheeking"
- If giving liquid antipsychotics, use at least 60 ml of distilled water or fruit juice to mask taste; dilute and give immediately; take drug with food to minimize GI upset
- Keep patient quiet after injection, to prevent falls associated with postural hypotension
- For dry mouth, give chewing gum, hard candies, lip balm; monitor urinary output; check for bladder distention in inactive patients, older men, and patients on high doses
- Assist with ambulation, if patient is having blurred vision; dim room lights for photosensitivity
- Ensure safety with hypotension; sit on side of bed before rising, head-low position for dizziness, avoid hot showers, wear elastic stockings
- Check B/P (supine, sitting, standing) and pulse before and after each dose when possible; observe for side effects
- Monitor body temperature for indications of neuroleptic malignant syndrome, e.g., muscle rigidity, fever, depressed neurologic status; ensure adequate hydration, nutrition, and ventilation
- Protect patient from exposure to extreme hot or cold
- Recognize impending hypersensitivity: pruritis or jaundice with hepatitis; flu or coldlike symptoms, evidence of bleeding with blood dyscrasia
- Observe for involuntary movements

Teaching

- About benefits and potential harm of antipsychotic drugs; weigh need to know against causing apprehension
- To comply with drug treatment
- To avoid activities requiring clear vision for a few weeks after treatment starts; to report eye pain immediately
- About the importance of exercise, fluids, and fiber in diet
- To watch for symptoms of heart failure, e.g., weight gain, dyspnea, distended neck veins, tachycardia

- Possible male sexual performance failure; suggest relaxed, stress-free environment
- To avoid conception; women should practice effective contraception; phenothiazines may cause false-positive result in pregnancy tests
- To avoid exposure to sunlight; keep skin covered but with temperature-appropriate clothing
- That patient cannot become addicted to antipsychotic drugs

Evaluate

- Follows prescribed regimen, takes medications as ordered
- Avoids injury; reports dizziness or need for assistance
- Verbalizes reduced anxiety
- Experiences minimal or no adverse responses
- Uses appropriate interventions to minimize side effects
- Achieves improved mental status

Lab Test Interferences

Increase: Liver function tests, cardiac enzyme levels, cholesterol, blood glucose, prolactin, bilirubin, PBI, cholinesterase, I-131 levels

Decrease: Hormones (blood, urine)

False positive: Pregnancy tests, PKU

False negative: Urinary steroids

Treatment of Overdose: Lavage, provide an airway; do not induce vomiting; control EPSEs and hypotension

Administration

- Psychosis: *Adult:* PO 50-100 mg tid, *maximum dose* 800 mg/day; dosage is gradually increased to desired response, then reduced to minimum maintenance dose
- Depression, behavioral problems: *Adult:* PO 25 tid, range from 10 mg bid-qid to 50 mg tid-bid; *child 2-12 yr;* PO 0.5-3 mg/kg/day in divided doses
- Mix concentrate in distilled water or orange or grapefruit juice
- Available forms include: Tabs 10, 15, 25, 50, 100, 150, 200 mg; conc 30, 100 mg/ml; susp 25, 100 mg/5 ml

Thiothixene

NAVANE

(thye-oh-thix'een) (Chapters 4, 15, 16)

Functional classifications: Antipsychotic, neuroleptic

Chemical classification: Thioxanthene

FDA pregnancy category: C

T U

Indications: Psychotic disorders

Contraindications: Hypersensitivity, blood dyscrasias, child <12 yr, bone marrow depression

Cautious use: Lactation, seizure disorders, hypertension, hepatic disease

Pharmacologic Effects: Antipsychotic drugs produce a neuroleptic effect characterized by sedation, emotional quieting, psychomotor slowing, and affective indifference; exact mode of action is not fully understood; Antipsychotics block dopamine receptors in the basal ganglia, hypothalamus, limbic system, brain stem, and medulla; antipsychotics are also thought to depress certain components of the reticular activating system that partially control body temperature, wakefulness, vasomotor tone, emesis, and hormonal balance; additionally, antipsychotics have significant anticholinergic and alpha-adrenergic blocking effects

Pharmacokinetics: PO onset slow, peak 2-8 hr, duration up to 12 hr; IM onset 15-30 min, peak 1-6 hr, duration up to 12 hr; metabolized by liver, excreted in urine, crosses placenta, enters breast milk, half-life 34 hr

Side Effects: *CNS:* Parkinsonism, akathisias, dystonias, tardive dyskinesia, oculogyric crisis; *Peripheral:* Blurred vision (cycloplegia or paralysis of accommodation), ocular pain, photophobia, mydriasis, impaired vision; intolerance of extreme heat or cold, possible heat stroke or fatal hyperthermia; nasal congestion, wheezing, dyspnea; **hypotension, especially orthostatic,** leading to dizziness, syncope; **tachycardia,** irregular pulse, arrhythmias; **dry mouth, constipation,** jaundice, abdominal pain; urinary retention, urinary hesitancy, galactorrhea, gynecomastia, impaired ejaculation, amenorrhea

Interactions

- Alcohol and other CNS depressants (barbiturates, antihistamines, antianxiety or antidepressant drugs): Increased CNS depression, increased risk of EPSEs
- Amphetamines: Possible decreased antipsychotic effect
- Antacids (magnesium and aluminum products): Possible decreased antipsychotic effect
- Anticholinergics (atropine, H_1-type antihistamines, antidepressants, etc.): Increased risk of excessive atropine-like side effects or toxic effects
- Benztropine: Possible decreased antipsychotic effect, increased risk of severity of peripheral anticholinergic side effects
- Diazoxide: Possible severe hyperglycemia, prediabetic coma
- Guanethidine: Poor control of hypertension by guanethidine
- Hypoglycemia drugs (insulin, oral hypoglycemia agents): Poor diabetic control
- Lithium: Poor control of psychosis with combined therapy; can mask lithium intoxication; neurotoxic effects with confusion, delirium, seizures, encephalopathy
- Meperidine, morphine: Increased risk of severe CNS depression, respiratory depression, hypotension
- Propranolol: Increased pharmacologic effects of either drug

Implications

Assess

- Establish baseline VS, laboratory values, to assess side effects, allergic or hypersensitivity reactions
- Physiologic and psychologic status before therapy, to determine needs and evaluate progress
- For early stages of tardive dyskinesia by use of abnormal involuntary movement scale
- Identify concurrent symptoms that may be aggravated by antipsychotics, e.g., glaucoma, diabetes

Planning/Implementation

- Ensure that drug has been taken; check mouth for "cheeking"
- If giving liquid antipsychotics, use at least 60 ml of compatible beverage to mask taste; dilute and give immediately; take drug with food to minimize GI upset; give IM injections in lateral thigh
- Keep patient quiet after injection, to prevent falls associated with postural hypotension
- For dry mouth, give chewing gum, hard candies, lip balm; monitor urinary output; check for bladder distention in inactive patients, older men, and patients on high doses
- Assist with ambulation, if patient is having blurred vision; dim room lights for photosensitivity
- Ensure safety with hypotension; sit on side of bed before rising, head-low position for dizziness, avoid hot showers, wear elastic stockings
- Check B/P (supine, sitting, standing) and pulse before and after each dose when possible; observe for side effects
- Monitor body temperature for indications of neuroleptic malignant syndrome, e.g., muscle rigidity, fever, depressed neurologic status; ensure adequate hydration, nutrition, and ventilation
- Protect patient from exposure to extreme hot or cold
- Recognize impending hypersensitivity: pruritus or jaundice with hepatitis; flu or coldlike symptoms, evidence of bleeding with blood dyscrasia
- Observe for involuntary movements

Teaching

- About benefits and potential harm of antipsychotic drugs; weigh need to know against causing apprehension
- To comply with drug treatment
- To avoid activities requiring clear vision for a few weeks after treatment starts; to report eye pain immediately
- About the importance of exercise, fluids, and fiber in diet
- To watch for symptoms of heart failure, e.g., Weight gain, dyspnea, distended neck veins, tachycardia
- Possible male sexual performance failure; suggest relaxed, stress-free environment
- To avoid conception; women should practice effective contraception
- To avoid exposure to sunlight; keep skin covered but with temperature-appropriate clothing

- That patient cannot become addicted to antipsychotic drugs

Evaluate

- Follows prescribed regimen; takes medications as ordered
- Avoids injury; reports dizziness or need for assistance
- Verbalizes reduced anxiety
- Experiences minimal or no adverse responses
- Uses appropriate interventions to minimize side effects
- Achieves improved mental status

Lab Test Interferences

- Increase: Liver function tests, cardiac enzyme levels, cholesterol, blood glucose, prolactin, bilirubin, PBI, cholinesterase, ^{131}I levels
- Decrease: Uric acid

Treatment of Overdose: Lavage, if orally ingested; provide an airway; do not induce vomiting

Administration

Adult: PO 2-5 mg bid-qid, depending on severity of condition; dose is gradually increased to 20-30 mg, if needed; IM 4 mg bid-qid, maximum dose is 30 mg qd; administer PO dose as soon as possible

- Mix concentrate in orange or grapefruit juice
- Available forms include: Caps 1, 2, 5, 10, 20 mg; conc 5 mg/ml; inj IM 2 mg/ml; powder for inj 5 mg/ml

Tranylcypromine Sulfate

PARNATE

(tran-ill-sip'roe-meen) (Chapter 5)

Functional classifications: Antidepressant, MAOI

Chemical classification: Nonhydrazine

FDA pregnancy category: C

Indications: Depression refractory to drug therapy

Contraindications: Hypersensitivity to MAOIs, elderly patients (>60 yr), children <16 yr, hypertension, CHF, severe hepatic disease, pheochromocytoma, severe renal disease, severe cardiac disease

Cautious use: Suicidal patients, convulsive disorders, schizophrenia, hyperactivity, diabetes mellitus, hypomania, agitation, hyperthyroidism

Pharmacologic Effect: Inhibits monoamine oxidase, thus increasing the concentration of endogenous epinephrine, norepinephrine, serotonin, dopamine in storage sites in CNS

Pharmacokinetics: Metabolized by liver, excreted by kidneys, excreted in breast milk, half-life not established

Side Effects: *CNS:* **Dizziness,** drowsiness, confusion, **headache,** anxiety, **tremors,** stimulation, weakness, **hyperreflexia,** mania, **insomnia, fatigue,** weight gain; *Peripheral:* Change in libido, **constipation, dry mouth,** nausea and vomiting, **anorexia,** diarrhea, rash, flushing, increased perspiration, jaundice, **orthostatic hypotension, hypertension, arrhythmias,** hypertensive crisis, blurred vision

Interactions

- Drug-drug: *Sympathomimetics (indirect or mixed acting):* Severe headache, hypertension, hyperpyrexia, and hypertensive crisis; sympathomimetic drugs include amphetamines, levodopa, tryptophan, methylphenidate, OTC compounds containing phenylpropanolamine, ephedrine, and pseudoephedrine; TCAs, other MAOIs, guanethidine, methyldopa, guanadrel, and reserpine; *Anticholinergic drugs:* Additive effect; *Antihypertensive drugs (diuretics, beta blockers, hydralazine, nitroglycerin, prazosin):* Hypotension
- Drug-food: *Tyramine-rich foods* (see text): Hypertensive crisis

Implications

Assess

- B/P (lying, standing), pulse; if systolic B/P drops 20 mm Hg, withhold drug, notify physician
- Blood studies: CBC, leukocyte count, cardiac enzyme levels (if patient is receiving long-term therapy)
- Hepatic studies: Hepatotoxicity may occur

Planning/Implementation:

- Increased fluids, bulk in diet, if constipation or urinary retention occurs
- With food or milk for GI symptoms

- Gum, hard candy, or frequent sips of water for dry mouth
- Phentolamine for severe hypertension
- Storage in tight container in cool environment
- Assistance with ambulation during beginning of therapy because drowsiness or dizziness occurs
- Safety measures, including side rails
- Checking to see that PO medication is swallowed

Teaching
- That therapeutic effects may take 2 days to 3 weeks
- To avoid driving or performing other activities that require alertness
- To avoid alcohol ingestion, CNS depressants or OTC medications for cold, weight, hay fever, cough
- Not to discontinue medication suddenly after long-term use
- To avoid high-tyramine foods like cheese (aged), caviar, dried fish, game meat, beer, wine, pickled products, liver, raisins, bananas, figs, avocados, meat tenderizers, chocolate, yogurt, increased caffeine, soy sauce
- Report headache, palpitations, neck stiffness

Evaluate
- Toxic effects: Increased headache, palpitation; discontinue drug immediately
- Mental status
- Urinary retention, constipation
- Withdrawal symptoms: Headache, nausea, vomiting, muscle pain, weakness

Treatment of Overdose: Lavage, activated charcoal, monitor electrolytes, VS, treat hypotension

Administration

Adult: 30 mg/day in divided doses; if no improvement after 2 weeks, increase by 10 mg/day in increments of 1-3 weeks, maximum dose 60 mg/day

- Available forms include: Tabs 10 mg

Trazodone HCl

DESYREL

(tray'zoe-done) (Chapter 5)

Functional classification: Tricyclic-like antidepressant
Chemical classification: Triazolopyridine
FDA pregnancy category: C

Indications: Depression
Unlabeled uses: Cocaine withdrawal, aggressive behavior, panic disorder

Contraindications: Hypersensitivity to trazodone, child <18 yr
Cautious use: Suicidal patients, hypotension, priapism, narrow-angle glaucoma, urinary retention, cardiac disease, hepatic disease, hyperthyroidism, ECT, elective surgery

Pharmacologic Effects: Selectively inhibits serotonin uptake in brain; therapeutic plasma levels 800-1600 ng/ml

Pharmacokinetics: Metabolized by liver, excreted by kidneys and feces; peak 1 hr without food; half-life 3-9 hr (biphasic)

Side Effects: *CNS:* Anger, ataxia, confusion, delirium; *Peripheral:* **Blurred vision,** photophobia, increased intraocular pressure, decreased tearing, orthostatic hypotension, arrhythmias, tachycardia, palpitations, dry mouth, constipation, diarrhea, decreased sweating, **priapism**

Interactions
- CNS depressants: Additive depressant effect
- MAOIs: Hypertensive crisis, atropine-like poisoning
- Phenytoin: May increase phenytoin level

Implications

Assess
- Establish baseline data, to aid recognition of adverse responses to medication, e.g., liver enzyme levels, VS, renal function, mental status, speech patterns, affect, weight
- For signs of noncompliance, e.g., poor therapeutic response
- Observe for major symptoms of depression, e.g., Apathy, sadness, sleep disturbances, hopelessness, guilt, decreased libido, spontaneous crying

- Review history for contraindicated conditions, e.g., glaucoma, CV disease, GI conditions, urologic conditions, seizures, pregnancy

Planning/Implementation
- Monitor for "cheeking" or hoarding; check drug dosage carefully, since a small overdose may cause toxic effects
- Monitor for suicidal ideations; suicidal thought content may increase as antidepressants begin to "energize" patient
- Monitor VS; if hypotension, tachycardia, or arrhythmias occur, withhold drug
- Observe for early signs of toxic effects, e.g., drowsiness, tachycardia, mydriasis, hypotension, agitation, vomiting, confusion, fever, restlessness, sweating
- If CNS overstimulation occurs, e.g., hypomania, delirium, discontinue drug

Teaching
- That this drugs has a lag time of up to 2-4 weeks
- To adhere to drug regimen
- To avoid alcohol and other depressants
- To avoid drugs listed in section on interactions
- About ways to deal with minor side effects, as follows: dry mouth, with hard candies, sips of water, mouth rinses; visual disturbances, with artificial tears, sunglasses, assistance with ambulation; constipation, with bulk-forming foods, increased fluids; urinary hesitancy, with adequate fluids, privacy; decreased perspiration, with appropriate clothing, avoidance of unnecessary exercise; orthostatic hypotension, with slow positional changes, avoidance of hot baths and showers; for drowsiness, take single dose hs with physician approval, avoid driving
- To notify physician and discontinue use of the drug if prolonged, painful erection occurs
- To take with food

Evaluate
- Desired therapeutic serum level
- Verbalize decrease in subjective symptoms
- Observe decrease in objective symptoms
- Minimal to no adverse drug effects
- Stable VS
- Less anxiety; sleep, talk, and feel better

Lab Test Interferences
Increases: Serum bilirubin, blood glucose, alkaline phosphatase levels
Decreases: VMA, 5-HIAA

Treatment of Overdose: Deaths have occurred as a result of use of trazodone and another drug (i.e., alcohol); there is no antidote; supportive care of hypotension and excessive sedation, gastric lavage

Administration
Adult: PO 150 mg/day in divided doses, may be increased by 50 mg/day q3-4d, not to exceed 600 mg/day
- Available forms include: Tabs 50, 100, 150, 300 mg

Triazolam
HALCION
(trye-ay'zoe lan) (Chapter 8)

Functional classifications: Sedative, hypnotic
Chemical classification: Benzodiazepine
Controlled substance schedule IV
FDA pregnancy category: X

Indications: Insomnia

Contraindications: Pregnancy, hypersensitivity to benzodiazepines, lactation
Cautious use: Depression, hepatic and renal disease, elderly patients, drug abuse, narrow-angle glaucoma, child <18 yr

Pharmacologic Effect: Produces CNS depression

Pharmacokinetics: PO onset 30-45 min, peak 0.5-2 hr, duration 6-8 hr, metabolized by liver, excreted by kidneys, crosses placenta, excreted in breast milk, half-life 1.5-5.5 hr

Side Effects: *CNS:* Anterograde amnesia, drowsiness, daytime sedation, dizziness, confusion, lightheadedness, headache, irritability; *Peripheral:* Nausea, vomiting, diarrhea, heartburn, abdominal pain, constipation, chest pain, palpitations

Interactions
- Cimetidine, disulfiram: Prolong half-life of benzodiazepines
- Alcohol, CNS depressants: CNS depression
- Antacids: Decrease effects of benzodiazepines
- Digoxin: Digoxin intoxication

Implications

Assess

- VS

Planning/Implementation

- For sleeplessness, ½ -1 hr before bedtime
- If GI symptoms occur, may be taken with food
- Assistance with ambulation
- Side rails, night light, call bell within easy reach
- Checking to see that medication has been swallowed

Teaching

- To avoid driving or other activities requiring alertness until drug is stabilized
- To avoid ingestion of alcohol or CNS depressants; serious CNS depression may result
- That it may take two nights to be able to sleep
- Triazolam should not be taken if a full night's rest cannot be obtained
- That hangover is common in elderly patients but less common than with barbiturates

Evaluate

- Therapeutic response: Ability to sleep at night, decreased amount of early morning awakening, if taking drug for insomnia
- Mental status: Mood, sensorium, affect, memory (long-term, short-term),
- Blood dyscrasias: Fever, sore throat, bruising, rash, jaundice, epistaxis (rare)
- Type of sleep problem: Falling asleep, staying asleep

Lab Test Interferences

Increase: ALT, AST, serum bilirubin level
Decrease: RAIU
False increase: Urinary 17-OHCS

Treatment of Overdose: Lavage, monitor electrolytes, VS, supportive care

Administration

Adult: PO 0.125-0.5 mg hs; *elderly patient:* PO 0.125-0.25 mg hs

- Available forms: Tabs 0.125, 0.25 mg

Trifluoperazine HCl

NOVOFLURAZINE,† SOLAZINE,† STELAZINE, TERFLUZINE,† TRIFLURIN†

(trye-floo-oh-per'a-zeen) (Chapters 4, 9, 17)

Functional classifications: Antipsychotic, neuroleptic
Chemical classifications: Phenothiazine, piperazine
FDA pregnancy category: C

Indications: Psychosis, anxiety

Contraindications: Hypersensitivity, coma, child <6 yr

Pharmacologic Effects: Antipsychotic drugs produce a neuroleptic effect characterized by sedation, emotional quieting, psychomotor slowing, and affective indifference; exact mode of action is not fully understood; antipsychotics block dopamine receptors in the basal ganglia, hypothalamus, limbic system, brain stem, and medulla; antipsychotics are also thought to depress certain components of the reticular activating system that partially control body temperature, wakefulness, vasomotor tone, emesis, and hormonal balance; additionally, antipsychotics have significant anticholinergic and alpha-adrenergic blocking effects

Pharmacokinetics: PO onset erratic, peak 2-4 hr, duration 4-6 hr; IM onset 15-30 min, peak 15-20 min, duration 4-6 hr; metabolized by liver, excreted in urine and feces, crosses placenta, enters breast milk

Side Effects: *CNS:* Parkinsonism, akathisias, dystonias, tardive dyskinesias, oculogyric crisis; *Peripheral:* Blurred vision (cycloplegia or paralysis of accommodation), ocular pain, photophobia, mydriasis, impaired vision; intolerance of extreme heat or cold, possible heat stroke or fatal hyperthermia; nasal congestion, wheezing, dyspnea; **hypotension, especially orthostatic,** leading to dizziness, syncope; **tachycardia,** irregular pulse, arrhythmias; **dry mouth,**

†Available in Canada only.

constipation, jaundice, abdominal pain; urinary retention, urinary hesitancy, galactorrhea, gynecomastia, impaired ejaculation, amenorrhea

Interactions

- Alcohol and other CNS depressants (barbiturates, antihistamines, antianxiety or antidepressant drugs): Increased CNS depression, increased risk of EPSEs
- Amphetamines: Possible decreased antipsychotic effect
- Antacids (magnesium and aluminum products): Possible decreased antipsychotic effect
- Anticholinergics (atropine, H_1-type antihistamines, antidepressants, etc.): Increased risk of excessive atropine-like side effects or toxic effects
- Benztropine: Possible decreased antipsychotic effect, increased risk of severity of peripheral anticholinergic side effects
- Diazoxide: Possible severe hyperglycemia, prediabetic coma
- Guanethidine: Poor control of hypertension by guanethidine
- Hypoglycemia drugs (insulin, oral hypoglycemia agents): Poor diabetic control
- Lithium: Poor control of psychosis with combined therapy; can mask lithium intoxication; neurotoxic effects with confusion, delirium, seizures, encephalopathy
- Meperidine, morphine: Increased risk of severe CNS depression, respiratory depression, hypotension
- Propranolol: Increased pharmacologic effects of either drug

Implications

Assess

- Establish baseline VS, laboratory values, to assess side effects, allergic or hypersensitivity reactions.
- Physiologic and psychologic status before therapy, to determine needs and evaluate progress
- For early stages of tardive dyskinesia by use of abnormal involuntary movement scale
- Identify concurrent symptoms that may be aggravated by antipsychotics, e.g., glaucoma, diabetes

Planning/Implementation

- Ensure that drug has been taken; check mouth for "cheeking"
- If giving liquid antipsychotics, use at least 60 ml of compatible beverage to mask taste; dilute and give immediately; take drug with food to minimize GI upset; give IM injections in lateral thigh
- Keep patient quiet after injection, to prevent falls associated with postural hypotension
- For dry mouth, give chewing gum, hard candies, lip balm; monitor urinary output; check for bladder distention in inactive patients, older men, and patients on high doses
- Assist with ambulation, if patient is having blurred vision; dim room lights for photosensitivity
- Ensure safety with hypotension; sit on side of bed before rising, head-low position for dizziness, avoid hot showers, wear elastic stockings
- Check B/P (supine, sitting, standing) and pulse before and after each dose when possible; observe for side effects
- Monitor body temperature for indications of neuroleptic malignant syndrome, e.g., muscle rigidity, fever, depressed neurologic status; ensure adequate hydration, nutrition, and ventilation
- Protect patient from exposure to extreme hot or cold
- Recognize impending hypersensitivity to pruritus or jaundice with hepatitis; flu or coldlike symptoms, evidence of bleeding with blood dyscrasia
- Observe for involuntary movements

Teaching

- About benefits and potential harm of antipsychotic drugs; weigh need to know against causing apprehension
- To comply with drug treatment
- To avoid activities requiring clear vision for a few weeks after treatment starts; to report eye pain immediately
- About the importance of exercise, fluids, and fiber in diet
- To watch for symptoms of heart failure, e.g., weight gain, dyspnea, distended neck veins, tachycardia
- Possible male sexual performance failure; suggest relaxed, stress-free environment

- To avoid conception; women should practice effective contraception; phenothiazines may cause false positive results in pregnancy tests
- To avoid exposure to sunlight; keep skin covered but with temperature-appropriate clothing
- That patient cannot become addicted to antipsychotic drugs

Evaluate

- Follows prescribed regimen, takes medications as ordered
- Avoids injury; reports dizziness or need for assistance
- Verbalizes reduced anxiety
- Experiences minimal or no adverse responses
- Uses appropriate interventions to minimize side effects
- Achieves improved mental status

Lab Test Interferences

Increase: Liver function tests, cardiac enzyme levels, cholesterol, blood glucose, prolactin, bilirubin, PBI, cholinesterase levels
Decrease: Hormones (blood and urine)
False positive: Pregnancy tests, PKU
False negative: Urinary steroids, 17-OHCS

Treatment of Overdose: Lavage, if orally ingested; provide an airway; do not induce vomiting, control EPSEs and hypotension

Administration

- Psychosis: *Adult:* PO 2-5 mg bid, usual range 15-20 mg/day, may require 40 mg/day or more; IM 1-2 mg q4-6h; *child* >6 *yr:* PO 1 mg qd or bid, maximum up to 15 mg/day; IM not recommended for children, but 1 mg may be given qd or bid
- Anxiety: *Adult:* PO 1-2 mg bid, not to exceed 6 mg/day; do not give for longer than 12 wk
- Available forms: Tabs 1, 2, 5, 10 mg; conc 10 mg/ml; inj IM 2 mg/ml

Triflupromazine*

VESPRIN

(trye-floo-proe'ma-zeen) (Chapter 7)

Functional classification: Antipsychotic
Chemical classification: Aliphatic phenothiazine
FDA pregnancy category: C

Indications: Infrequently used for psychosis, schizophrenia

Contraindications: Hypersensitivity, children <2½ yr

Pharmacologic Effects: See chlorpromazine

Pharmacokinetics: PO peak levels 2-4 hr, duration 4-6 hr, IM onset 15-30 min, peak levels 15-20 min, duration 4-6 hr; metabolized by liver, excreted in urine and feces, crosses placenta, enters breast milk

Side Effects: *CNS:* EPSEs, drowsiness, seizures; *Peripheral:* Respiratory depression, laryngospasm, blood dyscrasias, dry mouth, GI disturbances, blurred vision, nausea and vomiting, orthostatic hypotension, tachycardia, hypertension

Interactions: See chlorpromazine

Lab Test Interference: See chlorpromazine

Treatment of Overdose: See chlorpromazine

Administration

- Psychosis: *Adult:* IM: 60 mg, up to 150 mg/day; *child* >*2½ yr:* IM 0.2-0.25 mg/kg, up to a maximum dose of 10 mg/day
- Available forms: Inj 10, 20 mg/ml

*Infrequently used.

Trihexyphenidyl

ARTANE

(tyre-hex-ee-fen'i-dill)

Functional classification: Anticholinergic, antiparkinson
Chemical classification: Tertiary amine
FDA pregnancy category: C

Indications: Parkinsonism, EPSEs

Contraindications: Hypersensitivity, narrow-angle glaucoma, duodenal obstruction, peptic ulcer, prostatic hypertrophy, myasthenia gravis, megacolon

Pharmacologic Effects: Blocks cholinergic receptors, may inhibit the reuptake and storage of dopamine

Pharmacokinetics: Peak 1-1.3 hr, half-life 5.6-10.2 hr; little pharmacokinetic information is known

Side Effects: *CNS* : Depression develops in 19% to 30% of patients; disorientation, confusion, memory loss, hallucinations, psychoses, agitation, delusions, nervousness; *Peripheral:* **Tachycardia,** palpitations, hypotension, **orthostatic hypotension, dry mouth,** nausea, vomiting, constipation, paralytic ileus, **blurred vision,** mydriasis, diplopia, urinary retention and hesitancy, elevated temperature

Interactions

- Amantadine: Increased anticholinergic effect
- Digoxin: Increased digoxin serum levels
- Haloperidol: Worsening of schizophrenia, decreased haloperidol serum levels
- Levodopa: Possible reduction of levodopa efficacy
- Phenothiazines: Increased anticholinergic effect, decreased antipsychotic effect

Implications

Assess

- VS, B/P
- For glaucoma
- Mental status

Planning/Implementation

- Provide instructions for anticholinergic responses, i.e., dry mouth, constipation, urinary hesitancy, decreased sweating

Teaching

- Give with meals
- May cause drowsiness, blurred vision, dizziness: Emphasize safety
- Avoid alcohol and other CNS depressants
- For rapid or pounding heartbeat, notify physician
- Use caution in hot weather

Evaluate

- EPSE improvement
- For adverse effects
- Mental status: Confusion, delirium memory

Treatment of Overdose:
Emesis, lavage, activated charcoal, treat respiratory depression, hyperpyrexia

Administration

- Parkinsonism: *Adult:* PO initially, 1-2 mg first day, increase by 2-mg increments at 3- 5-day intervals, up to a daily dose of 6-10 mg in three divided doses at mealtime
- EPSEs: To start, 1 mg with 1 mg every few hours until symptoms controlled; maintenance or prophylactic use, 5-15 mg/day

Trimethadione*

TRIDIONE

(trye-meth-a-dye'one)

Functional classification: Antiepileptic
Chemical classification: Oxazolidinedione
FDA pregnancy category: D

Indications: Refractory absence seizures

Contraindications: Hypersensitivity, blood dyscrasias
Cautious use: Hepatic disease, renal disease

Pharmacologic Effects: Increases seizure threshold in cortex, basal ganglia; therapeutic serum level is 700 μg/ml

Pharmacokinetics: PO peak 30 min-2 hr, excreted in kidneys, half-life of 12-24 hr with a half-life of 6-13 days for the active metabolite dimethadione

Side Effects: *CNS:* **Drowsiness,** dizziness, fatigue, paresthesia, irritability, headache; *Peripheral:* Vaginal bleeding, albuminuria, nephrosis, abdominal pain,

*Infrequently used.

T U

weight loss, nausea, vomiting, bleeding gums, abnormal liver function test, **exfoliative dermatitis,** rash, alopecia, petechiae, erythema, photophobia, diplopia, epistaxis, retinal hemorrhage, hypertension, hypotension, thrombocytopenia, agranulocytosis, leukopenia, neutropenia, hemolytic anemia

Interactions: None known

Implications
Assess
- Blood studies: Hematocrit, hemoglobin level, Hct, RBCs, serum folate and vitamin D values, if on long-term therapy regimen
- Hepatic studies: ALT, AST, bilirubin and creatinine levels
- Skin: If rash occurs, withhold drug

Planning/Implementation
- Dilute oral solution with water
- Oral with juice or milk to cover taste and smell, to decrease GI symptoms

Teaching
- To take with food, if GI upset
- To carry MedicAlert identification bracelet
- To notify physician, if visual disturbances, sore throat, etc., occur
- To avoid driving and other activities that require alertness
- Not to discontinue medication abruptly after long-term use, since convulsions may result

Evaluate
- Mental status
- Renal and hematologic problems

Treatment of Overdose: Symptoms include nausea, drowsiness, dizziness, ataxia, visual disturbances; coma in cases of massive overdose; emesis, lavage, supportive care

Administration
Adult: PO 300 mg tid (900 mg/day), may increase by 300 mg/wk, not to exceed 600 mg qid (2400 mg/day); *child:* 300 to 900 mg/day in three or four equally divided doses
- Available forms include: Caps 300 mg, chew tabs 150 mg; oral sol 40 mg/ml

Trimipramine Maleate

SURMONTIL
(tri-mip′ra-meen) (Chapter 5)

Functional classification: TCA
Chemical classification: Tertiary amine
FDA pregnancy category: C

Indications: Depression

Contraindications: Hypersensitivity to TCAs, recovery phase of myocardial infarction, convulsive disorders, prostatic hypertrophy, children
Cautious use: Suicidal patients, severe depression, increased intraocular pressure, narrow-angle glaucoma, urinary retention, cardiac disease, hepatic disease, hyperthyroidism, ECT, elective surgery, MAOI therapy

Pharmacologic Effect: Inhibits serotonin and norepinephrine uptake; therapeutic plasma level 180 ng/ml

Pharmacokinetics: Metabolized by liver, excreted by kidneys, steady state 2-6 days; half-life 7-30 hr

Side Effects: *CNS:* **Sedation,** ataxia, confusion, delirium; *Peripheral:* **Blurred vision,** photophobia, increased intraocular pressure; decreased tearing, orthostatic hypotension, arrhythmias, tachycardia, palpitations, dry mouth, constipation, diarrhea, decreased sweating, **urinary retention, hesitancy**

Interactions
- Anticholinergic agents: Additive anticholinergic effects with atropine, antihistamines (H_1 blocker), antiparkinson drugs, antipsychotics, OTC cold and allergy drugs
- CNS depressants: Additive depressant effect
- Guanethidine, clonidine: Decreased antihypertensive effect
- MAOIs: Hypertensive crisis, atropine-like poisoning
- Oral contraceptives: Inhibit effects of TCAs
- Phenothiazines: May increase TCA serum level

- Quinidine: Additive effect, heart block possible
- Sympathomimetics: Potentiates sympathomimetic effects
- Thyroid preparations: Tachycardia, arrhythmias; may increase TCA effect

Implications

Assess

- Establish baseline data, to aid recognition of adverse responses to medication, e.g., liver enzyme levels, VS, renal function, mental status, speech patterns, affect, weight
- For signs of noncompliance, e.g., poor therapeutic response
- Observe for major symptoms of depression: Apathy, sadness, sleep disturbances, hopelessness, guilt, decreased libido, spontaneous crying
- Review history for contraindicated conditions, e.g., glaucoma, CV disease, GI conditions, urologic conditions, seizures, pregnancy

Planning/Implementation

- Monitor for "cheeking" or hoarding; check drug dosage carefully, since a small overdose may cause toxic effects
- Monitor for suicidal ideations; suicidal thought content may increase as antidepressants begin to "energize" patient
- Monitor VS; if hypotension, tachycardia, or arrhythmias occur, withhold TCAs
- Give most TCAs in a single dose hs
- Observe for early signs of toxic effects, e.g., drowsiness, tachycardia, mydriasis, hypotension, agitation, vomiting, confusion, fever, restlessness, sweating
- If CNS overstimulation occurs, e.g., hypomania, delirium, discontinue drug

Teaching

- That these drugs have a lag time of up to 1 month
- To adhere to drug regimen
- To avoid OTC drugs, particularly those containing sympathomimetics or anticholinergics
- To avoid drugs listed in section on interactions
- About ways to deal with minor side effects, as follows: dry mouth, with hard candies, sips of water, mouth rinses; visual disturbances, with artificial tears, sunglasses, assistance with ambulation; constipation, with bulk-forming foods, increased fluids; urinary hesitancy, with adequate fluids, privacy; decreased perspiration, with appropriate clothing, avoidance of unnecessary exercise; orthostatic hypotension, with slow positional changes, avoidance of hot baths and showers; for drowsiness, take single dose hs with physician approval, avoid driving
- That abrupt discontinuance may result in cholinergic rebound, e.g., nausea, vomiting, insomnia

Evaluate

- Desired therapeutic serum level
- Verbalize decrease in subjective symptoms
- Observe decrease in objective symptoms
- Minimal to no adverse drug effects
- Stable VS
- Less anxiety; sleep, talk, and feel better

Lab Test Interferences

Increase: Serum bilirubin, blood glucose, alkaline phosphatase levels
False increase: Urinary catecholamines
Decrease: VMA, 5-HIAA

Treatment of Overdose: ECG monitoring, induce emesis, lavage, activated charcoal, administer anticonvulsant; treat anticholinergic effects, if needed

Administration

Adult: PO 75 mg/day in divided doses, may be increased to 200 mg/day; *adolescent and geriatric:* 50 mg/day to start, gradually increase to 100 mg/day

- Available forms: Caps 25, 50, 100 mg

Valproic Acid and Derivatives

DEPAKENE SYRUP/DEPAKOTE/ DEPAKENE

(val-proe'ic) (Chapter 7)

Functional classification: Anticonvulsant
Chemical classification: Carboxylic acid derivative
FDA pregnancy category: D

Indications: Drug of choice for tonic-clonic and absence seizures; psychomotor seizures

Contraindications: Hypersensitivity to valproic acid; hepatic disease or significant hepatic dysfunction
Cautious use: Children with metabolic disorders, lactation, children <2 yr

Pharmacologic Effects: Mechanism not known but may be related to increased brain levels of GABA; therapeutic serum levels are 50-100 μg/ml

Pharmacokinetics: PO rapidly absorbed, peak levels 1-4 hr, time to steady state 2-4 days, half-life 6-16 hr

Side Effects: Serious side effects are *not* common; *CNS:* Sedation but usually dissipates; *Peripheral:* **Nausea, vomiting, indigestion,** other GI symptoms; emotional upset; minor elevation in SGOT and LDH; severe hepatotoxicity may occur; blood dyscrasias, **rash**

Interactions
- Alcohol and other CNS depressants: CNS depression
- Anticonvulsants: May increase serum levels of phenobarbital; clonazepam toxicity may be increased; phenytoin causes two opposite interactions: Increase in serum phenytoin and decrease in serum phenytoin levels
- Aspirin and warfarin: Prolonged bleeding time
- Chlorpromazine and aspirin: Increased valproic acid half-life
- Carbamazepine and phenytoin: Decreased valproic acid serum levels

Implications
Assess
- Blood studies, hepatic studies

Planning/Implementation
- Serious side effects are uncommon
- Do not dilute elixir with carbonated beverage

Teaching
- Take with food for GI upset
- Swallow tabs and caps whole, to avoid irritation
- Take hs to avoid drowsiness during day
- Notify that valproic acid alters blood and urine volume in diabetes
- Wear MedicAlert identification bracelet

Evaluate
- Efficacy of treatment

Treatment of Overdose: *Symptoms:* Coma and death have occurred; however, more typical symptoms of overdose include motor restlessness, visual hallucinations; supportive care, paying close attention to adequate urinary output

Administration
Adult and child: PO 15 mg/kg/day; increase at weekly intervals by 5 to 10 mg/kg/day until seizures are controlled or as side effects dictate; maximum dose 60 mg/kg/day; if total dose exceeds 250 mg/day, give in divided doses
- Available forms: *Valproic acid:* Caps 250 mg; syr 250 mg/5 ml; *Valproate sodium-valproic acid:* Tabs 125, 250, 500 mg

APPENDIX

Controlled Substance Chart

Drugs	United States	Canada
Heroin, LSD, peyote, marijuana, mescaline	Schedule I	Schedule H
Opiates such as morphine and meperidine, amphetamines, cocaine, short-acting barbiturates (amobarbital, secobarbital), hydromorphone	Schedule II	Schedule G
Glutethimide, paregoric, cerebral stimulants used to treat obesity (benzphetamine, phendimetrazine)	Schedule III	Schedule F
Chloral hydrate, benzodiazepines, cerebral stimulants used to treat obesity (mazindol, fenfluramine), meprobamate, mephobarbital, pemoline, phenobarbital	Schedule IV	Schedule F
Antidiarrheals with opium, antitussives	Schedule V	

FDA Pregnancy Categories

A No risk demonstrated to the fetus in any trimester

B No adverse effects in animals, no human studies available, or if adverse effects in animals, none demonstrated in human studies

C Only given after risks to the fetus are considered; animal studies have shown adverse reactions, no human studies available, or no animal studies and inadequate human studies

D Definite fetal risks, may be given in some situations because of mother's condition

X Absolute fetal abnormalities; risk outweighs potential benefit

Abbreviations

ac	Before meals
ADHD	Attention deficit hyperactivity disorder
ALT	Alanine aminotransferase, serum
AST	Aspartate aminotransferse, serum
bid	Twice a day
B/P	Blood pressure
BUN	Blood urea nitrogen
cap	Capsules
CBC	Complete blood cell count
CHF	Congestive heart failure
CNS	Central nervous system
conc	Concentrate
CPK	Creatinine phosphokinase
CV	Cardiovascular
ECG	Electrocardiogram
EEG	Electroencephalogram
ECT	Electroconvulsive therapy
elix	Elixir
EPSEs	Extrapyramidal side effects
ext rel	Extended release
5HT	5-hydroxytryptamine (serotonin receptor)
g	Gram
GABA	Gamma-aminobutyric acid
gr	Grain
GI	Gastrointestinal
GU	Genitourinary
5-HIAA	5-Hydroxyindoleacetic acid
hr	Hour
hs	At bedtime
I-131	Thyroid uptake
IM	Intramuscular
inj	Injection
I&O	Intake and Output
IV	Intravenous
kg	kilogram
L	Liter
LDH	Lactic dehydrogenase
MAOIs	Monoamine oxidase inhibitors
mEq	Milliequivalent
mg	Milligram
ml	Milliliter
μg	Microgram
mo	Month
Na	Sodium
ng	Nanogram
NMS	Neuroleptic malignant syndrome
NPO	Nothing by mouth
OTC	Over-the-counter
PBI	Protein-bound iodine
PDR	*Physicians' Desk Reference*
PKU	Phenylketonuia
PO	By mouth
PTSD	Posttraumatic stress disorder
prn	As needed
q	Every
qd	Every day
qh	Every hour
qid	Four times a day
qod	Every other day
q2h	Every 2 hours, and so forth
RAIU	Radioactive iodine uptake
RBC	Red blood cell count
REC	Rectal
r/t	Related to
SC	Subcutaneous
OHCS-17	17-hydroxycorticosteroids
SGOT	Serum glutamic-oxaloacetic transaminase
SMA-12	Sequential multiple-analysis-12
supp	suppository
susp	Suspension
Syr	Syrup
tabs	Tablets
TCA	Tricyclic antidepressant
tid	Three times daily
time-rel	Timed-release
UA	Urinalysis
VMA	Vanillylmandelic acid
VS	Vital signs
WBC	White blood cell count

General Index

I

R

S

Disorders Index

Drug Index

E

Q

R